MW01014468

Pediatric Neuropsychology

PEDIATRIC NEUROPSYCHOLOGY
MEDICAL ADVANCES AND LIFESPAN OUTCOMES

Edited by
Ida Sue Baron, Ph.D.
and
Celiane Rey-Casserly, Ph.D.

OXFORD
UNIVERSITY PRESS

Oxford University Press is a department of the University of Oxford.
It furthers the University's objective of excellence in research, scholarship,
and education by publishing worldwide.

Oxford   New York
Auckland   Cape Town   Dar es Salaam   Hong Kong   Karachi
Kuala Lumpur   Madrid   Melbourne   Mexico City   Nairobi
New Delhi   Shanghai   Taipei   Toronto

With offices in
Argentina   Austria   Brazil   Chile   Czech Republic   France   Greece
Guatemala   Hungary   Italy   Japan   Poland   Portugal   Singapore
South Korea   Switzerland   Thailand   Turkey   Ukraine   Vietnam

Oxford is a registered trade mark of Oxford University Press
in the UK and certain other countries.

Published in the United States of America by
Oxford University Press
198 Madison Avenue, New York, NY 10016

Pediatric neuropsychology : medical advances and lifespan outcomes /
edited by Ida Sue Baron, Celiane Rey-Casserly.
p. cm.
Includes bibliographical references and index.
ISBN 978–0–19–982932–3
1. Pediatric neuropsychology.   I. Baron, Ida Sue.   II. Rey-Casserly, Celiane.
RJ486.5.P434 2013
362.198928–dc23
2012030196

Contents

Section II Impact on Educational Systems

Section III Methodological and Lifespan Developmental
              Considerations

Preface

The genesis of this book was in a moment of great appreciation for the numerous advances in medicine and psychology that have occurred over several decades and brought us to this truly remarkable era of patient care. As a result of the gains that have been made in assessment, diagnosis, treatment, and rehabilitation and through rigorous research across disciplines, the prognosis for infants and children with systemic and central nervous system diseases and disorders has been substantially and favorably altered. Most of these steps forward have been incremental over a long period of time. Thus, it might be easy to overlook the fact that today's medical care and outcomes for infants and children are substantially improved from past eras and that many pediatric patients will now survive and live a full lifespan. If the patients described in this volume had been cared for in earlier eras, they likely would have had an early mortality or suffered severe incapacitation and lifelong disability. That course is no longer inevitable for patients today, and a number of populations that have been beneficiaries of these advances are the focus of this volume.

Pediatric care in past eras included aspects that now seem archaic. For example, best practices included pneumoencephalograms and their painful aftermath, in which air was injected to visualize the ventricular system as a means to diagnose hydrocephalus; early radiologic images that were not as finely detailed as they are today; high-dose radiation treatments that reduced the risk of mortality from childhood leukemia but had the unintended consequence of producing associated late neuropsychological deficits in survivors; an absence of successful protocols for cardiac, liver, and kidney transplant surgeries in children; a lack of recognition that some adult conditions, such as multiple sclerosis, might also affect children; a far more restricted armamentarium of medications than currently exists; fewer genetic tests and more limited understanding of rare disorders, such as phenylketonuria; and an expectation that many survivors of premature birth would inevitably suffer brain damage and lifelong complications such as severe sensorineural deficits, cerebral palsy, and severe intellectual disability. When pediatric neuropsychology was just emerging as a viable area of clinical practice, human immunodeficiency virus had not been discovered and the incidence of autism spectrum disorders was far below current estimates. Some treatment protocols once eschewed, such as cooling to limit the effects of neonatal encephalopathy, have been reintroduced. In those earlier decades, survival was often the deserved measurement of success, and neuropsychological outcomes were justifiably secondary to the imperative of survival.

When one compares past standards of care, diagnostic procedures, surgical techniques, and treatment protocols with those presently available for the wider pediatric population, it is evident that both quality of life and duration of lifespan have improved for many of these children. However, survival may be accompanied by morbidities that were either unknown or unexpected when the lifespan was predictably short. Transitioning through stages of development—infancy, childhood, adolescence into young adulthood—was unanticipated in the past for many of these pediatric patients. Today a full lifespan is now a reality and an expectation. Diseases and conditions that resulted in early death or severe disability are now often successfully treated and managed as chronic disorders that often provide an opportunity for a relatively healthy functional status throughout a normal length of lifespan.

These developments have had far-reaching societal implications. To accommodate the gains made in caring for children who will mature into young adulthood and even age normally, multiple systems have had to adjust and adapt in order to better serve these children and their families. In healthcare, the transition to adult-oriented care for adolescents and young adults with chronic medical conditions must be carefully planned because these individuals often face multiple barriers as they attempt to access coordinated care. School systems have also been challenged to meet the needs of children and adolescents with complex medical diagnoses and associated learning disabilities. For example, according to US federal law and guidelines, public schools must provide a "free and appropriate public education" to individuals with disabilities, ensuring they are given the opportunity for academic and vocational proficiency. Psychological and vocational systems have also been altered by the survival of many who in earlier years would not have survived to adulthood and led full adult lives. Thus, adult practitioners who are unfamiliar with developmental disabilities and the effects of severe childhood illness may now find that they are involved in the care of these individuals. Yet, these practitioners are unfamiliar with how their clients' early-appearing disease or injury will affect their functioning in adulthood. Consequently, adult practitioners increasingly need to expand their knowledge about neurodevelopmental and other childhood medical disorders in order to formulate treatment strategies or effectively counsel these individuals as they face these once unexpected challenges, including vocational choice, partnering for a family, individual health needs, and aging.

This volume was envisioned as one that would be of interest and importance for both pediatric and adult practitioners and merge pediatric and adult neuropsychological methods and theory to provide a broader perspective of specific clinical populations. For pediatric/child practitioners, this volume may enhance appreciation for the obstacles their patients might encounter as they mature into young adulthood. For adult practitioners, it may serve as a reference that will provide information about select patient groups with which they have limited familiarity but whose pediatric experiences have allowed them to reach adulthood. A confluence of pediatric and adult foundational knowledge is necessary to understand the trajectory of development as it relates to specific pediatric medical conditions over the individual's lifespan.

We asked the authors of chapters in Section I, *Medical Disorders*, to summarize historical and current knowledge. Our hope is that the trajectory of diagnosis and care for each specific condition or disease will be placed in a meaningful context for the reader. Each chapter in this section presents central features of a particular diagnosis or condition, reviews the historical and current pediatric literature, and provides an updated summary of what is known about outcomes in adolescence/young adulthood. Included are chapters on acute lymphocytic leukemia (Krull and Brinkman), autism spectrum disorders (Joseph, Black, and Thurm), brain tumors (Rey-Casserly), cerebral palsy (Warschausky, Kaufman, and Felix), congenital heart disease (Bellinger and Newburger), human immunodeficiency virus (Nichols, Kammerer, and Patton), neonatal encephalopathy (Kline, Leonberger, and Baron), kidney disease (Hooper and Gerson), liver disease (Sorensen), multiple sclerosis (MacAllister and Harder), phenylketonuria (Waisbren and Antshel), prematurity (Baron, Leonberger, and Ahronovich), sickle cell disease (Wills), spina bifida/hydrocephalus(Zabel, Jacobson, and Mahone), and traumatic brain injury (Kirkwood, Peterson, and Yeates).

We asked the authors of Section II, *Impact on Educational Systems*, to address related academic changes and accommodations that have taken place as a consequence of the impact of modern medical advances on the educational system that serves these survivors. Chapter 16 (Goldberger, Meier, and Panarelli) describes relevant educational modifications and practice in the elementary school years and the changes faced by public elementary schools that are attempting to meet the needs of medically challenged children. Chapter 17 (Wolf and Kroesser) addresses the transitioning of youth with disabilities into higher education settings.

Section III, *Methodological and Developmental Considerations*, addresses a broader perspective on changes in statistical methodology as well as lifespan theoretical considerations. Chapter 18 (Weiss) focuses on the transition from statistical significance testing to the use of effect sizes and includes other methodological concerns. Chapter 19 (Bernstein and Rey-Casserly) covers the important linkages between pediatric and adult practice, and Chapter 20 (Ris and Hiscock) extends this focus and provides a perspective related to modeling cognitive aging following early central nervous system injury, with particular emphasis on the concepts of reserve and the Flynn effect.

We hope this contribution to the literature serves our readers and patients and their families well across a full and rewarding lifespan.

Ida Sue Baron, Ph.D.
Potomac, MD, and Fairfax, VA

Celiane Rey-Casserly, Ph.D.
Boston, MA

Acknowledgments

We are deeply grateful for the invaluable assistance and support of all at Oxford University Press who helped bring this book from concept to reality, with special thanks to Joan Bossert, Vice President/Editorial Director in the Medical Division; Miles Osgood, Assistant Editor in the Academic Division; and Papitha Ramesh our Project Manager.

We also express gratitude to the children and families we work with and for the privilege of sharing their stories and journey to adulthood.

Contributors

Margot D. Ahronovich, M.D.
Fairfax Neonatal Associates, P.C.
Fairfax, VA

Kevin M. Antshel, Ph.D.
Department of Psychiatry and
Behavioral Sciences
SUNY—Upstate Medical University
Syracuse, NY

Ida Sue Baron, Ph.D.
Independent Private Practice
Potomac, MD and Fairfax, VA and
Departments of Neurosciences and
Pediatrics
Inova Children's Hospital
Falls Church, VA

David C. Bellinger, Ph.D., M.Sc.
Department of Neurology
Boston Children's Hospital and Harvard
Medical School
Department of Environmental Health
Harvard School of Public Health
Boston, MA

Jane Holmes Bernstein, Ph.D.
Department of Psychiatry
Boston Children's Hospital and Harvard
Medical School
Boston, MA

David Black, Ph.D.
Pediatrics and Developmental
Neuroscience Branch
National Institute of Mental Health
Bethesda, MD

Tara Brinkman, Ph.D.
Department of Epidemiology and
Cancer Control
St. Jude Children's Research Hospital
Memphis, TN

Lindsey Felix, Ph.D.
Department of Physical Medicine and
Rehabilitation
University of Michigan
Ann Arbor, MI

Arlene C. Gerson, Ph.D.
Department of Pediatrics and
Epidemiology
Johns Hopkins University School of
Medicine and
Johns Hopkins Bloomberg School of
Public Health
Baltimore, MD

Ellen Goldberger, Ph.D.
School Psychologist
Fairfax County Public Schools
Fairfax, VA

Lana Harder, Ph.D.
Departments of Psychiatry and
Neurology
Children's Medical Center Dallas
University of Texas Southwestern
Medical School
Dallas, TX

Merrill Hiscock, Ph.D.
Clinical Psychology
Developmental Psychology
Center for Neuro-Engineering and
Cognitive Science
University of Texas at Austin
Austin, TX

Stephen R. Hooper, Ph.D.
Department of Psychiatry and The
Carolina Institute for Developmental
Disabilities
University of North Carolina School of
Medicine
Chapel Hill, NC

Lisa Jacobson, Ph.D.
Department of Neuropsychology
Kennedy Krieger Institute
Department of Psychiatry and
Behavioral Sciences
Johns Hopkins University School of
Medicine
Baltimore, MD

Lisa Joseph, Ph.D.
Pediatrics and Developmental
Neuroscience Branch
National Institute of Mental Health
Bethesda, MD

Betsy Kammerer, Ph.D.
Department of Psychiatry
Boston Children's Hospital/Harvard
Medical School
Boston, MA

Jacqueline N. Kaufman, Ph.D.
Department of Physical Medicine and
Rehabilitation
University of Michigan
Ann Arbor, MI

Michael W. Kirkwood, Ph.D.
Department of Physical Medicine and
Rehabilitation
Children's Hospital Colorado
University of Colorado Denver School of
Medicine
Aurora, CO

Alex Kline, M.D.
Fairfax Neonatal Associates, P.C.
Fairfax, VA

Sarah Kroesser, MS.Ed.
Graduate Research Assistant
Office of Disability Services
Boston University
Boston, MA

Kevin R. Krull, Ph.D.
Department of Epidemiology and
Cancer Control
St. Jude Children's Research Hospital
Memphis, TN

Katherine Ann Leonberger, M. Psy.
Professional Psychology Program
Columbian College of Arts and Sciences
The George Washington University
Washington, DC

William S. MacAllister, Ph.D.
Department of Neurology
New York University School of Medicine
New York, NY

E. Mark Mahone, Ph.D.
Department of Neuropsychology
Kennedy Krieger Institute
Department of Psychiatry and
Behavioral Sciences
Johns Hopkins University School of
Medicine
Baltimore, MD

Irene Meier, Ed.D.
Director, Special Education Instruction
Fairfax County Public Schools
Fairfax, VA

Jane W. Newburger, M.D., M.P.H.
Department of Cardiology
Boston Children's Hospital
Department of Pediatrics
Harvard Medical School
Boston, MA

Sharon L. Nichols, Ph.D.
Department of Neurosciences
University of California, San Diego
San Diego, CA

Mary Ann Panarelli, Ed.D.
Director, Intervention and Prevention
Services
Department of Special Services
Fairfax, VA

Doyle E. Patton, Ph.D.
Children's Diagnostic & Treatment
Center, Inc.
Fort Lauderdale, FL

Robin L. Peterson, Ph.D.
Department of Psychology
University of Denver
Denver, CO

Celiane Rey-Casserly, Ph.D.
Department of Psychiatry
Boston Children's Hospital
Boston, MA

M. Douglas Ris, Ph.D.
Department of Pediatrics
Baylor College of Medicine
Texas Children's Hospital
Houston, TX

Lisa G. Sorensen, Ph.D.
Department of Clinical Psychiatry and
Behavioral Sciences
Northwestern University's Feinberg
School of Medicine
Ann and Robert H. Lurie Children's
Hospital of Chicago
Chicago, IL

Audrey Thurm, Ph.D.
Pediatrics and Developmental
Neuroscience Branch
National Institute of Mental Health
Bethesda, MD

Susan E. Waisbren, Ph.D.
Department of Psychiatry
Department of Genetics
Boston Children's Hospital/Harvard
Medical School
Boston, MA

Seth Warschausky, Ph.D.
Department of Physical Medicine and
Rehabilitation
University of Michigan
Ann Arbor, MI

Brandi A. Weiss, Ph.D.
Department of Educational Leadership
The George Washington University
Washington, DC

Karen E. Wills, Ph.D.
Department of Psychology
Children's Hospitals and Clinics of
Minnesota
Minneapolis, MN

Lorraine E. Wolf, Ph.D.
Department of Medicine
Department of Rehabilitation Sciences
Boston University
Boston, MA

Keith Owen Yeates, Ph.D.
Department of Pediatrics
The Ohio State University
Center of Biobehavioral Health
The Research Institute at Nationwide
Children's Hospital
Columbus, OH

T. Andrew Zabel, Ph.D.
Department of Neuropsychology
Kennedy Krieger Institute
Department of Psychiatry and
Behavioral Sciences
Johns Hopkins University School of
Medicine
Baltimore, MD

SECTION I
MEDICAL DISORDERS

1 Childhood Acute Lymphoblastic Leukemia

A Lifespan Perspective

Kevin R. Krull and Tara Brinkman

HISTORICAL MEDICAL PERSPECTIVE

Acute lymphoblastic leukemia (ALL) is the most common form of childhood cancer, accounting for roughly 30% of new cancer diagnoses (Howlander et al., 2010). Although the annual incidence of ALL is relatively low, that is, roughly 3000 new cases per year in the United States, advances in treatment have resulted in a remarkable increase in survival rates, leading to a substantial population of long-term survivors. The 5-year survival rate increased from roughly 20% in the 1960s to over 80% today (Pui, Robison, & Look, 2008). This success has contributed to an estimated 300,000 survivors in the United States, which is a prevalence of 1 in 640 (Ries et al., 2007). The rapid increase in survival for children diagnosed with ALL was, in large part, due to the recognition of the central nervous system (CNS) as a sanctuary for leukemic cells and the subsequent use of prophylactic treatment of the CNS to prevent relapse.

In addition to a combination of chemotherapy agents to attain remission, protocols in the 1960s and 1970s relied on CNS treatment with cranial radiation therapy (CRT). Early cumulative doses of CRT were established at 24 gray (Gy), applied to the entire brain and spinal cord and occasionally involved total body irradiation. Because late-occurring toxicities became apparent using this regimen, particularly neurocognitive sequelae, CRT doses were decreased to 18 Gy without a significant reduction in survival rates. With continued concern over radiation-induced CNS toxicity, chemotherapy-only protocols involving various agents injected directly into the spinal fluid (i.e., intrathecal [IT] injections) for prophylactic CNS treatment were emphasized. Currently, the vast majority of children diagnosed with low- or standard-risk ALL are successfully treated with chemotherapy alone, relying only on CRT for CNS relapse (Pui, 2009).

CURRENT MEDICAL FACTORS AND TREATMENT UPDATE

Treatment for childhood ALL is focused on risk-based therapy in order to achieve a balance between maximum survival and minimum toxicity. This balance involves stratification of children into treatment arms according to risk of relapse (i.e., low, standard, high), which generally dictates treatment intensity. Risk stratum is based on a combination of factors, including age, initial white blood cell count, immunophenotype (i.e., B-cell, T-cell), and cytogenetics (Pui, 2000).

Current therapeutic protocols for childhood ALL rely primarily on chemotherapy drugs delivered at different times and through different routes. The typical treatment protocol is broken into three phases: induction therapy, consolidation therapy, and continuation/maintenance therapy. Induction therapy is designed to bring about remission; typically involves the use of vincristine, corticosteroids, and L-asparaginase; and may include IT injection of methotrexate (MTX) alone or in conjunction with corticosteroids and cytarabine. Children identified on a high-risk protocol or with refractory CNS disease may also receive low-dose CRT (12–18 Gy), depending upon the particular protocol with which they are treated.

Induction typically continues for 6–7 weeks, after which the consolidation phase of therapy begins in order to reduce the number of cancer cells and obtain a complete remission. This phase usually lasts several months and includes systemic treatment as well as direct CNS therapy. Children on low- and standard-risk protocols are generally treated with intermediate- to high-dose intravenous (IV) MTX as well as numerous IT injections comprised of MTX, cytarabine, and hydrocortisone. The doses used in the IT injections are typically standardized to the child's age and body surface area. Children on high-risk protocols are also treated with IV and IT chemotherapy, though they usually receive higher doses of IV MTX and a higher total number of IT injections.

Consolidation therapy is followed by continuation therapy, which lasts for roughly 2 years of continuous and complete remission. Continuation therapy usually involves oral, IV, and IT MTX at specified intervals as well as regular pulses of vincristine and corticosteroids. Many current protocols also include one or two cycles of delayed intensification. These cycles include treatment similar to that given during the induction phase, that is, IV and IT MTX, and are designed to prevent delayed relapse. Additional classes of chemotherapeutic drugs administered during one or more of the phases of treatment include anthracyclines, platinum-based agents, and additional antimetabolites.

Following the completion of continuation therapy, children regularly visit their oncologist who monitors for relapse. Although many children may experience acute toxicities during the course of treatment for ALL, including fever, seizures, and infections, many of these toxicities are apparently transient. However, exposure-specific late effects, defined as morbidity occurring ≥5 years postdiagnosis or ≥2 years following the completion of therapy, are well documented. Late effects include increased risk of cardiac morbidity with exposure to anthracyclines (Hudson, 2007), peripheral neuropathy associated with vincristine exposure (Parasole et al., 2010), ototoxicity associated with exposure to platinum-based agents such as cisplatin (Al-Khatib, Cohen, Carret, & Daniel, 2010), and osteonecrosis associated with exposure to corticosteroids (Burger et al., 2005). Neurocognitive late effects have also been commonly reported (Krull, Okcu, et al., 2008).

EARLY PSYCHOLOGICAL AND NEUROPSYCHOLOGICAL FINDINGS

Neurocognitive impairment is one of the most common late effects in long-term survivors of childhood ALL, with 20%–40% of survivors demonstrating deficits in one or more domains of function (Krull, Okcu, et al., 2008; Moleski, 2000; Mulhern, Fairclough, & Ochs, 1991). Intellectual and academic functions have been a common focus of early studies. Children who survive ALL are more likely to need special education services and are rated lower on academic skills when compared with referenced controls (Christie, Leiper, Chessells, & Vargha-Khadem, 1995). Deficits in mathematics calculation and applied arithmetic problem solving are frequently noted, and reading difficulties have also been reported (Kaemingk, Carey, Moore, Herzer, & Hutter, 2004; Peterson et al., 2008). This impact on academics, as well as on global cognitive abilities, may not fully emerge until at least 5 years after diagnosis, with a steady decline in functions over time (Brown & Madan-Swain, 1993; Kingma, Rammeloo, van Der Does-van den Berg, Rekers-Mombarg, & Postma, 2000). This altered pattern of functioning may lead to a reduction in academic and vocational success as well as lowered self-esteem and behavioral dysfunction. Long-term survivors of childhood ALL are at increased risk for lower ultimate levels of academic attainment.

In addition to intellectual functioning and academics, abnormalities in specific neurocognitive skills are reported, particularly processing speed, attention, and memory functions (Moore, 2005). Behavioral attention problems, which are common, correspond to reduced school performance and teacher-rated math difficulties (Buizer, de Sonneville, van den Heuvel-Eibrink, & Veerman, 2006; Krull, Brouwers, et al., 2008). In a survey of 2979 parents of long-term adolescent survivors of childhood cancer, children with ALL were identified as having significantly higher rates of attention problems compared with sibling controls (Schultz et al., 2007). Early-onset attention deficits can have a major impact on the development of functional academic skills as well as on higher-level cognitive functions.

Higher cumulative doses of cranial radiation and younger age at the time of radiation are associated with general intellectual dysfunction and reduced academic performance. Children treated with 24 Gy CRT are at increased risk for impairment compared with those treated with 18 Gy CRT (Mulhern et al., 1991). The impact of CRT on intellectual function appears to emerge over time and may progress as the child ages. Deficits in specific neurocognitive processes appear to be implicated in reduced global intellectual functioning over time. Specifically, deficits in processing speed, attention and working memory appear to precede the deficits in intelligence (Schatz, Kramer, Ablin, & Matthay, 2000). Risk is further exacerbated when treatment is given when the child is <6 years (Kadan-Lottick et al., 2010). Gender has also been observed to interact with the impact of CRT, with females demonstrating higher rates of impairment than males (Waber et al., 1995). Females children treated with high-dose CRT when <6 years are noted to be at particularly high risk.

In addition to the clear effects of CRT, high-dose chemotherapy has also been implicated as contributing to neurocognitive impairment. In an early study of childhood ALL patients treated at St. Jude Children's Research Hospital, children who received only chemotherapy treatment had neurotoxic effects similar to those experienced by patients who received 18 Gy of CRT (Ochs et al., 1991). Neurocognitive problems included decreases in intelligence as well as arithmetic achievement. In fact, roughly

25% of the children who received no radiation experienced clinically apparent deterioration in neurocognitive function during the follow-up period (median 7.4 years; Mulhern et al., 1991). In a recent meta-analysis of 13 studies examining ALL survivors treated with chemotherapy only, moderate to large effect sizes were consistently identified for measures of intelligence and academic achievement (Peterson et al., 2008).

Although a number of chemotherapeutic agents may contribute to the development of neurocognitive impairment, most attention has focused on MTX. In children with ALL, MTX has been linked to reduced intelligence, visual–motor decline, and academic problems, particularly in mathematics (Montour-Proulx et al., 2005; Peterson et al., 2008). Deficits in performance-based intelligence have been associated with cumulative IT MTX (Montour-Proulx et al., 2005). In addition, attention deficits appear to be particularly common in children treated with MTX (Buizer, de Sonneville, van den Heuvel-Eibrink, & Veerman, 2005), and the intensity of high-dose IV MTX has been correlated with the degree of attention and working memory problems (Buizer et al., 2005; Carey et al., 2007).

The neurotoxic impact of chemotherapeutic treatment of ALL is further reflected through brain imaging studies. In a large retrospective multicenter study, pathological brain magnetic resonance imaging (MRI) scans were reported in 52% of ALL survivors (Hertzberg et al., 1997). Although rates of MRI abnormality were higher in children who received cranial irradiation, 39% of the children who received only chemotherapy also displayed abnormal MRI scans. In a subsequent prospective MRI study of childhood ALL survivors, 16.7% of those treated with chemotherapy only were identified as having white matter changes, which occurred predominantly in the frontal lobes (Paakko et al., 2000). Reddick and colleagues examined change in white matter integrity during active therapy for ALL. Rates of leukoencephalopathy were reported at 86% in children treated on a high-risk protocol immediately following consolidation therapy, though rates decreased to roughly 40% by the end of continuation therapy (Reddick et al., 2005). Furthermore, these investigators demonstrated associations between white matter abnormalities and problems in sustained attention (Reddick et al., 2006). Specifically, 112 ALL survivors were compared with 33 healthy siblings who participated as a control group. Within the ALL group, 84 patients received chemotherapy treatment only, while 28 also received cranial irradiation. Neurocognitive measures of sustained attention, intelligence, and academic achievement were performed and MRI was obtained. Those patients treated with CRT displayed reduced development of academic functions, including mathematics and reading skills, as well as problems with sustained attention. For the chemotherapy-only group, sustained attention was the single task that was significantly reduced. Furthermore, in both groups, smaller white matter volumes were significantly associated with impaired sustained attention. Reduced frontal white matter volume in ALL survivors has also been associated with reduced performance on measures of math calculation and vocabulary (Carey et al., 2008).

Early reports of psychological functioning following treatment for childhood ALL indicated few, if any, difficulties. Although children may experience emotional and behavioral problems during active therapy, either due to pain or distress associated with an invasive procedure or due to acute side effects of CRT (e.g., fatigue) or corticosteroid therapy (e.g., agitation), research studies have not consistently reported persistence of these problems during the first few years following completion of therapy (Eiser, Vance, & Seamark, 2000; Kupst & Schulman, 1988; Kupst et al., 1983; Patenaude

& Kupst, 2005). On the other hand, parents of survivors of childhood ALL have been identified as at increased risk for persistent psychological distress, including symptoms of posttraumatic stress (Alderfer, Cnaan, Annunziato, & Kazak, 2005; Kazak et al., 2004). Such parental distress may impact parental reporting of child adjustment and behavior and should be considered as a source of variability in child outcomes.

RECENT PSYCHOLOGICAL AND NEUROPSYCHOLOGICAL FINDINGS

More recent studies of childhood ALL survivors have focused on understanding the course, etiology, and variability in outcomes during and following treatment. These include the specific onset and evolution of deficits from young children undergoing active treatment to outcomes in long-term survivors during adulthood. The process of MTX toxicity and that of other potentially neurotoxic agents are being more closely examined. In addition, other direct and indirect sources of variability in outcomes are being explored, including chronic health conditions and health behaviors, as well as genetic predispositions. This active research will not only help clarify the risks experienced by long-term survivors but also provide insight for new treatment approaches.

The impact of chemotherapeutic agents on neurocognitive function is not universal, and most investigations have found significant individual variability in outcomes. Some investigators have reported no neurocognitive deficits in groups of children treated on recent chemotherapy-only protocols and have questioned whether chemotherapy truly impacts brain functions. Using a prospective-longitudinal design, Kingma and colleagues (2002) reported few neurocognitive problems in children exposed to chemotherapy alone, with survivors only demonstrating impairment on a measure of sustained attention several years following the end of therapy. However, some children displayed large declines in functioning, while others appeared relatively unaffected.

In an examination of patients treated with CRT, high-dose IV MTX, or standard-dose IV MTX, Spiegler and colleagues (2006) reported few neurocognitive deficits by 5 years postdiagnosis. Of the many measures included, again only a measure of sustained attention demonstrated reduction in the non-CRT group. These results may demonstrate an increased threshold for chemotherapeutic impact or a more gradual decline in function that may not be fully demonstrated until more than 5 years postdiagnosis.

Waber and colleagues (2007) also reported fewer problems associated with chemotherapy treatment. In comparing standard-risk patients randomly assigned to 18 Gy CRT or chemotherapy only, no impacts of treatment on standard measures of intelligence, academic skills, or memory storage and retrieval were reported in either group 6 years after diagnosis. However, children treated with CRT exhibited slowed information processing and diminished adaptability. Additionally, roughly 30% of the ALL survivors scored below the 10th percentile on indices of the Rey-Osterrieth Complex Figure, suggesting executive function may be impacted in a subset of survivors.

In a subsequent study, these investigators reported that high-risk patients treated with 18 Gy CRT performed significantly worse on measures of memory, working memory, and visual learning compared with standard-risk patients, two-thirds of whom were treated with chemotherapy alone (Waber et al., 2011). Importantly, performance of both risk groups approximated the expected population mean for most neurocognitive measures, though weaknesses in verbal working memory and processing of complex visual–spatial information were observed.

These differences in study outcomes raise questions about sample representation and individual variability as well as methodological differences. Recruitment strategies that focus on samples of convenience (e.g., patients who show up in the long-term survivor clinic) may result in either over- or underrepresentation of pathology. Those patients lost to follow-up may not experience the same degree of problems as those seeking medical evaluations. Unfortunately, many studies do not include sufficient data to determine whether the results can be generalized to the patient population. When more representative samples are included, the impact of chemotherapy-only treatment is often more localized to specific processes (i.e., sustained attention, cognitive fluency) or to a specific subset of patients at higher risk. In addition, neurocognitive impairment in long-term survivors appears to emerge with time.

The greatest risk for morbidity appears to begin 5 years following diagnosis, while many early and current studies include samples with shorter follow-up times. This fact is inherently related to the first point since many clinics do not include systematic follow-up of survivors beyond 5 years. To further complicate matters, not all children appear to be at risk, and those children who appear unaffected are often noted to be functioning in the above-average range. According to national demographics, childhood ALL does not appear to be randomly distributed throughout the population, rather it tends to occur at higher rates in Caucasians and middle to upper socioeconomic samples (Ries et al., 2007). This pattern will impact estimated rates of impairment when using nationally representative norms, particularly when focused only on group means. As such, many investigators have begun reporting rates of impairment as a primary outcome.

When taking these considerations into account, neurocognitive problems associated with chemotherapy treatment appear more specific and may be focused in the areas of attention deficits and executive dysfunction. A recent meta-analysis supports this finding by demonstrating that attention problems were most common, with moderate to large effect sizes, though problems in executive functions were also consistently reported, with moderate effect sizes (Peterson et al., 2008). Deficits in cognitive flexibility and cognitive fluency appear relatively more common in long-term survivors of ALL (Krull, Okcu, et al., 2008), though the onset of problems is uncertain.

Sex of the survivor may influence the specific profile of neurocognitive deficits following chemotherapy. Although females appear to demonstrate higher sensitivity to CRT, this does not appear to be the case with chemotherapy-only treatment. Rather, the treatment may interact with typical patterns of white matter development. In a recent report of 103 survivors of childhood ALL, all of whom were more than 5 years postdiagnosis, Jain and colleagues (2009) noted that female survivors demonstrated more problems with shifting and sustained attention, while male survivors demonstrated more problems with working memory and inhibitory control. This pattern may be mediated by typical sexual dimorphism in the brains of boys and girls. Throughout maturation, boys tend to display more age-related decreases in gray matter and increases in white matter volume compared with girls (De Bellis et al., 2001). This results in girls having a higher relative percentage of gray matter than white matter (Cosgrove, Mazure, & Staley, 2007). This may predispose girls to neurocognitive deficits that are dependent on subcortical white matter integrity, whereas boys may be more impacted by disruption of cortical gray matter integrity (Schmithorst, Holland, & Dardzinski, 2007).

Routes and intensity of MTX administration have also been examined as a source of variability in outcomes. Recently, Kadan-Lottick and colleagues (2009) compared single IT chemotherapy (i.e., MTX only) with triple IT chemotherapy (i.e., MTX combined with cytarabine and hydrocortisone), the latter of which continues to be the current process for IT therapy. When comparing 82 children treated with IT MTX with 89 children receiving triple IT therapy, all of whom were at least 1 year postcompletion of chemotherapy, no significant group differences were apparent. Still, roughly 30% of children in both groups demonstrated elevated impairment in attention and visual–motor integration. However, because only 32% of patients treated on the specific protocols were successfully recruited for neurocognitive testing, it is unclear as to whether these rates are over- or underestimations of impairment.

One area of additional consideration related to MTX neurotoxicity is the role of leucovorin rescue. MTX is an antimetabolite used to suppress cellular reproduction. Its effects are not specific to cancer cells, and it will suppress cell division in normal cells as well. Leucovorin is a form of folate usually given within 24 hours of MTX to protect normal cellular function. The dose and timing of leucovorin rescue may impact neurocognitive outcomes in long-term survivors.

Research in neurocognitive outcomes of long-term survivors of childhood ALL has also begun to address concerns over the potential neurotoxic effects of corticosteroids. Neurocognitive impairment following corticosteroid treatment has been reported in noncancer patients (Bender, Ikle, DuHamel, & Tinkelman, 1998; Lupien, Gillin, & Hauger, 1999). Dexamethasone, a particularly potent corticosteroid with relatively high CNS penetrance (Bostrom et al., 2003), is of particular concern; given its efficacy in cancer therapy, it is currently the preferred steroid. Compared with prednisone, treatment with dexamethasone has been reported to result in memory problems and reduced visual–spatial organization in children with ALL (Waber et al., 2000). However, this early study employed historical cohorts treated in different decades, making direct comparison difficult.

More recently, a study of long-term outcomes in 51 children treated with dexamethasone compared with 41 children treated with prednisone reported no significant differences on measures of attention, memory, visual–motor integration, math, and spelling (Kadan-Lottick, Brouwers, Breiger, Kaleita, Dziura, Liu, et al., 2009). Patients in both groups demonstrated increased rates of attention problems, and those treated with dexamethasone did score 5 standard score points (one-third of a standard deviation) lower on a measure of word reading. However, only 42% of eligible patients treated on the various protocols were evaluated, again limiting the potential for generalization.

Treatment with corticosteroids has also been linked to acute adverse neurobehavioral side effects, including difficulties with emotional control, mood lability, behavior regulation, and executive functions, with more adverse effects reported in preschoolers compared with school-aged children (Mrakotsky et al., 2011). Dexamethasone has also been associated with altered sleep and fatigue during active treatment (Hinds et al., 2007); these are symptoms that may also contribute to neurocognitive dysfunction.

In addition to variability in follow-up duration, specific neurocognitive processes examined, route and combination of chemotherapeutic agents, and representativeness of the sample of long-term survivors, outcomes associated with chemotherapeutic treatment may be influenced by genetic predispositions. Given the impact of MTX on folate metabolism, polymorphisms in the folate pathway have the potential to influence neurocognitive outcomes. Folate, which acts as a carrier of single carbon fragments for the conversion of homocysteine to methionine, has a role in purine and thymidine synthesis (Robien & Ulrich, 2003). Reduced-folate carrier is responsible for cellular uptake of folate and MTX (Ganapathy, Smith, & Prasad, 2004). The primary mechanism of action of MTX is inhibition of dihydrofolate reductase, the enzyme primarily responsible for the conversion of dihydrofolates to the active tetrahydrofolate (Goldman & Matherly, 1985). Another key enzyme in folate metabolism is methylenetetrahydrofolate reductase, which plays a role in the remethylation of homocysteine to methionine (Robien, Boynton, & Ulrich, 2005). Deficiency in this process can result in hyperhomocysteinemia. Alterations in the function of folate pathway enzymes may impact CNS folate levels, which will be further impacted by MTX chemotherapy and potentially result in synergistic toxic effects. Additional classes of polymorphisms to consider include those commonly associated with glucocorticoids, drug metabolism, and oxidative stress. Polymorphisms in the glucocorticoid receptor gene, nuclear receptor subfamily 3, can influence sensitivity to corticosteroids (van Rossum et al., 2004).

Glutatione S-transferase genes (GSTs) belong to a family of enzymes that catalyze the glutathione conjugation of a variety of compounds, including carcinogens, mutagens, cytotoxic drugs and their metabolites, and products of reactive oxidation (Hayes & Pulford, 1995). They catalyze detoxification of alkylating agents and platinum compounds used in cancer chemotherapy (Dirven, van Ommen, & van Bladeren, 1994). Furthermore, GSTs also detoxify free oxygen radicals, which are formed spontaneously or by chemotherapy drugs, and can sequester alkylating agents and steroids by direct binding (Hayes & Pulford, 1995).

A final class of polymorphisms to consider includes those related to impairment in attention and executive function, which appear to be involved in the typical neurocognitive phenotype seen in ALL survivors. Polymorphisms in dopamine receptor genes and monoamine oxidase A genes have been reported in children with attention deficits (Bobb et al., 2005; Fan, Fossella, Sommer, Wu, & Posner, 2003; Rueda, Rothbart, McCandliss, Saccomanno, & Posner, 2005; Shaw et al., 2007; Thapar, O'Donovan, & Owen, 2005; Todd & Lobos, 2002). In addition, polymorphisms in catechol-O-methyltransferase have been linked to the development of impaired executive function in a variety of populations (Barnett, Jones, Robbins, & Muller, 2007; Kramer et al., 2007; Lipsky et al., 2005; MacDonald, Carter, Flory, Ferrell, & Manuck, 2007; Weiss et al., 2007).

We recently examined the association between polymorphisms in these classes of genes and neurocognitive outcomes in ALL survivors. In a sample of 48 long-term survivors of pediatric leukemia, attention problems reported on a parental questionnaire were related to polymorphisms in the methylenetetrahydrofolate reductase enzyme, with a 7.4-fold increase in risk of attention problems (Krull, Brouwers, et al., 2008). In a sample of 72 survivors of ALL, polymorphisms in the methionine synthase enzyme were related to lower performance on direct measures of shifting attention and processing speed (Kamdar et al., 2011). Additionally, survivors with more than five folate pathway risk alleles demonstrated significantly lower performance on measures of processing speed and shifting attention compared with survivors who had fewer than six risk alleles.

More recently, we confirmed the association between polymorphisms in methi-onine synthase and attention problems, as measured on a continuous performance task in a validation sample of 243 survivors treated on a uniform chemotherapy protocol; this was a sample consisting of 70.4% of all eligible patients treated on the protocol (Krull, Bhojwani, et al., 2012). Controlling for age, sex, and treat-ment intensity, survivors with polymorphisms in methionine synthase, glutathione S-transferase, and monoamine oxidase were significantly more likely to demon-strate impaired sustained attention by the end of therapy. Furthermore, those with polymorphisms in apolipoprotein E4 were more likely to be reported by their par-ents as having significant attention and learning problems at the end of therapy. Although the novel associations with glutathione S-transferase, monoamine oxi-dase, and apolipoprotein E4 require validation, these associations would suggest the presence of general underlying risk factors that may not be dependent on the specific neurotoxic agent.

The studies discussed previously suggest that neurocognitive impairment in sur-vivors of childhood cancer emerge over time, though subtle deficits may appear rela-tively early in the course of survivorship. There are relatively few reported studies of neurocognitive changes during active therapy for childhood leukemia. In a feasibil-ity study with a sample of 50 ALL patients, Jansen and colleagues (2005) reported no impairment in IQ, language, memory, or attention when patients were evaluated within 2 weeks of starting therapy. However, in a prospective longitudinal study with a slightly larger cohort of 82 consecutive leukemia patients, Hockenberry and colleagues (2007) reported declines in processing speed detected within 2 months of diagnosis. These deficits predicted reduced development of higher-level visual–motor and per-ceptual reasoning abilities 1 year after the completion of chemotherapy. In this study, survivors demonstrated mean processing speed scores that were 0.8 standard devia-tions below the national mean. As therapy continued into the second and third years of treatment, visual–motor integration and perceptual problem-solving skills steadily declined. Significant positive correlations between initial performance on processing speed and subsequent visual–motor integration were found ($r = .54$, $p < .001$) as well as between the initial processing speed and subsequent perceptual problem solving ($r = .33$, $p < .007$).

In a related study, processing speed and working memory performance during the first year of chemotherapy were found to be associated with treatment intensity. Children treated with lower doses of IV MTX show improved performance during the first year of chemotherapy, while the performance of children treated with higher doses declined over time (Carey et al., 2007). By the end of the second year of ther-apy, 10.5% of the children treated with low-dose IV MTX and 38.5% of the children treated with high-dose IV MTX fell more than 1 standard deviation below the mean on a measure of nonverbal working memory.

These early changes in neurocognitive performance have been associated with markers of oxidative stress in cerebral spinal fluid (CSF). Using CSF samples collected prior to IT injections, we demonstrated an increased concentration of oxidized phos-pholipids following induction and consolidation therapy (Caron et al., 2009; Krull, Hockenberry, Miketova, Carey, & Moore, 2011), suggesting oxidized injury to CNS membrane integrity. The increases in oxidized phospholipids following induction and consolidation therapy were associated with decreased working memory, organ-izational abilities, and verbal fluency at the end of chemotherapy (Caron et al., 2009).

Consistent with previous reports, younger age at diagnosis was associated with both increased oxidative stress and decreased executive function.

More recently, we demonstrated that increases in phospholipids specific to myelin integrity (i.e., sphingomyelin and lysophosphatidylcholine) following induction and consolidation therapy preceded and predicted the onset of processing speed and working memory performance deficits, which were demonstrated by the end of the continuation phase of chemotherapy (Krull, Hockenberry, et al., 2011).

The studies mentioned above demonstrate a relatively early change in CNS integrity during chemotherapy, manifested through reduced processing speed and attention and through various biomarkers, including MRI and CSF evidence of white matter injury as early as the end of consolidation therapy. Although the neurocognitive impairment is subtle, it is correlated with these biomarkers and involves basic skills associated with the development of higher-order brain functions. However, given some of the difficulties with retention of participants in follow-up studies that extend beyond 5 years, little is known about very long-term outcomes. Two prospective cohort studies have been recently utilized to examine such outcomes in adult survivors of childhood cancer: the Childhood Cancer Survivor Study (CCSS) and the St. Jude Lifetime Cohort Study (SJLIFE).

The CCSS is a retrospective cohort study designed to evaluate the impact of childhood cancer and its treatment on long-term function and health. Eligible participants were treated for one of eight cancer diagnoses at 26 institutions between 1970 and 1986 when <21 years. Cohort entry was limited to those individuals who survived for at least 5 years after their original diagnosis. More than 14,000 cancer survivors and 5000 randomly selected siblings have completed multiple questionnaires since enrollment. Compared with siblings, adult survivors of ALL are more likely to be unemployed (Kirchhoff et al., 2010), less likely to be employed in a professional or managerial occupation (Kirchhoff et al., 2011), and less likely to live independently (Kunin-Batson et al., 2011) or to marry (Janson et al., 2009). The reduced social attainment is likely associated with the increased risk for these survivors to experience chronic health conditions (Oeffinger et al., 2006), though continued neurocognitive and psychological limitations also likely play an important role.

Although overall rates of emotional problems do not differ from national norms, adult survivors of childhood ALL are 1.6 and 2.0 times more likely to report problems with mental health and functional impairment, respectively, compared with sibling controls (Mody et al., 2008). Female survivors who are treated at an older age with more intensive treatment procedures are also at increased risk for posttraumatic stress disorder as adults (Stuber et al., 2010). Because such distress is not apparent shortly after completion of therapy, increased risk for emotional problems may reflect a developed response to persistent stress associated with functional limitations and chronic health conditions.

The CCSS cohort has also completed a neurocognitive questionnaire that assesses task efficiency, memory, organization, and emotional regulation (Krull, Gioia, et al., 2008). Of those completing this measure, 1792 were adult survivors of childhood ALL: 624 treated only with chemotherapy and 1168 treated with CRT. Those treated with CRT were significantly more likely to report neurocognitive problems compared with sibling controls (Kadan-Lottick et al., 2010). Conversely, ALL survivors treated with only chemotherapy did not differ significantly from sibling controls, which is somewhat inconsistent with previous reports. However, the results of the CCSS study are based entirely on self-reported neurocognitive deficits in a cohort that was an average of 24 years postdiagnosis, a diagnosis that occurred during childhood. It is entirely plausible that survivors may adjust their expectations such that their persistent symptoms are no longer considered "problems" as often defined in patient-reported measures. Conversely, if the symptoms cause major limitations in life events or the symptoms occur following a period of normal development of which the survivor is aware, survivors may be less likely to adjust expectations. Survivors who have experienced attention or processing-speed problems since early childhood may be less aware or troubled by such deficits as adults.

Harila and colleagues (2009) used direct assessment to compare neurocognitive the outcomes of 64 adult survivors of ALL at least 10 years after diagnosis with those of 45 healthy controls. Survivors treated with cranial irradiation performed significantly worse on measures of verbal reasoning, nonverbal reasoning, memory, and attention compared with both nonirradiated survivors and healthy controls. Previous neuropsychological testing data were available for a subsample of survivors. These data demonstrated a significant decline in verbal and performance intelligence scores over time for irradiated survivors, while nonirradiated survivors only demonstrated a decline in verbal IQ. However, these findings must be interpreted with caution given the small sample size and concerns over the representativeness of the sample.

The SJLIFE is a prospective cohort study designed to examine long-term functional outcomes in adults treated for childhood cancer at St. Jude Children's Research Hospital (Hudson et al., 2011). Eligibility criteria for inclusion in the SJLIFE study include the following: (1) diagnosis of childhood malignancy treated at SJCRH; (2) survival ≥10 years from diagnosis; and (3) current age ≥18 years. Three levels of participation are offered: (1) comprehensive on-campus evaluations; (2) limited home evaluation; or (3) completion of health surveys only. To date, 92% of more than 4000 survivors treated since 1962 have been successfully contacted, of whom 91% have agreed to participate. Among participants, 89% agreed to an on-campus evaluation.

We recently examined neurocognitive function in 653 adult survivors of childhood ALL included in this cohort, representing 83% of eligible ALL survivors contacted to date. Survivors completed a comprehensive battery of neurocognitive measures, and analysis was restricted to survivors who have not experienced a relapse or second cancer that required additional CNS therapy. Eligible participants were on average 35 years old and were 29 years postdiagnosis. Two hundred and thirty-nine survivors (36%) were treated with 24 Gy CRT, 187 (29%) were treated with 18 Gy CRT, and 227 (35%) were treated with chemotherapy only. Elevated rates of significant impairment, defined as a score falling below the 2nd percentile, were observed on measures of vocabulary (Wechsler Abbreviated Scale of Intelligence - Vocabulary; 12.5%), mathematics (Woodcock-Johnson Tests of Academic Achievement III Calculation; 8.9%), sustained and/or focused attention (Conners Continuous Performance Test or Trail Making A; 21.5%), memory (California Verbal Learning Test; 19.8%), fine motor dexterity (Grooved Pegboard; 19.3%), cognitive flexibility (Trail Making B; 20.1%), and verbal fluency (Controlled Oral Word Association; 9.3%). Self-rating of executive function (i.e., Behavior Rating Inventory of Executive Function [BRIEF]-Adult) suggested problems with shifting (11.1%), emotional control (11.9%), and working memory (21.0%). Although CRT was clearly related to impairments in all neurocognitive functions, patients treated with only chemotherapy demonstrated significant impairment on measures of attention, long-term memory, and executive function, with the latter being most prevalent. Controlling for academic and intellectual functions, those survivors with executive function deficits were 35% more likely to not complete college, and those with attention problems were 35% more likely to not be employed.

These results provide strong support for the notion that long-term survivors of childhood ALL are at continued risk for neurocognitive impairment. Although survivors treated with high-dose CRT are at risk for impairment in multiple domains, those treated with lower doses of CRT and those treated only with chemotherapy are at risk for impairment in attention and executive function, which is associated with limitations in ultimate educational attainment and employment.

INTERVENTION AND TREATMENT GAINS

Although significant effort has been directed at characterizing neurocognitive late effects, considerably less attention has focused on remediation or prevention of such deficits. One area of intervention that has received attention is the use of psychostimulants to treat attention problems in survivors. Early studies with small samples of survivors of childhood ALL and brain tumors suggested the promise of methylphenidate in the short-term treatment of primary attention problems, based on a continuous performance measure of sustained attention (Thompson et al., 2001), as well as on parent and teacher ratings of attention and teacher ratings of social skills (Mulhern et al., 2004). In a recent double-blind, placebo-controlled, cross-over trial, methylphenidate treatment was associated with acute improvement on a measure of cognitive interference control, though not attention or processing speed (Conklin et al., 2007). Using a subset of survivors from the placebo trial, a 12-month open-label trial of methylphenidate demonstrated significantly improved performance based on a continuous performance test, as well as on parent, teacher, and self-ratings of attention (Conklin, Reddick, et al., 2010). To date, none of these trials have reported an impact on higher-order cognitive skills. It is important to consider that improvement demonstrated while participants are actively taking methylphenidate may not be maintained following discontinuation of the drug. Further, a positive response rate to methylphenidate treatment appears substantially lower among cancer survivors compared with the rate observed in other populations (i.e., attention-deficit/hyperactivity disorder [ADHD]; Conklin, Helton, et al., 2010), Also, subgroups of survivors may be at increased risk for side effects (Conklin et al., 2009). Notably, deceleration of body mass index and height has been reported following methylphenidate treatment in childhood cancer survivors (Jasper et al., 2009).

Although attention deficits experienced by survivors have been described as being similar to those observed in children with ADHA–predominately inattentive type (ADHD-PI; Butler & Mulhern, 2005), a recent study yielded data that challenge the appropriateness of applying an ADHD phenotype to ALL survivors. In a study of 161 survivors of childhood ALL, Krull and colleagues (2011) reported that 10.5% met criteria for ADHD, though 25.5% of the entire sample reported attention symptoms that impaired functioning in multiple settings. This study raises important questions regarding the characteristic phenotype and potential treatment options for attention deficits in this population and further suggests that attention problems experienced by survivors of leukemia are not fully captured by the syndrome of ADHD.

Direct rehabilitation of neurocognitive deficits in childhood cancer survivors has also been investigated. Butler and colleagues (2008) conducted a multicenter, randomized clinical trial of a cognitive remediation program (CRP) with survivors of childhood cancer who were aged 6–17 years and who demonstrated significant attention problems, either by performance on a continuous performance test or on a behavior rating inventory. Of 173 eligible survivors, 109 were randomized to the intervention while 54 were randomized to a wait-list control group. The intervention was delivered over 20 two-hour sessions over a 4- to 5-month period and included hierarchically graded mass practice, strategy training, and cognitive–behavioral therapy. Eighty survivors in the intervention group completed 60% of the scheduled sessions. Survivors in the intervention group demonstrated significant improvement in academic achievement (effect size = 0.15), working memory (effect size = 0.28), an assessment of learning strategies (effect size = 0.98), and teacher-reported attention problems (effect size = 0.33). Both groups demonstrated significant improvements in focused attention (effect size = 0.30, control group; effect size = 0.31, intervention), memory recall (effect size = 0.41, control; effect size = 0.29, intervention), vigilance (effect size = 0.52, control; effect size = 0.42, intervention), and parent-reported attention problems (effect size = 0.22, control; effect size = 0.70, intervention). These results provide support for small improvement in specific cognitive skills and large improvement in learning strategies with an intensive intervention. However, this intervention demands significant resources, and issues with feasibility have limited its generalization.

Computerized cognitive training may be a more practical approach, and two recent pilot studies reported positive effects of such training in survivors of childhood cancer. The first study involved survivors of childhood ALL (n = 3) and brain tumors (n = 6), aged 10–17 years, with documented deficits in attention and working memory (Hardy, Willard, & Bonner, 2011). Participants completed baseline and follow-up neurocognitive testing, separated by a 12-week home-based computerized cognitive training program. Significant improvements on a measure of short-term memory and parent-reported attention problems were observed from baseline through a 3-month follow-up. Although an increase in standard scale points was observed for working memory tasks, these improvements did not reach statistical significance. The intervention was associated with good feasibility and acceptability.

Kesler and colleagues (2011) reported on the feasibility and efficacy of an 8-week home-based computerized cognitive rehabilitation program. Participants included 23 survivors of ALL (n = 14) and brain tumors (n = 9), aged 7–19 years, with documented executive function deficits. Results revealed significant improvements in processing speed, cognitive flexibility, and visual and verbal declarative memory. In addition, functional neuroimaging revealed significantly increased activation in the dorsolateral prefrontal cortex following completion of the rehabilitation program. Compliance with the cognitive rehabilitation program was 83%.

Importantly, both studies were limited by small sample sizes; improvement was limited primarily to specific cognitive processes targeted by the training programs, with no reported evidence of generalization of gains to daily activities. Further, the long-term maintenance of improvement is unclear.

The limited effect sizes and generalization of past rehabilitation efforts may be associated with the fact that they were initiated following the onset of documented dysfunction. Neurocognitive impairment associated with treatment for ALL is somewhat predictable, unlike impairment following traumatic brain injury or epilepsy. As discussed above, although subtle changes begin to occur within months of diagnosis, impairments in attention and working memory processes generally do not become clinically significant until 3–5 years following diagnosis. Given this window of opportunity, it may be feasible and more efficacious to implement cognitive stimulation approaches with the aim of preventing or mitigating neurocognitive dysfunction.

Recently, Moore and colleagues (2011) evaluated the efficacy of a preventive intervention for patients newly diagnosed with ALL. Patients were randomized to either a mathematics intervention (n = 15) or standard care (n = 17) for a 1-year period during the latter portion of consolidation therapy. The intervention group received roughly 50 hours of individualized intervention using multimodalities (i.e., pictures, abstract symbols, mathematical language, concrete manipulatives) to teach transferable problem-solving approaches. Each child received an individualized curriculum based on an assessment of current mathematical knowledge, with content and process consistent with that recommended by the National Council of Teachers of Mathematics. The standard care group received a written report with recommendations they could take to their school. Neurocognitive evaluations were conducted at baseline, at the end of chemotherapy, and 1 year following the completion of chemotherapy. The intervention group demonstrated significant improvements in calculation and applied mathematics from baseline to postintervention (effect size = 0.51, calculation; effect size = 0.61, applied mathematics). More importantly, visual working memory improved from baseline to the 1-year postchemotherapy follow-up (effect size = 0.62). Significant between-group differences were observed for applied mathematics and visual working memory, with the intervention group demonstrating steady improvement and the standard care group demonstrating a gradual decline. These results, when applied prior to the onset of neurocognitive impairment, provide preliminary evidence for generalization from teaching educational strategies to working memory skills.

In sum, growing evidence suggests that cognitive training may yield short-term improvements in specific neurocognitive processes. Yet questions remain regarding the long-term maintenance of such gains as well as generalization to functional daily activities. An increased focus on preventive efforts is warranted.

CURRENT RESOURCES

Resources specially designed for survivors of childhood cancer are not well integrated into the public education system. Unlike conditions such as traumatic brain injury or autism, childhood ALL is a relatively rare condition, and schools may not have sufficient experience with the unique needs of survivors. With proper documentation, children who experience neurocognitive or psychological problems or mobility limitations, including excessive fatigue, can receive services under an individualized education plan. Resource guidelines have been developed by a variety of organizations to assist with monitoring and healthy development.

The Children's Oncology Group (COG) is a multidisciplinary organization funded by the National Cancer Institute to organize and implement clinical trials in childhood cancer. COG has established guidelines for the standard of care in monitoring the late effects on long-term survivors of pediatric cancer (www.survivorshipguidelines.org). These guidelines are updated every 2 years by a multidisciplinary committee that conducts a comprehensive annual review of the published literature. Recommendations for screening and follow-up care are made according to specific treatment exposures, supported by findings in the peer-reviewed literature. It is recommended that survivors exposed to high-dose IV or IT antimetabolites (i.e., cytarabine or MTX), cranial radiation, or neurosurgery receive a formal neuropsychological evaluation. This evaluation is recommended at entry into long-term follow-up (i.e., 5 years following diagnosis or 2 years following completion of therapy) and then periodically as clinically indicated. It is recommended that these survivors be referred to a school liaison, psychologist, or social worker for facilitation of access to educational resources and support. Consideration for use of psychotropic medication is also recommended, as is vocational rehabilitation for those transitioning into adulthood. It is recommended that survivors with any cancer experience, as well as symptoms of depression, anxiety, posttraumatic stress, fatigue, and social withdrawal, have an annual psychosocial assessment to obtain history of educational and/or vocational progress. Patient-oriented individual health links (available in English and Spanish) are also available on the COG Web site.

The CCSS is funded by the National Cancer Institute as a resource for professionals interested in cancer survivorship. The CCSS Web site (http://ccss.stjude.org/) provides open access to survivorship statistics, research questionnaires, and study publications. It also provides guidance for investigators seeking access to the data on more than 35,000 long-term survivors and 8000 siblings who participate in regular follow-up surveys.

Additional resources are available through the National Cancer Institute (http://www.cancer.gov/) and their Office of Cancer Survivorship (http://dccps.nci.nih.gov/ocs/) and the American Cancer Society (http://www.cancer.org/index). Resources specific to ALL are also available through the Leukemia Lymphoma Society (http://www.lls.org/).

FUTURE AIMS AND RESEARCH OPPORTUNITIES

In addition to further characterizing progression of neurocognitive problems in long-term survivors as they age, future research is needed to elucidate risk factors for poor outcomes following cancer therapy. These risk factors not only include the environmental and genetic predispositions outlined above but also chronic health conditions that may cause or exacerbate neurocognitive dysfunction. Hopefully, such efforts will also stimulate new and novel research focused on rehabilitation and preventative interventions.

As survivors of childhood cancer age, they are at increased risk for chronic health conditions. Roughly 70% of ALL survivors will experience a chronic condition within the first 30 years of survival, with 20% experiencing a severe, life-threatening, or disabling condition (Oeffinger et al., 2006). These conditions include congestive heart failure, coronary artery disease, cerebrovascular accident, renal failure, and pulmonary morbidity. Currently, the contribution of these chronic conditions to neurocognitive and psychological functioning in ALL survivors is unknown. One could surmise that a survivor who has already experienced neurotoxicity would be particularly susceptible to the effects of chronic health problems.

Neurocognitive and psychological issues may also increase the risk for health problems in long-term survivors. Children who demonstrate social withdrawal as long-term survivors are less likely to engage in regular exercise as adults, even when controlling for body mass index and exercise levels as a child (Krull et al., 2010). In addition, survivors with significant attention problems are less likely to demonstrate proper sunscreen use (Krull et al., 2010). These poor health behaviors increase the risk of a second cancer, the treatment of which may add to the cumulative neurotoxicity profile. Further adding to this long-term risk is the fact that adults who demonstrate neurocognitive problems following their treatment for childhood cancer are less likely to engage in routine and recommended health screening exams, which help detect second cancers (Krull, Annett, et al., 2011). Thus, in addition to enhancing educational and vocational attainment and quality of life, addressing neurocognitive and psychological problems in cancer survivors may have an indirect impact on survival.

Research has examined the association between cancer therapy and fatigue in long-term survivors (Hinds et al., 2007; Meeske, Siegel, Globe, Mack, & Bernstein, 2005). However, only recently has it been reported that these behaviors impact neurocognitive function in survivors as well (Clanton et al., 2011). If fatigue and sleep difficulties exacerbate neurocognitive deficits in ALL survivors, treatment of fatigue and enhanced sleep behavior may improve neurocognitive function. A randomized clinical trial exploring this question is currently underway at St. Jude Children's Research Hospital.

The established risk for chronic health problems in cancer survivors may be associated with increased rates of pharmacologic treatment for symptom management. In fact, a forthcoming report from CCSS indicates that survivors are significantly more likely to report using prescription psychoactive medications compared with siblings, with more than 40% of adult survivors reporting such use over a 16-year period (Brinkman et al., 2012). This raises important questions regarding health-status impact on medication efficacy in patients at risk for cardiopulmonary, renal, neurologic, and metabolic conditions following cancer-directed therapies. There is a need to better understand the use of psychoactive medications in cancer survivors because underlying medical vulnerabilities may increase the risk for adverse medication side effects, including reduced quality of life and neurocognitive dysfunction.

Given the success in treatment of childhood ALL, there exists an aging cohort of long-term survivors. This cohort, combined with the organized tracking resources of COG and CCSS, provides opportunities for research that did not previously exist. New research questions include the following: Are adults who experience neurotoxic effects of CRT or chemotherapy as young children at risk for early-onset dementia as they age? Does a traumatic medical event as a young child sensitize adults to psychological problems following medical illness as adults, or does the successful survival of a life-threatening illness provide them an emotional buffer against such future events? These are just some of the many areas that warrant future investigation.

In summary, with the tremendous success in the treatment of childhood ALL, we are confronted with a large population of long-term survivors who are at risk for a variety of medical, neuropsychological, and psychological late effects. Over the next several decades, major clinical advances will not come from enhanced survival because there is little room for improvement in that area. Rather the next frontier to master is enhanced quality of life and functional outcomes, areas where much work still needs to be done. Strategies may include adjustments to treatment protocols and supportive care to prevent morbidity as well as rehabilitative approaches to enhance recovery and promote healthy aging. Neuropsychologists can play a pivotal role in these future efforts.

REFERENCES

Al-Khatib, T., Cohen, N., Carret, A. S., & Daniel, S. (2010). Cisplatinum ototoxicity in children, long-term follow up. *International Journal of Pediatric Otorhinolaryngology, Int J Pediatr Otorhi, 74,* 913–919. doi: 10.1016/j.ijporl.2010.05.011

Alderfer, M. A., Cnaan, A., Annunziato, R. A., & Kazak, A. E. (2005). Patterns of post-traumatic stress symptoms in parents of childhood cancer survivors. [*Journal of Family Psychology, 19,* 430–440. doi: 10.1037/0893-3200.19.3.430

Barnett, J. H., Jones, P. B., Robbins, T. W., & Muller, U. (2007). Effects of the catechol-O-methyltransferase Val158Met polymorphism on executive function: a meta-analysis of the Wisconsin Card Sort Test in schizophrenia and healthy controls. *Molecular Psychiatry, 12,* 502–509.

Bender, B. G., Ikle, D. N., DuHamel, T., & Tinkelman, D. (1998). Neuropsychological and behavioral changes in asthmatic children treated with beclomethasone dipropionate versus theophylline. *Pediatrics, 101,* 355–360.

Bobb, A. J., Addington, A. M., Sidransky, E., Gornick, M. C., Lerch, J. P., Greenstein, D. K.,...Rapoport, J. L. (2005). Support for association between ADHD and two candidate genes: NET1 and DRD1. *American Journal of Medical Genetics Part B: Neuropsychiatric Genetics, 134,* 67–72.

Bostrom, B. C., Sensel, M. R., Sather, H. N., Gaynon, P. S., La, M. K., Johnston, K.,...Trigg, M. E. (2003). Dexamethasone versus prednisone and daily oral versus weekly intravenous mercaptopurine for patients with standard-risk acute lymphoblastic leukemia: a report from the Children's Cancer Group. *Blood, 101,* 3809–3817.

Brinkman, T. M., Zhang, N., Ullrich, N. J., Brouwers, P., Green, D. M., Srivastava, D. K.,...Krull, K. R. (2012). Psychoactive medication use and neurocognitive function in adult survivors of childhood cancer: A report from the childhood cancer survivor study. *Pediatric Blood & Cancer.* doi: 10.1002/pbc.24255.

Brown, R. T., & Madan-Swain, A. (1993). Cognitive, neuropsychological, and academic sequelae in children with leukemia. *Journal of Learning Disabilities, 26,* 74–90.

Buizer, A. I., de Sonneville, L. M., van den Heuvel-Eibrink, M. M., & Veerman, A. J. (2005). Chemotherapy and attentional dysfunction in survivors of childhood acute lymphoblastic leukemia: effect of treatment intensity. *Pediatric Blood & Cancer, 45,* 281–290.

Buizer, A. I., de Sonneville, L. M., van den Heuvel-Eibrink, M. M., & Veerman, A. J. (2006). Behavioral and educational limitations after chemotherapy for childhood acute lymphoblastic leukemia or Wilms tumor. *Cancer, 106,* 2067–2075.

Burger, B., Beier, R., Zimmermann, M., Beck, J. D., Reiter, A., & Schrappe, M. (2005). Osteonecrosis: a treatment related toxicity in childhood acute lymphoblastic leukemia (ALL)—experiences from trial ALL-BFM 95. *Pediatric Blood & Cancer, 44,* 220–225. doi: 10.1002/pbc.20244

Butler, R. W., Copeland, D. R., Fairclough, D. L., Mulhern, R. K., Katz, E. R., Kazak, A. E.,...Sahler, O. J. (2008). A multicenter, randomized clinical trial of a cognitive remediation program for childhood survivors of a pediatric malignancy. *Journal of Consulting & Clinical Psychology, 76,* 367–378. doi: 2008-06469-002 [pii]10.1037/0022-006X.76.3.367

Butler, R. W., & Mulhern, R. K. (2005). Neurocognitive interventions for children and adolescents surviving cancer. *Journal of Pediatric Psychology, 30,* 65–78.

Carey, M. E., Haut, M. W., Reminger, S. L., Hutter, J. J., Theilmann, R., & Kaemingk, K. L. (2008). Reduced frontal white matter volume in long-term childhood leukemia survivors: a voxel-based morphometry study. *American Journal of Neuroradiology, 29,* 792–797.

Carey, M. E., Hockenberry, M. J., Moore, I. M., Hutter, J. J., Krull, K. R., Pasvogel, A., & Kaemingk, K. L. (2007). Brief report: effect of intravenous methotrexate dose and infusion rate on neuropsychological function one year after diagnosis of acute lymphoblastic leukemia. *Journal of Pediatric Psychology, 32,* 189–193.

Caron, J. E., Krull, K. R., Hockenberry, M., Jain, N., Kaemingk, K., & Moore, I. M. (2009). Oxidative stress and executive function in children receiving chemotherapy for acute lymphoblastic leukemia. *Pediatric Blood & Cancer, 53,* 551–556. doi: 10.1002/pbc.22128

Christie, D., Leiper, A. D., Chessells, J. M., & Vargha- Khadem, F. (1995). Intellectual performance after presymptomatic cranial radiotherapy for leukaemia: effects of age and sex. *Archives of Diseases in Childhood, 73,* 136–140.

Clanton, N. R., Klosky, J. L., Li, C., Jain, N., Srivastava, D. K., Mulrooney, D.,... Krull, K. R. (2011). Fatigue, vitality, sleep, and neurocognitive functioning in adult survivors of childhood cancer: A report from the Childhood Cancer Survivor Study. *Cancer.* doi: 10.1002/cncr.25797

Conklin, H. M., Helton, S., Ashford, J., Mulhern, R. K., Reddick, W. E., Brown, R.,... Khan, R. B. (2010). Predicting methylphenidate response in long-term survivors of childhood cancer: a randomized, double-blind, placebo-controlled, crossover trial. *Journal of Pediatric Psychology, 35,* 144–155. doi: jsp044 [pii]10.1093/jpepsy/jsp044

Conklin, H. M., Khan, R. B., Reddick, W. E., Helton, S., Brown, R., Howard, S. C.,... Mulhern, R. K. (2007). Acute neurocognitive response to methylphenidate among survivors of childhood cancer: a randomized, double-blind, cross-over trial. *Journal of Pediatric Psychology, 32,* 1127–1139.

Conklin, H. M., Lawford, J., Jasper, B. W., Morris, E. B., Howard, S. C., Ogg, S. W.,... Khan, R. B. (2009). Side effects of methylphenidate in childhood cancer survivors: a randomized placebo-controlled trial. *Pediatrics, 124,* 226–233. doi: 124/1/226 [pii]10.1542/peds.2008-1855

Conklin, H. M., Reddick, W. E., Ashford, J., Ogg, S., Howard, S. C., Morris, E. B.,... Khan, R. B. (2010). Long-term efficacy of methylphenidate in enhancing attention regulation, social skills, and academic abilities of childhood cancer survivors. *Journal of Clinical Oncology, 28,* 4465–4472. doi: 10.1200/JCO.2010.28.4026

Cosgrove, K. P., Mazure, C. M., & Staley, J. K. (2007). Evolving knowledge of sex differences in brain structure, function, and chemistry. *Biological Psychiatry, 62,* 847–855.

De Bellis, M. D., Keshavan, M. S., Beers, S. R., Hall, J., Frustaci, K., Masalehdan, A.,... Boring, A. M. (2001). Sex differences in brain maturation during childhood and adolescence. *Cerebral Cortex, 11,* 552–557.

Dirven, H. A., van Ommen, B., & van Bladeren, P. J. (1994). Involvement of human glutathione S-transferase isoenzymes in the conjugation of cyclophosphamide metabolites with glutathione. *Cancer Research, 54,* 6215–6220.

Eiser, C., Vance, Y. H., & Seamark, D. (2000). The development of a theoretically driven generic measure of quality of life for children aged 6–12 years: a preliminary report. *Child: Care, Health and Development, 26,* 445–456.

Fan, J., Fossella, J., Sommer, T., Wu, Y., & Posner, M. I. (2003). Mapping the genetic variation of executive attention onto brain activity. *Proceedings of the National Academy of Sciences, 100,* 7406–7411.

Ganapathy, V., Smith, S. B., & Prasad, P. D. (2004). SLC19: The folate/thiamine transporter family. *Pflügers Archiv European Journal of Physiology, 447,* 641–646.

Goldman, I. D., & Matherly, L. H. (1985). The cellular pharmacology of methotrexate. *Pharmacological Therapy, 28,* 77–102.

Hardy, K. K., Willard, V. W., & Bonner, M. J. (2011). Computerized cognitive training in survivors of childhood cancer: a pilot study. *Journal of Pediatric Oncology Nursing, 28,* 27–33. doi: 1043454210377178 [pii] 10.1177/1043454210377178

Harila, M. J., Winqvist, S., Lanning, M., Bloigu, R., & Harila-Saari, A. H. (2009). Progressive neurocognitive impairment in young adult survivors of childhood acute lymphoblastic leukemia. *Pediatric Blood & Cancer, 53*, 156–161. doi: 10.1002/pbc.21992

Hayes, J. D., & Pulford, D. J. (1995). The glutathione S-transferase supergene family: regulation of GST and the contribution of the isoenzymes to cancer chemoprotection and drug resistance. *Critical Reviews in Biochemistry and Molecular Biology, 30*, 445–600.

Hertzberg, H., Huk, W. J., Ueberall, M. A., Langer, T., Meier, W., Dopfer, R.,... Beck, J. D. (1997). CNS late effects after ALL therapy in childhood. Part I: Neuroradiological findings in long-term survivors of childhood ALL—an evaluation of the interferences between morphology and neuropsychological performance. The German Late Effects Working Group. *Medical and Pediatric Oncology, 28*, 387–400.

Hinds, P. S., Hockenberry, M. J., Gattuso, J. S., Srivastava, D. K., Tong, X., Jones, H.,... Pui, C. H. (2007). Dexamethasone alters sleep and fatigue in pediatric patients with acute lymphoblastic leukemia. *Cancer, 110*, 2321–2330.

Hockenberry, M., Krull, K., Moore, K., Gregurich, M. A., Casey, M. E., & Kaemingk, K. (2007). Longitudinal evaluation of fine motor skills in children with leukemia. *Journal of Pediatric Hematology/Oncology, 29*, 535–539.

Howlander, N., Noone, A. M., Krapcho, M., Neyman, N., Aminou, R., Waldron, W.,... Edwards, B. K. (2010). *SEER Cancer Statistics Review, 1975-2008*. Bethesda, MD: Retrieved from http://seer.cancer.gov/csr/1975_2008/, based on November 2010 SEER data submission, posted to the SEER web site, 2011.

Hudson, M. M. (2007). Anthracycline cardiotoxicity in long-term survivors of childhood cancer: The light is not at the end of the tunnel. *Pediatric Blood &Cancer, 48*, 649–650. doi: 10.1002/pbc.21165

Hudson, M. M., Ness, K. K., Nolan, V. G., Armstrong, G. T., Green, D. M., Morris, E. B.,... Robison, L. L. (2011). Prospective medical assessment of adults surviving childhood cancer: study design, cohort characteristics, and feasibility of the St. Jude Lifetime Cohort study. *Pediatric Blood & Cancer, 56*, 825–836. doi: 10.1002/pbc.22875

Jain, N., Brouwers, P., Okcu, M. F., Cirino, P. T., & Krull, K. R. (2009). Sex-specific attention problems in long-term survivors of pediatric acute lymphoblastic leukemia. *Cancer, 115*, 4238–4245. doi: 10.1002/cncr.24464

Jansen, N. C., Kingma, A., Tellegen, P., van Dommelen, R. I., Bouma, A., Veerman, A., & Kamps, W. A. (2005). Feasibility of neuropsychological assessment in leukaemia patients shortly after diagnosis: directions for future prospective research. *Archives of Diseases in Childhood, 90*, 301–304.

Janson, C., Leisenring, W., Cox, C., Termuhlen, A. M., Mertens, A. C., Whitton, J. A.,... Kadan-Lottick, N. S. (2009). Predictors of marriage and divorce in adult survivors of childhood cancers: a report from the Childhood Cancer Survivor Study. *Cancer Epidemiology, Biomarkers & Prevention, 18*, 2626–2635. doi: 18/10/2626 [pii]10.1158/1055-9965.EPI-08-0959

Jasper, B. W., Conklin, H. M., Lawford, J., Morris, E. B., Howard, S. C., Wu, S.,... Khan, R. B. (2009). Growth effects of methylphenidate among childhood cancer survivors: a 12-month case-matched open-label study. *Pediatric Blood & Cancer, 52*, 39–43. doi: 10.1002/pbc.21770

Kadan-Lottick, N. S., Brouwers, P., Breiger, D., Kaleita, T., Dziura, J., Liu, H.,... Neglia, J. P. (2009). A comparison of neurocognitive functioning in children previously randomized to dexamethasone or prednisone in the treatment of childhood acute lymphoblastic leukemia. *Blood, 114*, 1746–1752. doi: blood-2008-12-186502 [pii]10.1182/blood-2008-12-186502

Kadan-Lottick, N. S., Brouwers, P., Breiger, D., Kaleita, T., Dziura, J., Northrup, V.,...Neglia, J. P. (2009). Comparison of neurocognitive functioning in children previously randomly assigned to intrathecal methotrexate compared with triple intrathecal therapy for the treatment of childhood acute lymphoblastic leukemia. *Journal of Clinical Oncology, 27*, 5986–5992. doi: JCO.2009.23.5408 [pii]10.1200/JCO.2009.23.5408

Kadan-Lottick, N. S., Zeltzer, L. K., Liu, Q., Yasui, Y., Ellenberg, L., Gioia, G.,...Krull, K. R. (2010). Neurocognitive functioning in adult survivors of childhood non-central nervous system cancers. *Journal of the National Cancer Institute, 102*, 881–893. doi: djq156 [pii] 10.1093/jnci/djq156

Kaemingk, K. L., Carey, M. E., Moore, I. M., Herzer, M., & Hutter, J. J. (2004). Math weaknesses in survivors of acute lymphoblastic leukemia compared to healthy children. *Child Neuropsychology, 10*, 14–23.

Kamdar, K. Y., Krull, K. R., El-Zein, R. A., Brouwers, P., Potter, B. S., Harris, L. L.,...Okcu, M. F. (2011). Folate pathway polymorphisms predict deficits in attention and processing speed after childhood leukemia therapy. *Pediatric Blood & Cancer, 57*, 454–460. doi: 10.1002/pbc.23162

Kazak, A. E., Alderfer, M., Rourke, M. T., Simms, S., Streisand, R., & Grossman, J. R. (2004). Posttraumatic stress disorder (PTSD) and posttraumatic stress symptoms (PTSS) in families of adolescent childhood cancer survivors. *Journal of Pediatric Psychology, 29*, 211–219.

Kesler, S. R., Lacayo, N. J., & Jo, B. (2011). A pilot study of an online cognitive rehabilitation program for executive function skills in children with cancer-related brain injury. *Brain Injury, 25*, 101–112. doi: 10.3109/02699052.2010.536194

Kingma, A., Rammeloo, L. A., van Der Does-van den Berg, A., Rekers-Mombarg, L., & Postma, A. (2000). Academic career after treatment for acute lymphoblastic leukaemia. *Archives of Diseases in Childhood, 82*, 353–357.

Kingma, A., Van Dommelen, R. I., Mooyaart, E. L., Wilmink, J. T., Deelman, B. G., & Kamps, W. A. (2002). No major cognitive impairment in young children with acute lymphoblastic leukemia using chemotherapy only: a prospective longitudinal study. *Journal of Pediatric Hematology/Oncology, 24*, 106–114.

Kirchhoff, A. C., Krull, K. R., Ness, K. K., Park, E. R., Oeffinger, K. C., Hudson, M. M.,...Leisenring, W. (2011). Occupational outcomes of adult childhood cancer survivors: a report from the childhood cancer survivor study. *Cancer, 117*, 3033–3044. doi: 10.1002/cncr.25867

Kirchhoff, A. C., Leisenring, W., Krull, K. R., Ness, K. K., Friedman, D. L., Armstrong, G. T.,...Wickizer, T. (2010). Unemployment among adult survivors of childhood cancer: a report from the childhood cancer survivor study. *Medical Care, 48*, 1015–1025. doi: 10.1097/MLR.0b013e3181eaf880

Kramer, U. M., Cunillera, T., Camara, E., Marco-Pallares, J., Cucurell, D., Nager, W.,...Munte, T. F. (2007). The impact of catechol-O-methyltransferase and dopamine D4 receptor genotypes on neurophysiological markers of performance monitoring. *Journal of Neuroscience, 27*, 14190–14198.

Krull, K. R., Annett, R. D., Pan, Z., Ness, K. K., Nathan, P. C., Srivastava, D. K.,...Hudson, M. M. (2011). Neurocognitive functioning and health-related behaviours in adult survivors of childhood cancer: A report from the Childhood Cancer Survivor Study. *European Journal of Cancer, 47*, 1380–1388. doi: S0959-8049(11)00145-6 [pii] 10.1016/j.ejca.2011.03.001

Krull, K. R., Bhojwani, D., Pei, D., Conklin, H., Cheng, C., Reddick, W. E.,...Pui, C. H. (2012). Genetic Mediators of Neurocognitive Outcomes in Childhood Acute Lymphoblastic Leukemia. *Journal of Clinical Oncology.* (in press).

Krull, K. R., Brouwers, P., Jain, N., Zhang, L., Bomgaars, L., Dreyer, Z., . . . Okcu, M. F. (2008). Folate pathway genetic polymorphisms are related to attention disorders in childhood leukemia survivors. *Journal of Pediatrics, 152*, 101–105.

Krull, K. R., Gioia, G., Ness, K. K., Ellenberg, L., Recklitis, C., Leisenring, W., . . . Zeltzer, L. (2008). Reliability and validity of the Childhood Cancer Survivor Study Neurocognitive Questionnaire. *Cancer, 113*, 2188–2197.

Krull, K. R., Hockenberry, M. J., Miketova, P., Carey, M., & Moore, I. M. (2012). Chemotherapy-related changes in central nervous system phospholipids and neurocognitive function in childhood acute lymphoblastic leukemia. *Leukemia & Lymphoma.* doi: 10.3109/10428194.2012.717080

Krull, K. R., Huang, S., Gurney, J. G., Klosky, J. L., Leisenring, W., Termuhlen, A., . . . Hudson, M. M. (2010). Adolescent behavior and adult health status in childhood cancer survivors. *Journal of Cancer Survivorship, 4*, 210–217. doi: 10.1007/s11764-010-0123-0

Krull, K. R., Khan, R. B., Ness, K. K., Ledet, D., Zhu, L., Pui, C. H., . . . Morris, E. B. (2011). Symptoms of attention-deficit/hyperactivity disorder in long-term survivors of childhood leukemia. *Pediatric Blood & Cancer, 57*, 1191–1196. doi: 10.1002/pbc.22994

Krull, K. R., Okcu, M. F., Potter, B., Jain, N., Dreyer, Z., Kamdar, K., & Brouwers, P. (2008). Screening for neurocognitive impairment in pediatric cancer long-term survivors. *Journal of Clinical Oncology, 26*, 4138–4143.

Kunin-Batson, A., Kadan-Lottick, N., Zhu, L., Cox, C., Bordes-Edgar, V., Srivastava, D. K., . . . Krull, K. R. (2011). Predictors of independent living status in adult survivors of childhood cancer: A report from the Childhood Cancer Survivor Study. *Pediatric Blood & Cancer.* doi: 10.1002/pbc.22982

Kupst, M. J., & Schulman, J. L. (1988). Long-term coping with pediatric leukemia: a six-year follow-up study. *Journal of Pediatric Psychology, 13*, 7–22.

Kupst, M. J., Schulman, J. L., Maurer, H., Morgan, E., Honig, G., & Fochtman, D. (1983). Psychosocial aspects of pediatric leukemia: from diagnosis through the first six months of treatment. *Medical and Pediatric Oncology, 11*, 269–278.

Lipsky, R. H., Sparling, M. B., Ryan, L. M., Xu, K., Salazar, A. M., Goldman, D., & Warden, D. L. (2005). Association of COMT Val158Met genotype with executive functioning following traumatic brain injury. *Journal of Neuropsychiatry & Clinical Neurosciences, 17*, 465–471.

Lupien, S. J., Gillin, C. J., & Hauger, R. L. (1999). Working memory is more sensitive than declarative memory to the acute effects of corticosteroids: a dose-response study in humans. *Behavioral Neuroscience, 113*, 420–430.

MacDonald, A. W., 3rd, Carter, C. S., Flory, J. D., Ferrell, R. E., & Manuck, S. B. (2007). COMT val158Met and executive control: a test of the benefit of specific deficits to translational research. *Journal of Abnormal Psychology, 116*, 306–312.

Meeske, K. A., Siegel, S. E., Globe, D. R., Mack, W. J., & Bernstein, L. (2005). Prevalence and correlates of fatigue in long-term survivors of childhood leukemia. *Journal of Clinical Oncology, 23*, 5501–5510.

Mody, R., Li, S., Dover, D. C., Sallan, S., Leisenring, W., Oeffinger, K. C., . . . Neglia, J. P. (2008). Twenty-five-year follow-up among survivors of childhood acute lymphoblastic leukemia: A report from the Childhood Cancer Survivor Study. *Blood, 111*, 5515–5523. doi: 10.1182/blood-2007-10-117150

Moleski, M. (2000). Neuropsychological, neuroanatomical, and neurophysiological consequences of CNS chemotherapy for acute lymphoblastic leukemia. *Archives of Clinical Neuropsychology, 15*, 603–630.

Montour-Proulx, I., Kuehn, S. M., Keene, D. L., Barrowman, N. J., Hsu, E., Matzinger, M. A., . . . Halton, J. M. (2005). Cognitive changes in children treated for acute lymphoblastic leukemia with chemotherapy only according to the Pediatric Oncology Group 9605 protocol. *Journal of Children Neurology, 20,* 129–133.

Moore, B. D., 3rd. (2005). Neurocognitive outcomes in survivors of childhood cancer. *Journal of Pediatric Psychology, 30,* 51–63.

Moore Ki, I. M., Hockenberry, M. J., Anhalt, C., McCarthy, K., & Krull, K. R. (2011). Mathematics intervention for prevention of neurocognitive deficits in childhood leukemia. *Pediatric Blood & Cancer, 59,* 278–284. doi: 10.1002/pbc.23354

Mrakotsky, C. M., Silverman, L. B., Dahlberg, S. E., Alyman, M. C., Sands, S. A., Queally, J. T.,...Waber, D. P. (2011). Neurobehavioral side effects of corticosteroids during active treatment for acute lymphoblastic leukemia in children are age-dependent: report from Dana-Farber Cancer Institute ALL Consortium Protocol 00–01. [Research Support, Non-U.S. Gov't]. *Pediatric Blood & Cancer, 57,* 492–498. doi: 10.1002/pbc.23060

Mulhern, R. K., Fairclough, D., & Ochs, J. (1991). A prospective comparison of neuropsychologic performance of children surviving leukemia who received 18-Gy, 24-Gy, or no cranial irradiation. *Journal of Clinical Oncology, 9,* 1348–1356.

Mulhern, R. K., Khan, R. B., Kaplan, S., Helton, S., Christensen, R., Bonner, M.,...Reddick, W. E. (2004). Short-term efficacy of methylphenidate: a randomized, double-blind, placebo-controlled trial among survivors of childhood cancer. *Journal of Clinical Oncology, 22,* 4795–4803. doi: 22/23/4743 [pii] 10.1200/JCO.2004.04.128

Ochs, J., Mulhern, R., Fairclough, D., Parvey, L., Whitaker, J., Ch'ien, L.,...Simone, J. (1991). Comparison of neuropsychologic functioning and clinical indicators of neurotoxicity in long-term survivors of childhood leukemia given cranial radiation or parenteral methotrexate: a prospective study. *Journal of Clinical Oncology, 9,* 145–151.

Oeffinger, K. C., Mertens, A. C., Sklar, C. A., Kawashima, T., Hudson, M. M., Meadows, A. T.,...Robison, L. L. (2006). Chronic health conditions in adult survivors of childhood cancer. *New England Journal of Medicine, 355,* 1572–1582.

Paakko, E., Harila-Saari, A., Vanionpaa, L., Himanen, S., Pyhtinen, J., & Lanning, M. (2000). White matter changes on MRI during treatment in children with acute lymphoblastic leukemia: correlation with neuropsychological findings. *Medical and Pediatric Oncology, 35,* 456–461.

Parasole, R., Petruzziello, F., Menna, G., Mangione, A., Cianciulli, E., Buffardi, S.,...Poggi, V. (2010). Central nervous system complications during treatment of acute lymphoblastic leukemia in a single pediatric institution. *Leukemia Lymphoma, 51,* 1063–1071. doi: 10.3109/10428191003754608

Patenaude, A. F., & Kupst, M. J. (2005). Psychosocial functioning in pediatric cancer. *Journal of Pediatric Psychology, 30,* 9–27.

Peterson, C. C., Johnson, C. E., Ramirez, L. Y., Huestis, S., Pai, A. L., Demaree, H. A., & Drotar, D. (2008). A meta-analysis of the neuropsychological sequelae of chemotherapy-only treatment for pediatric acute lymphoblastic leukemia. *Pediatric Blood & Cancer, 51,* 99–104.

Pui, C. H. (2000). Acute lymphoblastic leukemia in children. *Current Opinion in Oncology, 12,* 3–12.

Pui, C. H. (2009). Prophylactic cranial irradiation: going, going, gone. *Lancet Oncology, 10,* 932–933. doi: S1470-2045(09)70239-6 [pii] 10.1016/S1470-2045(09)70239-6

Pui, C. H., Robison, L. L., & Look, A. T. (2008). Acute lymphoblastic leukaemia. *Lancet, 371,* 1030–1043.

Reddick, W. E., Glass, J. O., Helton, K. J., Langston, J. W., Xiong, X., Wu, S., & Pui, C. H. (2005). Prevalence of leukoencephalopathy in children treated for acute lymphoblastic leukemia with high-dose methotrexate. *AJNR American Journal of Neuroradiology, 26,* 1263–1269.

Reddick, W. E., Shan, Z. Y., Glass, J. O., Helton, S., Xiong, X., Wu, S.,...Mulhern, R. K. (2006). Smaller white-matter volumes are associated with larger deficits in attention and learning among long-term survivors of acute lymphoblastic leukemia. *Cancer, 106,* 941–949.

Ries, L. A. G., Melbert, D., Krapcho, M., Mariotto, A., Miller, B. A., Feuer, E. J.,...Edwards, B. K. (2007). SEER Cancer Statistics Review, 1975–2004. (http://seer.cancer.gov/csr/1975_2004/). Bethesda, MD: National Cancer Institute.

Robien, K., Boynton, A., & Ulrich, C. M. (2005). Pharmacogenetics of folate-related drug targets in cancer treatment. *Pharmacogenomics, 6,* 673–689.

Robien, K., & Ulrich, C. M. (2003). 5,10-methylenetetrahydrofolate reductase polymorphisms and leukemia risk: a HuGE minireview. *American Journal of Epidemiology, 157,* 571–582.

Rueda, M. R., Rothbart, M. K., McCandliss, B. D., Saccomanno, L., & Posner, M. I. (2005). Training, maturation, and genetic influences on the development of executive attention. *Proceedings of the National Academy of Science USA, 102,* 14931–14936.

Schatz, J., Kramer, J. H., Ablin, A., & Matthay, K. K. (2000). Processing speed, working memory, and IQ: A developmental model of cognitive deficits following cranial radiation therapy. *Neuropsychology, 14,* 189–200.

Schmithorst, V. J., Holland, S. K., & Dardzinski, B. J. (2007). Developmental differences in white matter architecture between boys and girls. *Human Brain Mapping, 29,* 696–710.

Schultz, K. A., Ness, K. K., Whitton, J., Recklitis, C., Zebrack, B., Robison, L. L.,...Mertens, A. C. (2007). Behavioral and social outcomes in adolescent survivors of childhood cancer: a report from the childhood cancer survivor study. *Journal of Clinical Oncology, 25,* 3649–3656.

Shaw, P., Gornick, M., Lerch, J., Addington, A., Seal, J., Greenstein, D.,...Rapoport, J. L. (2007). Polymorphisms of the dopamine D4 receptor, clinical outcome, and cortical structure in attention-deficit/hyperactivity disorder. *Archives of General Psychiatry, 64,* 921–931.

Spiegler, B. J., Kennedy, K., Maze, R., Greenberg, M. L., Weitzman, S., Hitzler, J. K., & Nathan, P. C. (2006). Comparison of long-term neurocognitive outcomes in young children with acute lymphoblastic leukemia treated with cranial radiation or high-dose or very high-dose intravenous methotrexate. *Journal of Clinical Oncology, 24,* 3858–3864.

Stuber, M. L., Meeske, K. A., Krull, K. R., Leisenring, W., Stratton, K., Kazak, A. E.,...Zeltzer, L. K. (2010). Prevalence and predictors of posttraumatic stress disorder in adult survivors of childhood cancer. *Pediatrics, 125,* e1124–1134. doi: 125/5/e1124 [pii] 10.1542/peds.2009-2308

Thapar, A., O'Donovan, M., & Owen, M. J. (2005). The genetics of attention deficit hyperactivity disorder. *Human Molecular Genetics, 14 Spec No. 2,* R275–282.

Thompson, S. J., Leigh, L., Christensen, R., Xiong, X., Kun, L. E., Heideman, R. L.,...Mulhern, R. K. (2001). Immediate neurocognitive effects of methylphenidate on learning-impaired survivors of childhood cancer. *Journal of Clinical Oncology, 19,* 1802–1808.

Todd, R. D., & Lobos, E. A. (2002). Mutation screening of the dopamine D2 receptor gene in attention-deficit hyperactivity disorder subtypes: Preliminary report of a research strategy. *American Journal of Medical Genetics, 114,* 34–41.

van Rossum, E. F., Roks, P. H., de Jong, F. H., Brinkmann, A. O., Pols, H. A., Koper, J. W., & Lamberts, S. W. (2004). Characterization of a promoter polymorphism in the glucocorticoid receptor gene and its relationship to three other polymorphisms. *Clinical Endocrinology (Oxford), 61,* 573–581.

Waber, D. P., Carpentieri, S. C., Klar, N., Silverman, L. B., Schwenn, M., Hurwitz, C. A.,...Sallan, S. E. (2000). Cognitive sequelae in children treated for acute lymphoblastic leukemia with dexamethasone or prednisone. *Journal of Pediatric Hematology/Oncology*, *22*, 206–213.

Waber, D. P., Queally, J. T., Catania, L., Robaey, P., Romero, I., Adams, H.,...Silverman, L. B. (2011). Neuropsychological outcomes of standard risk and high risk patients treated for acute lymphoblastic leukemia on Dana-Farber ALL consortium protocol 95-01 at 5 years post-diagnosis. *Pediatric Blood & Cancer*, *58*, 758–765. doi: 10.1002/pbc.23234

Waber, D. P., Tarbell, N. J., Fairclough, D., Atmore, K., Castro, R., Isquith, P.,...Sallon, S. E. (1995). Cognitive sequelae of treatment in childhood acute lymphoblastic leukemia: cranial radiation requires an accomplice. *Journal of Clinical Oncology*, *13*, 2490–2496.

Waber, D. P., Turek, J., Catania, L., Stevenson, K., Robaey, P., Romero, I.,...Silverman, L. B. (2007). Neuropsychological outcomes from a randomized trial of triple intrathecal chemotherapy compared with 18 Gy cranial radiation as CNS treatment in acute lymphoblastic leukemia: findings from Dana-Farber Cancer Institute ALL Consortium Protocol 95-01. *Journal of Clinical Oncology*, *25*, 4914–4921.

Weiss, E. M., Stadelmann, E., Kohler, C. G., Brensinger, C. M., Nolan, K. A., Oberacher, H.,...Marksteiner, J. (2007). Differential effect of catechol-O-methyltransferase Val158Met genotype on emotional recognition abilities in healthy men and women. *Journal of International Neuropsychological Society*, *13*, 881–887.

2 Autism Spectrum Disorders

Lisa Joseph, David Black, and Audrey Thurm

Autism spectrum disorders (ASDs), currently referred to as pervasive developmental disorders in the *Diagnostic and Statistical Manual of Mental Disorders*, fourth edition, text revision (DSM-IV-TR; APA, 2000), are neurodevelopmental disorders characterized by impairments in reciprocal social interactions and communication and by the presence of restricted and repetitive behaviors. This chapter provides a historical medical perspective of ASDs, a summary of current medical factors, a treatment/ intervention update, early psychological and neuropsychological findings, more recent psychological and neuropsychological findings, intervention and treatment gains and long term outcomes. There are many very important active areas of autism research and treatment that this chapter does not cover; these include etiological research in genetics, genomics, gene–environment interactions, and epidemiology.

HISTORICAL MEDICAL PERSPECTIVE

Kanner's Autism

In 1943, psychiatrist Leo Kanner identified 11 pediatric patients with the following symptom presentations: lack of response to social overtures, language delays, and presence of repetitive behaviors. Kanner (1943) called these symptoms "autistic disturbances of affective content." These symptoms were observed in children before age 3 years, with parents reporting the presence of some symptoms from birth. Kanner noted that although the symptoms were similar to those of childhood schizophrenia, there were symptoms that differentiated the two disorders. Notably, in childhood schizophrenia, development was described as within normal limits up to 10 years of age, with the gradual presentation of symptoms including hallucinations.

There were several factors unique to Kanner's original cohort. The 11 children all came from "highly intelligent families"; he also observed that the "autistic aloneness" was present from birth. Kanner concluded that social isolation was the most defining symptom in these children, with their parents describing the children as "happiest when left alone," "acting as if people weren't there," and "like in a shell" (Kanner, 1943). The language impairments were characterized by the presence of echolalia, pronoun reversal, odd intonation, stereotyped language, and receptive language difficulties. Abnormalities in what is now termed "pragmatic language" were also described and included a problem with "literalness." Feeding issues and sensitivity to loud noises were observed; Kanner (1968) theorized that the children viewed these stimuli as intrusions from the outside world. Insistence on sameness was described as "an anxiously obsessive desire for the maintenance of sameness." Also reported was a fascination with objects, in which Kanner observed the children "handled with skill in fine motor movement" (Kanner & Eisenberg, 1955). Verbal rituals and difficulties with changes were other symptoms observed.

Kanner followed the 11 children in the original study for several years and was able to make observations about the course of the disorder. Increased use of language and decreased sensory sensitivities were documented over time. Additionally, the repetitive behaviors more resembled obsessive preoccupations as the children aged. Some children also began to engage in parallel play (Kanner, 1968). However, Kanner reported that social deficits continued to be one of the symptoms causing the most impairment. Even children who progressed in other areas lacked "social perceptiveness" (Kanner & Eisenberg, 1955). The children with the best prognoses were those who developed some language before age 5 years (Kanner, Rodriguez, & Ashenden, 1972).

Although Kanner is credited with first describing autism, the origins of Asperger's disorder were noted during the same time frame. In 1944, the year after Kanner published his paper on autism, Hans Asperger also used the term "autism" to describe children with similar deficits in social interaction and stereotyped behavior. However, in Asperger's descriptions, the children did not demonstrate communicative or cognitive impairments (Asperger & Frith, 1991). Preserved cognitive functioning and lack of language delays continue to distinguish Asperger's disorder from autism in the DSM-IV-TR, however Asperger himself thought there were other distinctions between the clinical symptoms he observed and those observed by Kanner, such as social impairments that were apparent from as early as 2 years (Wing, 1997). However, Asperger surmised that intact cognitive functioning allowed these patients to function well in work environments; and, like Kanner, he viewed the social deficits to be a lifelong impairment (Wolff, 2004).

Early Psychoanalytic Theories of Autism

Many of Kanner's initial observations of symptoms remain core to the framework of the diagnostic criteria of autism. However, other observations have since been discounted or updated. Although he did believe there was a biological problem inherent in the disorder, Kanner theorized that inadequate parenting was a cause of the disorder. He believed that a history of parental obsessiveness was present and characterized the parents as aloof, theorizing such lack of affection and emotional coldness from parents as causal (Kanner & Eisenberg, 1955). Bettelheim (1967) developed the "refrigerator mother" concept soon after (1967). He theorized that the symptoms of autism were the child's defense against cold and detached mothers. He argued that the treatment for these children was to provide them with nurturing that would cure their "autistic defenses." Bettelheim claimed that his treatment cured 85% of his patients; however, it was later revealed that these patients were not autistic and that some of the reports he published were fabricated (Herbert, Sharp, & Gaudiano, 2002). Although credence to Bettelheim's theories was not long-standing in the scientific community (see below), his book *Empty Fortress* was widely read and created an unfortunate legacy that may have impacted how professionals and families approached autism research (Baker, 2010).

Biological Theories

While psychodynamic theories predominated in the 1950s and 1960s, both biological theories and clinical observations of the disorder began to surface. Some early biological theories maintained that autism was due to organic brain disease, brain damage that occurred during pregnancy or birth, problems with the reticular system, or over-arousal (Rutter, 1968). Although these early disease models were later discredited, biological and clinical observations provided some of the most important empirical evidence against the early psychoanalytic theories of autism.

Early electroencephalogram (EEG) studies indicated a high prevalence of seizures in children with autism (Creak & Pampiglione, 1969). Other studies presented evidence for the influence of genetic factors in autism. In one early study to examine the genetic link to autism, high rates of concordance in monozygotic twins indicated a strong heritability for the disorder (Folstein & Rutter, 1977). Physical abnormalities were also observed in some children (Campbell, Geller, Small, Petti, & Ferris, 1978). Along with the increase in biologic research, studies began examining psychosocial factors that earlier psychodynamic theories had highlighted as problematic. However, studies of parent-child interaction that compared children with autism to typically developing children found no significant differences in interactions (Byassee & Murrell, 1975; Cantwell, Baker, & Rutter, 1978).

Broadening Definitions: A Spectrum of Disorders

One of the first epidemiological studies of autistic disorder was initiated in 1966 by the epidemiologist Victor Lotter. He used the characteristics defined by Kanner to determine the diagnoses of children between 8 years and 10 years in England. Lotter also collected the children's social and medical histories and obtained estimates of cognitive and language development. Results indicated that 5 in 10,000 children met Kanner's criteria for autism (Lotter, 1966). Studies also indicated that the disorder was more likely to occur in males than in females (Rutter & Bartak, 1971).

In 1979, Wing and Gould studied a broadened spectrum that included children who had some, but not necessarily all, of the features described by Kanner. As a result of this broadened diagnostic criteria, the study determined that 20 in 10,000 children had some features of autistic disorder. In this study, children with symptoms similar to those described by Asperger were identified (Wing, 1981). Figure 2.1 graphically captures findings from more recent epidemiologic studies, indicating a rapid increase in prevalence of ASDs in recent years (Autism Speaks, 2009).

Descriptions of autism in DSM have evolved over time, first considered within the context of childhood schizophrenia, later becoming an independent disorder, and ultimately placed in a spectrum of similar disorders. In the first two editions of the DSM,

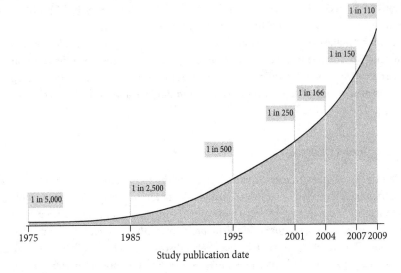

FIGURE 2.1

Autism Prevalence on the Rise. Reprinted with permission from Autism Speaks.

only descriptions for childhood schizophrenia existed. In the third edition (DSM-III; APA, 1980), the category of pervasive developmental disorders (PDDs) was introduced. In this group of disorders, autism (termed "infantile autism") was a diagnosis with its own distinct criteria. In the DSM-III revision (APA, 1987), there was a change in the diagnostic criteria for autism that allowed inclusion of children with fewer overt symptoms of social withdrawal. In that edition of the DSM, PDDs were defined as a group of related disorders, under which autism, then changed to "autistic disorder," was defined. The diagnosis Pervasive Developmental Disorder–not otherwise specified (PDD-NOS) was also introduced, allowing individuals with a core impairment in reciprocal social interaction, but not meeting the full criteria for autistic disorder, to be captured diagnostically. In 1994, the DSM-IV broadened the diagnostic criteria for autistic disorder. In addition, Asperger's disorder and Rett syndrome were included as separate disorders. Figure 2.2 describes the proposed changes to diagnostic categorization in DSM-5, which is scheduled for publication in May 2013 (see www.dsm5.org).

Pervasive Developmental Disorders: Current

In DSM-IV-TR, autistic disorder, Asperger's disorder, and PDD-NOS are grouped together as PDDs, colloquially referred to as autism spectrum disorders. The core features of ASDs are marked impairment in social interaction and the presence of repetitive and restricted behaviors and interests (APA, 2000). In autistic disorder and PDD-NOS, impairment in communication is also present, while the current criteria for Asperger's disorder exclude history of delayed language development or the presence of significant other communication symptoms (e.g., repetitive or echolalic speech, impaired conversation skills, or diminished imaginative play skills). The remainder of this chapter will focus on autistic disorder, Asperger's disorder, and PDD-NOS, termed ASD, however we indicate when findings are specific to a certain disorder, for example using the term autism when discussing findings regarding autistic disorder. Brief descriptions of the two other disorders described under the PDD section are described below.

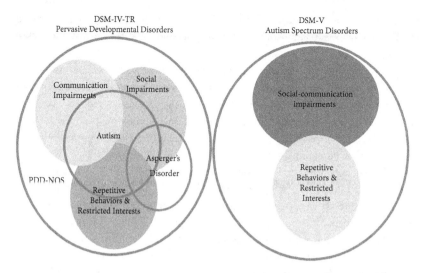

DSM-IV-TR
Pervasive Developmental Disorders

Communication Impairments

Social Impairments

Autism

Asperger's Disorder

PDD-NOS

Repetitive Behaviors & Restricted Interests

DSM-V
Autism Spectrum Disorders

Social-communication impairments

Repetitive Behaviors & Restricted Interests

FIGURE 2.2
Diagnostic Criteria for Autism Spectrum Disorders: Current and Future.

Rett syndrome and childhood disintegrative disorder (CDD) are included under the label of PDD in DSM-IV-TR. However, the presentation, known etiology, and course of these disorders differ from those of the other ASDs such that it has been proposed that both be removed from DSM-5 (Volkmar, State, & Klin, 2009).

Rett syndrome is characterized by typical development in the first 6 months of life, followed by the loss of purposeful motor functioning of the hands and development of repetitive hand wringing. Loss of language skills and decelerated head growth are also present. In 1999, the disorder was identified to be associated with a mutation in the methyl CpG binding protein 2 (MECP2) gene, which is on the X chromosome (Amir et al., 1999). Predominantly observed in females, the prevalence of the disorder is approximately 1 in 15,000 for females; to date, there have been only 18 published cases of the disorder in males (Condie, Goldstein, & Wainwright, 2010).

Originally termed "disintegrative psychosis," CDD is currently defined by a period of normal development of language, social, and motor skills, followed by a regression of skills between the ages of 2 years and 10 years in at least two of the of the following areas: social and play skills, receptive or expressive language, adaptive behavior, and motor skills. The following two onset patterns have been reported: (1) over a period of weeks and months or (2) rapid onset presenting over the course of a few days (Malhotra & Gupta, 1999). The prevalence of the disorder is reported to be 2 in 10,000 (Fombonne, 2009). Very little research has been published regarding this disorder's specific phenotype or natural history.

Autism

As currently defined in the DSM-IV-TR, the core features of autistic disorder, or autism, are marked impairments in social interaction, impairments in communication, and the presence of repetitive and restricted behaviors and interests. In addition, the onset of symptoms must occur before age 3 years. The social impairments that define the disorder include deficits in the use of nonverbal behaviors, lack of or impairment in peer relationships, lack of social–emotional reciprocity, and lack of shared enjoyment.

Communication impairments include the delay or lack of verbal communication, without the use of compensatory communication strategies such as gestures; impairment in reciprocal communication; the presence of stereotyped or repetitive language; and impaired age-appropriate imaginative and social imitative play (APA, 2000). Concerns regarding delays in this domain are among the first to be reported by parents (De Giacomo & Fombonne, 1998).

Restricted, repetitive, and stereotyped patterns of behavior and interests comprise the third domain of symptoms. These behaviors include preoccupations with stereotyped interests, insistence on maintaining nonfunctional routines, repetitive motor mannerisms such as hand flapping, and preoccupation with parts of objects (APA, 2000). Repetitive behaviors are not specific to ASDs because they are symptoms observed in some anxiety disorders, other developmental disorders, and in typically developing children. However, studies have indicated that the type and severity of repetitive behaviors can distinguish ASD from other disorders (Bodfish, Symons, Parker, & Lewis, 2000).

The clinical presentation of PDD-NOS is similar to that of autistic disorder because it is marked by impairment in reciprocal social interaction and communication as well as the presence of repetitive behaviors and interests. However, it differs from autistic disorder, which requires six symptoms for diagnosis, in that no specific number of deficits in any of the three domains is required. Thus, the symptom presentation is milder and the prognosis over time is reported to be better (Gillberg, 1991). The vagueness of the criteria has been grounds for confusion and has raised concerns of the possibility of both over- and underdiagnosis.

Unlike autistic disorder, the DSM-IV-TR diagnostic criteria for Asperger's disorder requires no significant delays in language development; however the presence of both social impairments and repetitive behaviors are required. Additionally individuals with Asperger's disorder cannot have significant delays in cognitive development or adaptive behaviors. Over the last decade, researchers have examined the degree to which the diagnosis and traits of this disorder have overlapped with autistic disorder, and whether the current criteria are sufficient for a separate diagnostic phenotype.

EARLY PSYCHOLOGICAL AND NEUROPSYCHOLOGICAL FINDINGS

Early Neuropsychological Findings

Autism was described as a disorder involving the frontal and temporal lobes as early as 1978 (Damasio & Maurer, 1978). Numerous studies have examined the neuropsychology of ASDs, often focusing on language, executive functioning, and cognitive flexibility. Regarding language, Tager-Flusberg (1981) argued that the development of semantic and pragmatic aspects of language were clearly aberrant in ASDs, while structural language development (e.g., syntax, phonology) was generally intact in children with ASDs and average-range intellectual abilities. In contrast, she noted deficits in structural language among children with ASDs and intellectual delays. Baron-Cohen, Leslie, and Frith (1985) demonstrated that individuals with ASDs have deficits in theory of mind (ToM), that is, the ability to appreciate the mental state of oneself and others. As early as 1985, Rumsey and colleagues (1985) demonstrated that individuals with autism have significant trouble with cognitive flexibility based on findings from a card-sorting task. However, subsequent research has suggested that social demands of the task (i.e., the examiner gives verbal feedback concerning performance after each trial) may have contributed to deficient performance (Ozonoff & Miller, 1995).

RECENT PSYCHOLOGICAL AND NEUROPSYCHOLOGICAL FINDINGS

Behavioral Research Findings

The neuropsychological profile of ASD is now known to be complex and highly variable. Depending on the study, 40%–70% of individuals diagnosed with ASDs are also diagnosed with intellectual disability (ID), with strictly defined autistic disorder associated with the higher end of this range (Baird et al., 2006; Fombonne, 2005). Among those with and without ID, many individuals with ASDs have discrete areas of cognitive competence and a variable profile of strengths and weaknesses among nonverbal and verbal domains (Munson et al., 2008). There is general agreement in the literature that among those with ASDs who do not have ID, deficits in structural and pragmatic language, theory of mind/social cognition, and executive functioning are common (Hill, 2004; Kenworthy, Yerys, Anthony, & Wallace, 2008). In addition, given overall cognitive abilities, deficits in adaptive functioning or practical daily living skills are routinely demonstrated to be 1 or 2 standard deviations lower than predicted (Gilotty, Kenworthy, Sirian, Black, & Wagner, 2002; Klin et al., 2007).

A focus on neuropsychological deficits in preschoolers with autism has resulted in the finding that joint attention may be seen as a precursor to later neuropsychological deficits such as in ToM and may be considered a core deficit in autism (Mundy, Sigman, Ungerer, & Sherman, 1987). Impairments in precursors to joint attention, including visual tracking, may be observed as early as 12 months in children who are later diagnosed with autism (Zwaigenbaum et al., 2005). Imitation skills have also been found to be deficient in children with autism (Rogers, Hepburn, Stackhouse, & Wehner, 2003).

Neuropsychological Findings

The following sections provide a brief summary of some recent neuropsychological findings in language, social cognition, and executive functions found with ASDs.

Language

Numerous studies have examined language development in ASDs. Many children with autism or PDD-NOS are delayed or deficient in the acquisition of speech and language skills. Study results are quite varied; however, recent findings from a sample of 9-year-old children indicated that approximately 70% of individuals with autism develop at least single words and up to 25% may be considered "fluent" (Anderson, Oti, Lord, & Welch, 2009). This same study found that more than 95% of children diagnosed with PDD-NOS attained single words. Similar studies have corroborated these findings, indicating that 80%–90% of individuals with autism or PDD-NOS develop functional speech by age 9 years (Turner, Stone, Pozdol, & Coonrod, 2006). Although previously controversial, it is currently held that once language develops, deficits in structural language (phonology, morphology, syntax) persist for a subset of children with autism, while deficits in pragmatic language are nearly universal (Kjelgaard & Tager-Flusberg, 2001).

For the purpose of this chapter, pragmatic language is defined as aspects of language that include semantics and the use of language in social contexts. The study of pragmatic language in ASDs has been quite varied. In addition to difficulties on standardized language tests (Volden, Coolican, Garon, White, & Bryson, 2009), other specific findings include diminished differentiation of intonation in preschoolers (Kuhl, Coffey-Corina, Padden, & Dawson, 2005), decreased description of mental states by children with autism compared with mental age-matched peers (Tager-Flusberg, 1992), and multiple types of conversational deficits in verbal individuals with ASDs (de Villiers, 2007).

Social Perception and Social Cognition

Research into social perception and social cognition has grown increasingly complex and sophisticated over the past decade. In particular, the field has made strides in its ability to use experimental tasks to evaluate individuals with ASDs who are not severely impaired. Prior research has demonstrated that individuals with ASDs have difficulty accurately reading facial expressions. Following the initial findings of deficits in first-order ToM, accurately inferring what another person is thinking (e.g., Baron-Cohen et al., 1985), and in second-order ToM (Baron-Cohen, 1989), a wide range of research studies have demonstrated deficits in various other aspects of social cognition. For example, Castelli and colleagues (2002) found that adults with Asperger's disorder had difficulty attributing mental states to inanimate figures. Other studies have suggested weaknesses in deception (Happe, 1994) and in recognizing social misjudgments (Baron-Cohen, O'Riordan, Stone, Jones, & Plaisted, 1999). More recent research has shown that ToM can be taught, to some extent (Begeer et al., 2011), and is highly variable among individuals with autism over time (Pellicano, 2010).

A series of studies by Klin and colleagues (e.g., Klin et al., 2009), which used eye tracking among toddlers (2-year-olds), preschoolers, adolescents, and adults with an ASD, demonstrated deficits in their attention to socially salient, relevant information in naturalistic settings. They theorized that the basis of this deficiency may be a biologically predisposed, chronic lack of attention to social cues beginning within the first year of life, which in turn leads to understimulation of brain regions essential to understanding the social world. Klin and colleagues (2003) argue that without an accurate perception of the social world, individuals with ASDs will naturally struggle to make accurate social inferences and social attributions.

Executive Functioning

Considerable research has focused on executive functioning (EF), also referred to as cognitive control, in ASDs. Regarded as the most complex human behavior, EF can be conceptualized as higher-order cognition required for goal-oriented problem solving.

It involves attention, inhibition, planning, organization, working memory, cognitive flexibility, and monitoring of progress toward goals (Kenworthy et al., 2008).

Pennington and Ozonoff (1996) identified weaknesses in flexibility (set shifting), planning, and working memory in individuals with autism. More recent reviews also reflect deficits in flexibility and planning in those with ASDs (Hill, 2004), while studies examining working memory and inhibition have produced inconsistent results (Sergeant, Geurts, & Oosterlaan, 2002). In addition, Geurts, Corbett, and Solomon (2009) argue that the literature on cognitive flexibility in autism is far from conclusive. Although much of the research on EF in ASDs has relied on higher-functioning individuals (i.e., typically defined as having cognitive abilities that approach the average range), one recent study examined cognitive flexibility in "lower-functioning" individuals with an ASD (i.e., those categorized as intellectually disabled). Reed and colleagues (2011) demonstrated, relative to a cognitively matched control sample, weaknesses in set-shifting among a sample of 15 children with autism who were on average 2 ½ years cognitively delayed. A handful of studies have examined EF in preschool children with ASDs with mixed results. Although some studies have not found deficits relative to controls (e.g., Yerys, Hepburn, Pennington, & Rogers, 2007), Pellicano (2007) reported trouble with inhibitory control, planning, and set-shifting relative to healthy controls in 4- to 7-year-olds with ASDs.

Ozonoff and colleagues (1991) found that performance on two EF measures of planning and flexibility (the Tower of Hanoi and the Wisconsin Card Sorting Test) effectively discriminated children with autism from a non-autism control group that included children with attention-deficit/hyperactivity disorder (ADHD), learning disorders, and mild intellectual disability. Such striking group differences may have contributed to initial theories of EF as one of many necessary causal factors in the manifestation of autism. However, more recent research has cast doubt on EF as a causal factor in autism (Hill, 2004). Stronger performance on computer-administered versions of the Wisconsin Card Sorting Test and Tower of Hanoi tasks among individuals with an ASD has raised questions about the role of the examiner, who is an inherent social component of traditional EF tasks, in the modest performance of children with an ASD when the task is administered in person (e.g., Kenworthy et al., 2008; Ozonoff & Miller, 1995).

Assessment of EF in the laboratory has been criticized as lacking sufficient ecological validity, in part, because in vivo EF involves the simultaneous juggling of multiple unpredictable factors that laboratory measures explicitly attempt to control (see Kenworthy et al., 2008, for a discussion). An alternative approach has been to develop EF measures that better reflect the real world. Much of this research has relied on informant-report measures of EF in daily activities. In general, results from these measures suggest that individuals with autism have generalized trouble carrying out unstructured tasks and also have specific deficits in flexibility and organization (Kenworthy et al., 2005). These types of deficits in parent-reported EF have also been associated with poor adaptive functioning (Gilotty et al., 2002).

Neuropsychological deficits in autism have been studied in parallel to their underlying neural substrates, most recently in studies linking brain–behavior relationships. One of the first central nervous system investigations in autism was a neuropathology study by Bauman and Kemper (1985), followed by several other postmortem reports by the same researchers. These studies revealed several areas of potential abnormality that include core limbic structures (hippocampus and amygdala) as well as subiculum, entorhinal cortex, mamillary body, septum, and anterior cingulate cortex. Cerebellum and related inferior olive abnormalities were also found (Kulesza, Lukose, & Stevens, 2011).

Brain–Behavior Findings

Contemporary understanding of the neural basis of autism is largely informed by neuroimaging studies at different age and functioning levels. However, in these studies, older individuals and those with more advanced cognitive and language abilities are overrepresented. This is explained by difficulties inherent in the types of studies used in this area, such as functional magnetic resonance imaging (fMRI); younger and more impaired individuals often cannot comprehend and/or withstand the procedures of sitting still for prolonged imaging. Notwithstanding, structural MRI, fMRI, and head circumference studies have begun to identify structural and functional abnormalities that include overgrowth in brain volume in at least some young children (2–4 years) (Nordahl et al., 2011), differences in cortical gray matter volume (cortical thickness; Hadjikhani, Joseph, Snyder, & Tager-Flusberg, 2006), and aberrant functional connectivity in autism (Minshew & Keller, 2010). Several studies now point to abnormalities in a collection of brain regions coined the "social brain" (Pelphrey, Shultz, Hudac, & Vander Wyk, 2011). Studies using fMRI have replicated many of the previous behavioral neuropsychological findings, demonstrating differences in various brain regions when solving social tasks such as social cuing and social decision making.

The number of imaging studies of younger individuals with autism is also increasing, but findings thus far have been quite limited. Structural studies have found conflicting results with respect to volumetric differences in the cortex (Hazlett et al., 2009; Muller, Pierce, Ambrose, Allen, & Courchesne, 2001). Functional studies of toddlers have found differences in response to auditory stimuli as well as reduced activity in several regions of the brain (Redcay & Courchesne, 2008).

Event-related potential (ERP) and magnetoencephalography (MEG) have also been used in several studies. Children with autism have been shown to differ from typically developing peers in ERP with respect to response to auditory stimuli (Roberts et al., 2010), facial perception (Kylliainen, Braeutigam, Hietanen, Swithenby, & Bailey, 2006), and visual processing (Neumann et al., 2011). In addition to the investigation of impaired processing that may underlie the core features of autism, studies have also investigated whether differential brain responses to specific stimuli can help elucidate autism subtypes such as those with additional language impairment (Roberts et al., 2010). Ultimately, it is hoped that this type of technology will advance the search for potential specific biomarkers for autism, or specific subtypes, and also enhance understanding of the brain–behavior relationships that relate to core features of the disorder.

CURRENT MEDICAL FACTORS AND TREATMENT AND INTERVENTION UPDATE

Comorbid Disorders/Associated Symptoms

Knowledge about medical problems that co-occur with autism is quite limited because individuals with autism are often unable to report medical symptoms such as pain.

Thus, most of the literature on this topic is based on parental reporting. Several medical, neurological, and psychiatric disorders have been reported to co-occur with ASDs. The presence of these disorders can sometimes complicate the symptom presentation of the disorder and make diagnosis and treatment more challenging. One of the most frequently reported comorbid medical disorders is epilepsy. As some of the earliest studies indicate, EEG abnormalities are frequently observed in ASD populations (Rutter, Greenfeld, & Lockyer, 1967). A review of the literature on epilepsy in ASDs found rates that ranged from 5% to 46%. In addition, age, gender, and the intellectual disability are all factors that relate to the prevalence of epilepsy in ASDs (Spence & Schneider, 2009).

Several other problems are commonly reported in individuals with ASD, including sleep disturbances. Children with ASDs are reported to have more difficulty with sleep than children with other developmental disorders (DeVincent, Gadow, Delosh, & Geller, 2007). Motor delays (Ghaziuddin & Butler, 1998) and sensory processing abnormalities (Rogers, Hepburn, & Wehner, 2003) are also prevalent. Gastrointestinal (GI) problems, with diarrhea, constipation, and abdominal pain among the most commonly occurring problems, have been reported in ASDs. However, there have been inconsistent findings regarding prevalence of these problems, with rates ranging from 9% (Buie et al., 2010) to 70% (Valicenti-McDermott et al., 2006). Differences in methodology as well as difficulties in assessing the extent of GI problems contribute to the inconsistent findings.

Estimates of the prevalence of comorbid psychiatric disorders in children with ASDs are quite variable, with rates ranging from approximately 10% (Levy et al., 2010) to 71% (Simonoff et al., 2008). Symptoms indicative of ADHD, anxiety disorders, and mood disorders are commonly reported comorbid psychiatric disorders in this population. In a review of studies of children and adolescents with ASDs, White and colleagues (2009) found that the rate of anxiety-related problems ranged from 11% to 84%. Despite the current preclusion of the DSM for the comorbid diagnosis of ADHD in individuals with ASDs, based on symptom presentation, there has been a high prevalence of co-occurrence of the disorders (Gadow, DeVincent, & Pomeroy, 2006). The presentation of mood and anxiety disorders varies with both age and developmental level because the ability to have insight into symptoms can affect presentation. Although identification of these co-occurring problems is now increasing with the availability of specialty multidisciplinary clinics (Coury, Jones, Klatka, Winklosky, & Perrin, 2009), evidence-based treatment of these co-occurring problems is progressing slowly.

Interventions

There are numerous approaches to intervention for individuals with ASDs. This brief review will not summarize or even mention all types of interventions utilized. This section briefly describes models and specific treatments within the domains of behavioral interventions, interventions carried out by allied health professionals, educational interventions, complementary and alternative interventions, and pharmacological interventions. Brief summaries of the state of the research on each are also provided.

Behavioral Interventions

There are primarily two types of behavioral interventions: interventions that adhere to a behavioral treatment approach, and interventions that encompass a developmental focus (Howlin, Magiati, & Charman, 2009). Additionally, there are several intervention programs that combine aspects of different approaches. Within and between the various models, there are variations in the setting of treatment services, the type and focus of services, and the intensity and frequency of treatment. For example, home-based settings are often used for preschool-aged children, while educational settings are more commonly used for school-aged children. The focus of interventions also varies; some interventions focus on the core behavioral symptoms of the disorder, others have a more broad-based approach to treatment.

Applied Behavioral Interventions and Modern Variants

Applied behavior analysis (ABA), which is the clinical field derived from behavioral analysis, has the most empirical evidence for treatment of ASDs (Levy, Mandell, & Schultz, 2009). Based on the model developed by Lovaas (1987), ABA interventions focus on analyzing behaviors and understanding the environment's role in the development and maintenance of behaviors. Teaching is used to manage behaviors. The original Lovaas therapy was based on a specific curriculum and included up to 40 hours per week of learning with the use of an individual, discrete trial setting. Several more recent variants of ABA exist including pivotal response training (PRT) (Koegel & Frea, 1993), which utilizes a more natural setting compared with Lovaas's therapy and includes the child's interests in creating rewards for exhibiting specific behaviors. Based on Skinner's original behavioral work, verbal behavior is another such variant that focuses on language development through the use of discrete trials (Sundberg & Michael, 2001). Although such approaches are now used more often in a group setting and in more natural settings, rather than traditional "table time," the utility of these approaches is limited by the cost of training and staffing such time-intensive treatment. Research continues to explore the efficacy of these techniques in specific settings. Investigation of moderators and mediators of treatment effects with these models is also lacking.

Developmental Models

Developmental models of intervention use an individual's current skill set to develop specific treatment goals. The treatment plan is developed once clinical observations and a developmental history and assessment of current developmental functioning are completed. The developmental Individual-Difference, Relationship-Based (DIR), or Floor Time, Model is one such developmentally based model that focuses on the emotional development of the child, individual differences in sensory processing, and relationships and interactions (Greenspan & Wieder, 1998). The Denver Model is one of the most empirically tested developmental models (Vismara & Rogers, 2010). An early intervention approach for children as young as 2 years, the Early Start Denver Model was also developed (Dawson et al., 2010); it utilizes a structured curriculum and behavioral principles but focuses on development in the areas of imitation, play, communication, and language (Rogers & Dawson, 2010).

Educational Interventions

In many real-world educational settings, including classrooms with a specific autism focus, aspects of multiple models of autism treatment are utilized and integrated.

Some models are explicitly stated as such. For example, the Treatment and Education of Autistic and Communication Handicapped Children Model (Mesibov, Shea, & Schopler, 2005) and the Daily Life Therapy Program (Howlin et al., 2009) use a combined approach to intervention.

Allied Health Interventions

Speech and language therapy is very often administered to individuals with ASDs because of the communication deficits that are inherent with the disorder. However, communication-focused interventions may be thought of separately and are developed based on the individual's language level. For children who are predominantly nonverbal, interventions focus primarily on the acquisition of skills to communicate basic wants and needs through augmentative communication (e.g., the picture exchange communication system [Bondy & Frost, 1994]). In contrast, the goal of therapy for verbal individuals may be to develop reciprocal communication skills and improve pragmatic language (Rogers & Vismara, 2008). Other interventions carried out by allied health professionals include music therapy, occupational therapy, and sensory-integration therapy.

Complementary and Alternative Interventions

Perhaps due to the intractable nature and complicated presentation, the autism spectrum disorders have attracted a widely varied canon of medical interventions. In addition to traditional medications (summarized below), complementary and alternative medical (CAM) treatments, that is, products and procedures that are generally considered to be outside the realm of traditional medicine, have become popular in the autism community. Five major areas of CAM treatment have been identified (Hanson et al., 2007): alternative medical systems, mind–body interventions (e.g., meditation), biologically based therapies (e.g., vitamin megadoses), manipulative and body-based methods (e.g., massage), and energy-based methods (e.g., Reiki). Although many of these treatments have been used in clinical practice and efficacy is reported anecdotally, very few have been tested rigorously with masked randomized controlled trials (Warren et al., 2011). Fewer have focused on core symptoms of autism as the primary outcome.

Despite extremely limited research on the efficacy of CAM, the use is widespread. A 2007 survey of 112 parents of children with developmental disabilities (including ASDs) showed that 74% engaged in a CAM treatment, with 54% of the sample using a biologically based therapy (Hanson et al., 2007). Another recent survey of parents of children with autism indicates that biomedical treatments are frequently utilized to treat children with autism (Interactive Autism Network, 2008). According to these recent surveys, the most commonly reported CAM interventions include special diets, such as a gluten-free/casein-free diet, and the use of dietary supplements including essential fatty acids and probiotics.

Psychopharmacological Treatment

The majority of children with ASDs will be prescribed psychopharmacological medication by the time they reach adolescence (Rosenberg et al., 2010). However, current pharmacological treatments for autism are aimed not at the core symptoms of ASDs but at comorbid symptoms such as hyperactivity and irritability. Most often, the medications used to treat these symptoms have been empirically supported in other psychiatric disorders with similar presentations. Neuroleptic (or antipsychotic) medications, used to treat psychosis, aggressive behavior, and self-injury in schizophrenia, are commonly used to treat children with ASDs. Of all classes, two atypical antipsychotics are the only medications to have a US Food and Drug Administration indication for autism: aripiprazole and risperidone; both are indicated for specific irritability symptoms. Decreased repetitive behavior was a secondary outcome for these drugs (McPheeters et al., 2011). Selective serotonin reuptake inhibitors (SSRIs), used in typically developing populations to treat anxiety and depressive disorders, are often used to treat the repetitive behaviors seen in ASDs. However, recent studies have shown mixed efficacy for SSRIs in autism (King et al., 2009). To treat inattention and hyperactivity in ASDs, stimulant medications are sometimes prescribed, with mixed results reported (Posey et al., 2007).

Despite the fact that few medications have been determined to be efficacious, the prescription of medications for use in ASDs has increased over the past decade. Reviews of the literature indicate that the number and type of prescribed medications change as individuals age (Rosenberg et al., 2010). In a longitudinal study of adolescents and adults on psychotropic medication, Esbensen and colleagues (2009) found that psychotropic use increased over a 4.5-year period. Other studies have found that older age and the presence of comorbid symptoms were predictors of medication use (Aman, Lam, & Van Bourgondien, 2005).

Although children with autism engage in a variety of educational, behavioral, biomedical, and pharmacological interventions, research into the efficacy of treatments and for whom (moderators) and how (mediators) treatments work is quite limited. Two factors that limit intervention trials in ASDs are the heterogeneity of the disorder itself and the lack of sensitive outcome measures to assess change over time (Spence & Thurm, 2010). A trial with a negative outcome may not be ineffective; rather it may have been effective for only a subset of patients with specific symptoms. The small sample size and consequent lack of power in treatment studies of ASDs may be to blame for the lack of exploration of moderators in this context. The paucity of reliable and valid measures of change in core autism symptoms severely inhibits the ability of the field to evaluate adequately the efficacy of treatment interventions.

INTERVENTION AND TREATMENT GAINS

There are few reports of significant symptom improvement in autism. This may be due, in part, to ineffective treatment, particularly when rigorous randomized controlled trials have produced null results. However, it is also true that most treatment trials have not targeted the core symptoms (and thus have not reported improvement).

It is important to emphasize that although movement across diagnostic categories does occur, longitudinal studies of children with autism typically report that very few individuals show such significant improvement that they move to a diagnostic classification outside of the autism spectrum. Given the small proportion of individuals, it is difficult to fully characterize this group. Data have recently emerged on children whose symptoms improve dramatically, that is they have "recovered," "remitted," or achieved an "optimal outcome." (Helt et al., 2008). These studies proposed that some children may lose their autism diagnosis by failing to meet DSM-IV criteria, with only subtle difficulties in pragmatic language distinguishing this "recovered" group from typically developing controls on standardized tests. As reports of cases with such improvement emerge in the literature (Granpeesheh, Tarbox, Dixon, Carr, & Herbert, 2009), it will be important to explore both early symptom patterns and current neurocognitive and psychiatric profiles of these individuals.

Recovery does raise questions about whether some individuals simply "mature" over time, growing out of an autism diagnosis, even with minimal treatment (Turner & Stone, 2007) and whether individuals are benefitting from specific treatments or combinations of treatments that are proving effective in treating core symptoms of autism. Cross-sectional and retrospective case reports are informative but of limited utility in deriving predictors of optimal outcome. Longitudinal studies are critical in examining early predictors of the most favorable prognoses.

In general, studies of optimal outcome in autism have identified few predictors of treatment response. Prior research has indicated that stronger pretreatment cognitive and language skills and severity of autism symptoms are good predictors of treatment response (Eikeseth, Smith, Jahr, & Eldevik, 2002; McGovern & Sigman, 2005). More recently, Sutera and colleagues (2007), using a prospective design, attempted to identify which children diagnosed with an ASD at 24–30 months would no longer be on the autism spectrum 2 ½ years later, following early intensive community-based intervention. With measures of intellectual functioning, autism symptoms, and adaptive functioning, they found that overall cognitive level and motor skill development were predictive of outcome. The authors emphasized that many children who continued to meet criteria for an autism diagnosis at follow-up exhibited a similar pretreatment neurocognitive profile. Sherer and Schreibman (2005) found that among 3-year-olds with autism, more toy play, less social avoidance, and more verbal self-stimulatory behaviors were associated with better response to a specific behavioral treatment intervention (PRT).

To date, there are few data on children who fully "recover" that describe this group's functioning or early features. Data from larger prospective, longitudinal studies of children with autism have been used to explore predictors of best outcome, though not on remission. Such studies of larger samples with smaller time intervals between follow-ups, many of which are ongoing, may provide information on how the patterns of symptoms in autism change over time and may even begin to give clues about predictors and different outcomes. However, full interpretation of this literature remains difficult, due to incomparability of results stemming from varying definitions of best outcome and discrepant assessment methods.

LONG-TERM OUTCOMES

In the earliest observations by Kanner, autism is described as a developmental disorder in which the impairments can be observed throughout the life course. Several longitudinal studies have examined how the disorder changes and, as mentioned above, the predictors of improvement in later life. Although early diagnostic stability in autism is high (Daniels et al., 2011), symptom presentation may change over time. For example, Taylor and Seltzer (2010) reported symptom improvement in most areas from high school into young adulthood among a cohort of 242 adults with ASDs.

Some pioneers of autism research have completed the initial studies of adult outcome. Rutter and colleagues (1967) reported that over half of a group of adolescents and adults they followed were hospitalized, and the majority had what was rated as poor social outcomes. Lotter (1974) found similar social outcomes in the patients he followed. Howlin and colleagues (2004) used several measures to assess outcome in a follow-up study of 68 adults; measures included education, jobs, friendships, and autism symptoms. Although there is variability in what different studies determined to be a positive outcome (e.g., employment or independent living), several predictors of positive prognosis continue to emerge in the literature.

Cognitive functioning is associated with core symptom expression (Bishop, Richler, & Lord, 2006), decrease in symptom severity over time (Richler, Huerta, Bishop, & Lord, 2010), and related areas of functioning such as adaptive behavior (Baghdadli et al., 2011). Often cited as a differentiating factor between Asperger's disorder and autism, cognitive functioning has also been used within autism to distinguish individuals as "high functioning" or "low functioning." In studies that have examined autism in adulthood, better cognitive functioning was shown to be predictive of positive outcome (Howlin et al., 2004). Language is also predictive of prognosis. Individuals with early language acquisition (before age 5 years) have been reported to have a better quality of life and improved reciprocal communication as adults (Billstedt, Gillberg, & Gillberg, 2007). Farley and colleagues (2009) found that practical daily living skills predicted outcome (e.g., capacity for independent living) better than other factors. Not surprisingly, diagnosis itself is predictive of outcome; one study showed that when cognitive functioning was controlled for, autism was associated with worse outcome than was PDD-NOS (Mordre et al., 2011).

Overall, although some individuals were employed, many continued to be highly dependent on parents, and the majority of individuals were viewed as having poor outcomes (Howlin et al., 2004). More recently, Taylor and Seltzer (2011) reported that in a sample of young adults with ASDs, only a small percentage was employed without the support of adult day services; and of those in the sample with ID, an even smaller percentage was employed.

CURRENT RESOURCES

Autism is typically a lifelong neurodevelopmental disorder, and care for individuals with ASDs has several unique features not typically considered in the treatment of other psychiatric and medical conditions. Because autism is a *pervasive* disorder that affects all aspects of life, daily living and academic skills (in addition to social and communication domains) are often significantly compromised. Further, given the medical comorbidities described earlier, healthcare needs are often specific and specialized for individuals with autism across the lifespan.

The study of services in ASDs is a rapidly growing field. Recent findings indicate that healthcare needs are frequently unmet for individuals with autism, even when compared with other children with special needs (Chiri & Warfield, 2011). Further, there is substantial evidence indicating significant disparity in access to many types of services, from diagnostic assessments (Mandell et al., 2009) to autism-specific types of therapies (Thomas, Ellis, McLaurin, Daniels, & Morrissey, 2007). Specific programs are now being developed to mitigate such disparities, including use of technologies to accomplish tasks such as educating parents about how to implement early intervention for autism and training professionals in methods for screening for the disorder (Kobak et al., 2011). However, these types of programs are only beginning to fill the gaps in service accessibility. It is clear that such innovative strategies are necessary to improve access to assessment and intervention services.

The educational system is often the treatment home of many interventions for children with autism because the identification and treatment of ASDs often occurs prior to school entrance (Thomas, Morrissey, & McLaurin, 2007). Also, children with ASDs benefit from ancillary services provided by educational systems (e.g., speech therapy, occupational therapy) and often require specialized academic placements in order to acquire academic skills as well as socialization skills. Thus, families of children with autism often rely on the school system, particularly for the development of an individualized educational plan, so that these children can be placed in an appropriate setting and be provided with optimal interventions for core autism symptoms.

Reliance on the school system for interventions requires different demands and expectations for families when compared with disorders that rely more exclusively on private ancillary treatment providers. School interventions may also be difficult to integrate with other ancillary interventions (e.g., private social skills training), which is often quite important for children with ASDs, who benefit greatly from consistent language and behavioral strategies used in interventions. These factors necessitate that families actively manage and integrate all aspects of their child's therapy into a cohesive treatment package.

Because prognosis for ASDs is mixed and often does not include full integration of the individual into all aspects of society (e.g., workforce, independent living), societal adjustments are often required for individuals and, in particular, adults with ASDs. Currently, the trend is for adults with ASDs who cannot live independently to live with the family of origin or in a group home. However, societal accommodations need to be made for adults when these optimal living circumstances are not feasible.

It is becoming apparent that autism is a disorder that affects individuals in multiple medical domains. Therefore an essential part of care for individuals with autism is a "medical home." The search for biomarkers for the disorder is laced with the hope that discovery of biological underpinnings of the disorder can lead to earlier diagnosis and more targeted treatment and that a true medical home, including treatment provision, can be developed for the disorder.

Finally, because children with autism are widely varied in presentation of many aspects of cognitive, developmental, and medical functioning, the impact of the disorder upon their lives and the lives of their families also varies. The evolution of the literature on autism from sparse to overwhelmingly vast may be daunting for families attempting to determine the level of empirical support for a given treatment or theory.

FUTURE AIMS AND RESEARCH OPPORTUNITIES

Current and future research in autism appears to be increasingly focused on delineating meaningful subtypes. In this context, meaningful subtypes may be defined as subgroups that have distinct phenotypes that relate to specific etiologies, wherein mechanisms of pathways to phenotypes are identified, leading to treatments that confer significant clinical improvement. While this research is still in its infancy with respect to the majority of the autism spectrum, such progress is underway for genetic disorders known to confer significant risk for ASDs. For instance, in fragile X research, knowledge of the proteins expressed differentially by the gene disruption has led to the development of novel agents that are now being tested in clinical trials for improvement of behavioral as well as physiological symptoms of fragile X (Berry-Kravis, Knox, & Hervey, 2011). Moving forward, the challenge of the field will be translating findings into clinically meaningful contexts for families, and for science.

REFERENCES

Aman, M. G., Lam, K. S., & Van Bourgondien, M. E. (2005). Medication patterns in patients with autism: temporal, regional, and demographic influences. *Journal of Child and Adolescent Psychopharmacology, 15*, 116–126. doi: 10.1089/cap.2005.15.116

American Psychiatric Association (1980). *Diagnostic and Statistical Manual of Mental Disorders*, 3rd edition, American Psychiatric Association, Washington, DC.

American Psychiatric Association (1987). *Diagnostic and Statistical Manual of Mental Disorders*, 3rd edition, Revision, American Psychiatric Association, Washington, DC.

American Psychiatric Association (2000). *Diagnostic and Statistical Manual of Mental Disorders*, 4th edition, Text Revision, American Psychiatric Association, Washington, DC.

Amir, R. E., Van Den Veyver, I. B., Wan, M., Tran, C. Q., Francke, U., & Zoghbi, H. Y. (1999). Rett syndrome is caused by mutations in X-linked MECP2, encoding methyl-CpG-binding protein 2. *Nature Genetics, 23*, 185–188.

Anderson, D. K., Oti, R. S., Lord, C., & Welch, K. (2009). Patterns of growth in adaptive social abilities among children with autism spectrum disorders. *Journal of Abnormal Child Psychology, 37*, 1019–1034. doi: 10.1007/s10802-009-9326-0

Asperger, H., & Frith, U. (1991). "Autistic psychopathy" in childhood. In U. Frith (Ed.), *Autism and Asperger syndrome* (pp. 37–92). New York, NY: Cambridge University Press.

Autism Speaks.(2009). [Graph illustration Autism Prevalence on the Rise, 2009]. *The Year of Autism Epidemiology*. Retrieved from http://www.autismspeaks.org/science/science-news/year-autism-epidemiology

Baghdadli, A., Assouline, B., Sonie, S., Pernon, E., Darrou, C., Michelon, C.,...Pry, R. (2011). Developmental Trajectories of Adaptive Behaviors from Early Childhood to Adolescence in a Cohort of 152 Children with Autism Spectrum Disorders. *Journal of Autism and Developmental Disorders*. doi: 10.1007/s10803-011-1357-z

Baird, G., Simonoff, E., Pickles, A., Chandler, S., Loucas, T., Meldrum, D., & Charman, T. (2006). Prevalence of disorders of the autism spectrum in a population cohort of children in South Thames: the Special Needs and Autism Project (SNAP). *Lancet, 368*, 210–215. doi: 10.1016/s0140-6736(06)69041-7

Baker, J. P. (2010). Autism in 1959: Joey the mechanical boy. *Pediatrics, 125*, 1101–1103. doi: 10.1542/peds.2010-0846

Baron-Cohen, S. (1989). The theory of mind hypothesis of autism: a reply to Boucher. *British Journal of Disorders of Communication, 24*, 199–200.

Baron-Cohen, S., Leslie, A. M., & Frith, U. (1985). Does the autistic child have a "theory of mind"? *Cognition, 21*, 37–46.

Baron-Cohen, S., O'Riordan, M., Stone, V., Jones, R., & Plaisted, K. (1999). Recognition of faux pas by normally developing children and children with Asperger syndrome or high-functioning autism. *Journal of Autism and Developmental Disorders, 29*, 407–418.

Bauman, M., & Kemper, T. L. (1985). Histoanatomic observations of the brain in early infantile autism. *Neurology, 35*, 866–874.

Begeer, S., Gevers, C., Clifford, P., Verhoeve, M., Kat, K., Hoddenbach, E., & Boer, F. (2011). Theory of Mind training in children with autism: a randomized controlled trial. *Journal of Autism and Developmental Disorders, 41,* 997–1006. doi: 10.1007/s10803-010-1121-9

Berry-Kravis, E., Knox, A., & Hervey, C. (2011). Targeted treatments for fragile X syndrome. *Journal of Neurodevelopmental Disorders, 3,* 193–210. doi: 10.1007/s11689-011-9074-7

Bettelheim, B. (1967). *The empty fortress: Infantile autism and the birth of the self.* New York: Free Press.

Billstedt, E., Gillberg, I. C., & Gillberg, C. (2007). Autism in adults: symptom patterns and early childhood predictors. Use of the DISCO in a community sample followed from childhood. *Journal of Child Psychology and Psychiatry, 48,* 1102–1110. doi: JCPP1774 [pii] 10.1111/j.1469-7610.2007.01774.x

Bishop, S. L., Richler, J., & Lord, C. (2006). Association between restricted and repetitive behaviors and nonverbal IQ in children with autism spectrum disorders. *Child Neuropsychology, 12,* 247–267. doi: 10.1080/09297040600630288

Bodfish, J. W., Symons, F. J., Parker, D. E., & Lewis, M. H. (2000). Varieties of repetitive behavior in autism: Comparisons to mental retardation. *Journal of Autism and Developmental Disorders, 30,* 237–243. doi: 10.1023/a:1005596502855

Bondy, A. S., & Frost, L. A. (1994). The Picture Exchange Communication System. *Focus on Autistic Behavior, 9,* 1–19.

Buie, T., Campbell, D. B., Fuchs, G. J., 3rd, Furuta, G. T., Levy, J., Vandewater, J., . . . Winter, H. (2010). Evaluation, diagnosis, and treatment of gastrointestinal disorders in individuals with ASDs: a consensus report. *Pediatrics, 125 Suppl* 1, S1–18. doi: 125/Supplement_1/S1 [pii] 10.1542/peds.2009-1878C

Byassee, J. E., & Murrell, S. A. (1975). Interaction patterns in families of autistic, disturbed, and normal children. *American Journal of Orthopsychiatry, 45,* 473–478.

Campbell, M., Geller, B., Small, A. M., Petti, T. A., & Ferris, S. H. (1978). Minor physical anomalies in young psychotic children. *American Journal of Psychiatry, 135,* 573–575.

Cantwell, D., Baker, L., & Rutter, M. (1978). A comparative study of infantile autism and specific developmental receptive language disorder—IV. Analysis of syntax and language function. *Journal of Child Psychology and Psychiatry, 19,* 351–362.

Castelli, F., Frith, C., Happe, F., & Frith, U. (2002). Autism, Asperger syndrome and brain mechanisms for the attribution of mental states to animated shapes. *Brain, 125*(Pt 8), 1839–1849.

Chiri, G., & Warfield, M. E. (2011). Unmet Need and Problems Accessing Core Health Care Services for Children with Autism Spectrum Disorder. *Maternal Child Health Journal.* doi: 10.1007/s10995-011-0833-6

Condie, J., Goldstein, J., & Wainwright, M. S. (2010). Acquired microcephaly, regression of milestones, mitochondrial dysfunction, and episodic rigidity in a 46,XY male with a de novo MECP2 gene mutation. *Journal of Child Neurology, 25,* 633–636. doi: 10.1177/0883073809342004

Coury, D., Jones, N. E., Klatka, K., Winklosky, B., & Perrin, J. M. (2009). Healthcare for children with autism: the Autism Treatment Network. *Current Opinion in Pediatrics, 21,* 828–832. doi: 10.1097/MOP.0b013e328331eaaa

Creak, M., & Pampiglione, G. (1969). Clinical and EEG studies on a group of 35 psychotic children. *Developmental Medicine and Child Neurology, 11,* 218–227.

Damasio, A. R., & Maurer, R. G. (1978). A neurological model for childhood autism. *Archives of Neurololgy, 35,* 777–786.

Daniels, A. M., Rosenberg, R. E., Law, J. K., Lord, C., Kaufmann, W. E., & Law, P. A. (2011). Stability of initial autism spectrum disorder diagnoses in community settings. *Journal of Autism and Developmental Disorders, 41,* 110–121. doi: 10.1007/s10803-010-1031-x

Dawson, G., Rogers, S., Munson, J., Smith, M., Winter, J., Greenson, J.,...Varley, J. (2010). Randomized, controlled trial of an intervention for toddlers with autism: the Early Start Denver Model. *Pediatrics, 125,* e17–23. doi: 10.1542/peds.2009-0958

De Giacomo, A., & Fombonne, E. (1998). Parental recognition of developmental abnormalities in autism. *European Child and Adolescent Psychiatry, 7,* 131–136.

de Villiers, J. (2007). The Interface of Language and Theory of Mind. *Linguistics, 117,* 1858–1878. doi: 10.1016/j.lingua.2006.11.006

DeVincent, C. J., Gadow, K. D., Delosh, D., & Geller, L. (2007). Sleep disturbance and its relation to DSM-IV psychiatric symptoms in preschool-age children with pervasive developmental disorder and community controls. *Journal of Child Neurology, 22,* 161–169.

Eikeseth, S., Smith, T., Jahr, E., & Eldevik, S. (2002). Intensive behavioral treatment at school for 4- to 7-year-old children with autism. A 1-year comparison controlled study. *Behavior Modification, 26,* 49–68.

Esbensen, A. J., Greenberg, J. S., Seltzer, M. M., & Aman, M. G. (2009). A longitudinal investigation of psychotropic and non-psychotropic medication use among adolescents and adults with autism spectrum disorders. *Journal of Autism and Developmental Disorders, 39,* 1339–1349. doi: 10.1007/s10803-009-0750-3

Farley, M. A., McMahon, W. M., Fombonne, E., Jenson, W. R., Miller, J., Gardner, M.,...Coon, H. (2009). Twenty-year outcome for individuals with autism and average or near-average cognitive abilities. *Autism Research, 2,* 109–118. doi: 10.1002/aur.69

Folstein, S., & Rutter, M. (1977). Genetic influences and infantile autism. *Nature, 265,* 726–728.

Fombonne, E. (2005). Epidemiology of autistic disorder and other pervasive developmental disorders. *Journal of Clinical Psychiatry, 66, Suppl* 10, 3–8.

Fombonne, E. (2009). Epidemiology of pervasive developmental disorders. *Pediatric Research, 65,* 591–598. doi: 10.1203/PDR.0b013e31819e7203

Gadow, K. D., DeVincent, C. J., & Pomeroy, J. (2006). ADHD symptom subtypes in children with pervasive developmental disorder. *Journal of Autism and Developmental Disorders, 36,* 271–283. doi: 10.1007/s10803-005-0060-3

Geurts, H. M., Corbett, B., & Solomon, M. (2009). The paradox of cognitive flexibility in autism. *Trends in Cognitive Science, 13,* 74–82. doi: 10.1016/j.tics.2008.11.006

Ghaziuddin, M., & Butler, E. (1998). Clumsiness in autism and Asperger syndrome: A further report. *Journal of Intellectual Disability Research, 42,* 43–48. doi: 10.1046/j.1365-2788.1998.00065.x

Gillberg, C. (1991). Debate and argument: is autism a pervasive developmental disorder? *Journal of Child Psychology and Psychiatry, 32,* 1169–1170.

Gilotty, L., Kenworthy, L., Sirian, L., Black, D. O., & Wagner, A. E. (2002). Adaptive skills and executive function in autism spectrum disorders. *Child Neuropsychology, 8,* 241–248. doi: 10.1076/chin.8.4.241.13504

Granpeesheh, D., Tarbox, J., Dixon, D. R., Carr, E., & Herbert, M. (2009). Retrospective analysis of clinical records in 38 cases of recovery from autism. *Annals of Clinical Psychiatry, 21,* 195–204. doi: acp_2104a [pii]

Greenspan, S. I., & Wieder, S. (1998). *The child with special needs: Encouraging intellectual and emotional growth.* Reading, MA: Addison-Wesley.

Hadjikhani, N., Joseph, R. M., Snyder, J., & Tager-Flusberg, H. (2006). Anatomical differences in the mirror neuron system and social cognition network in autism. *Cerebral Cortex, 16,* 1276–1282. doi: bhj069 [pii]10.1093/cercor/bhj069

Hanson, E., Kalish, L. A., Bunce, E., Curtis, C., McDaniel, S., Ware, J., & Petry, J. (2007). Use of complementary and alternative medicine among children diagnosed with autism spectrum disorder. *Journal of Autism and Developmental Disorders, 37,* 628–636. doi: 10.1007/s10803-006-0192-0

Happe, F. G. (1994). An advanced test of theory of mind: understanding of story characters' thoughts and feelings by able autistic, mentally handicapped, and normal children and adults. *Journal of Autism and Developmental Disorders, 24,* 129–154.

Hazlett, H. C., Poe, M. D., Lightbody, A. A., Gerig, G., MacFall, J. R., Ross, A. K.,...Piven, J. (2009). Teasing apart the heterogeneity of autism: Same behavior, different brains in toddlers with fragile X syndrome and autism. *Journal of Neurodevelopmental Disorders, 1,* 81–90. doi: 10.1007/s11689-009-9009-8

Helt, M., Kelley, E., Kinsbourne, M., Pandey, J., Boorstein, H., Herbert, M., & Fein, D. (2008). Can children with autism recover? If so, how? *Neuropsychology Review, 18,* 339–366. doi: 10.1007/s11065-008-9075-9

Herbert, J. D., Sharp, I. R., & Gaudiano, B. A. (2002). Separating fact from fiction in the etiology and treatment of autism: A scientific review of the evidence. *The Scientific Review of Mental Health Practice: Objective Investigations of Controversial and Unorthodox Claims in Clinical Psychology, Psychiatry, and Social Work, 1,* 23–43.

Hill, E. L. (2004). Executive dysfunction in autism. *Trends in Cognitive Science, 8,* 26–32. doi: S1364661303003152 [pii]

Howlin, P., Goode, S., Hutton, J., & Rutter, M. (2004). Adult outcome for children with autism. *Journal of Child Psychology and Psychiatry, 45,* 212–229.

Howlin, P., Magiati, I., & Charman, T. (2009). Systematic review of early intensive behavioral interventions for children with autism. *American Journal on Intellectual and Developmental Disabilities, 114,* 23–41.

Interactive Autism Network (2008, February 26). *IAN Research Report #5: Autism Treatment Overview—February 2008.* Retrieved from http://www.iancommunity.org/cs/ian_research_reports/ian_research_report_feb_2008

Kanner, L. (1943). Autistic disturbances of affective contact. *Nervous Child, 2,* 217–250.

Kanner, L. (1968). Autistic disturbances of affective contact. *Acta Paedopsychiatrica, 35,* 100–136.

Kanner, L., & Eisenberg, L. (1955). Review of psychiatric progress 1954; child psychiatry and mental deficiency. *American Journal of Psychiatry, 111,* 520–523.

Kanner, L., Rodriguez, A., & Ashenden, B. (1972). How far can autistic children go in matters of social adaptation? *Journal of Autism and Childhood Schizophrenia, 2,* 9–33.

Kenworthy, L., Yerys, B. E., Anthony, L. G., & Wallace, G. L. (2008). Understanding executive control in autism spectrum disorders in the lab and in the real world. *Neuropsychology Review, 18,* 320–338. doi: 10.1007/s11065-008-9077-7

Kenworthy, L. E., Black, D. O., Wallace, G. L., Ahluvalia, T., Wagner, A. E., & Sirian, L. M. (2005). Disorganization: the forgotten executive dysfunction in high-functioning autism (HFA) spectrum disorders. *Developmental Neuropsychology, 28,* 809–827. doi: 10.1207/s15326942dn2803_4

King, B. H., Hollander, E., Sikich, L., McCracken, J. T., Scahill, L., Bregman, J. D.,...Ritz, L. (2009). Lack of efficacy of citalopram in children with autism spectrum disorders and high levels of repetitive behavior: citalopram ineffective in children with autism. *Archives of General Psychiatry, 66,* 583–590.

Kjelgaard, M. M., & Tager-Flusberg, H. (2001). An Investigation of Language Impairment in Autism: Implications for Genetic Subgroups. *Language and Cognitive Processes, 16,* 287–308. doi: 10.1080/01690960042000058

Klin, A., Jones, W., Schultz, R., & Volkmar, F. (2003). The enactive mind, or from actions to cognition: lessons from autism. *Philosophical Transactions of the Royal Society of London, Series B, Biological Sciences, 358,* 345–360. doi: 10.1098/rstb.2002.1202

Klin, A., Lin, D. J., Gorrindo, P., Ramsay, G., & Jones, W. (2009). Two-year-olds with autism orient to non-social contingencies rather than biological motion. *Nature, 459,* 257–261. doi: 10.1038/nature07868

Klin, A., Saulnier, C. A., Sparrow, S. S., Cicchetti, D. V., Volkmar, F. R., & Lord, C. (2007). Social and communication abilities and disabilities in higher functioning individuals with autism spectrum disorders: The Vineland and the ADOS. *Journal of Autism and Developmental Disorders, 37*, 748–759. doi: 10.1007/s10803-006-0229-4

Kobak, K. A., Stone, W. L., Wallace, E., Warren, Z., Swanson, A., & Robson, K. (2011). A web-based tutorial for parents of young children with autism: results from a pilot study. *Telemedicine Journal and E Health, 17*, 804–808. doi: 10.1089/tmj.2011.0060

Koegel, R. I., & Frea, W. D. (1993). Treatment of social behavior in autism through the modification of pivotal social skills. *Journal of Applied Behavior Analysis, 26*, 369–377. doi: 10.1901/jaba.1993.26-369

Kuhl, P. K., Coffey-Corina, S., Padden, D., & Dawson, G. (2005). Links between social and linguistic processing of speech in preschool children with autism: behavioral and electrophysiological measures. *Developmental Science, 8*, F1-F12. doi: 10.1111/j.1467-7687.2004.00384.x

Kulesza, R. J., Jr., Lukose, R., & Stevens, L. V. (2011). Malformation of the human superior olive in autistic spectrum disorders. *Brain Research, 1367*, 360–371. doi: 10.1016/j.brainres.2010.10.015

Kylliainen, A., Braeutigam, S., Hietanen, J. K., Swithenby, S. J., & Bailey, A. J. (2006). Face- and gaze-sensitive neural responses in children with autism: a magnetoencephalographic study. *European Journal of Neuroscience, 24*, 2679–2690. doi: 10.1111/j.1460-9568.2006.05132.x

Levy, S. E., Giarelli, E., Lee, L. C., Schieve, L. A., Kirby, R. S., Cunniff, C.,...Rice, C. E. (2010). Autism spectrum disorder and co-occurring developmental, psychiatric, and medical conditions among children in multiple populations of the United States. *Journal of Developmental and Behavioral Pediatrics, 31*, 267–275. doi: 10.1097/DBP.0b013e3181d5d03b

Levy, S. E., Mandell, D. S., & Schultz, R. T. (2009). Autism. *The Lancet, 374*, 1627–1638. doi: 10.1016/s0140-6736(09)61376-3

Lotter, V. (1966). Epidemiology of autistic conditions in young children. *Social Psychiatry and Psychiatric Epidemiology, 1*, 124–135.

Lotter, V. (1974). Factors related to outcome in autistic children. *Journal of Autism and Childhood Schizophrenia, 4*, 263–277.

Lovaas, O. I. (1987). Behavioral treatment and normal educational and intellectual functioning in young autistic children. *Journal of Consulting and Clinical Psychology, 55*, 3–9. doi: 10.1037/0022-006x.55.1.3

Malhotra, S., & Gupta, N. (1999). Childhood disintegrative disorder. *Journal of Autism and Developmental Disorders, 29*, 491–498.

Mandell, D. S., Wiggins, L. D., Carpenter, L. A., Daniels, J., DiGuiseppi, C., Durkin, M. S.,...Kirby, R. S. (2009). Racial/ethnic disparities in the identification of children with autism spectrum disorders. *American Journal of Public Health, 99*, 493–498. doi: 10.2105/ajph.2007.131243

McGovern, C. W., & Sigman, M. (2005). Continuity and change from early childhood to adolescence in autism. *Journal of Child Psychology and Psychiatry, 46*, 401–408. doi: JCPP361 [pii] 10.1111/j.1469-7610.2004.00361.x

McPheeters, M. L., Warren, Z., Sathe, N., Bruzek, J. L., Krishnaswami, S., Jerome, R. N., & Veenstra-Vanderweele, J. (2011). A systematic review of medical treatments for children with autism spectrum disorders. *Pediatrics, 127*, e1312–1321. doi: 10.1542/peds.2011-0427

Mesibov, G. B., Shea, V., & Schopler, E. (2005). *The TEACCH approach to autism spectrum disorders*: New York, NY, US: Springer Science + Business Media.

Minshew, N. J., & Keller, T. A. (2010). The nature of brain dysfunction in autism: functional brain imaging studies. *Current Opinions in Neurology, 23*, 124–130. doi: 10.1097/WCO.0b013e32833782d4

Mordre, M., Groholt, B., Knudsen, A. K., Sponheim, E., Mykletun, A., & Myhre, A. M. (2011). Is Long-Term Prognosis for Pervasive Developmental Disorder Not Otherwise Specified Different from Prognosis for Autistic Disorder? Findings from a 30-Year Follow-Up Study. *Journal of Autism and Developmental Disorders*. doi: 10.1007/s10803-011-1319-5

Muller, R. A., Pierce, K., Ambrose, J. B., Allen, G., & Courchesne, E. (2001). Atypical patterns of cerebral motor activation in autism: a functional magnetic resonance study. *Biological Psychiatry, 49*, 665–676.

Mundy, P., Sigman, M., Ungerer, J., & Sherman, T. (1987). Nonverbal communication and play correlates of language development in autistic children. *Journal of Autism and Developmental Disorders, 17*, 349–364.

Munson, J., Dawson, G., Sterling, L., Beauchaine, T., Zhou, A., Koehler, E.,…Abbott, R. (2008). Evidence for latent classes of IQ in young children with autism spectrum disorder. *American Journal on Mental Retardation, 113*, 439–452. doi: 10.1352/2008.113:439-452

Neumann, N., Dubischar-Krivec, A. M., Poustka, F., Birbaumer, N., Bolte, S., & Braun, C. (2011). Electromagnetic evidence of altered visual processing in autism. *Neuropsychologia, 49*, 3011–3017. doi: 10.1016/j.neuropsychologia.2011.06.028

Nordahl, C. W., Lange, N., Li, D. D., Barnett, L. A., Lee, A., Buonocore, M. H.,…Amaral, D. G. (2011). Brain enlargement is associated with regression in preschool-age boys with autism spectrum disorders. *Proceedings of the National Academy of Science USA, 108*, 20195-20200. doi: 10.1073/pnas.1107560108

Ozonoff, S., & Miller, J. N. (1995). Teaching theory of mind: a new approach to social skills training for individuals with autism. *Journal of Autism and Developmental Disorders, 25*, 415–433.

Ozonoff, S., Pennington, B. F., & Rogers, S. J. (1991). Executive function deficits in high-functioning autistic individuals: relationship to theory of mind. *Journal of Child Psychology and Psychiatry, 32*, 1081–1105.

Pellicano, E. (2007). Links between theory of mind and executive function in young children with autism: clues to developmental primacy. *Developmental Psychology, 43*, 974–990. doi: 2007-09251-014 [pii] 10.1037/0012-1649.43.4.974

Pellicano, E. (2010). The development of core cognitive skills in autism: A 3-year prospective study. *Child Development, 18*, 1400–1416. doi: 10.1111/j.1467-8624.2010.01481.x

Pelphrey, K. A., Shultz, S., Hudac, C. M., & Vander Wyk, B. C. (2011). Research review: Constraining heterogeneity: the social brain and its development in autism spectrum disorder. *Journal of Child Psychology and Psychiatry, 52*, 631–644. doi: 10.1111/j.1469-7610.2010.02349.x

Pennington, B. F., & Ozonoff, S. (1996). Executive functions and developmental psychopathology. *Journal of Child Psychology and Psychiatry, 37*, 51–87.

Posey, D. J., Aman, M. G., McCracken, J. T., Scahill, L., Tierney, E., Arnold, L. E.,…McDougle, C. J. (2007). Positive effects of methylphenidate on inattention and hyperactivity in pervasive developmental disorders: an analysis of secondary measures. *Biological Psychiatry, 61*, 538–544. doi: 10.1016/j.biopsych.2006.09.028

Redcay, E., & Courchesne, E. (2008). Deviant functional magnetic resonance imaging patterns of brain activity to speech in 2–3-year-old children with autism spectrum disorder. *Biological Psychiatry, 64*, 589–598. doi: S0006-3223(08)00667-7 [pii]10.1016/j.biopsych.2008.05.020

Reed, P., Watts, H., & Truzoli, R. (2011). Flexibility in young people with autism spectrum disorders on a card sort task. *Autism*. doi: 10.1177/1362361311409599

Richler, J., Huerta, M., Bishop, S. L., & Lord, C. (2010). Developmental trajectories of restricted and repetitive behaviors and interests in children with autism spectrum disorders. *Development and Psychopathology, 22,* 55–69. doi: 10.1017/s0954579409990265

Roberts, T. P., Khan, S. Y., Rey, M., Monroe, J. F., Cannon, K., Blaskey, L.,…Edgar, J. C. (2010). MEG detection of delayed auditory evoked responses in autism spectrum disorders: towards an imaging biomarker for autism. *Autism Research, 3,* 8–18. doi: 10.1002/aur.111

Rogers, S. J., & Dawson, G. (2010). *Early Start Denver Model for young children with autism: Promoting language, learning, and engagement:* New York, NY, US: Guilford Press.

Rogers, S. J., Hepburn, S., & Wehner, E. (2003). Parent reports of sensory symptoms in toddlers with autism and those with other developmental disorders. *Journal of Autism and Developmental Disorders, 33,* 631–642.

Rogers, S. J., Hepburn, S. L., Stackhouse, T., & Wehner, E. (2003). Imitation performance in toddlers with autism and those with other developmental disorders. *Journal of Child Psychology and Psychiatry, 44,* 763–781.

Rogers, S. J., & Vismara, L. A. (2008). Evidence-based comprehensive treatments for early autism. *Journal of Clinical Child and Adolescent Psychology, 37,* 8–38. doi: 10.1080/15374410701817808

Rosenberg, R. E., Mandell, D. S., Farmer, J. E., Law, J. K., Marvin, A. R., & Law, P. A. (2010). Psychotropic medication use among children with autism spectrum disorders enrolled in a national registry, 2007–2008. *Journal of Autism and Developmental Disorders, 40,* 342–351.

Rumsey, J. M., Rapoport, J. L., & Sceery, W. R. (1985). Autistic children as adults: psychiatric, social, and behavioral outcomes. *Journal of the American Academy of Child Psychiatry, 24,* 465–473.

Rutter, M. (1968). Concepts of autism: a review of research. *Journal of Child Psychology and Psychiatry, 9,* 1–25.

Rutter, M., & Bartak, L. (1971). Causes of infantile autism: some considerations from recent research. *Journal of Autism and Childhood Schizophrenia, 1,* 20–32.

Rutter, M., Greenfeld, D., & Lockyer, L. (1967). A five to fifteen year follow-up study of infantile psychosis. II. Social and behavioural outcome. *British Journal of Psychiatry, 113,* 1183–1199.

Sergeant, J. A., Geurts, H., & Oosterlaan, J. (2002). How specific is a deficit of executive functioning for attention-deficit/hyperactivity disorder? *Behavioral Brain Research, 130,* 3–28.

Sherer, M. R., & Schreibman, L. (2005). Individual behavioral profiles and predictors of treatment effectiveness for children with autism. *Journal of Consulting and Clinical Psychology, 73,* 525–538. doi: 2005-06517-015 [pii]10.1037/0022-006X.73.3.525

Simonoff, E., Pickles, A., Charman, T., Chandler, S., Loucas, T., & Baird, G. (2008). Psychiatric disorders in children with autism spectrum disorders: prevalence, comorbidity, and associated factors in a population-derived sample. *Journal of the American Academy of Child and Adolescent Psychiatry, 47,* 921–929. doi: 10.1097/CHI.0b013e318179964f

Spence, S. J., & Schneider, M. T. (2009). The role of epilepsy and epileptiform EEGs in autism spectrum disorders. *Pediatric Research, 65,* 599–606.

Spence, S. J., & Thurm, A. (2010). Testing autism interventions: trials and tribulations. *Lancet, 375,* 2124–2125.

Sundberg, M. L., & Michael, J. (2001). The benefits of Skinner's analysis of verbal behavior for children with autism. *Behavior Modification, 25,* 698–724.

Sutera, S., Pandey, J., Esser, E. L., Rosenthal, M. A., Wilson, L. B., Barton, M.,…Fein, D. (2007). Predictors of optimal outcome in toddlers diagnosed with autism spectrum disorders. *Journal of Autism and Developmental Disorders, 37*, 98–107. doi: 10.1007/s10803-006-0340-6

Tager-Flusberg, H. (1981). On the nature of linguistic functioning in early infantile autism. *Journal of Autism and Developmental Disorders, 11*, 45–56.

Tager-Flusberg, H. (1992). Autistic children's talk about psychological states: deficits in the early acquisition of a theory of mind. *Child Development, 63*, 161–172.

Taylor, J. L., & Seltzer, M. M. (2010). Changes in the autism behavioral phenotype during the transition to adulthood. *Journal of Autism and Developmental Disorders, 40*, 1431–1446. doi: 10.1007/s10803-010-1005-z

Taylor, J. L., & Seltzer, M. M. (2011). Employment and post-secondary educational activities for young adults with autism spectrum disorders during the transition to adulthood. *Journal of Autism and Developmental Disorders, 41*, 566–574. doi: 10.1007/s10803-010-1070-3

Thomas, K. C., Ellis, A. R., McLaurin, C., Daniels, J., & Morrissey, J. P. (2007). Access to care for autism-related services. *Journal of Autism and Developmental Disorders, 37*, 1902–1912. doi: 10.1007/s10803-006-0323-7

Thomas, K. C., Morrissey, J. P., & McLaurin, C. (2007). Use of autism-related services by families and children. *Journal of Autism and Developmental Disorders, 37*, 818–829.

Turner, L. M., & Stone, W. L. (2007). Variability in outcome for children with an ASD diagnosis at age 2. *Journal of Child Psychology and Psychiatry, 48*, 793–802. doi: JCPP1744 [pii] 10.1111/j.1469-7610.2007.01744.x

Turner, L. M., Stone, W. L., Pozdol, S. L., & Coonrod, E. E. (2006). Follow-up of children with autism spectrum disorders from age 2 to age 9. *Autism, 10*, 243–265. doi: 10.1177/1362361306063296

Valicenti-McDermott, M., McVicar, K., Rapin, I., Wershil, B. K., Cohen, H., & Shinnar, S. (2006). Frequency of gastrointestinal symptoms in children with autistic spectrum disorders and association with family history of autoimmune disease. *Journal of Developmental and Behavioral Pediatrics, 27*(2 Suppl), S128–136. doi: 00004703-200604002-00011 [pii]

Vismara, L. A., & Rogers, S. J. (2010). Behavioral treatments in autism spectrum disorder: What do we know? *Annual Review of Clinical Psychology, 6*, 447–468. doi: 10.1146/annurev.clinpsy.121208.131151

Volden, J., Coolican, J., Garon, N., White, J., & Bryson, S. (2009). Brief report: pragmatic language in autism spectrum disorder: relationships to measures of ability and disability. *Journal of Autism and Developmental Disorders, 39*, 388–393. doi: 10.1007/s10803-008-0618-y

Volkmar, F. R., State, M., & Klin, A. (2009). Autism and autism spectrum disorders: Diagnostic issues for the coming decade. *Journal of Child Psychology and Psychiatry, 50*, 108–115. doi: 10.1111/j.1469-7610.2008.02010.x

Warren, Z., Veenstra-VanderWeele, J., Stone, W., Bruzek, J. L., Nahmias, A. S., Foss-Feig, J. H.,…McPheeters, M. L. (2011). *Therapies for children with autism spectrum disorders.* Rockville, MD. US: AHRQ Comparative Effectiveness Reviews.

White, S. W., Oswald, D., Ollendick, T., & Scahill, L. (2009). Anxiety in children and adolescents with autism spectrum disorders. *Clinical Psychological Review, 29*, 216–229. doi: 10.1016/j.cpr.2009.01.003

Wing, L. (1981). Language, social, and cognitive impairments in autism and severe mental retardation. *Journal of Autism and Developmental Disorders, 11*, 31–44.

Wing, L. (1997). The autistic spectrum. *Lancet, 350*(9093), 1761–1766. doi: 10.1016/s0140-6736(97)09218-0

Wolff, S. (2004). The history of autism. *European Child and Adolescent Psychiatry, 13*, 201–208. doi: 10.1007/s00787-004-0363-5

Yerys, B. E., Hepburn, S. L., Pennington, B. F., & Rogers, S. J. (2007). Executive function in preschoolers with autism: evidence consistent with a secondary deficit. *Journal of Autism and Developmental Disorders, 37,* 1068–1079. doi: 10.1007/s10803-006-0250-7

Zwaigenbaum, L., Bryson, S., Rogers, T., Roberts, W., Brian, J., & Szatmari, P. (2005). Behavioral manifestations of autism in the first year of life. *International Journal of Developmental Neuroscience, 23,* 143–152. doi: S0736574804000553 [pii]10.1016/j.ijdevneu.2004.05.001

3 Childhood Brain Tumors

Celiane Rey-Casserly

Brain tumors are the most common solid tumors in children and second in incidence to leukemia with respect to overall pediatric malignancies (Ries et al., 2008). The overall incidence rate for brain and central nervous system (CNS) tumors for children aged 0–19 years is 5.05 per 100,000 person years (CBTRUS, 2012). Based on 2004–2008 data, it is estimated that 4,200 new cases of primary brain and CNS tumors will be diagnosed in the United States in 2012, with more than 70% of cases occurring in children <14 years (CBTRUS, 2012).

The etiology of childhood brain tumors is not well understood; specific genetic cancer predisposition syndromes associated with tumorigenesis include neurofibromatosis type 1 and type 2, Turcot syndrome, nevoid basal cell carcinoma (Gorlin syndrome), tuberous sclerosis, and Li-Fraumeni syndrome, but these only account for a small percentage of cases (Pollack & Jakacki, 2011). Exposure to ionizing radiation also increases risk of brain tumors (Preston-Martin, 1996), and secondary malignancy is a long-term risk factor for children treated for cancer with radiotherapy (Dickerman, 2007).

The incidence of different types of tumors varies by age group, histology, and location. Neuroepithelial tumors of embryonal origin (medulloblastoma, supratentorial primitive neuroectodermal tumors) are more common in children than in adults; glial tumors are more likely low grade (pilocytic astrocytoma) in children, whereas high-grade gliomas (glioblastoma multiforme) are more common in adults (Blaney et al., 2006). Location of tumors varies by age as well, with more than half of pediatric brain tumors occurring in the posterior fossa or brain stem (Fruhwald & Rutkowski, 2011), and adult tumors more likely in cortical regions (CBTRUS, 2008).

Survival rates have been increasing; deaths from brain and other CNS tumors fell at a rate of 1% per year from 1990 to 2004 (Centers for Disease Control and Prevention, 2007), and the youngest children (age 0–4 years) have shown the largest improvements in survival from 1975 to 2002 (Smith et al., 2010). Children are more likely to survive primary brain tumors than adults (see Table 3.1). With improvements in medical success in the treatment of CNS malignancies, attention increasingly turns to long-term outcomes and the quality of survival. For some childhood brain tumors

Table 3.1 Five-Year Survival Rates by Age Group

Age Group (years)	5-Year Survival Rate (%)
0–19	72.6
20–44	57.1
45–54	31.6
55–64	17.7
65–74	10.0
75+	5.6

Source: Central Brain Tumor Registry of the United States, 2012.

such as diffuse pontine gliomas, the prognosis remains very poor, but for most other neoplasms, survival rates have improved substantially. Research on neuropsychological and quality-of-life outcomes in survivors of childhood brain tumors has spurred changes in treatment protocols that seek to minimize toxicity and late consequences while improving or maintaining disease control.

The mainstays of treatment for childhood brain tumors are surgery, radiation, and chemotherapy. Each modality has associated complications or late effects that affect development and neuropsychological outcomes. Risk factors related to the tumor itself (location, infiltration/damage of brain structures, and complications such as hydrocephalus, endocrinopathies, and sensory/motor dysfunction) are also important in long-term outcome.

Location. Tumor location cannot be considered a single factor in outcome given that certain tumor types occur in specific areas of the brain and are associated with specific biological behaviors that require specific types of treatment. For example, infratentorial tumors are common in children and include both malignant tumors (medulloblastoma, anaplastic ependymoma), which are treated with intense multimodality therapy, and low-grade astrocytic tumors, which are generally controlled with surgery only. Tumor location in the sellar/suprasellar region is associated with endocrinopathies and vision loss, which have long-term consequences for neuropsychological and quality-of-life outcomes (Sands et al., 2005; Schroeder & Vezina, 2011).

Hydrocephalus. Children diagnosed with brain tumors often present with signs of increased intracranial pressure (Ullrich & Pomeroy, 2003; Wilne, Ferris, Nathwani, & Kennedy, 2006), which can be associated with tumor mass effects, are more often indicative of hydrocephalus because obstruction of cerebral spinal fluid (CSF) flow is frequent in childhood brain tumors. Hydrocephalus can damage periventricular white matter or cause vision deficits. Although tumor resection can remove the obstruction, in some cases, shunting is necessary to divert CSF flow. Medical complications, such as hydrocephalus at diagnosis, are associated with increased risk of neuropsychological deficits, even after effects of the tumor and treatment are taken into account (von Hoff et al., 2008).

Surgery. For most types of childhood brain tumors, gross total resection is the treatment of choice because the extent of resection is associated with positive outcome. In some situations, complete resection is not possible due to the location of the tumor and/or its adherence to vital structures. Because germ cell tumors respond to radiation and chemotherapy, the role of surgery may be limited for this type of tumor (Grondin, Scott, & Smith, 2009). Complications of neurosurgery include perioperative stroke, neurological deficits, changes in physical appearance, and damage to pituitary/hypo-thalamic structures. Neurological problems managed in the immediate postsurgical period include seizures, edema, and infection (Houdemont et al., 2011). Cerebellar surgery is associated with an increased risk of cerebellar mutism syndrome, also referred to as posterior fossa syndrome, which appears to be increasing in frequency since it was first identified in 1985 by Rekate (Rekate, Brugg, Aram, Hahn, & Ratcheson, 1985; Robertson et al., 2006). The syndrome emerges within 12 to 48 hours of posterior fossa surgery, following a period of normal functioning. Symptoms include mutism as well as a range of other manifestations. Pollack (2001) refers to it as a "complex neurobehavioral symptom complex" characterized by impairments in speech, initiation of voluntary movements, and emotional regulation as well as incontinence and personality changes. Ataxia and cranial nerve deficits are also commonly associated with this syndrome. Risk factors include brainstem involvement of the tumor and midline (vermal) location in the cerebellum (Gudrunardottir, Sehested, Juhler, & Schmiegelow, 2011). Recovery can occur over the course of days or weeks, but it has become increasingly apparent that residual difficulties remain over the long term (Gudrunardottir et al., 2011). In a prospective study of children who developed cerebellar mutism syndrome postsurgery for embryonal tumors, evaluations 12 months postsurgery noted more severe neurocognitive and academic deficits when compared with children with similar diagnoses and treatment who did not have cerebellar mutism (Palmer et al., 2010).

Radiation therapy. Radiation therapy is an essential modality in the treatment of brain tumors. Tumors with risk of dissemination require treatment to the whole brain and spine in order to prevent relapse in the neuroaxis. In the context of progressive disease or incomplete resection, radiotherapy can be very effective in disease control, though at what age one can begin to consider this treatment "safe" has not yet been determined (Packer, 2010). Radiation therapy can improve neurologic status and have a palliative role in children with tumors whose prognosis is poor (Cohen, Broniscer, & Glod, 2001). Whole-body radiation is used in conditioning protocols before bone marrow transplant in the treatment of young children (below 3 years of age) and in salvage protocols for relapsed disease (Marachelian, Butturini, & Finlay, 2008).

Radiation affects cells by damaging DNA, releasing free radicals, and causing apoptosis in proliferating cells (Georg Kuhn & Blomgren, 2011). Because radiation therapy targets rapidly dividing tumor cells, stem and progenitor cells, which are critical to brain development, are highly vulnerable to radiation-induced damage. Neoplastic cells are preferentially involved in replication, whereas normal tissue has more potential to repair radiation damage. Consequently, radiation therapy doses are divided into fractions and delivered over the course of several weeks; this allows for normal tissue repair while at the same time intensifying the effects on the tumor. In the context of small, circumscribed tumors, radiation can also be delivered in a single high dose through the use of stereotactic radiosurgery.

Vulnerability to radiation-induced damage varies in different tissues and at different stages in development, which explains some of the variability seen in late effects of treatment. Paulino and colleagues (2010) argue that the prevailing notion was that late effects of radiation were related to the radiosensitivity of the parenchymal cell population and its dysfunction as well as radiation-induced effects on microvasculature (Paulino et al., 2010). Currently, the understanding is of a more complex process, and late effects of radiation across the lifespan are conceptualized as stemming from multiple complex interactions that include cell-signaling processes affected by tissue microenvironments, immune system competence, and genetic factors. Differences between observed late effects in adults and children are likely related to more complex mechanisms, not just the degree of proliferative activity of the tissue targeted (Paulino et al., 2010). Furthermore, children are more vulnerable because they can sustain not only impairments in growth and maturation of systems undergoing active development but also damage to established systems due to dysfunction in repair processes.

Radiation can have both acute and short-term effects on cognitive function, mood, and well-being several weeks or months following treatment. Fatigue or frank somnolence syndrome can develop early in treatment. These symptoms typically resolve after therapy is completed. In contrast, late effects of radiation are likely not reversible and can be progressive (Armstrong, Gyato, Awadalla, Lustig, & Tochner, 2004). Toxic effects of radiation over the long term affect the endocrine system, growth and bone development, vision, hearing, neuropsychological development, and fertility (Fossati, Ricardi, & Orecchia, 2009). Cardiac and pulmonary toxicity, permanent hair loss, vasculopathies as well as increased risk of second cancers are also seen (Shih, Loeffler, & Tarbell, 2009). Younger age at treatment and higher radiation dose increase the risk of developing these late effects and the severity of impairments.

In children, radiation has been shown to affect developing white matter as well as stem and progenitor cells in the hippocampus (Monje, 2008; Monje, Mizumatsu, Fike, & Palmer, 2002; Reddick et al., 2005; Reddick et al., 2000). Damage to white matter is presumably related to effects on the oligodendrocyte precursor cell pool and microvasculature changes that compromise the blood–brain barrier (Sarkissian, 2005). These pathophysiological processes are presumed to underlie the progressive neurocognitive and learning impairments seen in children treated with radiation therapy.

Chemotherapy

Chemotherapy has a more prominent role in the treatment of brain tumors in children. Most chemotherapy agents are developed to incite cell death directly (cytoxans), though novel therapies that target cell signaling pathways and tumor angiogenesis are increasingly included in current protocols (Ali-Osman et al., 2005). Although chemotherapy has been added to many protocols in order to limit or avoid the toxicity associated with radiation, chemotherapy can also have an impact on long-term health and neuropsychological outcomes. Cancer chemotherapy has acute and chronic effects on a range of organ systems (cardiac, pulmonary, renal, reproductive, and central and peripheral nervous systems) (Gururangan, 2009). Late effects include changes in peripheral motor function, white matter integrity, leukoencephalopathy, seizures, hearing loss, cerebellar symptoms, and neurocognitive impairments (Ahles & Saykin, 2007; Dietrich, Han, Yang, Mayer-Proschel, & Noble, 2006). Hearing loss is a particularly challenging problem in the treatment of brain tumors. There seems to be a synergistic effect of the combination of platinum-based chemotherapy agents and radiation therapy on cochlear hair cells. As a result, progressive hearing loss can emerge over time (Gururangan, 2009; Schell et al., 1989). The cellular basis for chemotherapy toxicity to the CNS has been linked to damage to normal neural progenitor cells and oligodendrocytes (Dietrich et al., 2006). Increased neurotoxicity is associated with intrathecal administration, as opposed to intravenous delivery and with higher doses, and this is of concern for young children who are increasingly treated with chemotherapy alone at high doses (see Infant Brain Tumors, below). In addition, corticosteroids, which are often used in cancer treatment, can also affect memory or exacerbate other cognitive late effects (Krull, 2010; Mrakotsky & Waber, 2006).

HISTORICAL MEDICAL PERSPECTIVE

The management of childhood brain tumors has evolved considerably over the past three decades. The incidence of brain tumors was noted to increase from 1973 to 1994, which has been attributed to adoption of and advances in imaging techniques (computed tomography, magnetic resonance imaging [MRI]) that allow for earlier and more precise diagnosis (Baldwin & Preston-Martin, 2004; Smith et al., 2010). Treatment strategies have evolved over these years, contributing to increased survival and stepwise changes in treatment protocols. Postoperative craniospinal and focal radiation therapy, which was introduced in the 1950s, was responsible for substantial improvement in survival in children with malignant tumors. Before radiation therapy protocols were developed, children with tumors that had potential for dissemination, such as medulloblastoma, and who were treated only with surgery almost uniformly succumbed to their disease. These treatments included craniospinal radiation as well as focal radiation to the tumor bed because local treatment was not sufficient. In the 1970s, radiation therapy was used to treat young children with craniospinal doses much higher than those used in CNS prophylactic treatment for leukemia. Concerns about the adverse effects of radiation on the developing brain led to efforts to reduce treatment doses, develop alternative treatments, or defer radiation. Chemotherapy began to play a larger role in the treatment of brain tumors when it was recognized that certain tumors were chemosensitive. Inclusion of adjuvant chemotherapy in treatment protocols led to reductions in radiation therapy doses in the treatment of malignant tumors (Packer et al., 1999). In the treatment of medulloblastoma, the craniospinal irradiation dose has decreased from 36 gray (Gy) in the 1980s to 23.4 Gy. In the most recent treatment protocol for medulloblastoma, the proposed craniospinal dose is 18 Gy for children between the ages of 3 and 7 years with standard risk disease at diagnosis (Children's Oncology Group-ACNS0331).

Chemotherapy has also become increasingly important in the treatment of low-grade gliomas. Complete surgical resection is the treatment of choice, if possible, for low-grade tumors and is often curative (Packer, MacDonald, & Vezina, 2008). For deep-seated or infiltrative tumors that cannot be resected completely or are in locations not amenable to surgery, other treatment options are considered. Chemotherapy is often used as a first option in treatment, and the respective role of chemotherapy and radiation in low-grade gliomas is evolving (Abdullah, Qaddoumi, & Bouffet, 2008). Radiation is now more often avoided when treating children with neurofibromatosis (NF-1) with low-grade gliomas because it has been linked to vascular complications such as moyamoya disease (Ullrich et al., 2007) and an increased risk of secondary tumors.

CURRENT MEDICAL FACTORS AND TREATMENT AND INTERVENTION UPDATE

Major advances have been made in the diagnosis and treatment of childhood brain tumors. The current trend is toward increased individualization of treatment protocols through better understanding of tumor biology. More precise identification of different subtypes of tumors is possible through refinements in imaging techniques such as proton magnetic resonance spectroscopy, which can distinguish characteristics of higher-grade tumors (Grondin et al., 2009). Histological classification and grading are now informed by genomics research such that tumors with the same histology can be differentiated from each other on the basis of molecular characteristics (Dubuc et al., 2010). Using gene expression profiling, Pomeroy and colleagues (2002) not only distinguished different types of tumors but also identified subgroups of medulloblastoma and gene profiles that were more likely to respond to treatment. Different molecular subgroups with differing signaling pathways and prognostic implications have been identified (Gibson et al., 2010). Recent studies have discriminated molecular characteristics of primary tumors and their metastases, which have an impact on directing therapy (Wu et al., 2012). These advances have led to risk-adapted stratification and optimization of treatment informed by molecular biological characteristics of the tumor in addition to other clinical risk factors (Partap & Fisher, 2007; Pollack & Jakacki, 2011). This has allowed for reductions in treatment intensity for tumor subtypes that are more likely to respond to therapy.

Treatment and Intervention

In addition to more refined diagnosis and classification, treatment options have improved or expanded. Less invasive and more precise neurosurgical techniques as well as technological innovations have been introduced. Intraoperative MRI suites are becoming more available in pediatric hospital settings. Real-time intraoperative imaging provides repeat imaging during the surgical procedure, which enhances the ability to detect residual tumor, reduces the need for repeat surgery, and, when combined with navigation software, assists with more precise tumor localization (Grondin et al., 2009; Shah et al., 2012). Endoscopic third ventriculostomy is used more often to manage hydrocephalus, with fewer complications than conventional shunting procedures (Ruggiero et al., 2004).

Minimization of the use of radiation and limitation of toxicity to normal tissue drives new treatment efforts in radiation oncology. Techniques of radiation delivery developed from the early use of wide opposed lateral fields to more sophisticated three-dimensional plans and incorporation of more precise image-based radiation strategies such as intensity-modulated radiation therapy, which delivers a lower dose to critical structures adjacent to the tumor (Shih et al., 2009).

Radiotherapy with charged particles (protons) is increasingly used to treat childhood brain tumors. In proton beam radiotherapy, the charged particles deposit most of the radiation dose at the end of their range; consequently, the exit dose is expected to be lower than with photon-based radiation and avoids normal tissue (Yock & Tarbell, 2004). Multiple dosimetric studies clearly demonstrate superior normal tissue sparing in critical regions such as the temporal lobes, hypothalamus, and cochlea, as well as decreased integral dose, with proton radiotherapy (MacDonald et al., 2008). In addition, prediction studies suggest that the risk of secondary malignancies may be lower with the use of proton radiotherapy (Newhauser & Durante, 2011).

The study of radiogenomics seeks to develop genetic risk profiles to inform individualization of radiation doses in specific patients and in different contexts based on probabilities of developing toxicity (Barnett et al., 2009). This work, which is in its early stages, promises to contribute to optimization of therapy and to a decrease in morbidity associated with radiation therapy.

Chemotherapy for brain tumors has evolved with the increased understanding of biological systems involved in tumorigenesis at the molecular level. Finlay and colleagues (2007) note that dose intensification of traditional cytotoxic antineoplastic agents is not likely to contribute to advances in cure rates for childhood malignant or progressive tumors. Targeted therapies based on an understanding of cellular pathways that support tumor cell growth are being introduced in treatment protocols (Schor, 2009). Innovations in chemotherapy include biologic agents such as antiangiogenic therapies that target tumor vascular supply (Kieran, 2005) and molecular therapies that block activity of cancer-specific oncogenic proteins (Bouffet, Tabori, Huang, & Bartels, 2010; Nageswara Rao, Scafidi, Wells, & Packer, 2012). Immune-based targeted therapies are also under investigation.

Treatment and intervention strategies for pediatric brain tumors are evolving, and it is clear that future goals will include identifying specific subgroups of tumors and patients based on biological characteristics and genetic profiles of the tumor and the individual. Treatment protocols will be rationally developed for each individual, combining types of therapies in order to maximally benefit the specific individual and to minimize toxicity. This will require increased collaboration and cooperation among centers and a comprehensive catalogue of specific genetic profiles associated with specific tumors, response to treatment, and vulnerability to toxicity (Huse & Holland, 2010; Smith et al., 2010).

Infant Brain Tumors

Children diagnosed with brain tumors in infancy or early childhood (<5 years) present a significant challenge given the deleterious effect on brain development and cognition of life-saving treatments. Ten percent of all childhood tumors are diagnosed in the first year of life (Bishop, McDonald, Chang, & Esiashvili, 2010), and approximately 30% are diagnosed when the child is <3 years (Rickert, Probst-Cousin, & Gullotta, 1997). The rapidly developing brain of the very young child is more vulnerable to toxicity, and the long-term adverse effects of treatment and counseling families regarding treatment options can present ethical dilemmas (Levine, Cohen, & Wendler, 2012). Diagnosis in this group can be delayed because symptoms can be diffuse and nonspecific or difficult to ascertain because the infant skull can expand and accommodate increased intracranial pressure, which is a classic sign of brain malignancies in childhood (Bishop et al., 2010). Surgery can have a high risk of complications because infant tumors are very vascular, and complete resection can be difficult because tumors are often large and more likely to be high grade (Van Poppel et al., 2011).

For infants and young children, potentially curative radiation therapy needs to be deferred or avoided. In the past, treatment options were limited. However, protocols for this population have expanded over the past 30 years, with innovative regimens showing some promise of improved survival and disease control. Use of radiation therapy in young children has declined substantially since the 1980s with the introduction of these new treatment strategies (Bishop et al., 2010). Significant advances include development of new chemotherapy regimens and use of bone marrow transplantation to control disease so that radiation therapy can be avoided or deferred. Treatment options include myeloablative chemotherapy with autologous stem cell rescue after maximal surgery and conventional induction. Use of high-dose methotrexate (MTX) has been added to this regimen in more recent trials (Rutkowski et al., 2010). Outcomes have been promising with respect to overall survival, quality of life, and early neuropsychological status; however, treatment-related toxicity is high on the Head Start protocols (Dhall et al., 2008). In Germany, intraventricular chemotherapy was introduced instead of radiation therapy in a trial with 43 children (Rutkowski et al., 2005). This strategy included intensive systemic chemotherapy with high-dose MTX and intraventricular MTX delivered through an implanted reservoir. Five-year progression-free survival and overall survival were 82% and 93% for children without metastatic disease and without residual tumor, respectively. In contrast to the myeloablative chemotherapy studies, there were no treatment-related deaths. Imaging studies and neuropsychological assessments were included in follow-up studies. MRI scans performed on 23 of the children assessed leukoencephalopathy during and after treatment. Nineteen patients had evidence of leukoencephalopathy that ranged from mild to severe without related symptoms. Follow-up scans showed a decrease in severity of leukoencephalopathy in 10 patients and stable findings in 8. The cumulative dose of MTX was correlated with grade of leukoencephalopathy. Neuropsychological evaluation performed approximately 5 years after diagnosis using the Kaufman Assessment Battery for Children, Raven's Colored Progressive Matrices, and tests of visual–motor integration showed lower scores relative to controls; however, performance was significantly better than that of a group of children treated for medulloblastoma with radiotherapy (historical controls).

Advances in the management of infant brain tumors will result in a new group of survivors whose outcomes have yet to be elucidated. Although we have ideas about the role of specific risk factors such as intensity of treatment and timing of radiation on long-term outcome, we can only speculate about the impact of these new treatment protocols over the long term. Diffuse neuropsychological compromise and severe intellectual disability were commonly seen with radiation treatment at a young age. However, the way in which high-dose chemotherapy and bone marrow transplant can affect brain development in this newer cohort is unknown because late effects may not emerge until children are older and encounter more complex learning challenges. Very young children who present with brain tumors already evidence delays in development and cognition before treatment. The cumulative impact of tumor and treatment effects needs to be studied longitudinally in this emerging new group of survivors.

EARLY PSYCHOLOGICAL AND NEUROPSYCHOLOGICAL FINDINGS

There is an extensive literature regarding acute and long-term psychological and neuropsychological outcomes for children treated for brain tumors. Interpretation and generalization of findings are complicated by the wide heterogeneity of tumor types, small sample sizes, retrospective designs, samples of convenience, lack of comparable control groups, and failure to distinguish between different pathologies and treatments (Ris & Noll, 1994). For example, in many studies, different types of radiation treatment or doses (focal versus a combination of focal and craniospinal) are not differentiated. In an early review, Ris and Noll (1994) argued that more sophisticated methodologies and conceptualizations of factors affecting discrete outcomes would be needed to draw more specific conclusions regarding neurobehavioral and psychological outcomes.

Major findings in studies of this period noted greater neuropsychological impairment in children diagnosed at a young age and in those treated with radiation therapy.

As in many areas of pediatric neuropsychology, early psychological and neuropsychological studies focused on general cognitive ability (IQ), psychological adjustment, and overall quality of life. Studies of neurocognitive outcomes in children treated for medulloblastoma with surgery and radiation, with and without adjuvant chemotherapy, documented significant and progressive impairments in such functioning. In an early study of children treated for posterior fossa tumors with radiation and chemotherapy who had intelligence testing prior to diagnosis, the decline in IQ was 25 points posttreatment; there was evidence of significant cognitive deficits in all children in this study (intellectual disability, dementia) (Duffner, Cohen, & Thomas, 1983).

Packer and colleagues (1989) compared changes in cognitive function over 2 years after whole brain radiation therapy in 18 children treated for malignant brain tumors between the ages of 18 months and 18 years. Serial neuropsychological assessments were compared with those of a group of children treated for cerebellar tumors with surgery only. Overall change in IQ from baseline to year 2 was −13.8 points; children treated with radiation at age 7 years or younger had a 25-point drop in Full Scale IQ (FSIQ) over the 2 years. Degree of decline was correlated with age, with the youngest children showing the steepest decline. IQ scores were relatively stable in the surgery-only group. Another frequently cited study by Hoppe-Hirsch and colleagues (1995) compared intellectual outcomes in children treated for posterior fossa tumors with whole brain radiation with a group treated for ependymoma with focal radiation to the posterior fossa. Although outcomes were not different at short-term follow-up, over the long term more children in the whole brain radiation group were performing below average, with 20% scoring above 90 at 5 years and only 10% scoring above 90 at 10 years after treatment.

The adverse progressive impact of radiation therapy on young children was increasingly recognized. In a study of children <3 years diagnosed between 1985 and 1999, craniospinal and focal radiation therapy were associated with significant decline in IQ as well as endocrine dysfunction and placement in special education (Fouladi et al., 2005).

Adult Outcomes. In long-term outcome studies of adult survivors of childhood cancer, the brain tumor groups typically demonstrate increased risk of deficits in neurocognitive, health, quality of life, emotional, and educational/vocational functioning. International registry–based studies of the quality of survivorship note lower educational achievement, more limited employment, lower income, and lower likelihood of living independently in adults treated for CNS malignancies in childhood (Boman, Lindblad, & Hjern, 2010; Koch et al., 2006; Kuehni et al., 2012).

In the United States, the Childhood Cancer Survivor Study (CCSS) uses periodic surveys to track the outcomes of approximately 20,000 children treated for cancer between 1970 and 1986, comparing findings to sibling controls; more than 2000 are survivors of CNS malignancies (Robison et al., 2009; Robison et al., 2005). These adult survivors encounter multiple health risks including neurological (seizure disorder, strokes), endocrine, and sensory deficits (Bowers et al., 2006; Packer et al., 2003). Social–emotional, educational, and vocational outcomes are also poorer in this group compared with both survivors of other pediatric malignancies and sibling controls (Mitby et al., 2003; Zebrack et al., 2004; Zeltzer et al., 2009). Radiation therapy and treatment dose are consistently linked to more adverse outcomes, including medical late effects and neurocognitive deficits (Armstrong et al., 2009). Degree of neurocognitive impairment, as assessed by questionnaire, was correlated with dose of radiation, and radiation to the frontal or temporal regions was associated with lower rates of marriage and employment. In a subsequent study with this sample, impairments in memory as well as higher frequency of social and general health problems were linked to higher radiation dose to the temporal lobe; radiation to the frontal regions was associated with health problems and physical disabilities (Armstrong et al., 2010). Ellenberg and colleagues (2009) examined the types of cognitive issues seen in adult survivors of CNS malignancies in the CCSS cohort using the Childhood Cancer Survivor Study Neurocognitive Questionnaire (CCSS-NCQ), which is a 15-item version of the Behavior Rating Inventory of Executive Function. Survivors of CNS malignancies were more likely to report cognitive dysfunction, particularly in the domain of information processing and working memory; at least half of the respondents endorsed problems in at least one scale of the CCSS-NCQ. Individuals with neurological dysfunction (sensory/motor problems, stroke, hearing loss) were more likely to report neuropsychological impairment.

Reimers and colleagues (2003) report on long-term outcomes in survivors of childhood brain tumors diagnosed from 1970 to 1997; age at evaluation ranged from 7 to 40 years and mean length of follow-up was 13 years. This cohort included both child and adult survivors who likely experienced marked differences in treatment protocols over this timespan. Findings revealed lower IQ than expected in the group overall, and radiation therapy as well as hydrocephalus, tumor location in the cerebral hemispheres, and young age at diagnosis were associated with worse outcomes. Detailed assessment of memory function also revealed significant impairments in this group (Reimers, Mortensen, & Schmiegelow, 2007).

Long-term follow-up of survivors 10 years after treatment for medulloblastoma showed significant compromise of neuropsychological function and quality of life (Maddrey et al., 2005). Two-thirds of this sample showed significant impairment in cognitive ability, and the majority were unable to drive or live independently.

Cancer treatment success is typically discussed in terms of 5-year survival. Late-effects studies of adult survivors who are well beyond the 5-year mark note the enduring burden of CNS malignancies and their treatment over the lifespan. These findings provide a snapshot relevant to a particular epoch of care and support the notion of childhood brain tumors as a chronic disease with implications well into adult development.

RECENT PSYCHOLOGICAL AND NEUROPSYCHOLOGICAL FINDINGS

More recently, neuropsychological studies have focused on identifying risk profiles, describing specific cognitive domains affected in addition to IQ, elucidating mechanisms associated with types of compromise, and characterizing outcomes in a range of tumor diagnoses. For example, given their high risk of neurocognitive deficits, children treated for medulloblastoma have been the focus of numerous neuropsychological studies. Longitudinal studies document incremental decline in intelligence and academic progress as time from diagnosis increases (Mulhern et al., 2005; Palmer et al., 2001; Ris, Packer, Goldwein, Jones-Wallace, & Boyett, 2001; Spiegler, Bouffet, Greenberg, Rutka, & Mabbott, 2004). Palmer and colleagues (2001) demonstrated that loss of IQ points was related to slower acquisition of knowledge and skills, rather than deterioration in established ability. The case for progressive neurocognitive decline in children treated with craniospinal radiation for medulloblastoma is well documented; loss in IQ ranges from 2 to 4 points per year, with greater decline seen early in follow-up. Steeper declines are seen in children treated at younger ages and with higher doses of radiation (Palmer et al., 2001; Ris et al., 2001; Spiegler et al., 2004).

Advanced multidimensional techniques now allow for models that can predict neurocognitive outcome based on age, brain region, and radiation dosimetry. These studies find that exposure to supratentorial brain regions seems to have the most significant impact on cognitive function (Merchant et al., 2006; Merchant, Kiehna, Li, Xiong, & Mulhern, 2005). In a recent prospective study of stereotactic radiation therapy for residual or progressive low-grade or benign tumors, radiation therapy dose (>43.2 Gy) to the left temporal lobe was associated with a >10% drop in IQ in follow-up neuropsychological evaluation (Jalali et al., 2010), even though mean IQ remained stable for 2–3 years for the whole group studied.

Findings gradually emerged noting that radiation therapy is not the only important risk factor contributing to adverse neuropsychological outcomes in survivors of childhood brain tumors. Studies began to focus on the long-term outcomes of survivors who did not require extensive treatment. In our center, we studied the range of late effects experienced in survivors of low-grade brain tumors who did not receive any tumor-directed therapy after resection (Turner et al., 2009). Although these survivors were cured of their disease, 92% had at least one medical late effect. In addition, although IQ and adaptive function scores were in the average range, a higher than expected percentage of survivors scored below normative expectations. This was also seen on ratings of executive functions. In this group, executive function scores were a better predictor of overall adaptive function and level of independence than intelligence. Studies of other groups of children and adolescents treated for low-grade tumors in the cerebellum and outside the posterior fossa have reported similar results (Beebe & Ris, 2001; Ris et al., 2008), with more individuals than expected scoring below average on tests of intelligence, adaptive function, and academic achievement. Left hemisphere location was associated with an increased risk of compromised neuropsychological functioning. These studies served to highlight other factors contributing to long-term outcome.

Recent work is confirming the independent role of medical complications and tumor location in neuropsychological outcome. The role of the cerebellum in cognitive function has been an increasing focus of study over recent decades. Previously conceptualized as preferentially involved in balance, sensorimotor function, and motor planning/coordination, the cerebellum is now understood to be involved in a range of higher-order cognitive functions (Dum & Strick, 2003; Middleton & Strick, 1998; Riva & Giorgi, 2000). Studies of children treated for posterior fossa tumors document the impact of damage to the cerebellum and hydrocephalus, as well as postsurgical complications in neuropsychological outcomes (Cantelmi, Schweizer, & Cusimano, 2008; Di Rocco et al., 2010; Mabbott, Penkman, Witol, Strother, & Bouffet, 2008; Roncadin, Dennis, Greenberg, & Spiegler, 2008).

Neuropsychological studies are now focusing on specific cognitive processes affected by brain tumors and associated treatments. A triad of cognitive functions in attention, working memory, and processing speed constitute the core deficits seen in this population (Mabbott et al., 2008; Mulhern, Merchant, Gajjar, Reddick, & Kun,

2004; Steinlin et al., 2003). These deficits are noted at baseline before extensive treatment (Iuvone et al., 2011). Sustained attention and speed of processing were significantly impaired in children treated for lower-grade tumors, even though intelligence was normal (Aarsen et al., 2009). Attention deficits seen in survivors of childhood brain tumors are generally of the "inattentive" rather than impulsive/hyperactive type. Attention problems are noted to increase progressively when assessed longitudinally after treatment (Kiehna, Mulhern, Li, Xiong, & Merchant, 2006). In a study of 70 survivors of different types of brain tumors, the sample was divided into two groups defined by presence of attention problems (as seen on tests of auditory attention, working memory, and sequencing/switching; 29 children) or absence of attention problems. Age at diagnosis was significantly correlated with attention problems in this group. Children with attention problems were also rated higher on a scale of social problems.

Deficits in processing speed are common in children treated for brain tumors. In a study of children with localized brain tumors evaluated postsurgery but prior to radiation therapy, 36% scored below average on the Coding subtest, even though overall IQ was within the normal range (Carpentieri et al., 2003). Comparable findings were replicated in children treated with only surgery (Ris et al., 2008; Steinlin et al., 2003). In children treated with multimodality therapy, processing speed scores were lower than expected, and this finding was noted early on in follow-up and remained a significant deficit over time (Sands et al., 2012).

Studies of working memory in children treated for brain tumors are difficult to interpret because of differing definitions and assessment procedures used across studies. In some instances, measures categorized as assessing working memory in one study are the same as those used to assess attention in another. These constructs are very closely related, which contributes to this overlap. Working memory problems were seen in children treated with and without radiation therapy, with declining performance associated with radiation (Stargatt, Rosenfeld, Maixner, & Ashley, 2007). Spiegler and colleagues followed cohorts of children treated with radiation and studied changes in domains of cognitive function over time (Edelstein et al., 2011; Spiegler et al., 2004). In a study of 20 adult survivors of childhood medulloblastoma, all evidenced impairments in working memory, memory, executive function, academic achievement, and fine motor skills (Edelstein et al., 2011). Decline in intellectual ability was shown to stabilize years after treatment, but a progressive decline in working memory was seen over the course of the follow-up period. Functional life outcomes showed poorer educational, occupational, and social functioning as compared with expected outcomes for adults in the community.

Social and psychological functioning. Studies are now focusing on the combined impact of neuropsychological and social deficits on functional outcomes in survivors of childhood brain tumors. Although there are inconsistencies across studies, social functioning appears particularly affected. A recent review of studies in this area notes that both social adjustment, as assessed by rating scales or focus groups, and social competence are compromised relative to healthy controls as well as children with other cancers or chronic illness (Schulte & Barrera, 2010). In creative studies analyzing friendships in children treated for brain tumors, Vannata and colleagues demonstrated that these children were less likely to be included and less integrated with their peer group (Vannatta et al., 2008; Vannatta, Gartstein, Short, & Noll, 1998; Vannatta, Gerhardt, Wells, & Noll, 2007)

Imaging findings. Researchers at St. Jude Children's Research Hospital pioneered studies that linked neuropsychological outcomes with specific brain imaging findings in children treated for brain tumors with radiation therapy. Initial studies noted differences in volume of normal-appearing white matter in children treated with radiation; reductions in white matter were negatively correlated with radiation dose (Mulhern et al., 1999; Reddick et al., 2000). Regional analysis of white matter changes in 35 patients treated with craniospinal radiation showed that volume loss was most apparent in the posterior region of the corpus callosum (Palmer et al., 2002). Further studies clarified the relationship between white matter changes seen posttreatment and neuropsychological deficits, finding that IQ, learning, and attention deficits were associated with reductions in white matter volume (Reddick et al., 2003). The same group of researchers studied changes in hippocampal volume following craniospinal radiation treatment and found a pattern of declining volume in the hippocampus over the first 2–3 years after treatment (Nagel et al., 2004).

Recent studies have used diffusion tensor imaging (DTI) to study differences in the white matter of survivors of childhood brain tumors. Studies of children treated for medulloblastoma found reduced white matter diffusivity in a range of brain regions (temporal, parietal, and occipital periventricular) conforming to a posterior dominant pattern (Leung et al., 2004). Mabbott and colleagues (2006) compared fractional anisotropy (FA), apparent diffusion coefficient (ADC), and IQ measures in eight children treated with craniospinal radiation with a typically developing matched control group. Children treated with craniospinal radiation had evidence of reduced diffusivity in five of the six white matter regions studied, with the largest differences seen in the corpus callosum and internal capsule. In addition, reduced FA and increased ADC were associated with lower IQ, a finding that has been replicated by another group studying the association between cognitive deficits and white matter integrity in survivors of medulloblastoma (Khong et al., 2006). Imaging studies comparing different groups of survivors of posterior fossa tumors identified reductions in FA in patients treated with and without radiation and chemotherapy (Rueckriegel et al., 2010). For the medulloblastoma group, who had multimodality treatment, FA was reduced in the cerebellum, frontal lobes, and corpus callosum. Surprisingly, FA reductions were seen in the pilocytic astrocytoma group in not only the cerebellar hemispheres but also in supratentorial regions. The degree of reduction was not as great as that seen in the medulloblastoma group. The authors concluded that damage to the cerebellum and hydrocephalus also contributes to disruption in neuronal circuitry that leads to alterations in supratentorial white matter. Aukema and colleagues (2009) analyzed DTI findings in 17 survivors of childhood cancer: 6 treated for medulloblastoma and 11 treated for leukemia. The leukemia group was divided into high-dose and low-dose MTX groups. A control group of children was recruited from classmates of the participants. The children underwent MRI and neuropsychological studies of intellectual ability, processing speed, and fine motor skills. The patient group had decreased white matter FA compared with the control group, particularly in the right inferior fronto-occipital fasciculus and in the corpus callosum. Correlations between decreased FA and lower speed of processing were identified. This study had some significant limitations including small sample size, wide age differences, and a control group with somewhat lower IQ scores than expected. However, this study did support the notion that FA could be used as a biomarker of the progression of white matter injury in survivors at high risk for developing neurocognitive dysfunction (Palmer, 2008). As a whole, these imaging findings highlight the complex interrelationships of developmental and injury-related processes in children treated for brain tumors.

INTERVENTION AND TREATMENT GAINS

Interventions and treatments for survivors of childhood brain tumors are seen in a range of domains: educational modifications/accommodations, direct therapeutic services, psychological treatment, rehabilitation programs, and psychopharmacological interventions. Interventions for neuropsychological and learning problems are typically delivered in schools. Neuropsychologists play a critical role in evaluating each child's unique profile and in developing recommendations for treatment across domains of functioning. Recommendations can include educational accommodations or curriculum modifications and specialized therapies (e.g., speech/language, occupational, physical, vision, and mobility). Active communication with schools and teachers, as well as education around neuropsychological consequences of brain tumors and their treatment, are indispensable. Special educational support, transition services, and postsecondary accommodations need to be considered over the course of follow-up (Zelko & Sorensen, 2009). Family, group, and individual psychotherapy can be effective in addressing social–emotional adjustment issues.

Psychopharmacological interventions are important in the management of attention problems and other neurobehavioral symptoms. Stimulant medication has been used with good effect in subgroups of children and adolescents treated for brain tumors. Survivors of childhood cancer may present with attention problems, but their profiles generally do not meet formal criteria for attention-deficit/hyperactivity disorder (Kahalley et al., 2011). Conklin and colleagues are pursuing clinical trials of the efficacy of methylphenidate in treating attention issues in survivors of leukemia and brain tumors and have found that the medication is well tolerated and has some positive impact, with approximately half of the children studied showing a good response (Conklin, Helton, et al., 2010; Conklin et al., 2007). Parent and teacher ratings of attention improved with treatment, and treatment gains were maintained over a year; performance on measures of sustained attention improved as well, although there was no change noted in academic skills relative to untreated survivors (Conklin, Reddick, et al., 2010; Netson et al., 2011). Other pharmacological approaches include treatment of psychological symptoms of anxiety and depression with psychoactive medications. A current multicenter trial of modafanil is in progress to address arousal, attention, and fatigue problems in certain survivors. Researchers are also evaluating the benefit of medications traditionally used to treat cognitive dysfunction in older adults. In an open-label pilot trial of donepezil with children, preliminary findings showed improvements in executive functions on the Delis-Kaplan Executive Function System Tower Test and on the Behavior Rating Inventory of Executive Function (BRIEF) Plan/Organize scale with this medication in a group of survivors (Castellino et al., 2012). However, this study evaluated outcomes based on effect sizes of changes seen on test scores pre- and posttreatment, but did not use reliable change or repeated measures procedures to evaluate the significance of the findings.

There is increasing interest in the role of physical activity and exercise in promoting well-being after cancer treatment. Children treated for brain tumors are often deconditioned and less active during and after treatment. Nutrition issues and stamina problems can compromise overall energy. Re-engaging in an active life often requires support. The benefits of exercise in this population may improve cognitive as well as physical functioning. Naylor and colleagues (2008) reported that in rodent models, exercise (voluntary running) increases neurogenesis in the hippocampus, which is associated with improvements in learning. In irradiated mice provided with opportunities for voluntary running, neurogenesis could be partially restored and with positive effect on memory. Naylor and colleagues proposed that physical exercise might be a beneficial component of rehabilitation programs for childhood cancer survivors.

Cognitive remediation programs have been developed using strategies developed in traumatic brain injury rehabilitation. Programs such as Attention Process Training and Pay Attention! have been used to treat attention problems in survivors of leukemia (Kerns, Mateer, & Vernescu, 2008; Penkman, 2004; Sohlberg & Mateer, 2001). There is growing interest in using computer-based remediation programs that target working memory deficits in survivors of brain tumors and leukemia (Hardy, Willard, & Bonner, 2011; Klingberg et al., 2005). Butler and colleagues developed the Cognitive Remediation Program, which includes three components: massed practice, training in use of metacognitive strategies, and cognitive behavioral therapy (Butler et al., 2008; Nazemi & Butler, 2011). A multicenter trial of the program showed improvements in parental ratings of attention and achievement scores; however, there were no changes seen in measures of specific cognitive domains. The program demands a great deal of resources because it involves regular coaching and frequent training sessions. Future study will be needed to identify the active components of the program that result in improvements, as well as specific patient and family environmental factors that promote optimal gains. Factors that contribute to differences in response to training and rehabilitation are complex in developing children, and we need to know more about mechanisms that underlie success and effective learning (Jolles & Crone, 2012).

CURRENT RESOURCES

A number of organizations and foundations provide information, resources, and advocacy in the area of childhood brain tumors (see Table 3.2). These groups raise public awareness, provide grants, host conferences, raise funds for research, organize support groups, and develop educational materials, among other activities. They also sponsor special events and camps for children, adolescents, and families. Through their external Web pages, childhood cancer centers provide useful information and educational resources related to specific tumors, treatments, enrollment in clinical trials, and available services for patients and families. In addition, many have school re-entry programs or provide educational advocacy services to assist families in accessing needed services and accommodations and to educate the academic community about childhood cancer and learning needs.

The Children's Oncology Group (COG) formed from four cooperative groups studying childhood cancer in the United States (www.childrensoncologygroup.org). It is supported by the National Cancer Institute and sponsors clinical trials as well as studies in a range of areas including translational research, epidemiology, behavioral sciences, and survivorship. It developed follow-up guidelines for surveillance and ongoing healthcare for childhood cancer survivors. These guidelines (available at www.survivorshipguidelines.org) raise awareness of the increased health risks over the lifespan with specific types of cancers and their treatments (Landier, Wallace, & Hudson, 2006). The COG Long-term Follow-up Guidelines Task Force on Neurocognitive and

Table 3.2 Resources for Patients, Survivors, Families, and Caregivers

Organization
National Brain Tumor Society
www.braintumor.org
Brain Tumor Foundation for Children, Inc. www.braintumorkids.org
Childhood Brain Tumor Foundation www.childhoodbraintumor.org
Children's Brain Tumor Foundation
www.cbtf.org
Pediatric Brain Tumor Foundation of the United States www.pbtfus.org
Pediatric Low-Grade Astrocytoma Foundation (PLGA) www.fightplga.org
We Can Brain Tumor Network
www.wecan.cc
CureSearch for Children's Cancer
www.curesearch.org
Candlelighters Childhood Cancer Foundation
www.candlelighters.org
Children's Tumor Foundation (focus on neurofibromatosis)
www.ctf.org
American Cancer Society
www.cancer.org
Lance Armstrong Foundation
www.livestrong.org

Behavioral Complications after Childhood Cancer produced a set of recommendations regarding follow-up care for survivors at increased risk for neurocognitive and behavioral late effects (Nathan et al., 2007). The report also addresses advocacy, access to care, and the need for timely evaluation and intervention.

The Pediatric Oncology Group of Ontario (www.pogo.ca) is a collaborative organization that coordinates a system of care for children with cancer across the province and works with the Ontario Ministry of Health and Long-Term Care. It supports professional healthcare resources as well as education and services for families, including a vocational and educational transition program for adolescents and young adults.

Late-effects programs and clinics are increasingly available for survivors of childhood brain tumors. These programs not only provide needed care and surveillance but also educate survivors regarding their medical and behavioral health needs (Dilley & Lockart, 2009). In addition, efforts to educate primary care providers in the community about long-term management of late effects are expanding. Oeffinger, Nathan, and Kramer (2008) proposed a tiered strategy in a shared care model (cancer center and primary care) that stratifies groups of survivors based on risk of late effects, concentrating resources and increasing surveillance in the groups with the highest level of concern.

FUTURE AIMS AND RESEARCH OPPORTUNITIES

Future research efforts addressing neuropsychological development and outcomes will need to incorporate more complex models and include close collaboration with other specialties working in this area. Molecular biological studies have tended to focus on differentiating genetic profiles of specific tumors; this work will need to expand to incorporate understanding of unique host genetic polymorphisms that may play a role in increased vulnerability to toxicity. For neuropsychology, next steps will entail moving beyond a focus on characterizing the phenotype of neurobehavioral outcomes to incorporating a systems biological approach. Studies will need to continue to focus on understanding the trajectories of specific cognitive processes that are affected by brain tumors and their treatment and to link these studies to changes in imaging and other possible biomarkers of injury.

In the same way that cancer treatments are being individualized based on genetic profiles, future studies will need to delineate risks based on understanding of specific vulnerabilities and resilience factors that influence individual outcomes. Work in the area of outcomes after traumatic brain injury documents the role of environmental and family factors in mediating outcomes after injury. Examination of these variables should be a standard component of studies of survivors of brain tumors and will contribute to developing targeted intervention efforts for high-risk groups.

Intervention studies are in early development in childhood brain tumor research. Although neuropsychologists make detailed recommendations based on an understanding of a child's neuropsychological profile and medical history, we have not studied the nature, efficacy, or delivery of these recommended interventions systematically. Cognitive rehabilitation programs that demonstrate improvements in neuropsychological functioning will need to be examined in order to determine the relative contribution of contextual and treatment factors in outcome.

As more children survive their disease and grow into adulthood, transition of care and assured access to needed services becomes increasingly important. Models for transition of care need to be developed and their efficacy evaluated with respect to impact on health and facilitation of optimal outcomes (Henderson, Friedman, & Meadows, 2010). Survivors of childhood brain tumors face unique challenges that need to be addressed in the transition period. Neuropsychological deficits affecting attention, executive functions, and memory can compromise management of complex healthcare needs; neuropsychologists can work with their medical and psychosocial colleagues to help address these issues. Social difficulties can affect level of independence, psychological well-being, and understanding of social/community expectations. Preparation for transition needs to be an intentional and individualized process that begins in early adolescence and takes into account barriers to care and psychological factors that affect utilization of healthcare services (Granek et al., 2012).

The need for neuropsychological follow-up of survivors of childhood brain tumors is clearly established. Comprehensive multidisciplinary management is needed to address the range of late effects and ensure timely interventions. Neuropsychologists can collaborate with the team to develop a risk-based management plan to address neurocognitive, academic/vocational, and psychosocial issues (Palmer & Leigh, 2009). Each cohort of survivors carries a unique risk profile and trajectory. Current treatments increasingly involve multidimensional therapies and combinations of conventional and novel targeted chemotherapy agents. Patients will require close longitudinal follow-up to ensure an understanding of the long-term impact of these new therapies.

REFERENCES

Aarsen, F. K., Paquier, P. F., Arts, W. F., Van Veelen, M. L., Michiels, E., Lequin, M., & Catsman-Berrevoets, C. E. (2009). Cognitive deficits and predictors 3 years after diagnosis of a pilocytic astrocytoma in childhood. *Journal of Clinical Oncology, 27*, 3526–3532. doi: 10.1200/jco.2008.19.6303

Abdullah, S., Qaddoumi, I., & Bouffet, E. (2008). Advances in the management of pediatric central nervous system tumors. *Annals of the New York Academy of Sciences, 1138*, 22–31. doi: 10.1196/annals.1414.005

Ahles, T. A., & Saykin, A. J. (2007). Candidate mechanisms for chemotherapy-induced cognitive changes. *Nature Reviews Cancer, 7*, 192–201.

Ali-Osman, F., Friedman, H. S., Antoun, G. R., Reardon, D., Bigner, D. D., & Buolamwini, J. K. (2005). Rational design and development of targeted brain tumor therapeutics. In F. Ail-Osman (Ed.), *Contemporary cancer research: Brain tumors* (pp. 359–381). Totowa, N.J.: Humana Press.

Armstrong, C. L., Gyato, K., Awadalla, A. W., Lustig, R., & Tochner, Z. A. (2004). A critical review of the clinical effects of therapeutic irradiation damage to the brain: The roots of controversy. *Neuropsychology Review, 14*, 65–86.

Armstrong, G. T., Jain, N., Liu, W., Merchant, T. E., Stovall, M., Srivastava, D. K.,... Krull, K. R. (2010). Region-specific radiotherapy and neuropsychological outcomes in adult survivors of childhood CNS malignancies. *Neuro-Oncology, 12*, 1173–1186. doi: 10.1093/neuonc/noq104

Armstrong, G. T., Liu, Q., Yasui, Y., Huang, S., Ness, K. K., Leisenring, W.,... Packer, R. J. (2009). Long-term outcomes among adult survivors of childhood central nervous system malignancies in the childhood cancer survivor study. *Journal of the National Cancer Institute, 101*, 946–958. doi: djp148 [pii] 10.1093/jnci/djp148

Aukema, E. J., Caan, M. W. A., Oudhuis, N., Majoie, C. B. L. M., Vos, F. M., Reneman, L.,... Schouten-van Meeteren, A. Y. N. (2009). White matter fractional anisotropy correlates with speed of processing and motor speed in young childhood cancer survivors. *International Journal of Radiation Oncology, Biology, Physics, 74*, 837–843. doi: 10.1016/j.ijrobp.2008.08.060

Baldwin, R. T., & Preston-Martin, S. (2004). Epidemiology of brain tumors in childhood—a review. *Toxicology and Applied Pharmacology, 199*, 118–131.

Barnett, G. C., West, C. M. L., Dunning, A. M., Elliott, R. M., Coles, C. E., Pharoah, P. D. P., & Burnet, N. G. (2009). Normal tissue reactions to radiotherapy: Towards tailoring treatment dose by genotype. *Nature Reviews Cancer, 9*, 134–142. doi: 10.1038/nrc2587

Beebe, D., & Ris, M. D. (2001). Contributors to neuropsychological outcome in low grade astrocytoma. *Journal of the International Neuropsychological Society, 7*, 214.

Bishop, A. J., McDonald, M. W., Chang, A. L., & Esiashvili, N. (2010). Infant brain tumors: Incidence, survival, and the role of radiation based on surveillance, epidemiology, and end results (seer) data. *International Journal of Radiation Oncology, Biology, Physics, 82*, 341–347. doi: S0360-3016(10)03066-X [pii]10.1016/j.ijrobp.2010.08.020

Blaney, S. M., Kun, L. E., Hunter, J., Rorke-Adams, L. B., Lau, C., Strother, D., & Pollack, I. F. (2006). Tumors of the central nervous system. In P. A. Pizzo & D. G. Poplack (Eds.), *Principles and practice of pediatric oncology* (5th ed., pp. 787–863). Philadelphia: Lippincott Williams & Wilkins.

Boman, K. K., Lindblad, F., & Hjern, A. (2010). Long-term outcomes of childhood cancer survivors in Sweden: A population-based study of education, employment, and income. *Cancer, 116*, 1385–1391. doi: 10.1002/cncr.24840

Bouffet, E., Tabori, U., Huang, A., & Bartels, U. (2010). Possibilities of new therapeutic strategies in brain tumors. *Cancer Treatment Reviews, 36,* 335–341. doi: S0305-7372(10)00029-0 [pii] 10.1016 /j.ctrv.2010.02.009 [doi]

Bowers, D. C., Liu, Y., Leisenring, W., McNeil, E., Stovall, M., Gurney, J. G.,... Oeffinger, K. C. (2006). Late-occurring stroke among long-term survivors of childhood leukemia and brain tumors: A report from the childhood cancer survivor study. *Journal of Clinical Oncology, 24,* 5277–5282. doi: 10.1200/JCO.2006.07.2884

Butler, R. W., Copeland, D. R., Fairclough, D. L., Mulhern, R. K., Katz, E. R., Kazak, A. E.,... Sahler, O. J. Z. (2008). A multicenter, randomized clinical trial of a cognitive remediation program for childhood survivors of a pediatric malignancy. *Journal of Consulting and Clinical Psychology, 76,* 367–378.

Cantelmi, D., Schweizer, T. A., & Cusimano, M. D. (2008). Role of the cerebellum in the neurocognitive sequelae of treatment of tumours of the posterior fossa: An update. *Lancet Oncology, 9,* 569–576.

Carpentieri, S. C., Waber, D. P., Pomeroy, S. L., Scott, R. M., Goumnerova, L. C., Kieran, M. W.,... Tarbell, N. J. (2003). Neuropsychological functioning after surgery in children treated for brain tumor. *Neurosurgery, 52,* 1348–1356; discussion 1356–1347.

Castellino, S. M., Tooze, J. A., Flowers, L., Hill, D. F., McMullen, K. P., Shaw, E. G., & Parsons, S. K. (2012). Toxicity and efficacy of the acetylcholinesterase (ache) inhibitor donepezil in childhood brain tumor survivors: A pilot study. *Pediatric Blood & Cancer, 59,* 540–547. doi: 10.1002/pbc.24078

CBTRUS. (2008). Statistical report: Primary brain tumors in the United States, 2000–2004: Central Brain Tumor Registry of the United States. Retrieved from www.cbtrus.org

CBTRUS. (2012). CBTRUS statistical report: Primary brain and central nervous system tumors diagnosed in the united states in 2004–2008 (March 23, 2012 revision). Central Brain Tumor Registry of the United States. Retrieved from www.cbtrus.org

Centers for Disease Control and Prevention. (2007). Trends in childhood cancer mortality—United States, 1990–2004. *Morbidity and Mortality Weekly Report (MMWR), 56,* 1257–1261.

Central Brain Tumor Registry of the United States. Fact sheet Retrieved March 20, 2012, from http://www.cbtrus.org/factsheet/factsheet.html

Children's Oncology Group. A study evaluating limited target volume boost irradiation and reduced dose craniospinal radiotherapy (18.00 Gy) and chemotherapy in children with newly diagnosed standard risk medulloblastoma: A phase III double randomized trial.

Cohen, K. J., Broniscer, A., & Glod, J. (2001). Pediatric glial tumors. *Current Treatment Options in Oncology, 2,* 529–536.

Conklin, H. M., Helton, S., Ashford, J., Mulhern, R. K., Reddick, W. E., Brown, R.,... Khan, R. B. (2010). Predicting methylphenidate response in long-term survivors of childhood cancer: A randomized, double-blind, placebo-controlled, crossover trial. *Journal of Pediatric Psychology, 35,* 144–155. doi: jsp044 [pii]10.1093/jpepsy/jsp044 [doi]

Conklin, H. M., Khan, R. B., Reddick, W. E., Helton, S., Brown, R. T., Howard, S. C.,... Mulhern, R. K. (2007). Acute neurocognitive response to methylphenidate among survivors of childhood cancer: A randomized, double-blind, cross-over trial. *Journal of Pediatric Psychology, 32,* 1127–1139.

Conklin, H. M., Reddick, W. E., Ashford, J., Ogg, S., Howard, S. C., Morris, E. B.,... Khan, R. B. (2010). Long-term efficacy of methylphenidate in enhancing attention regulation, social skills, and academic abilities of childhood cancer survivors. *Journal of Clinical Oncology, 28,* 4465–4472. doi: JCO.2010.28.4026 [pii]10.1200/JCO.2010.28.4026 [doi]

Dhall, G., Grodman, H., Ji, L., Sands, S., Gardner, S., Dunkel, I. J.,... Finlay, J. L. (2008). Outcome of children less than three years old at diagnosis with non-metastatic medulloblastoma treated with chemotherapy on the "Head Start" I and II protocols. *Pediatric Blood & Cancer, 50*, 1169–1175. doi: 10.1002/pbc.21525

Di Rocco, C., Chieffo, D., Pettorini, B. L., Massimi, L., Caldarelli, M., & Tamburrini, G. (2010). Preoperative and postoperative neurological, neuropsychological and behavioral impairment in children with posterior cranial fossa astrocytomas and medulloblastomas: The role of the tumor and the impact of the surgical treatment. *Child's Nervous System, 26*, 1173–1188. doi: 10.1007/s00381-010-1166-2 [doi]

Dickerman, J. D. (2007). The late effects of childhood cancer therapy. *Pediatrics, 119*, 554–568. doi: 119/3/554 [pii] 10.1542/peds.2006-2826

Dietrich, J., Han, R., Yang, Y., Mayer-Proschel, M., & Noble, M. (2006). CNS progenitor cells and oligodendrocytes are targets of chemotherapeutic agents in vitro and in vivo. *Journal of Biology, 5*, 22.

Dilley, K., & Lockart, B. (2009). The pediatric brain tumor late effects clinic. In S. Goldman & C. D. Turner (Eds.), *Late effects of treatment for brain tumors* (pp. 97–109). New York: Springer.

Dubuc, A. M., Northcott, P. A., Mack, S., Witt, H., Pfister, S., & Taylor, M. D. (2010). The genetics of pediatric brain tumors. *Current Neurology and Neuroscience Reports, 10*, 215–223. doi: 10.1007/s11910-010-0103-9 [doi]

Duffner, P. K., Cohen, M. E., & Thomas, P. (1983). Late effects of treatment on the intelligence of children with posterior fossa tumors. *Cancer, 51*, 233–237.

Dum, R. P., & Strick, P. L. (2003). An unfolded map of the cerebellar dentate nucleus and its projections to the cerebral cortex. *Journal of Neurophysiology, 89*, 634–639.

Edelstein, K., Spiegler, B. J., Fung, S., Panzarella, T., Mabbott, D. J., Jewitt, N.,…Hodgson, D. C. (2011). Early aging in adult survivors of childhood medulloblastoma: Long-term neurocognitive, functional, and physical outcomes. *Neuro-Oncology, 13*, 536–545. doi: 10.1093/neuonc/nor015

Ellenberg, L., Liu, Q., Gioia, G., Yasui, Y., Packer, R. J., Mertens, A.,…Zeltzer, L. K. (2009). Neurocognitive status in long-term survivors of childhood CNS malignancies: A report from the Childhood Cancer Survivor Study. *Neuropsychology, 23*, 705–717. doi: 10.1037/a0016674

Finlay, J. L., Erdreich-Epstein, A., & Packer, R. J. (2007). Progress in the treatment of childhood brain tumors: No room for complacency. *Pediatric Hematology and Oncology, 24*, 79–84. doi: 10.1080/08880010601001073

Fossati, P., Ricardi, U., & Orecchia, R. (2009). Pediatric medulloblastoma: Toxicity of current treatment and potential role of protontherapy. *Cancer Treatment Reviews, 35*, 79–96.

Fouladi, M., Gilger, E., Kocak, M., Wallace, D., Buchanan, G., Reeves, C.,…Mulhern, R. (2005). Intellectual and functional outcome of children 3 years old or younger who have CNS malignancies. *Journal of Clinical Oncology, 23*, 7152–7160.

Fruhwald, M. C., & Rutkowski, S. (2011). Tumors of the central nervous system in children and adolescents. *Deutsches Arzteblatt International, 108*, 390–397. doi: 10.3238/arztebl.2011.0390

Georg Kuhn, H., & Blomgren, K. (2011). Developmental dysregulation of adult neurogenesis. *The European Journal of Neuroscience, 33*, 1115–1122. doi: 10.1111/j.1460-9568.2011.07610.x

Gibson, P., Tong, Y., Robinson, G., Thompson, M. C., Currle, D. S., Eden, C.,…Gilbertson, R. J. (2010). Subtypes of medulloblastoma have distinct developmental origins. *Nature, 468*, 1095–1099. doi: 10.1038/nature09587

Granek, L., Nathan, P., Rosenberg-Yunger, Z., D'Agostino, N., Amin, L., Barr, R.,…Klassen, A. (2012). Psychological factors impacting transition from paediatric to adult care by childhood cancer survivors. *Journal of Cancer Survivorship, 6*, 260–269. doi: 10.1007/s11764-012-0223-0

Grondin, R. T., Scott, R. M., & Smith, E. R. (2009). Pediatric brain tumors. *Advances in Pediatrics, 56,* 249–269. doi: 10.1016/j.yapd.2009.08.006

Gudrunardottir, T., Sehested, A., Juhler, M., & Schmiegelow, K. (2011). Cerebellar mutism: Review of the literature. *Child's Nervous System, 27,* 355–363. doi: 10.1007/s00381-010-1328-2

Gururangan, S. (2009). Late effects of chemotherapy. In S. Goldman & C. D. Turner (Eds.), *Late effects of treatment for brain tumors* (pp. 43–65). New York: Springer.

Hardy, K. K., Willard, V. W., & Bonner, M. J. (2011). Computerized cognitive training in survivors of childhood cancer: A pilot study. *Journal of Pediatric Oncology Nursing, 28,* 27–33. doi: 10.1177/1043454210377178

Henderson, T. O., Friedman, D. L., & Meadows, A. T. (2010). Childhood cancer survivors: Transition to adult-focused risk-based care. *Pediatrics, 126,* 129–136. doi: 10.1542/peds.2009-2802

Hoppe-Hirsch, E., Brunet, L., Laroussinie, F., Cinalli, G., Pierre-Kahn, A., Renier, D.,... Hirsch, J. F. (1995). Intellectual outcome in children with malignant tumors of the posterior fossa: Influence of the field of irradiation and quality of surgery. *Child's Nervous System, 11,* 340–345; discussion 345–346.

Houdemont, S. P., De Carli, E., Delion, M., Ringuier, B., Chapotte, C., Jeudy, C.,... Rialland, X. (2011). Short-term neurological outcome of children after surgery for brain tumors: Incidence and characteristics in a pediatric intensive care unit. *Child's Nervous System, 27,* 933–941. doi: 10.1007/s00381-010-1373-x

Huse, J. T., & Holland, E. C. (2010). Targeting brain cancer: Advances in the molecular pathology of malignant glioma and medulloblastoma. [10.1038/nrc2818]. *Nature Reviews Cancer, 10,* 319–331.

Iuvone, L., Peruzzi, L., Colosimo, C., Tamburrini, G., Caldarelli, M., Di Rocco, C.,... Riccardi, R. (2011). Pretreatment neuropsychological deficits in children with brain tumors. *Neuro-Oncology, 13,* 517–524. doi: 10.1093/neuonc/nor013

Jalali, R., Mallick, I., Dutta, D., Goswami, S., Gupta, T., Munshi, A.,... Sarin, R. (2010). Factors influencing neurocognitive outcomes in young patients with benign and low-grade brain tumors treated with stereotactic conformal radiotherapy. *International Journal of Radiation Oncology, Biology, Physics, 77,* 974–979. doi: 10.1016/j.ijrobp.2009.06.025

Jolles, D. D., & Crone, E. A. (2012). Training the developing brain: A neurocognitive perspective. *Frontiers in Human Neuroscience, 6,* 76. doi: 10.3389/fnhum.2012.00076

Kahalley, L. S., Conklin, H. M., Tyc, V. L., Wilson, S. J., Hinds, P. S., Wu, S.,... Hudson, M. M. (2011). Adhd and secondary adhd criteria fail to identify many at-risk survivors of pediatric all and brain tumor. *Pediatric Blood & Cancer, 57,* 110–118. doi: 10.1002/pbc.22998

Kerns, K. A., Mateer, C. A., & Vernescu, R. (2008). Evidence based strategies for cognitive remediation in children. *Journal of the International Neuropsychological Society, 14*(Supplement S2). doi: doi:10.1017/S1355617708081071

Khong, P.-L., Leung, L. H. T., Fung, A. S. M., Fong, D. Y. T., Qiu, D., Kwong, D. L. W.,... Chan, G. C. F. (2006). White matter anisotropy in post-treatment childhood cancer survivors: Preliminary evidence of association with neurocognitive function. *Journal of Clinical Oncology, 24,* 884–890. doi: 10.1200/jco.2005.02.4505

Kiehna, E. N., Mulhern, R. K., Li, C., Xiong, X., & Merchant, T. E. (2006). Changes in attentional performance of children and young adults with localized primary brain tumors after conformal radiation therapy. *JournaloOf Clinical Oncology, 24,* 5283–5290.

Kieran, M. W. (2005). Anti-angiogenic therapy in pediatric neuro-oncology. *Journal of Neuro-Oncology, 75,* 327–334.

Klingberg, T., Fernell, E., Olesen, P. J., Johnson, M., Gustafsson, P., Dahlstrom, K.,...Westerberg, H. (2005). Computerized training of working memory in children with adhd—a randomized, controlled trial. *Journal of the American Academy of Child and Adolescent Psychiatry, 44*, 177–186.

Koch, S. V., Kejs, A. M. T., Engholm, G., Møller, H., Johansen, C., & Schmiegelow, K. (2006). Leaving home after cancer in childhood: A measure of social independence in early adulthood. *Pediatric Blood & Cancer, 47*, 61–70. doi: 10.1002/pbc.20827

Krull, K. (2010). Leukemia and lymphoma across the lifespan. In J. Donders & S. J. Hunter (Eds.), *Principles and practice of lifespan developmental neuropsychology* (pp. 379–391). Cambridge, UK: Cambridge University Press.

Kuehni, C. E., Strippoli, M.-P. F., Rueegg, C. S., Rebholz, C. E., Bergstraesser, E., Grotzer, M.,...for the Swiss Pediatric Oncology, G. (2012). Educational achievement in Swiss childhood cancer survivors compared with the general population. *Cancer, 118*, 1439–1449. doi: 10.1002/cncr.26418

Landier, W., Wallace, W. H., & Hudson, M. M. (2006). Long-term follow-up of pediatric cancer survivors: Education, surveillance, and screening. *Pediatric Blood & Cancer, 46*, 149–158. doi: 10.1002/pbc.20612

Leung, L. H., Ooi, G. C., Kwong, D. L., Chan, G. C., Cao, G., & Khong, P. L. (2004). White-matter diffusion anisotropy after chemo-irradiation: A statistical parametric mapping study and histogram analysis. *Neuroimage, 21*, 261–268.

Levine, D., Cohen, K., & Wendler, D. (2012). Shared medical decision-making: Considering what options to present based on an ethical analysis of the treatment of brain tumors in very young children. *Pediatric Blood & Cancer*. doi: 10.1002/pbc.24189

Mabbott, D. J., Noseworthy, M. D., Bouffet, E., Rockel, C., & Laughlin, S. (2006). Diffusion tensor imaging of white matter after cranial radiation in children for medulloblastoma: Correlation with IQ. *Neuro-Oncology, 8*, 244–252.

Mabbott, D. J., Penkman, L., Witol, A., Strother, D., & Bouffet, E. (2008). Core neurocognitive functions in children treated for posterior fossa tumors. *Neuropsychology, 22*, 159–168.

MacDonald, S. M., Safai, S., Trofimov, A., Wolfgang, J., Fullerton, B., Yeap, B. Y.,...Yock, T. (2008). Proton radiotherapy for childhood ependymoma: Initial clinical outcomes and dose comparisons. *International Journal of Radiation Oncology, Biology, Physics, 71*, 979–986. doi: S0360-3016(07)04758-X [pii]10.1016/j.ijrobp.2007.11.065

Maddrey, A. M., Bergeron, J. A., Lombardo, E. R., McDonald, N. K., Mulne, A. F., Barenberg, P. D., & Bowers, D. C. (2005). Neuropsychological performance and quality of life of 10 year survivors of childhood medulloblastoma. *Journal of Neuro-Oncology, 72*, 245–253.

Marachelian, A., Butturini, A., & Finlay, J. (2008). Myeloablative chemotherapy with autologous hematopoietic progenitor cell rescue for childhood central nervous system tumors. *Bone Marrow Transplantation, 41*, 167–172.

Merchant, T. E., Kiehna, E. N., Li, C., Shukla, H., Sengupta, S., Xiong, X.,...Mulhern, R. K. (2006). Modeling radiation dosimetry to predict cognitive outcomes in pediatric patients with cns embryonal tumors including medulloblastoma. *International Journal of Radiation Oncology, Biology, Physics, 65*, 210–221.

Merchant, T. E., Kiehna, E. N., Li, C., Xiong, X., & Mulhern, R. K. (2005). Radiation dosimetry predicts iq after conformal radiation therapy in pediatric patients with localized ependymoma. *International Journal of Radiation Oncology, Biology, Physics, 63*, 1546–1554.

Middleton, F. A., & Strick, P. L. (1998). The cerebellum: An overview. *Trends in Neurosciences, 21*, 367–369.

Mitby, P. A., Robison, L. L., Whitton, J. A., Zevon, M. A., Gibbs, I. C., Tersak, J. M.,...Mertens, A. C. (2003). Utilization of special education services and educational attainment among long-term survivors of childhood cancer: A report from the childhood cancer survivor study. *Cancer, 97,* 1115–1126.

Monje, M. L. (2008). Cranial radiation therapy and damage to hippocampal neurogenesis. *Developmental Disabilities Research Reviews, 14,* 238–242. doi: 10.1002/ddrr.26

Monje, M. L., Mizumatsu, S., Fike, J. R., & Palmer, T. D. (2002). Irradiation induces neural precursor-cell dysfunction. *Nature Medicine, 8,* 955–962.

Mrakotsky, C., & Waber, D. (2006). Chemotherapy agents for treatment of acute lympho-blastic leukemia. In D. Bellinger (Ed.), *Human developmental neurotoxicology* (pp. 131–147). New York: Taylor and Francis.

Mulhern, R. K., Merchant, T., Gajjar, A., Reddick, W. E., & Kun, L. E. (2004). Late neu-rocognitive sequelae in survivors of brain tumours in childhood. *The Lancet Oncology, 5,* 399–408.

Mulhern, R. K., Palmer, S. L., Merchant, T. E., Wallace, D., Kocak, M., Brouwers, P., . . . Gajjar, A. (2005). Neurocognitive consequences of risk-adapted therapy for childhood medullo-blastoma. *Journal of Clinical Oncology, 23,* 5511–5519.

Mulhern, R. K., Reddick, W., Palmer, S. L., Glass, J. O., Elkin, T. D., Kun, L. E., . . . Gajjar, A. (1999). Neurocognitive deficits in medulloblastoma survivors and white matter loss. *Annals of Neurology, 46,* 834–841.

Nagel, B. J., Palmer, S. L., Reddick, W. E., Glass, J. O., Helton, K. J., Wu, S., . . . Mulhern, R. K. (2004). Abnormal hippocampal development in children with medulloblastoma treated with risk-adapted irradiation. *AJNR. American Journal of Neuroradiology, 25,* 1575–1582. doi: 25/9/1575 [pii]

Nageswara Rao, A. A., Scafidi, J., Wells, E. M., & Packer, R. J. (2012). Biologically targeted therapeutics in pediatric brain tumors. *Pediatric Neurology, 46,* 203–211. doi: 10.1016/j.pediatrneurol.2012.02.005

Nathan, P. C., Patel, S. K., Dilley, K., Goldsby, R., Harvey, J., Jacobsen, C., . . . Armstrong, F. D. (2007). Guidelines for identification of, advocacy for, and intervention in neu-rocognitive problems in survivors of childhood cancer: A report from the Children's Oncology Group. *Archives of Pediatrics and Adolescent Medicine, 161,* 798–806.

Naylor, A. S., Bull, C., Nilsson, M. K., Zhu, C., Bjork-Eriksson, T., Eriksson, P. S., . . . Kuhn, H. G. (2008). Voluntary running rescues adult hippocampal neurogenesis after irradia-tion of the young mouse brain. Proceedings of the National Academy of Sciences of the United States of America, *105,* 14632–14637. doi: 10.1073/pnas.0711128105

Nazemi, K. J., & Butler, R. W. (2011). Neuropsychological rehabilitation for survivors of childhood and adolescent brain tumors: A view of the past and a vision for a promising future. *Journal of Pediatric Rehabilitation Medicine, 4,* 37–46. doi: 10.3233/prm-2011-0151

Netson, K. L., Conklin, H. M., Ashford, J. M., Kahalley, L. S., Wu, S., & Xiong, X. (2011). Parent and teacher ratings of attention during a year-long methylphenidate trial in children treated for cancer. *Journal of Pediatric Psychology, 36,* 438–450. doi: 10.1093/jpepsy/jsq102

Newhauser, W. D., & Durante, M. (2011). Assessing the risk of second malignancies after modern radiotherapy. *Nature Reviews Cancer, 11,* 438–448.

Oeffinger, K. C., Nathan, P. C., & Kremer, L. C. (2008). Challenges after curative treatment for childhood cancer and long-term follow up of survivors. *Pediatric Clinics of North America, 55,* 251–273.

Packer, R. J. (2010). Radiation therapy for pediatric low-grade gliomas: Survival and seque-lae. *Current Neurology and Neuroscience Reports, 10,* 10–13. doi: 10.1007/s11910-009-0084-8

Packer, R. J., Goldwein, J., Nicholson, H. S., Vezina, L. G., Allen, J. C., Ris, M. D., . . . Boyett, J. M. (1999). Treatment of children with medulloblastomas with reduced-dose craniospinal radiation therapy and adjuvant chemotherapy: A Children's Cancer Group study. *Journal of Clinical Oncology, 17*, 2127–2136.

Packer, R. J., Gurney, J. G., Punyko, J. A., Donaldson, S. S., Inskip, P. D., Stovall, M., . . . Robison, L. L. (2003). Long-term neurologic and neurosensory sequelae in adult survivors of a childhood brain tumor: Childhood Cancer Survivor Study. *Journal of Clinical Oncology, 21*, 3255–3261.

Packer, R. J., MacDonald, T., & Vezina, G. (2008). Central nervous system tumors. *Pediatric Clinics of North America, 55*, 121–145, xi. doi: S0031-3955(07)00153-8 [pii] 10.1016/j. pcl.2007.10.010

Packer, R. J., Sutton, L. N., Atkins, T. E., Radcliffe, J., Bunin, G. R., D'Angio, G., . . . Schut, L. (1989). A prospective study of cognitive function in children receiving whole-brain radiotherapy and chemotherapy: 2-year results. *Journal of Neurosurgery, 70*, 707–713. doi: 10.3171/jns.1989.70.5.0707

Palmer, S. L. (2008). Neurodevelopmental impact on children treated for medulloblastoma: A review and proposed conceptual model. *Developmental Disabilities Research Reviews, 14*, 203–210.

Palmer, S. L., Goloubeva, O., Reddick, W. E., Glass, J. O., Gajjar, A., Kun, L., . . . Mulhern, R. K. (2001). Patterns of intellectual development among survivors of pediatric medulloblastoma: A longitudinal analysis. *Journal of Clinical Oncology, 19*, 2302–2308.

Palmer, S. L., Hassall, T., Evankovich, K., Mabbott, D. J., Bonner, M., Deluca, C., . . . Gajjar, A. (2010). Neurocognitive outcome 12 months following cerebellar mutism syndrome in pediatric patients with medulloblastoma. *Neuro-Oncology, 12*, 1311–1317. doi: 10.1093/ neuonc/noq094

Palmer, S. L., & Leigh, L. (2009). Survivors of pediatric posterior fossa tumors: Cognitive outcome, intervention, and risk-based care. *European Journal of Oncology Nursing, 13*, 171–178. doi: 10.1016/j.ejon.2008.09.002

Palmer, S. L., Reddick, W. E., Glass, J. O., Gajjar, A., Goloubeva, O., & Mulhern, R. K. (2002). Decline in corpus callosum volume among pediatric patients with medulloblastoma: Longitudinal mr imaging study. *AJNR American Journal Neuroradiology, 23*, 1088–1094.

Partap, S., & Fisher, P. G. (2007). Update on new treatments and developments in childhood brain tumors. *Current Opinion in Pediatrics, 19*, 670–674.

Paulino, A. C., Constine, L. S., Rubin, P., & Williams, J. P. (2010). Normal tissue development, homeostasis, senescence, and the sensitivity to radiation injury across the age spectrum. *Seminars in Radiation Oncology, 20*, 12–20. doi: 10.1016/j.semradonc.2009.08.003

Penkman, L. (2004). Remediation of attention deficits in children: A focus on childhood cancer, traumatic brain injury and attention deficit disorder. *Pediatric Rehabilitation, 7*, 111–123.

Pollack, I. F. (2001). Neurobehavioral abnormalities after posterior fossa surgery in children. *International Review of Psychiatry, 13*, 302–312.

Pollack, I. F., & Jakacki, R. I. (2011). Childhood brain tumors: Epidemiology, current management and future directions. *Nature Reviews Neurology, 7*, 495–506. doi: 10.1038/ nrneurol.2011.110

Pomeroy, S. L., Tamayo, P., Gaasenbeek, M., Sturla, L. M., Angelo, M., McLaughlin, M. E., . . . Golub, T. R. (2002). Prediction of central nervous system embryonal tumour outcome based on gene expression. *Nature, 415*, 436–442.

Preston-Martin, S. (1996). Epidemiology of primary CNS neoplasms. *Neurologic Clinics, 14*, 273–290.

Reddick, W. E., Glass, J. O., Palmer, S. L., Wu, S., Gajjar, A., Langston, J. W., . . . Mulhern, R. K. (2005). Atypical white matter volume development in children following craniospinal irradiation. *Neuro-Oncology, 7*, 12–19.

Reddick, W. E., Russell, J. M., Glass, J. O., Xiong, X., Mulhern, R. K., Langston, J. W.,...Gajjar, A. (2000). Subtle white matter volume differences in children treated for medulloblastoma with conventional or reduced dose craniospinal irradiation. *Magnetic Resonance Imaging, 18,* 787–793.

Reddick, W. E., White, H. A., Glass, J. O., Wheeler, G. C., Thompson, S. J., Gajjar, A.,...Mulhern, R. K. (2003). Developmental model relating white matter volume to neurocognitive deficits in pediatric brain tumor survivors. *Cancer, 97,* 2512–2519.

Reimers, T. S., Ehrenfels, S., Mortensen, E. L., Schmiegelow, M., Sonderkaer, S., Carstensen, H.,...Muller, J. (2003). Cognitive deficits in long-term survivors of childhood brain tumors: Identification of predictive factors. *Medical and Pediatric Oncology, 40,* 26–34.

Reimers, T. S., Mortensen, E. L., & Schmiegelow, K. (2007). Memory deficits in long-term survivors of childhood brain tumors may primarily reflect general cognitive dysfunctions. *Pediatric Blood & Cancer, 48,* 205–212.

Rekate, H., Brugg, R., Aram, D., Hahn, J., & Ratcheson, R. (1985). Muteness of cerebellar origin. *Archives of Neurology, 42,* 697–698.

Rickert, C. H., Probst-Cousin, S., & Gullotta, F. (1997). Primary intracranial neoplasms of infancy and early childhood. *Child's Nervous System, 13,* 507–513.

Ries, L., Melbert, D., Krapcho, M., Stinchcomb, D., Howlader, N., Horner, M.,...Edwards, B. e. (2008). SEER cancer statistics review, 1975–2005, from http://seer.cancer.gov/csr/1975_2005/based on November 2007 SEER data submission, posted to the SEER web site, 2008.

Ris, M. D., Beebe, D. W., Armstrong, F. D., Fontanesi, J., Holmes, E., Sanford, R. A., & Wisoff, J. H. (2008). Cognitive and adaptive outcome in extracerebellar low-grade brain tumors in children: A report from the Children's Oncology Group. *Journal of Clinical Oncology, 26,* 4765–4770. doi: JCO.2008.17.1371 [pii]10.1200/JCO.2008.17.1371

Ris, M. D., & Noll, R. (1994). Long-term neurobehavioral outcome in pediatric brain-tumor patients: Review and methodological critique. *Journal of Clinical and Experimental Neuropsychology, 16,* 21–42.

Ris, M. D., Packer, R. J., Goldwein, J., Jones-Wallace, D., & Boyett, J. M. (2001). Intellectual outcome after reduced-dose radiation therapy plus adjuvant chemotherapy for medulloblastoma: A Children's Cancer Group study. *Journal of Clinical Oncology, 19,* 3470–3476.

Riva, D., & Giorgi, C. (2000). The cerebellum contributes to higher functions during development: Evidence from a series of children surgically treated for posterior fossa tumours. *Brain, 123,* 1051–1061.

Robertson, P. L., Muraszko, K. M., Holmes, E. J., Sposto, R., Packer, R. J., Gajjar, A.,...Allen, J. C. (2006). Incidence and severity of postoperative cerebellar mutism syndrome in children with medulloblastoma: A prospective study by the Children's Oncology Group. *Journal of Neurosurgery, 105,* 444–451.

Robison, L. L., Armstrong, G. T., Boice, J. D., Chow, E. J., Davies, S. M., Donaldson, S. S.,...Zeltzer, L. K. (2009). The childhood cancer survivor study: A National Cancer Institute-supported resource for outcome and intervention research. *Journal of Clinical Oncology, 27,* 2308–2318. doi: 10.1200/JCO.2009.22.3339

Robison, L. L., Green, D. M., Hudson, M., Meadows, A. T., Mertens, A. C., Packer, R. J.,...Zeltzer, L. K. (2005). Long-term outcomes of adult survivors of childhood cancer. *Cancer, 104,* 2557–2564.

Roncadin, C., Dennis, M., Greenberg, M. L., & Spiegler, B. J. (2008). Adverse medical events associated with childhood cerebellar astrocytomas and medulloblastomas: Natural history and relation to very long-term neurobehavioral outcome. *Child's Nervous System, 24,* 995–1002.

Rueckriegel, S. M., Driever, P. H., Blankenburg, F., Lüdemann, L., Henze, G., & Bruhn, H. (2010). Differences in supratentorial damage of white matter in pediatric survivors of posterior fossa tumors with and without adjuvant treatment as detected by magnetic resonance diffusion tensor imaging. *International Journal of Radiation Oncology, Biology, Physics, 76,* 859–866. doi: 10.1016/j.ijrobp.2009.02.054

Ruggiero, C., Cinalli, G., Spennato, P., Aliberti, F., Cianciulli, E., Trischitta, V., & Maggi, G. (2004). Endoscopic third ventriculostomy in the treatment of hydrocephalus in posterior fossa tumors in children. *Child's Nervous System, 20,* 828–833. doi: 10.1007/s00381-004-0938-y

Rutkowski, S., Bode, U., Deinlein, F., Ottensmeier, H., Warmuth-Metz, M., Soerensen, N.,... Kuehl, J. (2005). Treatment of early childhood medulloblastoma by postoperative chemotherapy alone. *The New England Journal of Medicine, 352,* 978–986.

Rutkowski, S., Cohen, B., Finlay, J., Luksch, R., Ridola, V., Valteau-Couanet, D.,... Grill, J. (2010). Medulloblastoma in young children. *Pediatric Blood & Cancer, 54,* 635–637. doi: 10.1002/pbc.22372

Sands, S., Milner, J. S., Goldberg, J., Mukhi, V., Moliterno, J. A., Maxfield, C., & Wisoff, J. H. (2005). Quality of life and behavioral follow-up study of pediatric survivors of craniopharyngioma. *Journal of Neurosurgery, 103,* 302–311.

Sands, S., Zhou, T., O'Neil, S. H., Patel, S. K., Allen, J., McGuire Cullen, P.,... Finlay, J. L. (2012). Long-term follow-up of children treated for high-grade gliomas: Children's Oncology Group 1991 final study report. *Journal of Clinical Oncology, 30,* 943–949. doi: 10.1200/jco.2011.35.7533

Sarkissian, V. (2005). The sequelae of cranial irradiation on human cognition. *Neuroscience Letters, 382,* 118–123.

Schell, M. J., McHaney, V. A., Green, A. A., Kun, L. E., Hayes, F. A., Horowitz, M., & Meyer, W. H. (1989). Hearing loss in children and young adults receiving cisplatin with or without prior cranial irradiation. *Journal of Clinical Oncology, 7,* 754–760.

Schor, N. F. (2009). New approaches to pharmacotherapy of tumors of the nervous system during childhood and adolescence. *Pharmacology and Therapeutics, 122,* 44–55. doi: S0163-7258(09)00003-5 [pii] 10.1016/j.pharmthera.2009.01.001

Schroeder, J. W., & Vezina, L. G. (2011). Pediatric sellar and suprasellar lesions. *Pediatric Radiology, 41,* 287–298. doi: 10.1007/s00247-010-1968-0

Schulte, F., & Barrera, M. (2010). Social competence in childhood brain tumor survivors: A comprehensive review. *Support Care Cancer, 18,* 1499–1513. doi: 10.1007/s00520-010-0963-1

Shah, M. N., Leonard, J. R., Inder, G., Gao, F., Geske, M., Haydon, D. H.,... Limbrick, D. D. (2012). Intraoperative magnetic resonance imaging to reduce the rate of early reoperation for lesion resection in pediatric neurosurgery. *Journal of Neurosurgery. Pediatrics, 9,* 259–264. doi: 10.3171/2011.12.PEDS11227

Shih, H. A., Loeffler, J. S., & Tarbell, N. (2009). Late effects of CNS radiation therapy. In S. Goldman & C. D. Turner (Eds.), *Late effects of treatment for brain tumors* (pp. 23–41). New York: Springer.

Smith, M. A., Seibel, N. L., Altekruse, S. F., Ries, L. A. G., Melbert, D. L., O'Leary, M.,... Reaman, G. H. (2010). Outcomes for children and adolescents with cancer: Challenges for the twenty-first century. *Journal of Clinical Oncology, 28,* 2625–2634. doi: 10.1200/jco.2009.27.0421

Sohlberg, M. M., & Mateer, C. A. (2001). *Cognitive rehabilitation: An integrative neuropsychological approach.* New York: Guilford Press.

Spiegler, B. J., Bouffet, E., Greenberg, M. L., Rutka, J. T., & Mabbott, D. J. (2004). Change in neurocognitive functioning after treatment with cranial radiation in childhood. *Journal of Clinical Oncology, 22,* 706–713.

Stargatt, R., Rosenfeld, J. V., Maixner, W., & Ashley, D. (2007). Multiple factors contribute to neuropsychological outcome in children with posterior fossa tumors. *Developmental Neuropsychology, 32*, 729–748.

Steinlin, M., Imfeld, S., Zulauf, P., Boltshauser, E., Lovblad, K. O., Ridolfi Luthy, A.,…Kaufmann, F. (2003). Neuropsychological long-term sequelae after posterior fossa tumour resection during childhood. *Brain, 126*, 1998–2008.

Turner, C. D., Chordas, C. A., Liptak, C. C., Rey-Casserly, C., Delaney, B. L., Ullrich, N. J.,…Kieran, M. W. (2009). Medical, psychological, cognitive and educational late-effects in pediatric low-grade glioma survivors treated with surgery only. *Pediatric Blood & Cancer, 53*, 417–423. doi: 10.1002/pbc.22081

Ullrich, N. J., & Pomeroy, S. L. (2003). Pediatric brain tumors. *Neurologic Clinics, 21*, 897–913.

Ullrich, N. J., Robertson, R., Kinnamon, D. D., Scott, R. M., Kieran, M. W., Turner, C. D.,…Pomeroy, S. L. (2007). Moyamoya following cranial irradiation for primary brain tumors in children. *Neurology, 68*, 932–938. doi: 68/12/932 [pii] 10.1212/01.wnl.0000257095.33125.48

Van Poppel, M., Klimo, P., Jr., Dewire, M., Sanford, R. A., Boop, F., Broniscer, A.,…Gajjar, A. J. (2011). Resection of infantile brain tumors after neoadjuvant chemotherapy: The St. Jude experience. *Journal of Neurosurgery Pediatrics, 8*, 251–256. doi: 10.3171/2011.6.PEDS11158

Vannatta, K., Fairclough, F., Farkas-Patenaude, A., Gerhardt, C., Kupst, M., Olshefski, R.,…Turner, C. (2008). Peer relationships of pediatric brain tumor survivors. *Paper presented at 13th International Symposium on Pediatric Neuro-Oncology.*

Vannatta, K., Gartstein, M. A., Short, A., & Noll, R. B. (1998). A controlled study of peer relationships of children surviving brain tumors: Teacher, peer, and self ratings. *Journal of Pediatric Psychology, 23*, 279–287.

Vannatta, K., Gerhardt, C. A., Wells, R. J., & Noll, R. B. (2007). Intensity of CNS treatment for pediatric cancer: Prediction of social outcomes in survivors. *Pediatric Blood and Cancer, 49*, 716–722.

von Hoff, K., Kieffer, V., Habrand, J. L., Kalifa, C., Dellatolas, G., & Grill, J. (2008). Impairment of intellectual functions after surgery and posterior fossa irradiation in children with ependymoma is related to age and neurologic complications. *BMC Cancer, 8*, 15.

Wilne, S. H., Ferris, R. C., Nathwani, A., & Kennedy, C. R. (2006). The presenting features of brain tumours: A review of 200 cases. *Archives of Diseases in Childhood, 91*, 502–506.

Wu, X., Northcott, P. A., Dubuc, A., Dupuy, A. J., Shih, D. J., Witt, H.,…Taylor, M. D. (2012). Clonal selection drives genetic divergence of metastatic medulloblastoma. *Nature, 482*, 529–533. doi: 10.1038/nature10825

Yock, T. I., & Tarbell, N. J. (2004). Technology insight: Proton beam radiotherapy for treatment in pediatric brain tumors. *Nature Clinical Practice Oncology, 1*, 97–103. Zebrack, B. J., Gurney, J. G., Oeffinger, K., Whitton, J., Packer, R. J., Mertens, A.,…Zeltzer, L. K. (2004). Psychological outcomes in long-term survivors of childhood brain cancer: A report from the childhood cancer survivor study. *Journal of Clinical Oncology, 22*, 999–1006.

Zelko, F. A. J., & Sorensen, L. G. (2009). Academic issues: Special education and related interventions. In S. Goldman & C. D. Turner (Eds.), *Late effects of treatment for brain tumors* (pp. 317–330). New York: Springer.

Zeltzer, L. K., Recklitis, C., Buchbinder, D., Zebrack, B., Casillas, J., Tsao, J. C.,…Krull, K. (2009). Psychological status in childhood cancer survivors: A report from the Childhood Cancer Survivor Study. *Journal of Clinical Oncology, 27*, 2396–2404. doi: JCO.2008.21.1433 [pii] 10.1200/JCO.2008.21.1433

4 Cerebral Palsy

Seth Warschausky, Jacqueline N.
Kaufman, and Lindsey Felix

HISTORICAL MEDICAL PERSPECTIVE

Descriptions of individuals with probable cerebral palsy (CP) can be found in images and mythology dating back thousands of years, including the perinatal spastic hemiplegia of the Greek blacksmith god Hephaistos (Obladen, 2011). Early explanations included magic, god's wrath, contact with the devil, and maternal "miswatching," or viewing others' deformities while pregnant. More physical/mechanistic explanations blamed inadequate swaddling and poor caregiving. Brain-based explanations came to the fore in the 19th century, including initial descriptions of periventricular leukomalacia (PVL; Bednar, 1851). William John Little, credited with identifying spastic diplegia, initially called Little's disease, described a series of cases with spastic rigidity that he correlated with birth complications including asphyxia (Little, 1861–1862). Freud subsequently found evidence of these types of birth complications in only 50% of cases of CP, challenging Little's causal explanations and foreshadowing today's more complex understandings of etiologies (Freud, 1897).

To date, although it is generally accepted that brain insults that result in CP often occur prenatally, the etiology of those insults remains controversial. Hypoxia-ischemia often is a presumptive cause of PVL and CP, though epidemiological studies suggest a less prominent role (Korzeniewski, Birbeck, DeLano, Potchen, & Paneth, 2008). At this point, inflammatory processes have been implicated in the etiology of lesions associated with cerebral palsy (Nelson, Dambrosia, Grether, & Phillips, 1998; Yoon et al., 2000).

Early definitions of CP were quite general, one describing CP as a "…disorder of movement or posture due to a defect or lesion of the immature brain" (Bax, 1964). Recent definitions have become more comprehensive and precise. The International Workshop on Definition and Classification of Cerebral Palsy, convened in 2004, recognized motor impairment as the central feature of CP but expanded the definition to include activity limitations and frequent disturbances of sensation, perception, cognition, communication, and behavior as well as epilepsy and secondary musculoskeletal problems (Rosenbaum et al., 2007). Motor impairments typically are noted before the age of 18 months. Until quite recently, subtypes of CP were classified by motor tone or movement into spastic, dyskinetic, ataxic, and mixed subtypes. Spasticity subtypes, which are characterized by hypertonicity, were identified based on affected limbs; that is, diplegic CP referred to hypertonicity primarily noted in the legs, quadriplegic CP to when all limbs were affected, and hemiplegic CP to when the arm and leg on one side of the body were affected. Dyskinetic CP is characterized by choreiform and athetoid movement and postural abnormalities. Ataxic CP includes hypotonicity and impairments in balance, coordination, and gait.

In 2007, the International Workshop on Definition and Classification of Cerebral Palsy (Rosenbaum et al., 2007), in parallel with the Surveillance of Cerebral Palsy in Europe (SCPE) recommendations (Cans et al., 2007), developed a new classification system for CP. In that system, CP is characterized with four dimensions. The first dimension is the motor abnormality, characterized by the nature and typology of the motor disorder and the functional motor abilities. The severity of the motor abnormalities can be graded with scales such as the Gross Motor Function Classification System (GMFCS; Palisano et al., 1997) and the Manual Ability Classification System (Eliasson et al., 2006) (Table 4.1). There is evidence to suggest that a subset of individuals with CP show change in GMFCS status in particular, including declines associated with comorbidities and aging (Bartlett, Hanna, Avery, Stevenson, & Galuppi, 2010).

The second dimension identifies type and severity of accompanying impairments including later developing musculoskeletal problems, impairments in cognition, communicative functions, sensory functions, and behavior as well as epilepsy. The third dimension, described as anatomical and neuroimaging findings, includes the anatomic

Table 4.1 Five-Level Classification Systems for Gross Motor Function and Manual Ability

System	Level and Descriptor
GMFCS (E&R)	Level I—Walks without limitations
	Level II—Walks with limitations
	Level III—Walks using hand-held mobility device
	Level IV—Self-mobility with limitation; may use powered mobility
	Level V—Transported in manual wheelchair
MACS	Level I—Handles objects easily and successfully
	Level II—Handles most objects but with somewhat reduced quality and/or speed of achievement
	Level III—Handles objects with difficulty; needs help to prepare and/or modify activities
	Level IV—Handles a limited selection of easily managed objects in adapted situations
	Level V—Does not handle objects and has severely limited ability to perform even simple actions

Note: GMFCS E&R, Gross Motor Function Classification System, Expanded and Revised (Palisano et al., 1997 Palisano, Rosenbaum, Bartlett, & Livingston, 2008); MACS, Manual Ability Classification System (Eliasson et al., 2006).

distribution affected by motor impairments or limitations and neuroimaging findings such as ventricular enlargement, white matter loss, and brain anomalies. The fourth dimension in CP classification identifies cause and timing including the presumed time frame in which the insult occurred, with the caveat that, in many cases, the cause will remain unknown.

CURRENT MEDICAL FACTORS AND TREATMENT AND INTERVENTION UPDATE

Epidemiology and Etiology

Worldwide prevalence of CP is approximately 2–3 per 1000 live births (Blair & Watson, 2006; Odding, Roebroeck, & Stam, 2006). In perhaps the most comprehensive study of the prevalence of CP subtypes in children, conducted by the collaborative group for the SCPE (Cans et al., 2002), 55% had bilateral spastic CP, 29% had unilateral spastic CP, 7% had dyskinetic CP, 4% had ataxic CP, and 4% had CP of unknown subtype. There is conflicting evidence regarding the stability of the prevalence of the dyskinetic subtype in children with CP and normal birth weight (Himmelmann et al., 2009; Sellier et al., 2010).

Etiology and antecedents differ in industrialized and developing nations. In industrialized nations, prematurity, low birth weight, and birth plurality are often associated with CP (Odding, Roebroeck, & Stam, 2006). In developing nations, where children who were born prematurely and with low birth weight are less likely to survive, the etiology of CP is thought to be more often associated with maternal complications and perinatal asphyxia as well as postnatal acquired CP (Blair & Watson, 2006).

Neuropathology

Brain abnormalities are detectable in approximately 80% of children with CP, with magnetic resonance imaging studies reporting more overall abnormalities than computed tomography studies (Korzeniewski et al., 2008). Brain abnormalities typically associated with CP include white matter damage, gray matter damage, ventriculomegaly, brain malformations, and postnatal injuries. White matter damage is the most common finding, occurring in approximately 38% of all cases; however, this is thought to be an underestimate due to imprecise reporting. Isolated gray matter damage is the least common finding, occurring in approximately 6% of cases. Historically, there was some controversy about including brain malformations in the neural substrates associated with CP, but recent definitions of CP include this substrate. Only a few neuroimaging studies are population based, and those studies tend to indicate more white matter abnormalities and more malformations (Bax, Tydeman, & Flodmark, 2006; Himmelmann, Hagberg, Beckung, Hagberg, & Uvebrant, 2005; Himmelmann & Uvebrant, 2011; Krageloh-Mann et al., 1995; Miller & Cala, 1989; Wiklund, Uvebrant, & Flodmark, 1990).

White matter damage associated with CP often is termed periventricular leukomalacia (PVL). Often accompanied by ventriculomegaly, PVL refers to the necrosis of white matter in the dorsal and lateral external angles of the lateral ventricles, centrum semiovale, and optic and acoustic radiation (Serdaroglu, Tekgul, Kitis, Serdaroglu, & Gokben, 2004). PVL, in turn, is associated with corpus callosal abnormalities, either with complete agenesis of the corpus callosum or hypogenesis of the splenium and rostrum. In hemiplegic CP, combined abnormalities in the white and gray matter are most common, occurring in 31% of these cases.

Neuroimaging findings may have implications for understanding the timing of brain insults and abnormalities in CP. However, caution is necessary because the timing of developmental neuroanatomical events has not been precisely determined. For example, until recently, neuronal migration disorders were assumed to have occurred in the first half of pregnancy, but there is now evidence of migration occurring in the last weeks of gestation. Thus, initial statements that suggested that approximately one-third of CP is associated with prenatal insult, 40% with perinatal insult, and the remainder occurring postnatally should be interpreted as gross estimates (Korzeniewski et al., 2008).

Accompanying Impairments

Apart from gross motor impairments and later-developing musculoskeletal problems, individuals with CP are at significant risk for epilepsy, sensory impairments, and impairments in communication and cognition. Prevalence of seizures has been reported in 15%–55% of children and adults with CP (Pruitt & Tsai, 2009). In those with comorbid mental retardation, prevalence is 71%. Partial seizures are the most common type of seizure, particularly in those with hemiplegic CP. Tonic-clonic seizures are more common in those with spastic diplegia. Risk factors for epilepsy in CP include history of a neonatal seizure and presence of abnormal brain structure, particularly atrophy (Zelnik, Konopnicki, Bennett Back, Castel Deutsch, & Tirosh, 2010). There are mixed findings regarding gestational age and risk of epilepsy in this population.

CP and prematurity independently increase the risk of sensorineural impairments, including visual and hearing impairments (Pruitt & Tsai, 2009). Regarding visual impairments, individuals at higher, more impaired GMFCS levels are at greater risk of lower visual acuity (Himmelmann, Beckung, Hagberg, & Uvebrant, 2006; Nordmark, Hagglund, & Lagergren, 2001). Those with higher GMFCS levels also are at greater risk of uncommon visual abnormalities, including high myopia, dyskinetic strabismus, and other oculomotor abnormalities (Ghasia, Brunstrom, Gordon, & Tychsen, 2008). Children with hemiplegic CP are at significant risk of visual field defects (Guzzetta et al., 2001). Cerebral visual impairments are found in up to 16% of children with CP (Ghasia et al., 2008).

Hearing abnormalities occur in 30%–40% of children with CP (Pruitt & Tsai, 2009), with recent population-based findings indicating 11.5% with severe auditory impairment (Shevell, Dagenais, & Hall, 2009). History of prematurity, low birth weight, congenital infections, hypoxic ischemic injury, and hyperbilirubinemia are risk factors for hearing impairments.

Other important accompanying impairments and comorbidities associated with CP include pain, reported in more than half of children and adults with CP (Parkinson, Gibson, Dickinson, & Colver, 2010; Vogtle, 2009), sleep disturbance (Sandella, O'Brien, Shank, & Warschausky, 2011), and gastrointestinal and nutritional problems (Pruitt & Tsai, 2009). Oromotor function is frequently impaired, leading to risk of dysphagia (Calis et al., 2008) and placing individuals with CP at risk for aspiration and respiratory infection.

EARLY PSYCHOLOGICAL AND NEUROPSYCHOLOGICAL FINDINGS

Initial studies of the psychological health of children with CP focused on personality assessment with descriptors that included emotional immaturity, lack of persistence, lack of socialization, and fatigability (Holden, 1952; Portenier, 1942). Findings in adults included greater social introversion, more depression, and less emotional stability (Holden, 1952; Tracht, 1946). By the 1950s, there was increasing emphasis on the role of parent–child interactions in the development of psychological health in this population.

Early studies of the cognitive profiles of children with cerebral palsy centered on intelligence test findings, with findings suggestive of high risk of mental retardation (Bice & Cruickshank, 1955; Hohman, 1953; Miller & Rosenfeld, 1952). Early estimates of rates of mental retardation (i.e., IQ <70) ranged from 44% to 63%. Concomitant with the study of intelligence in this population, there has been a long-standing concern about the inaccessibility of standardized test instruments (Eriksen, 1955; "Infantile cerebral palsies," 1953; Sigurdardottir et al., 2008; Warschausky et al., 2012).

Recent studies of cognitive profiles associated with CP have included the work of Sigurdardottir and colleagues (2008) with a complete national cohort between 4 and 6 1/2 years of age and using a variety of test instruments. Approximately 60% of the sample had an IQ or developmental quotient >70. Children with spastic hemiplegia or diplegia had better outcomes than children with spastic quadriplegia or dyskinetic CP. Children with spastic diplegia and quadriplegia had higher verbal IQ than performance IQ. Gestational age appeared to be a stronger predictor of verbal-performance IQ discrepancy than motor impairment. Epilepsy was the only associated impairment with an independent effect on IQ.

RECENT PSYCHOLOGICAL AND NEUROPSYCHOLOGICAL FINDINGS

Psychological and Social Perspectives

Although there is no longer a focus on the CP-specific personality traits noted in the early psychological research, there is clear evidence of significant psychological risks associated with CP. Population-based studies indicate that more than 40% of children aged 8–12 years show elevated risk (Parkes et al., 2008). The most common difficulties are with social adjustment, followed by hyperactivity and emotional difficulties. Pain and intellectual impairments are associated with higher psychological risk; the associations with functional impairments are less clear. Among children with spastic hemiplegic CP, the psychological risks are higher, with population-based estimates that 70% of children aged 8–12 years exhibit risk (Parkes, White-Koning, McCullough, & Colver, 2009). The most common difficulties in children with hemiplegic CP were similar to those seen in the general population of children with CP, and risk factors were similar but included higher risk in boys. That said, there is no evidence of lower self-concept among male adolescents with CP, although adolescent girls with CP do appear to be at risk in the areas of social acceptance and self-perceived competence (Shields, Murdoch, Loy, Dodd, & Taylor, 2006).

There is increasing interest in the social development and peer relations of persons with CP. Children with CP identify social relationships as one of the most salient determinants of their self-rated quality of life (Vinson, Shank, Thomas, & Warschausky, 2010). Importantly, functional abilities were not significant predictors of those self-ratings. There is evidence to suggest that in mainstream classes, females with CP, in particular, have fewer reciprocated friendships and are more isolated (Nadeau & Tessier, 2006). A mixed sample of children with CP and spina bifida self-reported smaller social networks and less validation and caring in their friendships than typically developing peers; however, this was not a gender-specific finding (Cunningham, Thomas, & Warschausky, 2007). Level of intelligence predicts social functioning, with lower intelligence associated with smaller social networks and lower social adjustment in children with CP (Cunningham, Warschausky, & Thomas, 2009).

The risk of limited social integration appears to persist into adulthood, with evidence of low rates of marriage or cohabitation (Michelsen, Uldall, Hansen, & Madsen, 2006). There are few studies of employment outcomes; however, a population-based study in Denmark found a 29% competitive employment rate overall, with a 12% rate among those with quadriplegic CP (Michelsen, Uldall, Kejs, & Madsen, 2005). Again, higher intelligence predicts higher likelihood of cohabitation and employment.

Neuropsychological Findings

Although recent studies of neuropsychological risks associated with CP have focused less on level of intelligence and more on specific cognitive domains, these studies typically utilize very small sample sizes and exclude children with more severe motor impairments due to the inaccessibility of instrumentation. Thus, many studies should be regarded as preliminary in nature.

Attention and Related Functions

Children with CP appear to be at risk for slowed processing speed (PS). Traditional clinical measures of PS require speeded motor responses and may lack validity in this population. Studies using tests that required speeded manual, oral, and ocular responses have found slowed PS in this population (Christ, White, Brunstrom, & Abrams, 2003; White, Craft, Hale, Schatz, & Park, 1995). In studies using inspection time measures that largely eliminate speeded motor response demands, children with CP who had average receptive vocabulary and only mild motor impairments also showed slowed PS (Shank, Kaufman, Leffard, & Warschausky, 2010).

Initial studies of visual attention, which examined event-related brain potentials using an oddball paradigm, show no significant differences in the latency and amplitude of the N2-P300 complex in children with mild spastic CP (Hakkarainen, Pirila, Kaartinen, Eriksson, & van der Meere, 2011). Thus, slowed PS may not stem from slowing in the fundamental orientation and evaluation of stimulus novelty but rather from slowing in higher-level processes. There is evidence to suggest risk of diminished inhibition of return, or diminished normal inhibition of attention to a previously inspected location, in a subset of children with CP who had evidence of anterior cerebral lesions, and this may have an adverse effect on development of higher-order functions including the ability to efficiently scan complex stimuli (Schatz, Craft, White, Park, & Figiel, 2001).

Executive Functions

Little is known about executive functions in those diagnosed with CP. There are mixed findings regarding working memory, with some evidence to suggest lower span of apprehension using digit and word span tasks (Jenks et al., 2007a) and other findings of performance comparable to peers (White et al., 1995). In what remains one of the more precise studies of inhibitory control in this population, Christ and colleagues (2003) found evidence of impairments in prepotent response inhibition while controlling for processing speed. Recent studies have been suggestive of impairments in other aspects of attention and executive functions in children with CP, including impairments in vigilance and divided attention. However, the effects of slowed PS have not been fully addressed (Bottcher, Flachs, & Uldall, 2010). Given the evidence of executive function and working memory impairments in other disorders with striatal dysfunction, including Parkinson's disease and Huntington's disease, it is surprising that individuals with dystonic CP do not appear to exhibit similar risks (Jahanshahi, Rowe, & Fuller, 2003), although findings have been suggestive of reduced verbal fluency and possible dual-task decrement.

There is some very interesting and potentially beneficial work emerging from the study of the interactions between attention and movement, including evidence to suggest that children with CP exhibit greater dual-task interference in postural control (Reilly, Woollacott, van Donkelaar, & Saavedra, 2008). Investigators have speculated that some of the positive effects of dorsal rhizotomy on cognition may stem from reducing the allocation of attentional resources needed for postural control (Craft et al., 1995).

With converging evidence of risk of impairments in attention and executive functions, it is not surprising that early population-based research indicates a high prevalence of hyperkinesis in children with CP, estimated at 25.5% (McDermott et al., 1996). Recent prevalence rates of attention-deficit/hyperactivity disorder (ADHD) in children with CP are estimated at 19% (Schenker, Coster, & Parush, 2005). Despite high prevalence rates, there is a limited understanding of the nature of ADHD symptoms in children with CP. Children with CP show elevated inattentiveness and hyperactive-impulsive ADHD symptoms on behavior rating scales, but there is concern about the validity of those behavior ratings in this population (Shank et al., 2010). There has been limited study of pharmacological treatment of ADHD symptoms in individuals with CP (Gross-Tsur, Shalev, Badihi, & Manor, 2002; Symons, Tervo, Kim, & Hoch, 2007). To date, there have been no studies of the relative contributions of prematurity, twinning, and specific medical factors on the risk for ADHD symptoms in children with CP.

Memory

There is a paucity of research on memory and CP, including limited focus on executive aspects of memory. White and Christ (2005) found no significant differences between children with CP and typically developing peers in initial learning on the California Verbal Learning Test for Children, but the children's learning across repetition trials was lower. Children with CP exhibited less use of semantic clustering, and younger children with CP exhibited more false-positive errors. Findings were interpreted as evidence of impairments in executive aspects of learning, while associative memory difficulties were less pronounced. In a separate study, paired-associate learning was poorer in children with CP on tasks that required visual/nonverbal responses, while performance on paired associate learning on tasks with verbal response demands was comparable to peers (Schatz, Craft, Koby, & Park, 1997). Comorbid epilepsy is associated with memory impairments in children with CP (Vargha-Khadem, Isaacs, van der Werf, Robb, & Wilson, 1992).

Visuospatial and Visuoperceptual Functions

There is long-standing recognition that children with CP are at risk for impairments In visuospatial and visuoperceptual functions. Preterm infants do not perform as well as infants carried to term on visuoperceptual tasks (Pagliano et al., 2007). Preterm children with CP and PVL have been shown to have greater risks for deficits in visual object recognition, imagery, and visual memory, even in the context of intact visual acuity, visual association, face and letter recognition, nonverbal intelligence, and verbal intelligence (Fazzi et al., 2009). Among children with CP, performance on non-verbal visual–perceptual tasks is worse for those with brain malformations and brain damage acquired after the first year of life than for those whose insult was acquired in utero (Stiers et al., 2002). In combination, these findings suggest that children with CP are vulnerable to visual–perceptual deficits and that performance is typically worse in children with CP who were born preterm or had hemorrhage/PVL acquired after birth compared with children carried to term without neurological complications.

Across diagnostic categories, performance on visual–spatial construction tasks (e.g., block design) has been found to be impaired (Barca, Cappelli, Di Giulio, Staccioli, & Castelli, 2010). These findings have been replicated even when strabismus was controlled for, suggesting that deficits may be in isolation from ophthalmological and visual–perceptual functions (Koeda, Inoue, & Takeshita, 1997) or problems in visual acuity (Stiers et al., 2002).

Speech and Language

Approximately 60% of children with CP have some degree of communication difficulty (Bax et al., 2006). Population-based findings suggest that approximately 16%–28% of children with CP are nonverbal communicators due to severe dysarthria or anarthria, with discrepancies in findings largely stemming from lack of agreed-upon metrics for degree of communicative impairment (Andersen et al., 2008; Sigurdardottir & Vik, 2011). Nonverbal status is associated with more severe motor impairments, including spastic quadriplegic and dyskinetic subtypes, as well as epilepsy, visual impairment, and severe feeding difficulty. In parallel with the development of classification systems for gross motor functioning and manual dexterity, there have been recent efforts to develop a Communication Function Classification System (Hidecker et al., 2011). Although severe dysarthria and anarthria are associated with significant risk of language impairments, the lack of speech does not preclude development of verbal cognition. Sigurdardottir and Vik (2011) found that among children with severe dysarthria who were able to participate in standardized testing, 24% had a verbal IQ >70. There has been limited study of specific aspects of language in this population; however, there is evidence to suggest that children with CP who are verbal communicators exhibit mild delays in narrative ability and difficulty with aspects of narrative discourse cohesion (Holck, Dahlgren Sandberg, & Nettelbladt, 2011; Soto & Hartmann, 2006). As discussed below, there appear to be complex associations between dysarthria and development of phonological processing.

Academic Functioning

For children with CP, the language precursors for reading acquisition are similar to those noted in typically developing children. Although phonological awareness and phonological short-term memory have been shown to be important precursors for decoding in typically developing children, in children with CP the most important precursor for word decoding is speech production (Peeters, Verhoeven, de Moor, & van Balkom, 2009). That said, the role of speech impairments such as dysarthria on reading acquisition appears to be complex; anarthria, in and of itself, does not preclude literacy. Among children with CP and dysarthria, those who can read have higher phonological processing skills than those who cannot read (Sandberg & Hjelmquist, 1997). Children with CP are at risk for lower phonological processing, including specific impairments in detecting rhyme in written words, segmenting syllables, and manipulating phonemes in those with dysarthria (Card & Dodd, 2006; Larsson & Sandberg, 2008; Peeters, Verhoeven, van Balkom, & de Moor, 2008).

Few have examined reading comprehension in children with CP (Dorman, 1987; Sandberg & Hjelmquist, 1997). Dorman (1987) examined predictors of reading comprehension in adolescents with CP, using the Peabody Individual Achievement Test, Reading Comprehension subtest. Multivariate analyses found that the sole predictor of reading comprehension was a measure of auditory perception. Asbell and colleagues (2010), in a study of predictors of reading comprehension in elementary school-age children with and without CP, found that phonemic awareness, receptive vocabulary, and general reasoning were significant predictors in both groups. Importantly, phonemic awareness mediated the association between functional communication level and reading comprehension in children with CP.

Risk for slowed acquisition of mathematics in children with CP may, in part, stem from initial limitations in subitizing or the ability to identify small quantities without counting (Arp, Taranne, & Fagard, 2006). More advanced arithmetic skills in children with CP and typically developing peers appear to be predicted by similar neuropsychological functions including nonverbal intelligence, working memory, and ability to mentally shift (Jenks, de Moor, & van Lieshout, 2009; Jenks et al., 2007b; van Rooijen, Verhoeven, & Steenbergen, 2011).

INTERVENTION AND TREATMENT GAINS

Apart from medical interventions to address motor impairments and such comorbidities as epilepsy, pain, and sensorineural impairments, much of a child's "treatment" will occur in an educational setting. Because so much early learning in infancy results from physical exploration, children with CP who have lowered mobility are at risk of decreased opportunities for critical exploration activity. Motor exploration has been particularly linked to infant visual–perceptual development (Bushnell & Boudreau, 1993; Franchak, van der Zalm, & Adolph, 2010), an area of known risk for children with CP. Early intervention services (EISs) are recommended (Majnemer, 1998). There is evidence that low-birth-weight preterm children, including those with cerebral injuries, show sustained benefit from early intervention programs, with positive effects more consistently found for those with higher birth weight (Brooks-Gunn et al., 1994; Hill, Brooks-Gunn, & Waldfogel, 2003; McCarton et al., 1997; McCormick et al., 2006) than those at lower-birth-weight. EIS programs for this population may also enhance parent–child interactions (Ohgi, Fukuda, Akiyama, & Gima, 2004).

Following EIS programming for families using public school education, enrollment in a school curriculum optimally occurs in the context of an individualized education plan (IEP) that is carefully designed to ensure a free and appropriate public education in the least restrictive environment. Determination of classroom setting commonly varies by the age of the child, the availability of specialized education within the school district, and the specific needs of the individual child. The issue of placement (i.e., special education versus mainstream/inclusive classrooms) has been a hotly debated issue (Kauffman & Hung, 2009; Smith, 2007). Those supporting inclusion models argue that children with disabilities should be fully mainstreamed in regular education classrooms and be able to participate in all aspects of learning with typically developing peers. Proponents of special education posit that tailored education can more readily be provided in a special education setting by teachers who have specialized training in this type of instruction. There is limited evidence-based research to show clear positive benefit of inclusion (Lindsay, 2007). Inclusion as a means of improving socialization and reducing isolation may not be supported (Vaughn, Elbaum, & Schumm, 1996), although this appears to be complex. Interestingly, a frequent argument against inclusion has been the potential deleterious effects on typically developing peers; however, a recent study in the Netherlands did not support this concern (Ruijs, Van der Veen, & Peetsma, 2010). Special education supporters cite research that children with learning disabilities make more gains when in special education settings than in general education settings (Fuchs, Fuchs, & Fernstrom, 1993). The key benefit ascribed to the special education model is the use of curriculum-based measurement, with routine measurement of performance over time to tailor the student's learning program. Given the tremendous heterogeneity of clinical concerns (physical and cognitive) for children with CP, it is recommended that inclusion and special education be viewed as a continuum, with classroom planning tailored for each child based on the location of necessary resources for that child. This may vary from full self-contained classroom settings, to partial mainstreaming with pull-out time, to full inclusion with support. Caution is encouraged when recommending the use of a paraprofessional aide to ensure that one-on-one learning is used only when necessary. Caution is also necessary to ensure that paraprofessionals are not used as primary educators and are not limiting opportunities for independent education, self-care, and socialization (Giangreco, 2010).

Classroom instruction ideally focuses on core academic topics for those children who are able to develop these skills, including reading, writing, and arithmetic. Reading instruction is essential given the role of literacy in independent living. A recent preliminary study by Peeters, de Moor, and Verhoeven (2011) found that Dutch children as young as 5 and 6 years who had CP may be at a disadvantage for exposure to emergent literacy activities in the classroom. In part, this was related to paramedical therapies outside of the classroom. Teacher and parental expectations of the capacity of children with CP to develop literacy skills may place barriers for children to develop these skills because expectations for reading success appear important for development of this skill (Peeters, Verhoeven, & de Moor, 2009; Peeters, Verhoeven, van Balkom, & de Moor, 2009). A subset of children with CP utilizes augmentative and alternative communication (AAC) systems, and these students are at risk for literacy difficulties due to limited opportunities for rich conversation and more restricted vocabulary options. However, the use of symbolic information to represent word concepts may aid in print awareness necessary for developing literacy (Hetzroni, 2004). Assistive technology via computerized presentation of books with the aid of switch systems has been shown to enhance emerging literacy skills (Hetzroni & Schanin, 2002), suggesting basic modifications may increase literacy opportunities in limited communicators. Speech and movement impairments in users of AAC should not be assumed to be associated with literacy acquisition deficits (Sandberg, Smith, & Larsson, 2010; Smith, Sandberg, & Larsson, 2009); rather, data suggest a heterogeneous population requiring individualized but accessible assessment of ability to delineate an educational plan. Assessing phonological awareness alone may not best predict reading in this population (Smith et al., 2009). Thus, care must be given to a comprehensive evaluation of all facets of reading. Relatively little is known about interventions for math and writing in this population, although concerns have been raised about the quality of specialized education planning for children with CP when remediation was needed (Jenks, de Moor, van Lieshout, & Withagen, 2010). Handwriting skills have been assessed in children with unilateral CP (Kavak & Eliasson, 2011). It was found that children developed their handwriting skills over a protracted period, with continued improvement over time, but with performance below that of typically developing peers. Research on building writing skill for those who use AAC suggests possible benefit from graphic organizer software for writing to aid in planning, word prediction software to fill in vocabulary, and teaching of reviewing and revision skills (Koppenhaver & Williams, 2010).

It is important for schools and families to be aware of options for using assistive technology, ensuring that both simple technologies and more advanced technologies are considered in the development of an IEP. For children with mild motor impairment, consideration can be given to supportive techniques, including keyboarding, to reduce unnecessary physical fatigue and distraction from core topics of instruction. Audiobooks for students with delayed reading and/or visual impairments can be used for content learning. Consultation with the assistive technology specialist to evaluate potential resources that reduce staff load and increase learning is appropriate. Adapted physical education resources are available, and participation in sports has positive psychosocial consequences. Children with CP should have physical education included in their school plan if medically cleared by their physician, taking into account common issues faced by children with cognitive and physical disabilities (Patel & Greydanus, 2002; Patel & Greydanus, 2010). Ancillary learning opportunities that occur in mainstream classrooms include sexual education, and special education curricula should include such curricula for children with disabilities. For children with greater intellectual disability, programs tailored to intellectual level have been shown to be effective at increasing sexuality-related decision making (Dukes & McGuire, 2009; Neufeld, Klingbeil, Bryen, Silverman, & Thomas, 2002).

Transition planning is an essential component of later planning during education and should include the student in decision making. Students transitioning to collegiate settings benefit from instruction about resources available in college including student disability centers and assistive technology labs. For students participating in vocational planning, consideration can be given to partial training in the high school setting where available. Students requiring more workshop training opportunities would benefit from considerable efforts to include independent living skills as part of the educational curriculum.

FUTURE AIMS AND RESEARCH OPPORTUNITIES

With simultaneous improvements in prenatal care and the ability to successfully treat high-risk infants, the prevalence of CP has remained relatively stable. However, there has been a tremendous increase in our understandings of the risks, capabilities, and needs associated with CP. Neuropsychological research has progressed from studies of intelligence that utilized partially accessible measures, to the study of specific cognitive domains that continue to utilize partially accessible instruments. A fundamental need in future neuropsychological research is to address the motor confound in typical response demands, including for manual dexterity and speeded motor response. This ongoing need is highlighted in the recent National Institutes of Health Toolbox project to develop neuropsychological instruments for use across populations. The instruments are largely inaccessible to those with significant motor and sensory impairments. It will be very important to conduct future research with adapted accessible standardized measures as well as relatively motor-free instruments utilized in the cognitive neurosciences.

To date, the vast majority of studies of the neuropsychology of CP use very small sample sizes. In contrast, studies of medical status, functional ability, and psychosocial status are being conducted on a large scale using population-based registries, including those in Europe and Australia. These registries are being developing in other countries as well and ultimately will be critical to the study of complex neuropsychological profiles. Children with CP often were preterm and had seizure disorders among other cognitive risk factors. Large-scale studies are required to identify the multivariate factors that predict specific neuropsychological risks.

Finally, it is only in recent years that there has been widespread recognition that children with CP grow up to be adults with CP. There are superb population-based studies of adult activity and participation being conducted largely in Europe; however, to date there is little focus on lifespan neuropsychological development in this population. We have come a long way since the historical statement that even among those with CP who had average intelligence, handicaps were frequently so severe that their intelligence would not be of any social or economic importance (Hohman, 1953). With population-based studies indicating that the majority of adults with CP do not have competitive employment, partners, and children (Michelsen, Uldall, Hansen, & Madsen, 2006), we have a long way to go.

REFERENCES

Andersen, G. L., Irgens, L. M., Haagaas, I., Skranes, J. S., Meberg, A. E., & Vik, T. (2008). Cerebral palsy in Norway: Prevalence, subtypes and severity. *European Journal of Paediatric Neurology, 12,* 4–13.

Arp, S., Taranne, P., & Fagard, J. (2006). Global perception of small numerosities (subitizing) in cerebral-palsied children. *Journal of Clinical and Experimental Neuropsychology, 28,* 405–419.

Asbell, S., Donders, J., Van Tubbergen, M., & Warschausky, S. (2010). Predictors of reading comprehension in children with cerebral palsy and typically developing children. *Child Neuropsychology, 16,* 313–325.

Barca, L., Cappelli, F. R., Di Giulio, P., Staccioli, S., & Castelli, E. (2010). Outpatient assessment of neurovisual functions in children with Cerebral Palsy. *Research and Development on Disabilities, 31,* 488–495.

Bartlett, D. J., Hanna, S. E., Avery, L., Stevenson, R. D., & Galuppi, B. (2010). Correlates of decline in gross motor capacity in adolescents with cerebral palsy in Gross Motor Function Classification System levels III to V: an exploratory study. *Developmental Medicine and Child Neurology, 52,* e155-e160.

Bax, M., Tydeman, C., & Flodmark, O. (2006). Clinical and MRI correlates of cerebral palsy: The European Cerebral Palsy Study. *Journal of American Medical Association, 296,* 1602–1608.

Bax, M. C. (1964). Terminology and Classification of Cerebral Palsy. *Developmental Medicine and Child Neurology, 6,* 295–297.

Bednar, A. (1851). *Die Krankheiten der Neugeborenen und Sauglinge vom clinicschen und pathologisch-anatomischen Standpunkte bearbeitet* (Vol. 2). Wien, Austria: Verlag von Carl Gerold.

Bice, H. V., & Cruickshank, W. M. (1955). The evaluation of intelligence. In W. M. Cruickshank & G. M. Raus (Eds.), *Cerebral palsy, its individual and community problems.* Syracuse: Syracuse University Press.

Blair, E., & Watson, L. (2006). Epidemiology of cerebral palsy. *Seminars in Fetal & Neonatal Medicine, 11,* 117–125.

Bottcher, L., Flachs, E. M., & Uldall, P. (2010). Attentional and executive impairments in children with spastic cerebral palsy. *Developmental Medicine and Child Neurology, 52,* e42–47.

Brooks-Gunn, J., McCarton, C. M., Casey, P. H., McCormick, M. C., Bauer, C. R., Bernbaum, J. C., & Meinert, C.L. for Phase II of the Infant Health and Development Program. (1994). Early intervention in low-birth-weight premature infants. Results through age 5 years from the Infant Health and Development Program. *Journal of American Medical Association, 272,* 1257–1262.

Bushnell, E. W., & Boudreau, J. P. (1993). Motor development and the mind: the potential role of motor abilities as a determinant of aspects of perceptual development. *Child Development, 64,* 1005–1021.

Calis, E. A. C., Veugelers, R., Sheppard, J. J., Tibboel, D., Evenhuis, H. M., & Penning, C. (2008). Dysphagia in children with severe generalized cerebral palsy and intellectual disability. *Developmental Medicine and Child Neurology, 50,* 625–630.

Cans, C., Dolk, H., Platt, M. J., Colver, A., Prasauskiene, A., Krageloh-Mann, I., & SCPE Collaborative Group (2007). Recommendations from the SCPE collaborative group for defining and classifying cerebral palsy. *Developmental Medicine and Child Neurology, 49,* 35–38.

Cans, C., Guillem, P., Arnaud, C., Baille, F., Chalmers, J., McManus, V., & SCPE Collaborative Group (2002). Prevalence and characteristics of children with cerebral palsy in Europe. *Developmental Medicine and Child Neurology, 44*(9), 633–640.

Card, R., & Dodd, B. (2006). The phonological awareness abilities of children with cerebral palsy who do not speak. *Augmentative and Alternative Communication, 22,* 149–159.

Christ, S. E., White, D. A., Brunstrom, J. E., & Abrams, R. A. (2003). Inhibitory control following perinatal brain injury. *Neuropsychology, 17,* 171–178.

Craft, S., Park, T. S., White, D. A., Schatz, J., Noetzel, M., & Arnold, S. (1995). Changes in Cognitive Performance in Children with Spastic Diplegic Cerebral-Palsy Following Selective Dorsal Rhizotomy. *Pediatric Neurosurgery, 23,* 68–74.

Cunningham, S. D., Thomas, P. D., & Warschausky, S. (2007). Gender differences in peer relations of children with neurodevelopmental conditions. *Rehabilitation Psychology, 52,* 331–337.

Cunningham, S. D., Warschausky, S., & Thomas, P. D. (2009). Parenting and social functioning of children with and without cerebral palsy. *Rehabilitation Psychology, 54,* 109–115.

Dorman, C. (1987). Verbal, perceptual and intellectual factors associated with reading achievement in adolescents with cerebral palsy. *Perceptual & Motor Skills, 64,* 671–678.

Dukes, E., & McGuire, B. E. (2009). Enhancing capacity to make sexuality-related decisions in people with an intellectual disability. *Journal of Intellectual Disability Research, 53,* 727–734.

Eliasson, A. C., Krumlinde-Sundholm, L., Rosblad, B., Beckung, E., Arner, M., Ohrvall, A. M., & Rosenbaum, P. (2006). The Manual Ability Classification System (MACS) for children with cerebral palsy: scale development and evidence of validity and reliability. *Developmental Medicine and Child Neurology, 48,* 549–554.

Eriksen, B. (1955). Intelligence tests in children suffering from cerebral palsy. *Acta Paediatrica, 44,* 24–28.

Fazzi, E., Bova, S., Giovenzana, A., Signorini, S., Uggetti, C., & Bianchi, P. (2009). Cognitive visual dysfunctions in preterm children with periventricular leukomalacia. *Developmental Medicine and Child Neurology, 51,* 974–981.

Franchak, J. M., van der Zalm, D. J., & Adolph, K. E. (2010). Learning by doing: Action performance facilitates affordance perception. *Vision Research, 50,* 2758–2765.

Freud, S. (Ed.). (1897). *Die infantile cerebrallahmung* (2nd ed.). Wien, Austria: Alfred Holder.

Fuchs, D., Fuchs, L. S., & Fernstrom, P. (1993). A Conservative Approach to Special-Education Reform—Mainstreaming through Transenvironmental Programming and Curriculum-Based Measurement. *American Educational Research Journal, 30,* 149–177.

Ghasia, F., Brunstrom, J., Gordon, M., & Tychsen, L. (2008). Frequency and severity of visual sensory and motor deficits in children with cerebral palsy: gross motor function classification scale. *Investigative Ophthalmology & Visual Science, 49,* 572–580.

Giangreco, M. F. (2010). One-to-One Paraprofessionals for students with disabilities in inclusive classrooms: Is conventional wisdom wrong? *Intellectual and Developmental Disabilities, 48,* 1–13.

Gross-Tsur, V., Shalev, R. S., Badihi, N., & Manor, O. (2002). Efficacy of methylphenidate in patients with cerebral palsy and attention-deficit hyperactivity disorder (ADHD). *Journal of Child Neurology, 17,* 863–866.

Guzzetta, A., Fazzi, B., Mercuri, E., Bertuccelli, B., Canapicchi, R., van Hof-van Duin, J., & Cioni, G. (2001). Visual function in children with hemiplegia in the first years of life. *Developmental Medicine and Child Neurology, 43,* 321–329.

Hakkarainen, E., Pirila, S., Kaartinen, J., Eriksson, K., & van der Meere, J. J. (2011). Visual attention study in youth with spastic cerebral palsy using the event-related potential method. *Journal of Child Neurology, 26,* 1525–1528.

Hetzroni, O. E. (2004). AAC and literacy. *Disability and Rehabilitation, 26,* 1305–1312.

Hetzroni, O. E., & Schanin, M. (2002). Emergent literacy in children with severe disabilities using interactive multimedia stories. *Journal of Developmental and Physical Disabilities, 14,* 173–190.

Hidecker, M. J., Paneth, N., Rosenbaum, P. L., Kent, R. D., Lillie, J., Eulenberg, J. B., & Taylor, K. (2011). Developing and validating the Communication Function Classification System for individuals with cerebral palsy. *Developmental Medicine and Child Neurology, 53,* 704–710.

Hill, J. L., Brooks-Gunn, J., & Waldfogel, J. (2003). Sustained effects of high participation in an early intervention for low-birth-weight premature infants. *Developmental Psychology, 39,* 730–744.

Himmelmann, K., Beckung, E., Hagberg, G., & Uvebrant, P. (2006). Gross and fine motor function and accompanying impairments in cerebral palsy. *Developmental Medicine and Child Neurology, 48*, 417–423.

Himmelmann, K., Hagberg, G., Beckung, E., Hagberg, B., & Uvebrant, P. (2005). The changing panorama of cerebral palsy in Sweden. IX. Prevalence and origin in the birth-year period 1995–1998. *Acta Paediatrica, 94*, 287–294.

Himmelmann, K., McManus, V., Hagberg, G., Uvebrant, P., Krageloh-Mann, I., & Cans, C. (2009). Dyskinetic cerebral palsy in Europe: trends in prevalence and severity. *Archives of Disease in Childhood, 94*, 921–926.

Himmelmann, K., & Uvebrant, P. (2011). Function and neuroimaging in cerebral palsy: A population-based study. *Developmental Medicine and Child Neurology, 53*, 516–521.

Hohman, L. B. (1953). Intelligence levels in cerebral palsied children. *American Journal of Physical Medicine, 32*, 282–290.

Holck, P., Dahlgren Sandberg, A., & Nettelbladt, U. (2011). Narrative ability in children with cerebral palsy. *Research in Developmental Disabilities, 32*, 262–270.

Holden, R. H. (1952). A Review of Psychological Studies in Cerebral Palsy: 1947 to 1952. *American Journal of Mental Deficiency, 57*, 92–99.

Infantile cerebral palsies. (1953). *Lancet, 1*, 429–430.

Jahanshahi, M., Rowe, J., & Fuller, R. (2003). Cognitive executive function in dystonia. *Movement Disorders, 18*, 1470–1481.

Jenks, K. M., de Moor, J., van Lieshout, E. C., Maathuis, K. G., Keus, I., & Gorter, J. W. (2007a). The effect of cerebral palsy on arithmetic accuracy is mediated by working memory, intelligence, early numeracy, and instruction time. *Developmental Neuropsychology, 32*, 861–879.

Jenks, K. M., de Moor, J., & van Lieshout, E. C. D. M. (2009). Arithmetic difficulties in children with cerebral palsy are related to executive function and working memory. *Journal of Child Psychology and Psychiatry, 50*, 824–833.

Jenks, K. M., de Moor, J., van Lieshout, E. C. D. M., Maathuis, K. G. B., Keus, I., & Gorter, J. W. (2007b). The effect of cerebral palsy on arithmetic accuracy is mediated by working memory, intelligence, early numeracy, and instruction time. *Developmental Neuropsychology, 32*, 861–879.

Jenks, K. M., de Moor, J., van Lieshout, E. C. D. M., & Withagen, F. (2010). Quality of arithmetic education for children with cerebral palsy. *International Journal of Rehabilitation Research, 33*, 19–25.

Kavak, S. T., & Eliasson, A. (2011). Development of handwriting skill in children with unilateral cerebral palsy (CP). *Disability and Rehabilitation, 33*, 2084–2091.

Kauffman, J. M., & Hung, L. Y. (2009). Special education for intellectual disability: current trends and perspectives. *Current Opinion in Psychiatry, 22*, 452–456.

Koeda, T., Inoue, M., & Takeshita, K. (1997). Constructional dyspraxia in preterm diplegia: isolation from visual and visual perceptual impairments. *Acta Paediatrica, 86*, 1068–1073.

Koppenhaver, D., & Williams, A. (2010). A conceptual review of writing research in augmentative and alternative communication. *Augmentative and Alternative Communication, 26*, 158–176.

Korzeniewski, S. J., Birbeck, G., DeLano, M. C., Potchen, M. J., & Paneth, N. (2008). A systematic review of neuroimaging for cerebral palsy. *Journal of Child Neurology, 23*, 216–227.

Krageloh-Mann, I., Petersen, D., Hagberg, G., Vollmer, B., Hagberg, B., & Michaelis, R. (1995). Bilateral spastic cerebral palsy—MRI pathology and origin. Analysis from a representative series of 56 cases. [Research Support, Non-U.S. Gov't Review]. *Developmental Medicine & Child Neurology, 37*, 379–397.

Larsson, M., & Sandberg, A. D. (2008). Phonological awareness in Swedish-speaking children with complex communication needs. *Journal of Intellectual and Developmental Disabilities, 33,* 22–35.

Lindsay, G. (2007). Educational psychology and the effectiveness of inclusive education/ mainstreaming. *British Journal of Educational Psychology, 77,* 1–24.

Little, W. J. (1861–1862). On the influence of abnormal purturition, difficult labours, premature birth and asphyxia neonatorum on the mental and physical condition of the child, especially in relation to deformities. *Transactions of the Obstetrical Society of London, 3,* 293–344.

Majnemer, A. (1998). Benefits of early intervention for children with developmental disabilities. *Seminars on Pediatric Neurology, 5,* 62–69.

McCarton, C. M., Brooks-Gunn, J., Wallace, I. F., Bauer, C. R., Bennett, F. C., Bernbaum, J. C., & Meinert, C. L. (1997). Results at age 8 years of early intervention for low-birth-weight premature infants. The Infant Health and Development Program. *Journal of American Medical Association, 277,* 126–132.

McCormick, M. C., Brooks-Gunn, J., Buka, S. L., Goldman, J., Yu, J., Salganik, M., & Casey, P. H. (2006). Early intervention in low birth weight premature infants: results at 18 years of age for the Infant Health and Development Program. *Pediatrics, 117,* 771–780.

McDermott, S., Coker, A. L., Mani, S., Krishnaswami, S., Nagle, R. J., Barnett-Queen, L. L., & Wuori, D. F. (1996). A population-based analysis of behavior problems in children with cerebral palsy. *Journal of Pediatric Psychology, 21,* 447–463.

Michelsen, S. I., Uldall, P., Hansen, T., & Madsen, M. (2006). Social integration of adults with cerebral palsy. *Developmental Medicine and Child Neurology, 48,* 643–649.

Michelsen, S. I., Uldall, P., Kejs, A. M., & Madsen, M. (2005). Education and employment prospects in cerebral palsy. *Developmental Medicine and Child Neurology, 47,* 511–517.

Miller, E., & Rosenfeld, M. D. (1952). The psychologic evaluation of children with cerebral palsy and its implications in treatment. *Journal of Pediatrics, 41,* 613–621.

Miller, G., & Cala, L. A. (1989). Ataxic cerebral-palsy—clinico-radiologic correlations. *Neuropediatrics, 20,* 84–89.

Nadeau, L., & Tessier, R. (2006). Social adjustment of children with cerebral palsy in mainstream classes: peer perception. *Developmental Medicine and Child Neurology, 48,* 331–336.

Nelson, K. B., Dambrosia, J. M., Grether, J. K., & Phillips, T. M. (1998). Neonatal cytokines and coagulation factors in children with cerebral palsy. *Annals of Neurology, 44,* 665–675.

Neufeld, J. A., Klingbeil, F., Bryen, D. N., Silverman, B., & Thomas, A. (2002). Adolescent sexuality and disability. *Physical Medicine and Rehabilitation Clinics of North America, 13,* 857–873.

Nordmark, E., Hagglund, G., & Lagergren, J. (2001). Cerebral palsy in southern Sweden II. Gross motor function and disabilities. *Acta Paediatrica, 90,* 1277–1282.

Obladen, M. (2011). Lame from birth: Early concepts of cerebral palsy. *Journal of Child Neurology, 26,* 248–256.

Odding, E., Roebroeck, M. E., & Stam, H. J. (2006). The epidemiology of cerebral palsy: Incidence, impairments and risk factors. *Disability and Rehabilitation, 28,* 183–191.

Ohgi, S., Fukuda, M., Akiyama, T., & Gima, H. (2004). Effect of an early intervention programme on low birthweight infants with cerebral injuries. *Journal of Paediatrics and Child Health, 40,* 689–695.

Pagliano, E., Fedrizzi, E., Erbetta, A., Bulgheroni, S., Solari, A., Bono, R., & Riva, D. (2007). Cognitive profiles and visuoperceptual abilities in preterm and term spastic diplegic children with periventricular leukomalacia. [Article]. *Journal of Child Neurology, 22,* 282–288.

Palisano, R., Rosenbaum, P., Walter, S., Russell, D., Wood, E., & Galuppi, B. (1997). Development and reliability of a system to classify gross motor function in children with cerebral palsy. *Developmental Medicine and Child Neurology, 39,* 214–223.

Palisano, R. J., Rosenbaum, P., Bartlett, D., & Livingston, M. H. (2008). Content validity of the expanded and revised Gross Motor Function Classification System. *Developmental Medicine and Child Neurology, 50,* 744–750.

Parkes, J., White-Koning, M., Dickinson, H. O., Thyen, U., Arnaud, C., Beckung, E., & Colver, A. (2008). Psychological problems in children with cerebral palsy: A cross-sectional European study. *Journal of Child Psychology and Psychiatry, 49,* 405–413.

Parkes, J., White-Koning, M., McCullough, N., & Colver, A. (2009). Psychological problems in children with hemiplegia: A European multicentre survey. *Archives of Disease in Childhood, 94,* 429–433.

Parkinson, K. N., Gibson, L., Dickinson, H. O., & Colver, A. F. (2010). Pain in children with cerebral palsy: A cross-sectional multicentre European study. *Acta Paediatrica, 99,* 446–451.

Patel, D. R., & Greydanus, D. E. (2002). The pediatric athlete with disabilities. *Pediatric Clinics North America, 49,* 803–827.

Patel, D. R., & Greydanus, D. E. (2010). Sport participation by physically and cognitively challenged young athletes. *Pediatric Clinics North America, 57,* 795–817.

Peeters, M., de Moor, J., & Verhoeven, L. (2011). Emergent literacy activities, instructional adaptations and school absence of children with cerebral palsy in special education. *Research in Developmental Disabilities, 32,* 659–668.

Peeters, M., Verhoeven, L., & de Moor, J. (2009). Teacher literacy expectations for kindergarten children with cerebral palsy in special education. *International Journal of Rehabilitation Research, 32,* 251–259.

Peeters, M., Verhoeven, L., de Moor, J., & van Balkom, H. (2009). Importance of speech production for phonological awareness and word decoding: the case of children with cerebral palsy. *Research in Developmental Disabilities, 30,* 712–726.

Peeters, M., Verhoeven, L., van Balkom, H., & de Moor, J. (2008). Foundations of phonological awareness in pre-school children with cerebral palsy: The impact of intellectual disability. *Journal of Intellectual Disability Researc, 52,* 68–78.

Peeters, M., Verhoeven, L., van Balkom, H., & de Moor, J. (2009). Home literacy environment: characteristics of children with cerebral palsy. *International Journal of Language & Communication Disorders, 44,* 917–940.

Portenier, L. G. (1942). Psychological factors in testing and training the cerebral palsied. *Physiotherapy Review, 22,* 301–303.

Pruitt, D., & Tsai, T. (2009). Common medical comorbidities associated with cerebral palsy. *Physical Medicine and Rehabilitation Clinics of North America, 20,* 453–467.

Reilly, D. S., Woollacott, M. H., van Donkelaar, P., & Saavedra, S. (2008). The interaction between executive attention and postural control in dual-task conditions: Children with cerebral palsy. *Archives of Physical Medicine and Rehabilitation, 89,* 834–842.

Rosenbaum, P., Paneth, N., Leviton, A., Goldstein, M., Bax, M., Damiano, D., & Jacobsson, B. (2007). A report: The definition and classification of cerebral palsy April 2006. *Developmental Medicine & Child Neurology - Supplement, 109,* 8–14.

Ruijs, N. M., Van der Veen, I., & Peetsma, T. T. D. (2010). Inclusive education and students without special educational needs. *Educational Research, 52,* 351–390.

Sandberg, A. D., & Hjelmquist, E. (1997). Language and literacy in nonvocal children with cerebral palsy. *Reading and Writing, 9,* 107–133.

Sandberg, A. D., Smith, M., & Larsson, M. (2010). An analysis of reading and spelling abilities of children using AAC: Understanding a continuum of competence. *Augmentative
and Alternative Communication*, *26*, 191–202.

Sandella, D. E., O'Brien, L. M., Shank, L. K., & Warschausky, S. A. (2011). Sleep and quality
of life in children with cerebral palsy. *Sleep Medicine*, *12*, 252–256.

Schatz, J., Craft, S., Koby, M., & Park, T. S. (1997). Associative learning in children with
perinatal brain injury. *Journal of the International Neuropsychological Society*, *3*,
521–527.

Schatz, J., Craft, S., White, D., Park, T. S., & Figiel, G. S. (2001). Inhibition of return in children with perinatal brain injury. *Journal of the International Neuropsychological Society*,
7, 275–284.

Schenker, R., Coster, W. J., & Parush, S. (2005). Neuroimpairments, activity performance,
and participation in children with cerebral palsy mainstreamed in elementary schools.
Developmental Medicine and Child Neurology, *47*, 808–814.

Sellier, E., Surman, G., Himmelmann, K., Andersen, G., Colver, A., Krageloh-Mann, I., &
Cans, C. (2010). Trends in prevalence of cerebral palsy in children born with a birthweight of 2,500 g or over in Europe from 1980 to 1998. *European Journal of Epidemiology*,
25, 635–642.

Serdaroglu, G., Tekgul, H., Kitis, O., Serdaroglu, E., & Gokben, S. (2004). Correlative value
of magnetic resonance imaging for neurodevelopmental outcome in periventricular
leukomalacia. *Developmental Medicine and Child Neurology*, *46*, 733–739.

Shank, L. K., Kaufman, J., Leffard, S., & Warschausky, S. (2010). Inspection time and
attention-deficit/hyperactivity disorder symptoms in children with cerebral palsy.
Rehabilitation Psychology, *55*, 188–193.

Shevell, M. I., Dagenais, L., & Hall, N. (2009). Comorbidities in cerebral palsy and their
relationship to neurologic subtype and GMFCS level. *Neurology*, *72*, 2090–2096.

Shields, N., Murdoch, A., Loy, Y., Dodd, K. J., & Taylor, N. F. (2006). A systematic review
of the self-concept of children with cerebral palsy compared with children without disability. *Developmental Medicine and Child Neurology*, *48*, 151–157.

Sigurdardottir, S., Eiriksdottir, A., Gunnarsdottir, E., Meintema, M., Arnadottir, U., & Vik, T.
(2008). Cognitive profile in young Icelandic children with cerebral palsy. *Developmental
Medicine and Child Neurology*, *50*, 357–362.

Sigurdardottir, S., & Vik, T. (2011). Speech, expressive language, and verbal cognition of
preschool children with cerebral palsy in Iceland. *Developmental Medicine and Child
Neurology*, *53*, 74–80.

Smith, M., Sandberg, A. D., & Larsson, M. (2009). Reading and spelling in children with
severe speech and physical impairments: a comparative study. *International Journal of
Language & Communication Disorders*, *44*, 864–882.

Smith, P. (2007). Have we made any progress? Including students with intellectual disabilities in regular education classrooms. *Intellectual and Developmental Disabilities*, *45*,
297–309.

Soto, G., & Hartmann, E. (2006). Analysis of narratives produced by four children who use
augmentative and alternative communication. *Journal of Communication Disorders*, *39*,
456–480.

Stiers, P., Vanderkelen, R., Vanneste, G., Coene, S., De Rammelaere, M., & Vandenbussche,
E. (2002). Visual-perceptual impairment in a random sample of children with cerebral
palsy. *Developmental Medicine and Child Neurology*, *44*, 370–382.

Symons, F. J., Tervo, R. C., Kim, O., & Hoch, J. (2007). The effects of methylphenidate on the
classroom behavior of elementary school-age children with cerebral palsy: A preliminary observational analysis. *Journal of Child Neurology*, *22*, 89–94.

Tracht, V. S. (1946). A comparative study of personality factors among cerebral palsied and non-handicapped persons. *Unpublished M.A. thesis, University of Chicago.*

van Rooijen, M., Verhoeven, L., & Steenbergen, B. (2011). Early numeracy in cerebral palsy: review and future research. *Developmental Medicine and Child Neurology, 53,* 202–209.

Vargha-Khadem, F., Isaacs, E., van der Werf, S., Robb, S., & Wilson, J. (1992). Development of intelligence and memory in children with hemiplegic cerebral palsy. The deleterious consequences of early seizures. *Brain, 115,* 315–329.

Vaughn, S., Elbaum, B. E., & Schumm, J. S. (1996). The effects of inclusion on the social functioning of students with learning disabilities. *Journal of Learning Disabilities, 29,* 598–608.

Vinson, J., Shank, L., Thomas, P. D., & Warschausky, S. (2010). Self-generated domains of quality of life in children with and without cerebral palsy. *Journal of Developmental and Physical Disabilities, 22,* 497–508.

Vogtle, L. K. (2009). Pain in adults with cerebral palsy: impact and solutions. *Developmental Medicine and Child Neurology, 51,* 113–121.

Warschausky, S., Van Tubbergen, M., Asbell, S., Kaufman, J., Ayyangar, R., & Donders, J. (2012). Modified test administration using assistive technology: Preliminary psychometric findings. *Assessment, 19,* 472–479.

White, D. A., & Christ, S. E. (2005). Executive control of learning and memory in children with bilateral spastic cerebral palsy. *Journal of the International Neuropsychological Society, 11,* 920–924.

White, D. A., Craft, S., Hale, S., Schatz, J., & Park, T. S. (1995). Working memory following improvements in articulation rate in children with cerebral palsy. *Journal of the International Neuropsychological Society, 1,* 49–55.

Wiklund, L. M., Uvebrant, P., & Flodmark, O. (1990). Morphology of cerebral lesions in children with congenital hemiplegia. A study with computed tomography. *Neuroradiology, 32,* 179–186.

Yoon, B. H., Romero, R., Park, J. S., Kim, C. J., Kim, S. H., Choi, J. H., & Han, T. R. (2000). Fetal exposure to an intra-amniotic inflammation and the development of cerebral palsy at the age of three years. *American Journal of Obstetrics & Gynecology, 182,* 675–681.

Zelnik, N., Konopnicki, M., Bennett-Back, O., Castel-Deutsch, T., & Tirosh, E. (2010). Risk factors for epilepsy in children with cerebral palsy. *European Journal of Paediatric Neurology, 14,* 67–72.

5 Late Neurodevelopmental Outcomes in Children with Congenital Heart Disease

David C. Bellinger and
Jane W. Newburger

HISTORICAL MEDICAL PERSPECTIVE

With an incidence of approximately 1 in 125 births (Hoffman & Kaplan, 2002), congenital heart disease (CHD) is the most common structural birth defect, accounting for approximately 30% of birth defect–related deaths. CHD includes a heterogeneous group of lesions. However, relatively simple septal defects of the ventricles or atria occur more frequently (3540/1,000,000 and 1043/1,000,000, respectively) than complex forms such as d-transposition of the great arteries (d-TGA; 315/1,000,000), tetralogy of Fallot (TOF; 421/1,000,000), and hypoplastic left heart syndrome (266/1,000,000). Approximately one-third of children with CHD require critical intervention in infancy if they are to survive.

The first repair of a congenital heart defect was performed in 1938, consisting of a ligation of patent ductus arteriosus. Since that time, remarkable strides have been made in pediatric cardiology and cardiac surgery. With the development of vital organ support techniques, such as cardiopulmonary bypass and total circulatory arrest, and the use of pharmacologic agents, such as prostaglandins, to maintain duct patency in children with cyanotic heart disease, the survival rate among children with complex forms of CHD now exceeds 90%. The reparative interventions that enable survival are relatively recent, however. The arterial switch operation for children with d-TGA was developed approximately 25 years ago, and the three-stage sequence of operations used to reconstruct the heart of a child with hypoplastic left heart syndrome (HLHS) dates only from the mid-1990s. As a result of the success of these interventions, the number of adult survivors of CHD now exceeds the number of children with CHD, and the ongoing care of survivors, called GUCH (Grown Ups with Congenital Heart Disease), is a subspecialty field within adult cardiology.

It is not surprising that children with CHD are at increased risk of neurodevelopmental impairments. The brain and heart share embryological origins, in part, both developing from neural crest tissue derived from ectoderm (although most cardiac tissue forms from lateral plate mesoderm). Because much of brain development involves activity-dependent processes that involve increased metabolism and substrate needs, abnormalities of blood flow to the brain might jeopardize the integrity of these processes. Most forms of CHD involve aberrations of the fetal cerebral circulation, resulting in reduced, abnormal, even reversed flow patterns and, thus, hemodynamic instability of varying severity. Using ^{1}H-magnetic resonance spectroscopy and magnetic resonance imaging (MRI), Limperopoulos and colleagues (2010) showed that by the third trimester, fetuses with CHD have smaller brain volumes and reduced N-acetyl-aspartate/choline ratios. At birth, term children with CHD have a delay in brain maturation estimated to be 4–5 weeks (Licht et al. 2009; Miller et al., 2007). On diffusion-tensor imaging, term infants with CHD have increased diffusivity and reduced fractional anisotropy (Miller et al., 2007). The immaturity of the brain might explain the increased risk of periventricular leukomalacia and other white matter injuries, both before (Miller et al., 2007) and after (Galli et al., 2004) cardiac surgery, presumably reflecting an increased vulnerability of white matter to hypoxic and oxidative injury. In one cohort, evidence of stroke was found on MRI in 10% of children with CHD; however, in half, the stroke had occurred preoperatively (Chen et al., 2009). In another cohort, 43% of children with CHD showed evidence of brain injury prior to surgery (stroke, white matter injury, intraventricular hemorrhage), and the injury severity was unchanged following surgery (Block et al., 2010). The injuries appear to be persistent. In a cohort of adolescents with a history of CHD, white matter abnormalities (e.g., cystic lesions, gliosis), periventricular and cortical regional volume losses, and poststroke changes were evident in a substantial percentage (~20%) (von Rhein et al., 2011).

The role of genetic abnormalities in the neurologic outcomes of children with CHD is significant. Approximately 30% of children with CHD have chromosomal anomalies (Fuller, 2010), and CHD can be one aspect of the phenotypic expression of many syndromes. For instance, approximately 75% of children with a 22q11.2 deletion syndrome (also known as DiGeorge syndrome) have a cardiac anomaly (e.g., TOF, truncus arteriosus, interrupted aortic arch, ventricular septal defect). TOF can also be part of many other genetic syndromes, including trisomy 21, VACTERL (vertebral anomalies, anal atresia, cardiovascular anomalies, tracheoesophageal fistula, renal anomalies, limb defects), and CHARGE (coloboma of the eye, heart defects, atresia of the choanae, retardation of growth and/or development, genital and/or urinary defects, ear anomalies and/or deafness). Other forms of CHD, such as simple d-TGA, rarely co-occur with extracardiac malformations. Even in CHD patients who are nonsyndromic, it is likely that genetic factors are important because genes that affect inflammatory, oxidative, and coagulation pathways, as well as response to hypoxia/ischemia, may impact neurodevelopmental outcomes. Among children with CHD, those with a genetic syndrome have been reported to have lower scores on the Bayley scales postsurgery (Forbess et al., 2002; Atallah et al., 2007; Zeltser et al., 2008; Tabbutt et al., 2008). Although the data are inconsistent, in some cohorts infants with the ε2 allele of the apolipoprotein gene have worse neurodevelopmental outcomes following reparative surgery than infants carrying other alleles (Gaynor et al., 2003; Gaynor et al., 2009).

As the population of CHD survivors has grown, increasing attention has been invested in understanding the nature and severity of the neurological and neuropsychological risks they face. Because medical advances are relatively recent, however, the number of studies in which patients have been followed beyond infancy or early childhood is limited. The importance of adopting a lifespan perspective is suggested by the results of two prospective studies of children with d-TGA. In one study, the percentage of patients who manifest neurodevelopmental impairment at age 8–14 years (55%) was 2-fold greater than it had been when the same children were assessed at age 5 years (26%; Hovels-Gurich, Seghaye, Dabritz, Messmer, & von Bernuth, 1997; Hovels-Gurich et al., 2002). In the second study, using the Child Behavior Check List, parents rated their children's behavior as being better than that of the standardization sample when the children were aged 2.5 years but as worse than that of the standardization sample when the same children were aged 8 years (Bellinger, Rappaport, Wypij, Wernovsky, & Newburger, 1997; Bellinger et al., 2009). These findings suggest important changes over time in the neurodevelopment of children with CHD, or at least in the ability to detect problems, as children age. On the basis of our work with this patient population, we hypothesize that neurodevelopmental limitations become more apparent over time. The impairments of higher-level organizational skills and executive functions that are central to their presentation become especially salient when the children face the challenges for self-regulation and metacognition that arise in later childhood and adolescence.

This chapter summarizes key findings of this nascent field, including the key risk factors for late impairments and the domains in which patients are at particular risk.

EARLY PSYCHOLOGICAL AND NEUROPSYCHOLOGICAL FINDINGS

The primary motivation behind many of the early studies was to identify modifiable aspects of medical and surgical management that predicted children's neurologic outcomes. As a result, the focus was on familiar outcomes that would be recognized as sufficiently important that an adverse effect might be considered a reasonable basis for changing clinical practice. Therefore, most studies focused on IQ and clinical signs of neurologic injury, including stroke and seizures. A variety of factors were evaluated as predictors, most notably the alternative methods used to support vital organs (e.g., brain and kidneys) during surgery (i.e., deep hypothermia with total circulatory arrest versus continuous low-flow cardiopulmonary bypass), other aspects of perfusion strategies, the duration of cardiopulmonary bypass, the duration of cooling prior to initiation of bypass, the strategy used to manage acid–base balance during surgery, and the degree of hemodilution used to prevent thromboembolic events during surgery. Studies also sought to identify postoperative factors that were useful prognostic indicators, such as seizures, length of intubation, and length of stay in the hospital.

With improvements in management, the incidence of serious neurologic injury has fallen to 1%–2% (Menache, duPlessis, Wessel, Jonas, & Newburger, 2002). In general, however, it has become apparent that efforts to identify intraoperative factors that predict children's outcomes have been largely disappointing. Some studies identified longer periods of deep hypothermic total circulatory arrest as a risk factor (e.g., Bellinger et al., 1995; Wypij et al., 2003). However, in one cohort of children with d-TGA followed prospectively, patient factors, including family socioeconomic status and presence of a ventricular septal defect, explained far more of the variance in children's neuropsychological outcomes than did intraoperative management factors (Bellinger et al., 2003). Moreover, just as abnormal brain development has been demonstrated in children with CHD before surgical correction, studies in which children were assessed prior to surgical correction of a CHD or heart transplantation have identified the presence of neuropsychological deficits (Wray & Radley-Smith, 2010). In addition, studies involving assessments both precorrection and 1 year after correction have failed to find decrements in the children's performance (van der Rijken et al., 2008; Quartermain et al., 2010). Children with neurologic abnormalities prior to heart transplantation tend to have worse neuropsychological outcomes posttransplantation than children without such abnormalities (Haavisto, Korkman, Jalanko, Holmberg, & Ovist, 2010). Similarly, late outcomes tend to be worse among children who have seizures postoperatively (Rappaport et al., 1998; Bellinger et al., in press).

It is only recently that studies have been conducted to characterize the nature and severity of the neuropsychological impairments in the population of children with CHD. The results of these studies are described in the following section.

RECENT PSYCHOLOGICAL AND NEUROPSYCHOLOGICAL FINDINGS

A meta-analysis (Karsdorp, Everaerd, Kindt, & Mulder, 2007) suggested that neuropsychological outcomes differ depending on the specific form of CHD. With regard to IQ, for instance, children with an atrial septal or ventricular septal defect (VSD) achieve scores near 100, while children with more complex forms of CHD have lower scores. It should be noted, however, that children with a VSD have been found to have specific deficits (e.g., visual memory, visual–motor ability) (Simons, Glidden, Sheslow, & Pizarro, 2010). In the meta-analysis conducted by Karsdorp and colleagues (2007), the mean full-scale IQ deficit was 2.1 points in children with d-TGA, 2.6 points in children with TOF, and 12.3 points in children with HLHS. This meta-analysis was not stratified according to the presence or absence of a genetic syndrome, however. As noted, this is an important consideration for the outcomes of children with TOF and HLHS and suggests that separate effect sizes should be reported for children with and without a syndrome.

Most children with CHD have an IQ within the low-average to average range, but it has become clear that IQ does not adequately capture their important neuropsychological weaknesses. In many studies, the standard deviation of IQ scores is greater than expected, which suggests the presence of subgroups within this population that differ in terms of risk. Factors that might contribute to increased variability include presence of a genetic syndrome, medical acuity, intraoperative events, postoperative events, and the degree of hemodynamic instability.

Various aspects of speech and language are impaired in CHD patients, and abnormal speech production may become evident early. In the Boston Circulatory Arrest Study (BCAS), a prospective study involving children with d-TGA, 24% met criteria for apraxia of speech at age 4 years (Bellinger et al., 1999) and 13% still met criteria at age 8 years (Bellinger et al., 2003). The oral–motor coordination and planning difficulties were expressed as reduced ability to imitate oral movements and speech sounds, phonological deviations (e.g., cluster reductions and simplifications, omission of medial and final consonants), and transposition of syllables. This resulted in reduced intelligibility of speech, particularly in the absence of contextual cues to aid the listener. Similar findings were reported in a cohort of children with TOF or a VSD (Hovels-Gurich et al., 2008). In the BCAS, in free play with a parent, children with d-TGA produced less symbolic talk than did controls, despite producing an equivalent amount of language and being engaged in fewer symbolic play episodes (Ovadia, Hemphill, Winner, & Bellinger, 2000). Whereas the control children took a major role in constructing and verbally elaborating play episodes (e.g., giving a doll a bath and putting it to bed), the verbal contributions of children with d-TGA more often consisted of sound effects or simple labeling of objects, leaving the parent to provide most of the verbal scaffolding for their play. These language production problems were not due to structural defects or to reduced hearing. Other aspects of language were also weak, including phonological awareness and processing, auditory analysis, letter fluency, and sentence formulation.

Some studies suggest that beyond weaknesses in building-block linguistic skills such as phonology, syntax, and semantics, children with CHD are also at risk of difficulties in the development of higher-order language skills, including the use of language to accomplish social goals. In the BCAS, children at both age 4 years and age 8 years had deficits in oral and written discourse. On an elicited narrative task that involved telling a personal anecdote on a specified topic (e.g., going to a beach, having a spilling accident), the children produced stories that were substantially less mature than those of control children in terms of narrative organization (e.g., orienting the listener, providing an opening and closing, use of temporal markers, insertion of character speech, description of a logical sequence of events) (Hemphill, Uccelli, Winner, Chang, & Bellinger, 2002). Interestingly, they also less frequently referred to participants' affective states or to their plans and intentions. Overall, their narratives placed greater demands on the listener regarding character identities, the physical setting of the event, and sequence of events that provided coherence to the story. At age 4 years, the elicited oral narratives of children with CHD resembled those of typically developing children at age 2–3 years, while their elicited oral and written narratives at age 8 years resembled those of typically developing children at age 5 years. These represent deficits in pragmatic language skills, specifically in the use of language to accomplish interpersonal goals. The children with d-TGA had difficulty tailoring their messages to address the listener's informational needs, suggesting that they might also have deficits in social cognition, as discussed later.

Visual–spatial skill is frequently noted to be a domain of weakness among children with CHD. This has been demonstrated on various design copying tasks, most strikingly with the Rey-Osterrieth Complex Figure (Bellinger et al., 2003). In the BCAS, at age 8 years, children with d-TGA tended to apply an extreme part-oriented approach in copying the figure, to the neglect of its overall structure. The frequency of copies that were scored at the lowest level of organization using the Developmental Scoring System (Holmes & Waber, 1986) was twice that observed in the standardization sample. Poorer quality of copy was significantly associated with children's performance on the Wechsler Individual Achievement Test math scales, and a clinical sort of copies into five groups showed that as quality declined, the percentage of children requiring academic aid in school increased monotonically.

Because the majority of studies of children with CHD have involved relatively brief follow-up periods, often assessing children only as infants, relatively few studies have focused on executive functions. However, the relatively limited data available suggest that use of a short follow-up interval may underestimate the risk in this domain. In two cohorts, Miatton and colleagues (2007a; 2007b) found that the patients performed worse than controls on the Tower subtest of the NEPSY. Calderon and colleagues (2010) found that, compared with controls, children with d-TGA scored significantly lower in cognitive inhibition (Stroop Test), behavioral control (NEPSY Statue), verbal working memory (digit span backward), spatial working memory (Corsi block-tapping task), and planning (Tower of London). Children in the BCAS scored poorly on tests that reflect, at least in part, various aspects of executive functions, such as the Wisconsin Card Sorting Test (percent conceptual responses, number of categories achieved), digit span (forward and backward) (Bellinger et al., 2003), and on several subtests of the Delis-Kaplan Executive Function System (Bellinger et al., 2011). At age 16 years, children's scores on the parent-completed Behavior Rating Inventory of Executive Function (BRIEF) and, to an even greater extent, the teacher-completed BRIEF were considerably higher (up to 1.5 standard deviations) than those of the standardization sample, particularly on the subscales contributing to the metacognition composite (Bellinger et al., 2011). Interestingly, the self-ratings provided by the children differed minimally from those of the standardization sample, suggesting that they lack insight into their limitations in terms of executive functions.

Parents consistently identify attention as one of the most prominent vulnerabilities of children with CHD. On the Behavior Assessment Scales for Children–2-, 5-, to 10-years-old, children with complex CHD were three to four times more likely than children in the standardization sample to have clinically significant elevations on the hyperactivity scale, and approximately 30% had high-risk scores for either inattention or hyperactivity on the Attention-Deficit-Hyperactivity Disorder Rating Scale-IV (Shillingford et al., 2008). Hovels-Gurich and colleagues (2007) administered the Attention Network Test to children with either TOF or a ventricular septal defect at age 7 years. The children with CHD scored worse than controls on the tasks in the battery that assess executive control (resolving conflicts between responses) but not on the tasks that assess alerting or orienting/reorienting. The authors speculated that this finding implicated the integrity of the anterior cingulate and lateral prefrontal cortex.

The weaknesses of children with CHD in pragmatic language skills led Bellinger (2008) to speculate that this might reflect, in part, a deficit in social cognition skills, specifically in the theory-of-mind skill that enables one to "read" other people. Calderon and colleagues (2010) found that children aged 7 years with d-TGA performed significantly worse than controls on both first- and second-order false belief stories. The children were unable to inhibit responding based on a salient perceptual feature of the story instead of on the basis of a story character's false belief. Bellinger and colleagues (2011) found that children at age 16 years with d-TGA were significantly worse than controls at decoding emotions from photographs on the Reading the Mind in the Eyes Test–Revised.

The constellation of deficits manifested by children with CHD suggests an underlying executive dysfunction. The children consistently have difficulty on tasks that require organization, pacing, and monitoring of output. They do not "see the big picture," instead tending to get lost in the details. This is not task specific in that it is evident in their storytelling, when they place substantial demands on the listener to organize the elements into a coherent narrative, as well as on figure copying tasks such as the Rey-Osterrieth Complex Figure, on which they tend to preserve individual details but not the organization that binds the details together. Low-level, building-block skills, such as word attack and decoding skills, are generally intact, but the children often encounter difficulty when required to integrate these skills in order to accomplish higher-order goals, such as using them to acquire information from written material (i.e., reading comprehension) or to tailor verbal messages that achieve pragmatic communication goals. It is often noted that children with various forms of cardiac lesions have a neuropsychological presentation similar to that described for children with a nonverbal learning disability (Tindall et al., 1999; Swillen et al., 1999).

Behavior and Psychosocial Outcomes

Many factors appear to influence the frequency and severity of difficulties in the domain of behavior, including the lesion (Birkeland et al., 2005), the age at which behavior is assessed (Karsdorp et al., 2007), and the relationship to the patient of the individual providing the reports (Bellinger et al., 2011). With regard to lesion, patients with 22q11.2 deletion syndrome are at greatly increased risk of psychiatric disorders such as schizophrenia and bipolar disorder (Gothelf et al., 2007; Stoddard et al., 2010; Papolos et al., 1996). In general, children with more complex forms of heart disease, such as TOF, HLHS, and other single ventricle lesions, and children requiring transplantation appear to be at greater psychiatric risk than children with acyanotic disease (Spurkland et al., 1993; Sharma et al., 2000; Chinnock et al., 2008; Hovels-Gurich et al., 2007).

Some data suggest that the likelihood of identifying behavior problems in children with CHD increases with age (Bellinger et al., 1997; Bellinger et al., 2009), although this trend is often based on parent ratings rather than on diagnostic evaluations. Therefore, it could reflect true changes in children's risk, changes over time in parents' perceptions that their child's behavior is problematic, or both. Teacher ratings can be expected to be less vulnerable to this reporting bias, and approximately 15%–25% of children with d-TGA are rated by their teachers on the Child Behavior Checklist as having either internalizing or externalizing behaviors in the range of clinical concern (Bellinger et al., 2009; Ellerbeck et al., 1998; Hovels-Gurich et al., 2002). In general, children with CHD tend to self-report better behavioral outcomes and psychosocial adjustment than do other observers (Latel et al., 2009 Spijkerboer et al., 2008; van Rijen et al., 2005; Chen et al., 2005; Miatton et al., 2007c). Whether this reflects limited insight into the magnitude of their difficulties is not clear. Some studies of children with CHD suggest that young boys are at greater risk of behavioral problems than are young girls (Spijkerboer et al., 2008), but this sex difference might be age dependent. van Rijen and colleagues (2003) reported that young adult females manifested greater psychiatric disorder than young adult males. One hypothesis is that activity restrictions on patients with CHD adversely impact the psychosocial status of boys to a greater extent than girls in childhood, whereas the potential adverse impact of CHD on reproductive options affects females more than males in young adulthood.

It is difficult to draw inferences about the long-term psychosocial prognosis of children with CHD. It is hoped that the recent interventions that permit children to survive to adulthood and the rapid pace of changes in medical management techniques (e.g., postoperative procedures in the intensive care unit) will improve patient outcomes. One study, however, reported similar outcomes among patients operated on before 1980 and those operated on between 1990 and 1995 (Spijkerboer et al., 2008). The available data suggest that adults with CHD remain at increased risk of psychosocial difficulties. Among adults assessed at age 32 years, 50% satisfied diagnostic criteria for at least one mood or anxiety disorder, and severity of the CHD did not predict risk (Spijkerboer et al., 2008). In another long-term follow-up study that was conducted when patients and referents were aged 20–32 years, patients reported greater reduction in psychopathology over the preceding 10-year period than did referents (van Rijen et al., 2005). Parents and partners of the patients, however, reported more symptoms in the patients than did the patients themselves, similar to the reporting bias observed in children and adolescents. Perhaps this is why social and emotional functioning in adults with CHD did not differ significantly from that of the comparison group in a study involving only patient self-reports (van Rijen et al., 2003).

Quality of Life

Considerable evidence has accumulated on the quality-of-life outcomes in children with CHD, and three instruments have been developed specifically to address the issues most germane to these children (Uzark et al., 2003; Macran et al., 2006; Marino et al., 2008). It is clear that the adverse impact of CHD on quality of life begins early in life. Majnemer and colleagues (2008) reported that functional limitations in socialization, daily living skills, communication, and adaptive behavior were evident in 11%–17% of 5-year-olds with CHD. Ratings provided by teachers and parents on the competence sections of the Child Behavior Checklist show that children with CHD experience difficulties in the areas of activities, social adaptation, and school performance. In the BCAS, 67% of children with d-TGA had scores in the borderline/clinical range on the Total Competence Scale (Bellinger et al., 2009). As many as one-third to one-half of children have been reported to be receiving remedial academic services, and grade retention is not infrequent (Miatton et al., 2007c; Shillingford et al., 2008; Bellinger et al., 2009). In one prospective study, children who were not performing at a satisfactory level in terms of academic skills at age 8 years by teacher report showed a greater increase in the problem behaviors between the ages of 4 and 8 years, with scores on some subscales of the Child Behavior Checklist increasing by as much as 1 standard deviation (Bellinger et al., 2009).

Quality of life is an inherently subjective outcome and can change over time depending on developmental stage. Severity of CHD is sometimes a predictor of quality of life (Latal et al., 2009) but not always. Ternestedt and colleagues (2001) found that children with TOF reported a better quality of life than did children with a simpler cardiac lesion (atrial septal defect). As with self-ratings of behavior, the children's self-ratings of quality of life sometimes do not differ from or are more optimal than the self-ratings of children without CHD (Lambert et al., 2009; Goldbeck & Melches, 2005; Hovels-Gurich et al., 2002; Teixeira et al., 2011). In most studies, however, children with CHD have a lower quality of life than children without CHD (Uzark et al., 2008; Landolt et al., 2008; McCrindle et al., 2006). For example, among 537 children aged 6–18 years who had undergone the Fontan procedure for a single ventricle lesion, the percentages who were reported to have anxiety, depression, attention, learning, or behavior problems on the Child Health Questionnaire–PF50) were as much as eightfold greater than the percentages of these problems in the referent group (McCrindle et al., 2006). Quality of life appears to be better when patients report that they have a strong social network available to support them (Teixeira et al., in press).

CONCLUSION

The results of recent research strongly support the conclusion that children with CHD should be under long-term surveillance for neurodevelopmental deficits. Although some deficits such as gross motor and expressive language delays are apparent in the early years, impairments in some skills with import for long-term well-being, including visual–spatial skills, pragmatic language skills, and the executive functions of planning and organization, become increasingly evident as children get older. The children tend to enjoy less academic success and, according to their parents and teachers, but not always the children themselves, to have poorer psychosocial adjustment and reduced quality of life. The factors that place children at increased risk, which include patient characteristics (e.g., cardiac lesion, severity of illness, abnormalities of brain development, genetics), usually predict a larger percentage of the variance in outcomes than do aspects of medical management, such as surgical interventions and postoperative care. It should be noted, however, that medical events such as stroke can have a devastating outcome. Relatively few consistent and enduring associations have been found between intraoperative factors and late outcomes.

Because of the increased neurodevelopmental risk of children with CHD, a cardiac neurodevelopment program (CNP) was recently established at Children's Hospital Boston (CHB) to provide a variety of assessment and intervention services for this patient population. Similar programs are being developed at Children's Hospital of Philadelphia and Emory University School of Medicine and will likely appear at other centers that provide care for large numbers of patients with CHD. The program at CHB is designed for children who have undergone cardiac surgery within the first year of life, children of any age who have been placed on extracorporeal membrane oxygenation, children of any age who are pre- or posttransplant or having heart/lung transplant, children of any age on a ventricular assist device, and children of any age diagnosed with velo-cardiofacial syndrome. It provides comprehensive psychological assessments to address cognitive, learning, behavioral, and social–emotional concerns, beginning prior to hospital discharge. It also includes guidance and support for expectant parents whose babies have been diagnosed with cardiac disease in utero; interventions for children and families to address regulatory disorders such as feeding, sleeping, and behavior difficulties; and school consultations to design and implement special education services. The CNP also includes a network of community resources, including psychoeducational seminars for parents, adjustment groups for children with ongoing medical needs (and their siblings), and a school consultation program to advocate for children. In addition to these clinical components, the CNP also includes a registry of children with CHD for whom a standard set of data is collected to support future clinical and research initiatives.

REFERENCES

Atallah, J., Joffe, A. R., Robertson, C. M. T., Leonard, N., Blakley, P. M., Nettel-Aguirre, A.,…Rebeyka, I. M. (2007). Two-year general and neurodevelopmental outcomes after neonatal complex surgery in patients with deletion 22q11.2: A comparative study. *Journal of Thoracic and Cardiovascular Surgery, 134*, 772–779.

Bellinger, D. C. (2008). Are children with congenital cardiac malformations at increased risk of deficits in social cognition? *Cardiology in the Young, 18*, 3–9.

Bellinger, D. C., Bernstein, J. H., Kirkwood, M. W., Rappaport, L. A., & Newburger, J. W. (2003). Visual-spatial skills in children after open-heart surgery. *Journal of Developmental and Behavioral Pediatrics, 24,* 169–179.

Bellinger, D. C., Jonas, R. A., Rappaport, L. A., Wypij, D., Wernovsky, G., Kuban, K. C.,...Newburger, J. W. (1995). Developmental and neurologic status of children after heart surgery with hypothermic circulatory arrest or low-flow cardiopulmonary bypass. *New England Journal of Medicine, 332,* 549–555.

Bellinger, D. C., Newburger, J. W., Wypij, D., Kuban, K. C. K., duPlessis, A. J., & Rappaport, L. A. (2009). Behavior at age 8 years in children with corrected transposition of the great arteries: the Boston Circulatory Arrest Trial. *Cardiology in the Young, 19,* 86–97.

Bellinger, D. C., Rappaport, L. A., Wypij, D., Wernovsky, G., & Newburger, J. W. (1997). Patterns of developmental dysfunction after surgery during infancy to correct transposition of the great arteries. *Journal of Developmental and Behavioral Pediatrics, 18,* 75–83.

Bellinger, D. C., Wypij, D., duPlessis, A. J., Rappaport, L. A., Jonas, R. A., Wernovsky, G., & Newburger, J. W. (2003). Neurodevelopmental status at eight years in children with dextro-transposition of the great arteries: the Boston Circulatory Arrest Trial. *Journal of Thoracic and Cardiovascular Surgery, 126,* 1385–1396.

Bellinger, D. C., Wypij, D., Kuban, K. C., Rappaport, L. A., Hickey, P. R., Wernovsky, G., Jonas, R. A., & Newburger, J. W. (1999). Developmental and neurological status of children at 4 years of age after heart surgery with hypothermic circulatory arrest or low-flow cardiopulmonary bypass. *Circulation, 100,* 526–532.

Bellinger, D. C., Wypij, D., Rivkin, M. J., DeMaso, D. R., Robertson, R. L., Rappaport, L. A.,...Newburger, J. W. (2011). Adolescents with d- transposition of the great arteries corrected with the arterial switch procedure: Neuropsychological assessment and structural brain imaging. *Circulation, 124,* 1361–1369.

Birkeland, A. L., Rydberg, A., & Hagglof, B. (2005). The complexity of the psychosocial situation in children and adolescents with heart disease. *Acta Pediatrica, 94,* 1495–1501.

Block, A. J., McQuillen, P. S., Chau, V., Glass, H., Poskitt, K. J., Barkovich, A. J.,...Miller, S. P. (2010). Clinically silent preoperative brain injuries do not worsen with surgery in neonates with congenital heart disease. *Journal of Thoracic and Cardiovascular Surgery, 140,* 550–557.

Calderon, J., Bonnet, D., Courtin, C., Concordet, S., Plumet, M. H., & Angeard, N. (2010). Executive function and theory of mind in school-aged children after neonatal corrective cardiac surgery for transposition of the great arteries. *Developmental Medicine and Child Neurology, 52,* 1139–1144.

Chen, C.W., Li, C.Y., & Wang, J.K. (2005). Self-concept: comparison between school-aged children with congenital heart disease and normal school-aged children. *Journal of Clinical Nursing, 14,* 394–402.

Chen, J., Zimmerman, R. A., Jarvik, G. P., Nord, A. S., Clancy, R. R., Wernovsky, G.,...Ichord, R. (2009). Perioperative stroke in infants undergoing open heart operations for congenital heart disease. *Annals of Thoracic Surgery, 88,* 823–829.

Chinnock, R. E., Freier, M. C., Ashwal, S., Pivonka-Jones, J., Shankel, T., Cutler, D., & Bailey, L. (2008). Developmental outcomes after pediatric heart transplantation. *Journal of Heart and Lung Transplantation, 27,* 1079–1084.

Ellerbeck, K. A., Smith, M. L., Holden, E. W., McMenamin, S. C., Badawi, M. A., Brenner, J. I.,...Human, S. L. (1998). Neurodevelopmental outcomes in children surviving d- transposition of the great arteries. *Journal of Developmental and Behavioral Pediatrics, 19,* 335–341.

Forbess, J. M., Visconti, K. J., Hancock-Friesen, C., Howe, R. C., Bellinger, D. C., & Jonas, R. A. (2002). Neurodevelopmental outcome after congenital heart surgery: results from an institutional registry. *Circulation, 106,* 195–202.

Fuller, S. (2010). Genetic factors are important determinants of neurodevelopmental outcomes after neonatal cardiac surgery. *Progress in Pediatric Cardiology, 29*, 73–77.

Galli, K. K., Zimmerman, R. A., Jarvik, G. P., Wernovsky, G., Kuypers, M. K., Clancy, R. R.,…Gaynor J. W. (2004). Periventricular leukomalacia is common after neonatal cardiac surgery. *Journal of Thoracic and Cardiovascular Surgery, 127*, 692–704.

Gaynor, J. W., Gerdes, M., Zackai, E. H., Bernbaum, J., Wernovsky, G., Clancy, R. R.,…Jarvik, G. P. (2003). Apolipoprotein E genotype and neurodevelopmental sequelae of infant cardiac surgery. *Journal of Thoracic and Cardiovascular Surgery, 126*, 1736–1745.

Gaynor, J. W., Nord, A., Wernovsky, G., Bernbaum, J., Solot, C. B., Burnham, N.,…Gerdes, M. (2009). Apolipoprotein E genotype modifies the risk of behavior problems after infant cardiac surgery. *Pediatrics, 124*, 241–250.

Goldbeck, L., & Melches, J. (2005). Quality of life in families of children with congenital heart disease. *Quality of Life Research, 14*, 1915–1924.

Gothelf, D., Aviram-Goldring, A., Burg, M., Steinberg, T., Mahajnah, M., Frisch, A.,…Weizman, A. (2007). Cognition, psychosocial adjustment and coping in familial cases of velocardiofacial syndrome. *Journal of Neural Transmission, 114*, 1495–1501.

Haavisto, A., Korkmanm, M., Jalankom, H., Holmbergm, C., & Ovist, E. (2010). Neurocognitive function of pediatric heart transplant recipients. *Journal of Heart and Lung Transplantation, 29*, 764–770.

Hemphill, L., Uccelli, P., Winner, K., Chang, C. J., & Bellinger, D. (2002). Narrative discourse in young children with histories of early corrective heart surgery. *Journal of Speech Language and Hearing Research, 45*, 318–331.

Hoffman, J. I. E., & Kaplan, S. (2002). The incidence of congenital heart disease. *Journal of the American College of Cardiology, 39*, 1890–1900.

Holmes, J. H., & Waber, D. P. (1986). *Developmental scoring system for the Rey-Osterrieth Complex Figure*. Odessa, FL: Psychological Assessment Resources, Inc.

Hövels-Gürich, H. H., Seghaye, M. C., Däbritz, S., Messmer, B. J., & von Bernuth, G. (1997). Cognitive and motor development in preschool and school-aged children after neonatal arterial switch operation. *Journal of Thoracic and Cardiovascular Surgery, 114*, 578–585.

Hövels-Gürich, H. H., Konrad, K., Wiesner, M., Minkenberg, R., Herpertz-Dahlmann, B., Messmer, B. J., & von Bernuth, G. (2002). Long term behavioural outcome after neonatal arterial switch operation for transposition of the great arteries. *Archives of Diseases in Children, 87*, 506–510.

Hovels-Gurich, H. H., Seghaye, M. C., Schnitker, R., Wiesner, M., Huber, W., Minkenberg, R.,…von Bernuth G. (2002). Long-term neurodevelopmental outcomes in school-aged children after neonatal arterial switch operation. *Journal of Thoracic and Cardiovascular Surgery, 124*, 448–458.

Hovels-Gurich, H. H., Konrad, K., Skorenski, D., Minkenberg, R., Herpertz-Dahlmann, B., Messmer, B. J., & Seghaye, M. C. (2007). Long-term behavior and quality of life after corrective cardiac surgery during infancy to correct transposition of the great arteries. *Journal of Developmental and Behavioral Pediatrics, 28*, 346–354.

Hovels-Gurich, H. H., Konrad, K., Skorenski, D., Herpertz-Dahlman, B., Messmer, B. J., & Seghaye, M. C. (2007). Attentional dysfunction in children after corrective cardiac surgery in infancy. *Annals of Thoracic Surgery, 83*, 1425–1430.

Hovels-Gurich, H. H., Bauer, S. B., Schnitker, R., Willmes-von Hinckeldey, K., Messmer, B. J.,…Huber, W. (2008). Long-term outcome of speech and language in children after corrective surgery for cyanotic or acyanotic cardiac defects in infancy. *European Journal of Paediatric Neurology, 12*, 378–386.

Karsdorp, P. A., Everaerd, W., Kindt, M., & Mulder, B. J. M. (2007). Psychological and cognitive functioning in children and adolescents with congenital heart disease: A meta-analysis. *Journal of Pediatric Psychology, 32*, 527–541.

Lambert, L. M., Minich, L. L., & Newburger, J. W. (2009). Parent- versus child-reported functional health status after the Fontan procedure. *Pediatrics, 124,* e942–e949.

Landolt, M. A., Valsangiacomo Buechel, E. R., & Latal, B. (2008). Health-related quality of life in children and adolescents after open-heart surgery. *Journal of Pediatrics, 152,* 349–355.

Latel, B., Helfricht, S., Fischer, J. E., Bauersfeld, U., & Landolt, M. A. (2009). Psychological adjustment and quality of life in children and adolescents following open-heart surgery for congenital heart disease: A systematic review. *BMC Pediatrics, 9,* 6.

Licht, D. J., Shera, D. M., Clancy, R. R., Wernovsky, G., Montenegro, L. M., Nicolson, S.C.,…Gaynor, J. W. (2009). Brain maturation is delayed in infants with complex congenital heart defects. *Journal of Thoracic and Cardiovascular Surgery, 137,* 529–536.

Limperopoulos, C., Tworetzky, W., McElhinney, D. B., Newburger, J. W., Brown, D. W., Robertson, R. L.,…duPlessis, A. J. (2010). Brain volume and metabolism in fetuses with congenital heart disease: evaluation with quantitative magnetic resonance imaging and spectroscopy. *Circulation, 121,* 26–33.

Macran, S., Birks, Y., Parsons, J., Sloper, P., Hardman, G., Kind, P.,…Lewin, R. (2006). The development of a new measure of quality of life for children with congenital heart disease. *Cardiology in the Young, 16,* 165–172.

Majnemer, A., Limperopoulos, C., Rohlicek, C., Rosenblatt, B., & Tchervenkov, C. (2008). Developmental and functional outcomes at school entry in children with congenital heart defects. *Journal of Pediatrics, 153,* 55–60.

Marino, B. S., Shera, D., Wernovsky, G., Tomlinson, R. S., Aguirre, A., Gallagher, M.,…Shea, J. A. (2008). The development of the pediatric cardiac quality of life inventory: a quality of life measure for children and adolescents with heart disease. *Quality of Life Research, 17,* 13–26.

McCrindle, B. W., Williams, R. V., Mitchell, P. D., Hsu, D., Paridon, S. M., Atz, A. M.,…Newburger, J. W. (2006). Relationship of patient and medical characteristics to health status in children and adolescents after the Fontan procedure. *Circulation, 113,* 1123–1129.

Menache, C. C., duPlessis, A. J., Wessel, D. L., Jonas, R. A., & Newburger, J. W. (2002). Current incidence of acute neurologic complications after open-heart operations in children. *Annals of Thoracic Surgery, 73,* 1752–1758.

Miatton, M., De Wolf, D., François, K., Thiery, E., & Vingerhoets, G. (2007a). Neuropsychological performance in school-aged children with surgically corrected congenital heart disease. *Journal of Pediatrics, 151,* 73–78.

Miatton, M., De Wolf, D., François, K., Thiery, E., & Vingerhoets, G. (2007b). Intellectual, neuropsychological, and behavioral functioning in children with tetralogy of Fallot. *Journal of Thoracic and Cardiovascular Surgery, 133,* 449–455.

Miatton, M., DeWolf, D., Francois, K., Thiery, E., & Vingerhoets G. (2007c). Behavior and self- perception in children with a surgically corrected congenital heart disease. *Journal of Developmental and Behavioral Pediatrics, 28,* 294–301.

Miller, S. P., McQuillen, P. S., Hamrick, S., Xu, D., Glidden, D. V., Charlton, N.,…Vigneron, D. B. (2007). Abnormal brain development in newborns with congenital heart disease. *New England Journal of Medicine, 357,* 1928–1938.

Ovadia, R., Hemphill, L., Winner, K., & Bellinger, D. (2000). Just pretend: Participation in symbolic talk by children with histories of early corrective heart surgery. *Applied Psycholinguistics, 21,* 321–340.

Papolos, D. F. Faedda, G. L., Veit, S., Goldberg, R., Morrow, B., Kucherlapati, R., & Shprintzen, R. J. (1996). Bipolar spectrum disorders in patients diagnosed with velo-cardio-facial syndrome: Does a hemizygous deletion of chromosome 22q11 result in bipolar affective disorder? *American Journal of Psychiatry, 153,* 1541–1547.

Quartermain, M. D., Ittenbach, R. F., Flynn, T. B., Gaynor, J. W., Zhang, X., Licht, D. J.,...Wernovsky, G. (2010). Neuropsychological status in children after repair of acyanotic congenital heart disease. *Pediatrics, 126,* e351–359.

Rappaport, L. A., Wypij, D., Bellinger, D. C., Helmers, S. L., Holmes, G. L., Barnes, P. D.,...Newburger, J. W. (1998). Relation of seizures after cardiac surgery in early infancy to neurodevelopmental outcome. *Circulation, 97,* 773–779.

Sharma, R., Choudhary, S. K., Mohan, M. R., Padma, M. V., Jain, S., Bhardwaj, M.,... Venugopal, P. (2000). Neurological evaluation and intelligence testing in the child with congenital heart disease. *Annals of Thoracic Surgery, 70,* 575–581.

Shillingford, A. J., Glanzman, M. M., Ittenbach, R. F., Clancy, R. R., Gaynor, J. W., & Wernovsky, G. (2008). Inattention, hyperactivity, and school performance in a population of school-age children with complex congenital heart disease. *Pediatrics, 121,* e759–e767.

Simons, J. S., Glidden, R., Sheslow, D., & Pizarro C. (2010). Intermediate neurodevelopmental outcome after repair of ventricular septal defect. *Annals of Thoracic Surgery, 90,* 1586–1591.

Spijkerboer, A. W., Utens, E. M., Bogers, A. J., Verhulst, F. C., & Helbing, W. A. (2008). Long-term behavioural and emotional problems in four cardiac diagnostic groups of children and adolescents after invasive treatment for congenital heart disease. *International Journal of Cardiology, 125,* 66–73.

Spijkerboer, A. W., Utens, E. M., Bogers, A. J., Helbing, W. A., & Verhulst, F. C. (2008). A historical comparison of long-term behavioral and emotional outcomes in children and adolescents after invasive treatment for congenital heart disease. *Journal of Pediatric Surgery, 43,* 534–539.

Spurkland, I., Bjornstad, P. G., Lindberg, H., & Seem E. (1993). Mental health and psychosocial functioning in adolescents with congenital heart disease. A comparison between adolescents born with severe heart defect and atrial septal defect. *Acta Pediatrica, 82,* 71–76.

Stoddard, J., Niendam, T., Hendren, R., Carter, C., & Simon, T. J. (2010). Attenuated positive symptoms of psychosis in adolescents with chromosome 22q11.2 deletion syndrome. *Schizophrenia Research, 118,* 118–121.

Swillen, A., Vanderpitte, L., Cracco, J., Maes, B., Ghesquiere, P., Devriendt, K., & Fryns, J. P. (1999). Neuropsychological, learning and psychosocial profile of primary school aged children with the velo-cardio-facial syndrome (22q11 deletion): Evidence for a nonverbal learning disability. *Child Neuropsychology, 5,* 230–241.

Tabbutt, S., Nord, A. S., Jarvik, G. P., Bernbaum, J., Wernovsky, G., Gerdes, M.,...Gaynor, J. W. (2008). Neurodevelopmental outcomes after staged palliation for hypoplastic left heart syndrome. *Pediatrics, 121,* 476–483.

Ternestedt, B. M., Wall, K., Oddsson, H., Riesenfeld, T., Grith, I., & Schollin J. (2001). Quality of life 20 and 30 years after surgery in patients operated on for tetralogy of Fallot and for atrial septal defect. *Pediatric Cardiology, 22,* 128–132.

Teixeira, F. M., Coelho, R. M., Proenca, C., Silva, A. M., Vieira, D., Vaz, C.,...Areias, M. E. (2011). Quality of life experienced by adolescents and young adults with congenital heart disease. *Pediatric Cardiology, 2011,* 1132–1138.

Tindall, S., Rothermel, R. R., Delamater, A., Pinsky, W., & Klein, M. D. (1999). Neuropsychological abilities of children with cardiac disease treated with extracorporeal membrane oxygenation. *Developmental Neuropsychology, 16,* 101–115.

Uzark, K., Jones, K., Burwinkle, T. M., & Varni, J. W. (2003). The pediatric quality of life inventory in children with heart disease. *Progress in Pediatric Cardiology, 18,* 141–148.

Uzark, K., Jones, K., Slusher, J., Limbers, C. A., Burwinkle, T. M., & Varni, J. W. (2008). Quality of life in children with heart disease as perceived by children and parents. *Pediatrics, 121,* e1060–e1067.

van Rijen, E. H., Utens, E. M., Roos-Hesselink, J. W., Meijboom, F. J., van Domburg, R. T., Bogers, A. J., & Verhulst, F. C. (2009). Longitudinal development of psychopathology in an adult congenital heart disease cohort. *International Journal of Cardiology*, *99*, 315–323.

van Rijen, E. H., Utens, E. M., Roos-Hesselink, J. W., Meijboom, F. J., van Domburg, R. T., Roelandt, J. R.,... Verhulst, F. C. (2003). Psychosocial functioning of the adult with congenital heart disease: A 20–33 years follow-up. *European Heart Journal*, *24*, 673–683.

van der Rijken, R., Hulstijn-Dirkmaat, G., Kraaimaat, F., Nabuurs-Kohrman, L., Nijveld, A., Maassen, B., & Daniels, O. (2008). Open-heart surgery at school age does not affect neurocognitive functioning. *European Heart Journal*, *29*, 2681–2688.

Von Rhein, M., Scheer, I., Loenneker, T., Huber, R., Knirsch, W., & Latal, B. (2011). Structural brain lesions in adolescents with congenital heart disease. *Journal of Pediatrics*, *158*, 984–989.

Wray, J., & Radley-Smith, R. (2010). Cognitive and behavioral functioning of children listed for heart and/or lung transplantation. *American Journal of Transplantation*, *10*, 2527–2535.

Wypij, D., Newburger, J. W., Rappaport, L. A., duPlessis, A. J., Jonas, R. A., Wernovsky, G.,... Bellinger, D. C. (2003). The effect of duration of deep hypothermic circulatory arrest in infant heart surgery on late neurodevelopment: the Boston Circulatory Arrest Trial. *Journal of Thoracic and Cardiovascular Surgery*, *126*, 1397–1403.

Zeltser, I., Jarvik, G. P., Bernbaum, J., Wernovsky, G., Nord, A. S., Gerdes, M.,... Gaynor, J. W. (2008). Genetic factors are important determinants of neurodevelopmental outcome after repair of tetralogy of Fallot. *Journal of Thoracic and Cardiovascular Surgery*, *135*, 91–97.

6 Neuropsychological Outcomes of HIV in Childhood and Adolescence

Sharon L. Nichols, Betsy Kammerer, and Doyle E. Patton

HISTORICAL MEDICAL PERSPECTIVE

In 1981, a retrovirus that would become known as human immunodeficiency virus (HIV) emerged onto the medical scene and brought with it sweeping health, societal, economic, and political impacts. It was soon discovered that HIV attacks specific blood cells, that is, $CD4^+$ T cells, that are crucial to helping the body fight diseases. In degrading the body's natural immune system, untreated HIV elevates the susceptibility of infected individuals to a variety of diseases and opportunistic infection (OIs), ultimately placing many at risk for acquired immune deficiency syndrome (AIDS) and death. Although HIV was first observed in adults, 1983 witnessed the first descriptions of pediatric AIDS and the beginning of a staggering global epidemic among infants and children (World Health Organization [WHO], 2010). The scope of the tragedy awaiting children of the world, particularly those in developing countries, was not appreciated at that time. Also not anticipated was that treatment advances would transform HIV into a chronically managed illness, with children surviving into adolescence and adulthood. This development and the large number of people being infected during adolescence have brought HIV directly into the purview of neuropsychologists and health psychologists who see adolescents and assist with their transition to adulthood.

Infection of infants, children, and adolescents by HIV occurs primarily through the following three mechanisms: (1) transfusion of infected blood products, (2) mother-to-child transmission (MTCT), and (3) behavioral means (e.g., sexual contact, sharing needles, and similar behaviors). Although numerous children with hemophilia or other disorders requiring administration of blood products were infected by HIV-tainted blood products early in the epidemic, this transmission route has been all but eliminated in high-resource settings through screening and heat treatment of blood products. Although 2%–4% of HIV transmission worldwide continues to result from transfusions (Donegan, 2003), the majority of pediatric and adolescent infections currently occur through MTCT and behavioral means.

MTCT can occur in utero, during birth, or via breastfeeding. Before the introduction of antiretroviral therapy (ART), MTCT rates were 25%–30%. In 1994, it was discovered that administration of ART to women during pregnancy and birth (Connor et al., 1994) and to the infant for 6 weeks postnatally could reduce MTCT rates to <2% (Cooper et al., 2002). Although this led to a dramatic drop in the incidence of infant HIV infection in resource-rich countries, pediatric HIV remains an epidemic with devastating broad consequences in countries with less access to ART.

HIV transmission can also occur in youth via risk behaviors such as unprotected sexual contact or needle sharing. In spite of large-scale campaigns to promote safer sexual practices, behavioral transmission of HIV continues with especially high rates among youth. Neuropsychologists who work with adolescents need to be aware of this significant risk for HIV, particularly in those with developmental or psychiatric disorders who are at greater risk for infection (Brown, Danovsky, Lourie, DiClemente, & Ponton, 1997).

Despite widespread attempts to disseminate information regarding HIV, many myths remain among the lay public. Misconceptions range from the belief that HIV is rapidly fatal or precludes any possibility of a "normal" life, to beliefs that medications can cure the disease or eliminate its effects, such that transmission precautions are unneeded. Stigma remains a major issue for people living with HIV; many people continue to believe casual contact can transmit the disease and/or that individuals with HIV have necessarily been infected through stigmatized behaviors. Knowledge about HIV is essential to support those living with HIV and to promote appropriate practices to decrease HIV transmission.

CURRENT MEDICAL FACTORS AND TREATMENT AND INTERVENTION UPDATE

Although the incidence of pediatric HIV has decreased in countries where ART is most available, pediatric HIV continues to be a significant worldwide issue, with 2.5 million children <15 years living with HIV in 2009 and an estimated 370,000 new infections occurring that year alone (WHO, 2010). There were 260,000 deaths of children from AIDS that year, a compelling demonstration that life-saving ART continues to be unavailable for many. Furthermore, youth aged 15–24 years continue to represent more than 40% of new HIV infections each year, with an estimated 1.2 million young people in this age group living with HIV as of 2007 (Wilson, Wright, Safrit, & Rudy, 2010).

Untreated, HIV is a progressive illness that gradually destroys the immune system, allows development of severe OIs, and directly attacks the organ systems. The laboratory measures used most commonly to monitor HIV disease progression are CD4 count or percentage and viral load. CD4 lymphocyte cells are the components of the immune system that serve as the primary targets of HIV. CD4 cell count or percentage

Table 6.1 Pediatric Human Immunodeficiency Virus Classification[a]

Immunologic Category	Clinical Category			
	N: No Signs/ Symptoms	A: Mild Signs/ Symptoms	B: Moderate Signs/ Symptoms[b]	C: Severe Signs/ Symptoms[b]
1: No evidence of suppression	N1	A1	B1	C1
2: Evidence of moderate suppression	N2	A2	B2	C2
3: Severe suppression	N3	A3	B3	C3

[a]Children whose human immunodeficiency virus infection status is not confirmed are classified by using the above grid with a letter E (for perinatally exposed) placed before the appropriate classification code (e.g., EN2).

[b]Both category C and lymphoid interstitial pneumonitis in category B are reportable to state and local health departments as acquired immunodeficiency syndrome.

is an indicator of degree of immune compromise that contributes to clinical monitoring, disease severity staging, and treatment initiation decisions. HIV viral load refers to the number of copies of HIV-1 RNA per milliliter of plasma and is a key indicator of the burden of viral replication. Although less closely linked to the development of symptoms, it is critical for monitoring response to ART.

Current schemes for classifying the severity of HIV disease consider both clinical status and laboratory indicators. For children <13 years (Centers for Disease Control and Prevention [CDC], 1994) (Table 6.1), categories N, A, B, and C represent increasing severity of disease, with category N (nonsymptomatic) denoting an absence of overt symptoms and category C (severely symptomatic) being equivalent to AIDS. A diagnosis of class C status requires the presence of 1 of 24 AIDS-defining conditions, which can include HIV encephalopathy or certain OIs of the brain such as toxoplasmosis, in addition to OIs involving other organ systems. A separate scheme used for adolescents and adults consists of three stages defined by CD4 count and, in some cases, presence of an AIDS-defining condition (Table 6.2). Individuals retain the most severe classification category applied even if immunological improvement or resolution of the AIDS-defining condition occurs.

The current scheme for HIV severity classification is complemented by a nosology for the diagnosis of HIV-associated neurocognitive disorder (HAND) in adolescents and adults (Antinori et al., 2007), defined by performance on standardized tests and impairment in activities of daily living (Table 6.3). A similar scheme proposed for children included definitions of HIV encephalopathy and the milder HIV-related central nervous system (CNS) compromise (see Wolters & Brouwers, 2005a). In formulating the scheme, the authors added to the definitions considerations of deviations from the typical developmental trajectory, including both loss of previously acquired skills and failure to gain new skills or to develop at the expected rate based on peer norms or on the child's own previous developmental progression.

Although early recommendations were to begin ART when an individual's CD4 count had declined to the point of no longer protecting from OIs, there is mounting

Table 6.2 CDC Classification System for Human Immunodeficiency Virus-Infected Adults and Adolescents

CD4 Cell Category	Clinical Category		
	A Asymptomatic, Acute HIV, or PGL	B[a] Symptomatic Conditions, not A or C	C[b] AIDS-Indicator Conditions
1. ≥500 cells/μL	A1	B1	C1
2. 200–499 cells/μL	A2	B2	C2
3. <200 cells/μL	A3	B3	C3

Abbreviations: HIV, human immunodeficiency virus; PGL, persistent generalized lymphadenopathy.
[a]Category B Symptomatic Conditions: Defined as symptomatic conditions occurring in an HIV-infected adolescent or adult who meets at least one of the following criteria: (1) They are attributed to HIV infection or indicate a defect in cell-mediated immunity and (2) they are considered to have a clinical course or management that is complicated by HIV infection. Examples include, but are not limited to, *Oropharyngeal candidiasis* (thrush), *Vulvovaginal candidiasis*, persistent or resistant, pelvic inflammatory disease, cervical dysplasia/cervical carcinoma in situ, *Herpes zoster* (shingles), constitutional symptoms (e.g., fever >38.5°C or diarrhea lasting >1 month), peripheral neuropathy.
[b]Category C AIDS-Indicator Conditions: One of 24 conditions. Examples include recurrent bacterial pneumonia, cryptococcosis (extrapulmonary), cytomegalovirus disease, encephalopathy (HIV-related), progressive multifocal leukoencephalopathy, toxoplasmosis of brain, wasting syndrome caused by HIV.

evidence that early initiation of treatment helps prevent neurocognitive decline and other complications. However, concerns remain regarding ART toxicity and possible long-term negative effects of ART on cardiovascular and other systems that may confer their own risks on the CNS later in life. These concerns are magnified for children and adolescents who may face many decades of ART and who are taking these powerful medications at the same time the brain and other systems are still developing. Lifelong

Table 6.3 Research Criteria for Human Immunodeficiency Virus-Associated Neurocognitive Disorders

Diagnosis	Level of Impairment in at Least Two Domains[a]	Interference With Everyday Functioning	Impairment Does Not Meet Criteria for:[b]
HIV-associated asymptomatic neurocognitive impairment	At least 1 SD below the mean	None	Delirium or dementia
HIV-associated mild neurocognitive disorder	At least 1 SD below the mean	Mild	Delirium or dementia
HIV-associated dementia	At least 2 SD below the mean, typically in multiple domains	Marked	Delirium

Source: Adapted from Antinori et al. (2007).
Abbreviations: HIV, human immunodeficiency virus; SD, standard deviation.
[a]As demonstrated using demographically corrected scores on standardized neuropsychological tests.
[b]There is no evidence for another preexisting cause for the diagnosis.

monitoring of cognitive and neurological functioning may be important for adult survivors of perinatal or adolescent HIV infection.

EARLY PSYCHOLOGICAL AND NEUROPSYCHOLOGICAL FINDINGS

Before ART came into use, severe neurocognitive and motor impairments were common and much feared complications of HIV for both adults and children; these impairments remain a critical problem in countries without access to ART. In children with symptomatic HIV disease, estimates of early encephalopathy incidence in the United States ranged from 16% to 60% (Belman, 2008). Children presented with encephalopathy as the first AIDS-defining illness more often than adults, and this pattern was particularly common in infants classified as "early progressors" (i.e., those who developed AIDS early and died typically within the first years of life) (Belman, 2008).

Several patterns of the natural progression of CNS symptoms in children occur in settings without access to ART or in children who have experienced treatment failure or poor adherence. The most severe pattern, HIV-associated progressive encephalopathy, tends to occur in infants with early disease progression or in children who have developed significant immune compromise and other symptoms of HIV disease (Belman, 2008). This pattern is defined by the following three features: (1) impaired brain growth, (2) motor impairments or abnormal muscle tone, and (3) loss of developmental milestones or cognitive decline.

A second pattern, termed "static encephalopathy," refers to delays in acquisition of milestones and cognitive and/or motor impairment but no loss of previously acquired milestones or cognitive functions, with prevalence estimates as high as 90% prior to the introduction of ART (Shanbhag et al., 2005). Youth infected with HIV through blood products or risk behaviors, as well as perinatally infected children classified as "slow progressors" (i.e., reached school age without AIDS), showed a slower, more insidious development of symptoms resembling the course seen in the fully developed brains of adults, with subtle deficits seen first in processing speed, attention, and memory, before ART came into wide use.

Early studies using magnetic resonance imaging (MRI) and computed tomographic (CT) examinations showed a pattern of cerebral atrophy and white matter abnormalities, with calcifications of the basal ganglia in some children. Pathological findings postmortem included reduced brain volume, enlarged ventricles, and white matter and inflammatory changes (Belman, 2008). However, the manner in which HIV produced the observed CNS damage and dysfunction was not well understood at that time.

RECENT PSYCHOLOGICAL AND NEUROPSYCHOLOGICAL FINDINGS

Neural System Involvement

A substantial literature now shows that HIV infiltrates the CNS early in the course of infection across age groups. Once in the CNS, HIV does not infect neurons directly but rather exerts its effects indirectly through infection of perivascular macrophages, microglia, and astrocytes. HIV is associated with a state of chronic inflammation and activation of immune components, including those in the brain (Gannon, Khan, & Kolson, 2011), as well as with changes to the endothelial cells lining blood vessels and thus to the blood-brain barrier (BBB), which can alter its permeability to the virus. The production of cytokines and other toxins by activated immune cells in the brain is hypothesized to underlie HIV-associated CNS damage and to partially account for the mild neurocognitive effects observed in adults on combinations of antiretroviral therapies (cART) with good viral control (Heaton et al., 2011). Other damage is associated with direct toxic effects of viral proteins. Both viral and host genetic factors and comorbid factors, such as substance abuse or other infections (e.g., hepatitis C), can affect the interaction of HIV with the CNS (Antinori et al., 2007; Ellis et al., 2011).

Not all parts of the brain are equally susceptible to the virus. In adults, imaging and autopsy studies have shown cortical atrophy and white matter abnormalities, with the greatest impact on the hippocampus and frontal-subcortical structures such as the basal ganglia (Tate et al., 2009). This pattern corresponds with the most commonly observed cognitive impairments in memory; motor speed and motor functioning; complex attention and working memory; and executive functions such as fluency, planning, abstraction, and inhibition (Reger, Welsh, Razani, Martin, & Boone, 2002). Studies using proton magnetic resonance spectroscopy (MRS) have shown changes in brain metabolic functions soon after infection, as well as associations between neurocognitive impairment and biological markers of disease activity (e.g., inflammation and immune activation) (Lentz et al., 2011).

The neuropathology of HIV in children differs from that of adults in some respects. Atrophy and white matter abnormalities are similarly observed in the subcortical and frontostriatal systems, including the basal ganglia (Sharer, 2005). Infants infected through MTCT can also show poor brain growth and small head circumference, and basal ganglionic calcifications have been noted on CT scans, particularly in children with presumed intrauterine infection (see Allison, Wolters, & Brouwers, 2009). MRS studies have demonstrated glial activation consistent with inflammatory processes (Prado, Escorsi-Rosset, Cervi, & Santos, 2011), neuronal loss in encephalopathic patients, and a lack of normal developmental metabolic changes in the hippocampus and frontal white matter (Keller et al., 2004).

The finding of a divergence from typical metabolic development raises a key point, namely, the potential interaction of HIV in youth with developmental changes occurring in the brain. The greatest changes occur prenatally and during the first year of life, with rapid brain growth and exuberant synaptic production in the late prenatal and early postnatal period (Stiles, 2008). Untreated HIV infection during this period can have devastating effects on the CNS. Changes in brain structure and cognition continue through childhood, adolescence, and into early adulthood, with a general pattern of a linear increase in white matter, while gray matter volume increases and then declines as pruning occurs. The frontal systems and executive functions subserved by them undergo substantial changes during late childhood and adolescence (Blakemore & Choudhury, 2006). Notably, brain regions undergoing continued myelination into and through adolescence are areas that have been shown to be vulnerable to HIV in adults (Pfefferbaum et al., 2009), raising the concern that the neurophysiological effects of HIV may be magnified in adolescents.

Antiretroviral Medications and the Brain

Although HIV is deleterious to brain structure and function, cART has imparted neuroprotective benefits and changed the landscape of HIV-associated neurocognitive effects among both children (Patel et al., 2009) and adults (Heaton et al., 2011), with significant drops in the rates of HIV-associated encephalopathy (Shanbhag et al., 2005). However, subtle HIV-associated neurocognitive effects persist, and a recent meta-analysis of adult studies suggested that test performance of most HIV patients receiving ART is comparable to those not receiving ART (Al-Khindi, Zakzanis, & Van Gorp, 2011). Among possible explanations for the stable or rising prevalence of continuing subtle neurocognitive effects of HIV during the era of cART are that (1) the reduced morbidity and mortality offered by cART result in greater long-term exposure to the deleterious neurological effects of HIV, (2) neuronal injury resulting from periods of immunosuppression are irreversible despite immune system improvement, (3) brain inflammatory states established early in infection are not responsive to cART, and (4) the possibility that some cART regimens may not adequately treat HIV infection sequestered in the CNS behind the BBB because antiretroviral medications (ARVs) vary in their ability to penetrate the BBB. In addition, although ART offers neuroprotective benefits, some ARVs (e.g., efavirenz) may also be associated with adverse CNS side effects such as attention problems, insomnia, and depression (Marzolini et al., 2001), and concerns about more subtle long-term toxicities of ARVs persist as well.

In addition to the direct effects of long-term exposure to HIV and ART on neurocognitive functioning, indirect effects on cognition may occur through secondary routes, including opportunistic infections of the CNS, hepatotoxicity, cardiovascular effects (e.g., metabolic syndrome), medication-related hypersensitivity reactions, and nephropathy, among others. The neuropsychologist who works with people who have HIV and are on ART should be alert not only to the direct effects that the disease and its treatment may exert on neurocognition but also to the indirect effects.

Neuropsychology of Children and Youth Affected by HIV

Infancy

Infants suffer the most rapid and devastating CNS effects of HIV, particularly when infection occurs in utero as opposed to during birth (McGrath et al., 2006). Assessment of neurodevelopmental status is critically important because interventions to reduce risks and support positive development are likely more effective in changing the developmental trajectory in these early years. In countries where ART is readily available to prevent MTCT, it is unusual for the clinician to encounter infants, toddlers, and preschool-age children with HIV. However, perinatal HIV infection remains a significant global problem and does still occur, at times, in developed countries.

The vast majority of babies born with HIV disease live in sub-Saharan Africa, where 22.5 million people with HIV live, including 2.3 million children (WHO, 2010). In a review of the neurodevelopmental status of these children, Abubakar and colleagues (2008) described severe and persistent deficits in motor development from early infancy, consistent with patterns in early studies in the United States. Moderate delays were noted in mental development, and language delays were noted by 24 months of age. Although motor deficits were most significant, the authors caution that other areas such as language are not as easily assessed in resource-limited countries with few normed tests.

Studies comparing perinatally HIV-exposed but uninfected (PHEU) infants or HIV-unexposed infants with infants with HIV have attempted to disentangle the effects of HIV from those of HIV exposure and the host of confounding risks for infected infants. A study in Kenya (Abubakar, Holding, Newton, Van Baar, & van de Vijver, 2009) showed that children 6–35 months of age with HIV infection had significant motor and psychomotor delays compared with PHEU or unexposed children, with the degree of delay related to weight-for-age and disease severity. In a small study conducted in the Democratic Republic of Congo, Van Rie

and colleagues (2008) found that many of the children aged 18–72 months with perinatally acquired HIV (PHIV) had severe delays in cognitive functioning (60%), language expression (85%), and comprehension (77%). Interestingly, PHEU children showed a higher rate of cognitive delays (40%) than did children unaffected by HIV (24.4%). McGrath and colleagues (2006) also found that both PHIV and PHEU infants in Tanzania demonstrated poorer cognitive and motor development and a slower developmental trajectory than HIV-unexposed children.

Several pertinent issues are raised by studies of infant HIV exposure and infection. First, the long-term effects of active HIV disease are of concern even when followed by immune system recovery; although an issue for adults and older children as well, this may be particularly true when it occurs while the brain is undergoing rapid development during infancy. Furthermore, it is possible that the impairments, particularly motor, have the potential for lasting impact, partly by affecting the major developmental tasks of infancy such as exploration and social interaction.

Second, the cause of the lower functioning in PHEU children compared with unexposed children remains a concern. In countries with less consistent access to optimal ART regimens, PHEU children have higher rates of morbidity and mortality and, possibly, neurodevelopmental deficits (Filteau, 2009). Certainly issues such as poverty, maternal mental and physical health, and early stress associated with poverty and caregiving disruption (Shonkoff et al., 2012) may play a role, but these variables are often well controlled in studies. Possible reasons for the vulnerability of PHEU children are prenatal exposure to HIV and the mother's response to the infection, exposure to ART, and the impact of related variables such as reduced breastfeeding (Filteau, 2009). Potential risks associated with prenatal exposure to ARVs have been controversial. There is highly variable evidence of an increased rate of mitochondrial disorders in children exposed to ART in utero, and some ARVs have been associated with other risks such as preterm delivery (see Heidari et al., 2011, for review). Fortunately, the largest study of PHEU infants to date, with well-controlled confounding and moderator variables, has shown no relationship between any tested ARVs and negative neurodevelopmental outcomes (Williams et al., 2010). Studies examining the relative short- and long-term risks associated with different ARVs are important to provide guidance for medical management and for pregnant women with HIV.

Childhood

The welcome decrease in neurological morbidities and increase in expected lifespan secondary to ART have brought increased concerns about the possible impact of neurocognitive deficits on long-term cognitive, behavioral, and functional outcomes for PHIV+ children. Studies showing effects of even mild deficits on functional areas such as driving (Marcotte et al., 1999) and medication management (Heaton et al., 2004) in adults with HIV reinforce this concern. The early detection of deficits and identification of factors that predict them are keys to instituting interventions or treatment changes to prevent poor functional outcomes. This may be particularly critical in middle childhood when the foundations for learning life skills are established and testing begins to become useful for identification of potential cognitive deficits.

Both global and specific neurocognitive impacts of HIV are noted in preschool and school-age children. The research literature of the cART era suggests that although children with HIV may differ from population norms in terms of global cognitive functioning, as a group they function in the average to low average range and do not differ from children with similar risk factors. This has been observed in children with hemophilia (Hooper et al., 1997) and in neonatal transfusion (Cohen et al., 1991), as well as PHIV. Studies of children with PHIV show specific HIV-related factors that impact level of functioning. Subgroups of PHIV+ children with either current immune compromise or past periods of severe HIV disease, even with subsequent immune recovery with ART, appear to be at risk for impairment in overall cognitive functioning. For example, children aged 3–7 years with a class C diagnosis had lower cognitive scores than either PHEU children or those with HIV and no class C diagnosis, and these differences remained stable over 4 years (Smith et al., 2006). Children with PHIV and CT abnormalities suggesting earlier HIV-related brain disease were also noted to have lower scores than those without abnormalities or uninfected children (Martin et al., 2006). Wood and colleagues (2009) also found that older children with a past class C diagnosis had significantly lower IQ than those without, even though both groups had comparable immune functioning at the time of testing. The results of these studies agree with those reported in the recent literature on adults in showing that past HIV disease severity can be a more potent predictor of global functioning than current immune functioning and that CNS effects resulting from periods of poorly controlled HIV may not recover fully with immune reconstitution.

Domain-specific deficits have also been described in children with HIV and provide clues to the CNS impact of HIV in addition to having clinical significance. Language was one of the first areas noted to be vulnerable to the effects of PHIV. The pattern often seen in children with encephalopathy included declines in expressive language, reduced vocalization, and muteness in the end stages. However, discrepancies with expressive language less developed than receptive language have also been described in children without encephalopathy (Wolters, Brouwers, Civitello, & Moss, 1997). In addition, abnormalities in specific components of language functioning such as semantic priming have been identified (Brouwers et al. 2001). The expressive–receptive language differences have been viewed as part of a general pattern of impairment in expressive behavior, including reduced motor functioning and affect (Moss, Wolters, Brouwers, Hendricks, & Pizzo, 1996).

Rice and colleagues (2012) compared the performance of 252 HIV+ and 105 PHEU children aged 7–17 years and found elevated rates of primary language impairment (LI) in both groups but no group differences. However, secondary LI (LI in the context of more global deficits, hearing deficit, or multilingual exposure) was more common in PHIV+ children who had current severe HIV disease or history of class C diagnosis and in children who had initiated ART before age 6 months, suggesting significant early HIV-related illness. On the whole, the literature suggests language as an area of risk, particularly in children with systemic and other CNS impacts of HIV during development.

Although deficits in visuoperceptual and visuospatial functioning have been noted (Boivin et al., 1995), impairments in these domains have been less generally observed and have received less emphasis in studies of children with HIV. However, problems with fine and gross motor functioning have been commonly observed (Blanchette, Smith, King, Fernandes-Penney, & Read, 2002; Brouwers & Wolters, 2003) and are among the defining features of progressive HIV encephalopathy (Belman, 2008). Psychomotor and processing speed are functions affected relatively early in the course of HIV's impact on the CNS in adults (Reger et al., 2002), and they may also be sensitive indicators of HIV's impact on the CNS in children (Blanchette et al., 2002; Koekkoek, de Sonneville, Wolfs, Licht, & Geelen, 2008; Martin et al., 2006).

Attention deficits in children with HIV have primarily been discussed in the context of attention-deficit/hyperactivity disorder (ADHD). Studies have shown high risk for ADHD in both infected and uninfected children with perinatal HIV exposure, suggesting an effect of demographic, birth, or familial psychiatric factors. Findings regarding increased risk of ADHD for infected children have varied as has the HIV epidemic itself, and methodological approaches to studying it have evolved (Mellins et al., 2003), with a recent study suggesting that youth with HIV are at greater risk for ADHD than PHEU youth (Mellins et al., 2009). A few studies have noted that some specific components of attention may be affected by HIV acquired perinatally (Koekkoek et al., 2008) or through blood products (Watkins et al., 2000), although findings are inconsistent (see Wolters & Brouwers, 2005b). Attention and working memory are areas for which computerized interventions have been developed, and preliminary studies in Africa have begun to suggest the utility of these programs for children with HIV (Boivin et al., 2010).

Memory has been described as one of the functional areas consistently impacted by HIV in adults, but few studies have addressed memory functioning in children with HIV. These studies suggest that children with HIV may differ from controls or normative groups in verbal and visual recall (Blanchette et al., 2002; Jeremy et al., 2005) and that children, like adults, may show the "subcortical" pattern of worse recall than recognition memory (see Allison et al., 2009). Most studies suggest that memory deficits across ages and transmission routes are associated with either current HIV severity or history of class C diagnosis (see Allison et al., 2009, for review). A study using MRS showed significantly lower performance in spatial learning and memory for children with HIV and demonstrated relationships between imaging findings and long-delay spatial memory (Keller et al., 2004). Memory functioning is an important area for future research for children and adolescents with HIV, both to elucidate effects of HIV on the CNS and to provide guidance for interventions to help youth with acquisition of life skills, academic knowledge, and possibly medication adherence.

Executive functioning (EF) is critical to meeting the more complex cognitive and behavioral demands of this age group. Frontosubcortical circuits underlying EF develop throughout childhood and adolescence, with different aspects of EF maturing at various points. The literature on adults has already shown that HIV-related EF deficits contribute to difficulties in essential tasks such as medication management (Heaton et al., 2004), but literature on EF in children with HIV is limited. To date, small studies have found EF impairments in children with HIV compared with controls, as well as relationships with measures of disease severity (Bisiacchi, Suppiej, & Laverda, 2000; Koekkoek et al., 2008). Martin and colleagues (2006) found that PHIV+ children on highly active antiretroviral therapy (HAART) with CT brain scan abnormalities had lower scores on measures of cognitive functioning that were likely to involve EF. They also found that a measure of working memory was related to CD4+ counts and CD4 %. Impairments in EF and their contribution to problems in everyday life are areas of active research for both children and adults with HIV.

A few studies have validated concerns over the ability of children with HIV to meet the cognitive and psychosocial demands of school and home, showing deficits in adaptive behavior in children with PHIV (Gosling, Burns, & Hirst, 2004) and hemophilia with HIV (Nichols et al., 2000), although a recent study demonstrated comparable adaptive functioning between PHIV+ and PHEU children (Smith et al., 2010). Children with HIV are also at risk for low academic achievement (see Brouwers & Wolters, 2003), although studies are mixed regarding whether their performance is lower than that of matched comparison children (e.g., Blanchette et al., 2002; Brackis-Cott, Kang, Dolezal, Abrams, & Mellins, 2009). Nevertheless, children with PHIV have a high rate of receiving special education services in school (Mialky, Vagnoni, & Rutstein, 2001). Both adaptive and academic skills can be affected by other HIV-related factors in addition to cognitive impairments, such as fatigue or missing school due to appointments or illness, and to other environmental, educational, and family influences common in populations affected by HIV.

In a review of studies on psychiatric disorders in children and adolescents with HIV, Scharko (2006) concluded that disorders such as ADHD, anxiety, and depression are common in this population. In a study using psychiatric interviews to make diagnoses according to *Diagnostic and Statistical Manual of Mental Disorders*, fourth edition, criteria, Mellins and colleagues (2006) found high rates of anxiety, attention deficit/hyperactivity, and conduct and oppositional disorders in children aged 9–16 years with PHIV. However, the study did not include a control group, and the authors noted that the rates were similar to those found in other children with demographic risks or chronic health conditions. Children and youth with HIV face numerous risks for emotional and behavioral disturbances, including high rates of familial mental illness and substance use, environmental stress, potential or actual death of a parent, and HIV-related stigma, in addition to living with a disease associated with illness, changes in appearance, pain, and potentially death. Studies comparing children with HIV with PHEU using behavioral rating scales have found similarly high (Gadow et al., 2010; Mellins et al., 2003) rates, and a recent large study found even higher rates of emotional and behavioral issues among the uninfected group (Malee, Tassiopoulos, et al., 2011). Youth with HIV, however, have a higher likelihood of receiving either psychotropic medications or behavioral treatments (Chernoff et al., 2009).

Adolescence.

Adolescence and emerging adulthood comprise challenging developmental periods characterized by experimentation, exploration, and instability in the context of dramatic brain changes. During this period, there is an increasing emphasis on becoming self-sufficient, accepting responsibility for oneself, and making independent decisions. These developmental tasks give greater weight to the fact that HIV infection among adolescents and emerging adults is a major problem; with more HIV infections occurring among those aged 13–29 years than any other age group (CDC, 2008; Hall et al., 2008). Although neurocognition of prepubescent children is particularly susceptible to the effects of HIV due to vulnerability of the young developing brain, adolescence and emerging adulthood are attended by their own combination of risk factors.

Though sparse, research involving adolescents with HIV has begun to shed some light on the effects of HIV in relation to general cognition, adaptive abilities, academic achievement, and language functioning. As reported by Souza and colleagues (2010), even when demonstrating good health and infection control (e.g., normal CD4 count, high rates of undetectable viral load) PHIV+ adolescents in Brazil may be at risk for school failure and drop out. In a study involving children and adolescents aged 9–16 years, PHIV+ youth scored lower than PHEU youth on measures of receptive language (Peabody Picture Vocabulary Test-third edition) and word recognition (Wide Range Achievement Test, third edition Word Reading), though both groups performed poorly, with one-third scoring below the 10th percentile (Brackis-Cott et al., 2009). These findings suggest continuing risk regarding academic performance, a major predictor of adult success, as PHIV+ youth progress through adolescence. In a study involving PHIV+ youth aged 17–23 years, Paramesparan and colleagues (2010) reported high rates (66.7%) of neurocognitive impairment (NCI) among six adolescents who were reportedly in good health (i.e., no active OI or hepatitis C, no history of drug use, and no neurological disease or symptoms). The authors point out that the high rate of NCI in this group exceeds the rate typically observed for behaviorally infected adults, suggesting additional neurocognitive risk among those who are perinatally infected, given that such youth undergo neurodevelopment and maturation in the presence of HIV and ART. There are even fewer reports of cognitive functioning in adolescents with behaviorally acquired HIV. Hosek and colleagues (2005) studied 42 behaviorally infected youth aged 16–25 years and reported that, on average, the youth performed in the borderline range on a test reflecting word knowledge and that 69% of the participants had not yet transitioned to formal or abstract reasoning.

That HIV preferentially attacks the frontal brain regions (Pfefferbaum et al., 2009), which undergo the greatest development during adolescence and emerging adulthood, implies that those infected with HIV are at increased risk for problems with associated functions during that period. Given a natural tendency for maturing youth to experiment and explore, as testing of limits occurs in the context of emerging independence and self-sufficiency, any existing HIV-related deficits in executive functions and social cognition, which might include deficiencies in impulse control and social judgment, could contribute to the display of risky sexual behavior, substance use, and other behaviors that carry significant risks to the HIV-infected individual, as well as others. Possible negative consequences include, for example, nonadherence to antiviral regimens and transmission of HIV to the previously uninfected. Nevertheless, research that specifically investigates neurocognition in adolescents and emerging adults with HIV is scant, and it can only be speculated that executive functions and social cognition may be at particular risk, given that these are functions that are under active development during this period (Blakemore & Choudhury, 2006). Additional research clearly is needed to provide greater depth of coverage, as well as to address areas where the research is nonexistent.

General issues

This brief overview of the literature on the cognitive and behavioral effects of
in children and youth raises several issues. Systematic reviews of the literature
Allison et al., 2009; Sherr, Mueller, & Varrall, 2009; Willen, 2006) highlight some of the
problems with drawing conclusions regarding the effects of HIV on cognitive functioning in children. Studies have used widely varying batteries, with few including
both global measures and either comprehensive or theoretically driven selections of
domain instruments. The development of test batteries that can be used across cultures and in resource limited settings where HIV is most prevalent, while underway, is
in its infancy. Choosing control groups is challenging; whereas comparison with other
perinatally exposed children allows for isolation of the effects of HIV infection itself,
exposure to HIV in utero and to ART pre- and perinatally may also have long-term
developmental effects. The development of more effective medications and drug combinations, as well as shifts in guidance regarding when to initiate treatment, introduce
significant cohort effects and present a constantly changing target for those attempting
to define the CNS effects of HIV during childhood. Longitudinal studies with comprehensive batteries and comparison to both HIV-exposed and unexposed children
are needed.

A general conclusion that can be drawn from the literature, for children as well
as adults, is that control of HIV from the time the person is infected may be critical to preventing later cognitive and neurological sequelae. Research findings consistently demonstrate poorer functioning in individuals who have experienced declines
in immune functioning, especially those significant enough to allow the development of OIs and encephalopathy in particular. Current trends are toward initiation
of treatment early in the course of the disease; in the case of children with perinatal
infection, this means during infancy. Early treatment initiation has the potential to
prevent long-term cognitive problems for children and adolescents and to dramatically increase their quality of life and success as adults in addition to their longev-
ity. Any negative implications of early treatment are, however, magnified for pediatric
and adolescent populations. These individuals face many decades of ART and a longer
period of any drug-related toxicities for the CNS and other systems that impact the
brain, such as the cardiovascular system. Interactions of ART with brain development
may be either positive or negative, or both. The success of ART critically depends on
adherence, which is complicated by stressed and unstable family systems for children
young enough to rely on caregivers for medication administration or its supervision
and by the general tendency of adolescents to display reduced adherence, among other
obstacles. Long-term research studies to evaluate the effects of early treatment initiation and guide the choice of medications are critical.

As with other developmental disorders, the neuropsychologist and others involved
with the child's cognitive and behavioral life should be aware of the general principle
that early insults to the child's brain such as from HIV encephalopathy can have what
appear to be delayed effects as the child ages and more complex cognitive systems and
environmental demands come into play. Relatively subtle chronic deficits can have
significant downstream effects as skills that rely on them are imperfectly mastered,
impacting other higher-level skills in their turn. An HIV-related decrease in cognitive
reserve may also put the individual at greater risk for decline in the face of other brain
insults, such as traumatic brain injury or dementia later in life.

The assessment of children and youth with HIV is complicated by the other cognitive risk factors that are common to populations affected by HIV. For example, substance use, depression (which has clinical features, such as psychomotor slowing, in common with HIV encephalopathy), and side effects of ARV and psychiatric medications may affect cognition adversely and are important differential diagnoses if a child or adolescent shows cognitive decline or a deviation from an expected developmental trajectory. Learning deficits and psychiatric disorders such as ADHD and anxiety disorders (e.g., posttraumatic stress disorder) occur commonly in this population, as do pre- and perinatal risks such as exposure to alcohol and illicit or treatment-related drugs, prematurity and low birth weight, and infections such as cytomegalovirus or malaria. In addition, many children and youth affected by HIV face additional developmental risks related to socioeconomic factors. A disproportionate percentage of their families live in poverty, with attendant housing instability and food insecurity, educational disadvantage and lack of enrichment experiences, exposure to violence and other traumas, reduced access to healthcare services, and greater likelihood of exposure to toxins such as lead. Caregivers may have limited social and family support, which is restricted even more when anticipated stigma discourages disclosure of their HIV status. Children may be affected by losses due to illness, death, and changes in caregiver and by caregiver psychiatric disorders and substance use. It is critical for the clinician or researcher to view the child in the context of his or her complete familial, societal, and biological environment.

The assessment of a child, adolescent, or emerging adult should ideally be completed in collaboration with the patient's HIV care providers. A team approach should include medical providers, psychologists, nurses, nutritionists, and case managers to conference all aspects of the patient's care and include assessment of the familial, social, and educational context of the patient, including important issues of medication adherence, general healthcare, and mental health management. Liaison with psychiatrists, neurologists, occupational and speech/language therapists as well as school personnel is often necessary.

In addition to the medical history that would typically be obtained, it is necessary to gather information about any periods of significant immune compromise, previous diagnoses of HIV encephalopathy, any systemic illnesses such as hepatitis C, or OIs such as encephalitis that could potentially affect cognition and related sequelae such as seizures. Birth history should take note of the mother's health and ART during the pregnancy and birth, as well as other pregnancy and birth complications such as maternal substance abuse and prematurity. Other relevant prenatal infections such as cytomegalovirus, which can impact hearing, should also be noted. The timing of early milestones and particularly any loss of skills should be assessed, and a comprehensive education history included. Previous testing is particularly relevant given potential declines in functioning.

Given the broad range of impairments that have been associated with HIV, administration of a comprehensive battery of tests is warranted. The battery should include measures of general cognitive functioning as well as specific measures of language, attention, working memory, processing speed, motor functioning, both verbal and visual learning and memory, visuospatial and constructional abilities, and executive functions such as planning, problem solving, concept formation, fluency, and inhibition. Tests that provide information about subtle deficits or that relate to potential interventions and accommodations, such as contrasting recall and recognition memory, are particularly useful. Information about behavioral and emotional symptoms related to anxiety, depression, and ADHD should be gathered through questionnaires with caregivers, teachers if possible, and the patient, if old enough, and through structured interviews. Assessment of academic achievement as well as adaptive functions such as daily living and social skills is critical. How the child or youth and family are doing with medication adherence and other healthcare-related tasks is an important area of inquiry for the neuropsychologist, who is able to contribute information to the treatment team regarding potential implications of the youth's cognitive and behavioral functioning and ability to manage his or her medications independently. Finally, contextual factors concerning family functioning and the child or youth's living circumstances and daily stresses may provide insight into points of intervention. Disease or treatment-related symptoms such as fatigue or nausea that may affect test or school performance and activities of daily living should also be assessed.

A careful evaluation of risk behaviors is essential for adolescents with HIV. Substance use, in addition to being common in this population, is relevant not only because of its independent impact on cognitive functioning but also because alcohol and drugs such as methamphetamine, marijuana, and opiates may interact with HIV to affect the central nervous and immune systems (e.g., Gannon et al., 2011). Youth with HIV may use drugs, particularly marijuana, not only to cope with the emotional stresses associated with their HIV infection but also to ameliorate physical symptoms such as nausea and pain associated with HIV and ARVs. Substance use should be a particular concern for differential diagnosis in youth who show cognitive decline. The youth's engagement in sexual risk behaviors and likelihood of HIV transmission or unintended pregnancy are likely to be central issues for the provider team. The neuropsychologist's input regarding the patient's ability to control impulses and manage social interactions such as condom negotiation may be important for counselors working with the youth on strategies to avoid and handle risky situations.

Several considerations can affect the choice of assessment instruments for evaluation of children and youth with HIV. As for any patient with a potentially progressive disease, repeated testing is recommended, particularly when there are reasons to suspect deterioration, because changes have been noted by caregivers, teachers, or care providers or because of HIV disease progression and worsening immune function. It may also be useful to document cognitive gains that can provide evidence of treatment effectiveness. For those reasons, tests with alternate forms or that are less susceptible to practice effects should be included where possible. Finally, more severe HIV disease may be accompanied by motor and sensory deficits that limit the ability of some tests to reflect the patient's functioning and that warrant assessment in their own right as well as appropriate referrals.

In the United States, children and youth affected by HIV are disproportionately members of minority groups and may have limited access to neurodevelopmental services. The degree to which a test is free of cultural bias and has norms based on a sample with appropriate demographic diversity is an important consideration. The issue of appropriate assessment instruments is particularly important in all developmental monitoring in international settings (Boivin & Giordani, 2009), where much of the research guiding patient care is occurring. The impact of culture on neuropsychological assessment in general has not been well studied (Byrd, Arentoft, Scheiner,

Westerveld, & Baron, 2008). Sternberg (2004) notes that adapting or even renorming tasks is inadequate because one cannot assume different cultures use the same neurocognitive process to solve a task. Sherr and colleagues (2009) note that the lack of systematic and appropriate measurements across studies makes interpretation of the data and implications for interventions impossible. Fortunately, standards for adapting assessment tools (Hambleton, 2005; Malda et al., 2008) are being created, including assessment toolkits for resource-limited countries (Fernald, Kariger, Engle, & Raikes, 2009) and adaptations for assessing young children affected by HIV (Kammerer, Isquith, & Lundy, in press). A goal for research and clinical practice across countries and cultures would be for reliable and valid universal assessment tools that measure important neurocognitive domains.

INTERVENTION AND TREATMENT GAINS

The gains in medical treatment of HIV since the early years of the epidemic have been enormous, transforming it, where ART is readily available, from a fatal illness associated with devastating CNS impacts to a chronic illness with more subtle effects on neurocognition. The development of more accurate indicators of viral activity and immune system functioning has allowed clinicians better optimization of treatment, both in deciding when to initiate ART and in targeting drugs based on resistance profiles and genetic characteristics of the patient.

Despite this progress, significant challenges remain. Thus far, studies of CNS-targeted medications have largely been disappointing (McArthur, Steiner, Sacktor, & Nath, 2010). The fact that the effects of HIV in the brain can differ from those in other body systems raises the possibility that cART is less effective in the CNS. However, direct measures of HIV activity in the brain have been elusive, and despite recent neuroimaging studies, assessment of cognitive functioning and neurological symptoms remains among the best indicators of CNS disease progression. As efforts continue to optimize ART regimens for better penetration across the BBB balanced with concerns related to toxicity and long-term side effects (Gannon et al., 2011; Letendre, 2011), sensitive neurocognitive measures of CNS functioning are likely to continue playing a role in combination with neuroimaging and other biomarkers. Similar issues for children and adolescents with HIV are magnified by the complexities of measuring disease progression and treatment gains against a background of developmental change. Such issues require the input of neuropsychologists with knowledge of brain development and training and experience in pediatric and adolescent assessment. The long-term risk of CNS problems in these young people may be affected by poorly understood interactions, with changes associated with aging and cardiovascular and other effects of ART and HIV.

In a similar vein, the ability to almost eliminate MTCT of HIV through ART has been an extraordinarily powerful intervention in the war against HIV. Access to ARVs for treatment or prevention of transmission must continue to be expanded in countries with limited resources. At the same time, the potential impact of ARV exposure on these PHEU children must continue to be researched to ensure the ARVs chosen are the safest for their physical health and neurocognitive outcomes.

Behavioral and cognitive interventions fall into the following two categories: (1) those with direct effects on functional outcomes and (2) those with indirect effects. For children and youth, educational interventions such as access to special education resources fall into the first category. Computerized programs designed to increase working memory or other cognitive functions are beginning to play a role in the treatment of children with HIV (Boivin et al., 2010). Interventions with indirect effects would include, for example, those designed to increase ART effectiveness through improved medication adherence, treatments for psychiatric disorders with cognitive impacts such as ADHD or depression, and treatment for abuse of alcohol or other substances that can themselves affect cognition or possibly interact with HIV to do so.

Neurocognitive impairments are, in their turn, an important consideration for interventions related to behavioral and emotional issues for children and adolescents with HIV, as well as for planning for transition to adulthood. Although the understanding of psychosocial needs of children and youth with HIV has shown strong advances, treatment programs for these issues need expansion both in resource-rich (Steele, Nelson, & Cole, 2007) and resource-limited (Earls, Raviola, & Carlson, 2008; Petersen et al., 2010) countries.

For children with HIV, developmental stage and delays are relevant in individual and family counseling for issues such as dealing with loss and, importantly, HIV disclosure. Disclosure of the parent or child's HIV status, or that of an adolescent exploring his or her emerging sexuality, is naturally a complex and highly emotional task, given the issues of stigma, lack of understanding, possibility of poor choices in sharing with others, and potential stress or depression, as well as possible rejection by a sexual partner. Yet, disclosure of HIV status has long been supported by the American Academy of Pediatrics (1999) due to the known eventual benefits for mental health and important issues such as adherence to medication and safe sexual practices (Mellins et al., 2002). In a review of the history and current status of HIV disclosure, Wiener and colleagues (2007) describe low rates of disclosure and find no consensus on the age or outcomes of disclosure but do note principles that should be employed in the disclosure process. Disclosure must be seen as a dynamic process that takes into account the status of the whole family, including child developmental status and health as well as family readiness (Lesch et al., 2007). Despite the importance of disclosure, little is written which accounts for potentially differing cultural needs and implications of disclosure in resource-limited countries (Vaz et al., 2011). For adolescents, discussion of strategies for disclosure to partners is recommended as part of transition to adult care (Dowshen & D'Angelo, 2011).

Frequently, youth with PHIV have been followed closely by a pediatric healthcare team specialized in HIV that has provided considerable structure for healthcare management. It is recommended that youth transition to adult healthcare providers by the early 20s. However, studies have documented barriers to accessing adult services, and these barriers must be addressed to facilitate this transition (Wiener, Kohrt, Battles, & Pao, 2011). In developing transition plans, it is necessary to consider the current youth needs (Andiman, 2011) and to follow best practices that account for the developmental needs of this population (Fair, Sullivan & Gato, 2010). A gradual, planned transition is necessary to ensure that necessary skills are in place but also because the youth with HIV often has strong attachments to the pediatric team.

For adolescents with HIV, acquisition of the skills necessary for a successful transition to adulthood can be complicated by the presence of cognitive impairments. These skills include those that are important for any adolescent, such as academic achievement and training and preparation for the job force. Adolescents with HIV who grew up in environments with economic disadvantage or with familial substance use or mental health disorders face additional challenges in accessing academic and skills training opportunities and may have low motivation to do so. Identification and intervention regarding sexual and substance use risk behaviors and counseling on pregnancy prevention also take on particular significance when the adolescent has HIV.

Learning to manage their own healthcare is critical for youth with HIV, and medication adherence, in particular, is both a key to their survival and an area of great difficulty for many adolescents. Adherence to ART is challenging for a variety of reasons, including significant adverse side effects, difficult dosing schedules or requirements, youth and/or family stress, substance use, psychiatric issues, youth behavioral problems, lack of clarity about who is responsible for adherence, and a desire not to be reminded of HIV or to have others notice the medication (Malee et al., 2011; Martin et al., 2007; Williams et al., 2006.) However, a high rate of adherence (≥95%) is necessary for treatment success and to reduce the likelihood of HIV transmission. For adults, cognitive impairment has been documented to contribute to poor adherence (Ettenhofer et al., 2010), with impairments in particular functions such as prospective memory, which is especially predictive of poor adherence. There is evidence of a reciprocal relationship wherein reduced cognitive functioning can lead to diminished medication adherence; this, in turn, leads to further neuropsychological declines (Ettenhofer et al., 2010). Although the relationship is less established for children and youth, it appears that cognitive and academic problems may also place them at risk for poor adherence in some cases (Malee et al., 2009; Williams et al., 2006). Transitioning responsibility for medication adherence to adolescents is a vital and complex process that can benefit from the input of the neuropsychologist.

CURRENT RESOURCES

Over the course of the HIV epidemic, a variety of resources related to HIV treatment and prevention have become available. Unfortunately, treatment and prevention resources do not have equal global distribution, and economic and societal factors prevent many people from accessing them. Accessing resources related to HIV care can be complicated by familial factors such as changes in caregivers, disorganization, stress, and psychiatric and substance use disorders. Consequently, community and mental health treatment resources may be a necessary first step. Youth with cognitive impairment or low educational achievement may require assistance in comprehending or reading resources if available. This is a factor that is not always considered when they are given written material or instructions. Nevertheless, the enormous strides in information technology that have occurred simultaneously with advances in HIV care now enable widespread access to information about HIV risks, prevention, effects, and treatment. Information can be shared through the Internet. In addition, such advances allow individuals with HIV to connect with others for support and social and political networking.

CONCLUSIONS

Since the time when HIV was first identified more than 30 years ago, our knowledge and treatment of this complex retrovirus have advanced to the point that many people are able to live with it as a chronic illness. Unfortunately, a vaccine to prevent HIV infection is not likely to be available soon, and HIV transmission continues to occur, despite interventions using information distribution, behavioral strategies, and prophylactic medications. On a global scale, the impact of HIV on children and adolescents remains enormous, and research has demonstrated that the population of youth affected by HIV is at high risk for cognitive, behavioral, and functional problems from a variety of etiologies. With an emerging focus on helping these youth gain the skills needed to perform self-care tasks necessary to survive and to make the transition to independent and successful adulthood, the need for contributions from neuropsychologists has not decreased but has, in fact, grown. The neuropsychologist's knowledge about the development of the child's brain, cognitive impairments that impede meeting the complex demands of adolescence and emerging adulthood, complexities of cultural and environmental influences, and the potential role of the many contributing factors other than HIV in producing the thinking and behaving youth seen in the clinic are invaluable.

REFERENCES

Abubakar, A., Holding, P., Newton, C. R., van Baar, A., & van de Vijver, F. J. (2009). The role of weight for age and disease stage in poor psychomotor outcome of HIV-infected children in Kilifi, Kenya. *Developmental Medicine and Child Neurology, 51,* 968–973.

Abubakar, A., Van Baar, A., Van de Vijver, F. J. R., Holding, P., & Newton, C. R. J. C. (2008). Paediatric HIV and neurodevelopment in sub-Saharan Africa: A systematic review. *Tropical Medicine & International Health, 13,* 880–887. doi: 10.1111/j.1365-3156.2008.02079.x

Al-Khindi, T., Zakzanis, K. K., & van Gorp, W. G. (2011). Does antiretroviral therapy improve HIV-associated cognitive impairment? A quantitative review of the literature. *Journal of the International Neuropsychological Society, 17,* 956–969. doi:10.1017/S1355617711000968

Allison, S., Wolters, P., & Brouwers, P. (2009). Youth with HIV/AIDS: Neurobehavioral consequences. In R. H. Paul, N. Sacktor, V. Valcour, & K. T. Tashima (Eds.), *HIV and the brain: New challenges in the modern era* (pp. 187–211). New York: Humana Press.

American Academy of Pediatrics Committee on Pediatrics AIDS. (1999). Disclosure of illness status to children and adolescents with HIV infection. *Pediatrics, 103,* 164–166.

Andiman, W. A. (2011). Transition from pediatric to adult healthcare services for young adults with chronic illnesses: The special case of human immunodeficiency virus infection. *Journal of Pediatrics, 159,* 714–719.

Antinori, A., Arendt, G., Becker, J. T., Brew, B. J., Byrd, D. A., Cherner, M., ... Wojna, V. E. (2007). Updated research nosology for HIV-associated neurocognitive disorders. *Neurology, 69,* 1789–1799. doi: 10.1212/01.WNL.0000287431.88658.8b

Belman, A. (2008). Pediatric neuro-AIDS. In K. Goodkin, P. Shapshak, & A. Verma (Eds.), *The spectrum of neuro-AIDS disorders: Pathophysiology, diagnosis, and treatment* (pp. 455–471). Washington, DC: ASM Press.

Bisiacchi, P. S., Suppiej, A., & Laverda, A. (2000). Neuropsychological evaluation of neurologically asymptomatic HIV-infected children. *Brain and Cognition, 43,* 49–52.

Blakemore, S., & Choudhury, S. (2006). Development of the adolescent brain: Implications for executive function and social cognition. *Journal of Child Psychology and Psychiatry, 47,* 296–312.

Blanchette, N., Smith, M. L., King, S., Fernandes-Penney, A., & Read, S. (2002). Cognitive development in school-age children with vertically transmitted HIV infection. *Developmental Neuropsychology, 21,* 223–241. doi: 10.1207/s15326942dn2103_1

Boivin, M. J., Busman, R. A., Parikh, S. M., Bangirana, P., Page, C. F., Opoka, R. O., & Giordani, B. (2010). A pilot study of the neuropsychological benefits of computerized cognitive rehabilitation in Ugandan children with HIV. *Neuropsychology, 24,* 667–673. doi: 10.1037/a0019312

Boivin, M. J. & Giordani, B. (2009). Neuropsychological assessment of African children: Evidence for a universal basis to cognitive ability. In J. Y. Chiao (Ed.), *Cultural neuroscience: Cultural influences on brain function* (pp. 113–135). New York: Elsevier Publications.

Boivin, M. J., Green, S. D., Davies, A. G., Giordani, B., Mokili, J. K., & Cutting, W. A. (1995). A preliminary evaluation of the cognitive and motor effects of pediatric HIV infection in Zairian children. *Health Psychology, 14,* 13–21.

Brackis-Cott, E., Kang, E., Dolezal, C., Abrams, E. J., & Mellins, C. A. (2009). The impact of perinatal HIV infection on older school-aged children's and adolescents' receptive language and word recognition skills. *AIDS Patient Care STDS, 23,* 415–421. doi: 10.1089/apc.2008.0197

Brouwers, P., & Wolters, P. (2003). HIV-induced central nervous system and developmental abnormalities in childhood. In W. Shearer & C. I. Hanson (Eds.), *Medication management of AIDS in children* (pp. 227–247). Philadelphia, PA: Saunders.

Brouwers, P., Van Engelen, M., Lalonde, F., Perez, L., De Haan, E., Wolters, P., & Martin, A. (2001). Abnormally increased semantic priming in children with symptomatic HIV-1 disease: Evidence for impaired development of semantics? *Journal of the International Neuropsychological Society, 7,* 491–501.

Brown, L. K., Danovsky, M. B., Lourie, K. J., DiClemente, R. J., & Ponton, L. E. (1997). Adolescents with psychiatric disorders and the risk of HIV. *Journal of the American Academy of Child and Adolescent Psychiatry, 36,* 1609–1617. doi: 10.1016/s0890-8567(09)66573-4

Byrd, D., Arentoft, A., Scheiner, D., Westerveld, M., & Baron, I. S. (2008). State of multicultural neuropsychological assessment in children: Current research issues. *Neuropsychology Review, 18,* 214–222.

Centers for Disease Control and Prevention (CDC). (1994). Revised classification system for human immunodeficiency virus infection in children less than 13 years of age. *Morbidity and Morality Weekly Report, 43,* 1–10.

Centers for Disease Control and Prevention (CDC). (August, 2008). CDC HIV/AIDS Fact Sheet: Estimates of New HIV Infections in the United States. Atlanta, GA: U.S. Department of Health and Human Services, Centers for Disease Control and Prevention.

Chernoff, M., Nachman, S., Williams, P., Brouwers, P., Heston, J., Hodge, J.,...Gadow, K. D.; and the IMPAACT P1055 Study Team. (2009). Mental health treatment patterns in perinatally HIV-infected youth and controls. *Pediatrics, 124,* 627–636.

Cohen, S. E., Mundy, T., Karassik, B., Lieb, L., Ludwig, D. D., & Ward, J. (1991). Neuropsychological functioning in human immunodeficiency virus type 1 seropositive children infected through neonatal blood transfusion. *Pediatrics, 88,* 58–68.

Connor, E. M., Sperling, R. S., Gelber, R., Kiselev, P., Scott, G., O'Sullivan, M. J.,...Balsley, J. (1994). Reduction of maternal-infant transmission of human immunodeficiency virus type with zidovudine treatment. *New England Journal of Medicine, 331,* 1173–1180.

Cooper, E. R., Charurat, M., Mofenson, L., Hanson, I. C., Pitt, J., Diaz, C.,...Blattner, W. (2002). Combination antiretroviral strategies for the treatment of pregnant HIV-1-infected women and prevention of perinatal HIV-1 transmission. *Journal of Acquired Immune Deficiency Syndrome, 29,* 484–494.

Donegan, E. (2003). Transmission of HIV by blood, blood products, tissue transplantation, and artificial insemination. HIV InSite Knowledge Base Chapter. Accessed: December 8, 2011. Available at: http://hivinsite.ucsf.edu/InSite?page=kb-07–02–09

Dowshen, N., & D'Angelo, L. (2011). Health care transition for youth living with HIV/AIDS. *Pediatrics, 128,* 762–771.

Earls, F., Raviola, G., & Carlson, M (2008). Promoting child and adolescent mental health in the context of the HIV pandemic with a focus on sub-Saharan Africa. *Journal of Child Psychology and Psychiatry, 49*, 295–312.

Ellis, R., Badiee, J., Vaida, F., Letendre, S., Heaton, R., Clifford, D.,…Grant, I., for the CHARTER Group. (2011). Nadir CD4 is a predictor of HIV neurocognitive impairment in the era of combination antiretroviral therapy. *AIDS, 25*, 1747–1751.

Ettenhofer, M. L., Foley, J., Behdin, N., Levine, A. J., Castellon, S. A., & Hinkin, C. H. (2010). Reaction time variability in HIV-positive individuals. *Archives of Clinical Neuropsychology, 25*, 791–798. doi: 10.1093/arclin/acq064

Fair, C. D., Sullivan, K., & Gatto, A. (2010). Best practices in transitioning youth with HIV: Perspectives of pediatric and adult infectious disease care providers. *Psychology, Health & Medicine, 15*, 515–527.

Fernald, L. C. H., Kariger, P., Engle, P., & Raikes, A. (2009). *Examining early child development in low-income countries: A toolkit for the assessment of children in the first five years of life*. Washington, DC: World Bank.

Filteau, S. (2009). The HIV-exposed, uninfected African child. *Tropical Medicine and International Health, 14*, 276–287.

Gadow, K. D., Chernoff, M., Williams, P. L., Brouwers, P., Morse, E., Heston, J.,…Nachman, S. (2010). Co-occuring psychiatric symptoms in children perinatally infected with HIV and peer comparison sample. *Journal of Developmental and Behavioral Pediatrics, 31*, 116–128.

Gannon, P., Khan, M. Z., & Kolson, D. L. (2011). Current understanding of HIV-associated neurocognitive disorders pathogenesis. *Current Opinion in Neurology, 24*, 275–283. doi: 10.1097/WCO.0b013e32834695fb

Gosling, A. S., Burns, J., & Hirst, F. (2004). Children with HIV in the UK: A longitudinal study of adaptive and cognitive Functioning. *Clinical Child Psychology and Psychiatry, 9*, 25–37. doi: 10.1177/1359104504039168

Hall, H.I., Song, R., Rhodes, P., Prejean, J., An, Q., Lee, L.M.,…Janssen, R. S.; and the HIV Incidence Surveillance Group. (2008). Estimation of HIV incidence in the United States. *Journal of the American Medical Association, 300*, 520–529.

Hambleton, R. K. (2005). Issues, designs and technical guidelines for adapting tests into multiple languages and cultures. In R. K. Hambleton, P. F. Merenda and C. D. Spielberger (Eds.), *Adapting psychological and educational tests for cross-cultural assessment* (pp. 3–38). Mahwah, NJ: Lawrence Erlbaum.

Heaton, R. K., Marcotte, T. D., Mindt, M. R., Sadek, J., Moore, D. J., Bentley, H.,…Grant, I.; and the HNRC Group. (2004). The impact of HIV-associated neuropsychological impairment on everyday functioning. *Journal of the International Neuropsychological Society, 10*, 317–331.

Heaton, R. K., Franklin, D. R., Ellis, R. J., McCutchan, J. A., Letendre, S. L., Leblanc, S.,…Grant, I. (2011). HIV-associated neurocognitive disorders before and during the era of combination antiretroviral therapy: Differences in rates, nature, and predictors. *Journal of Neurovirology, 17*, 3–16. doi: 10.1007/s13365-010-0006-1

Heidari, S., Mofenson, L., Cotton, M. F., Marlink, R., Cahn, P., & Katabira, E. (2011). Antiretroviral drugs for preventing mother-to-child transmission of HIV: A review of potential effects on HIV-exposed but uninfected children. *Journal of Acquired Immune Deficiency Syndrome, 57*, 290–296.

Hooper, S. R., Whitt, J. K., Tennison, M. B., Burchinal, M., Gold, S. H., & Hall, C. D. (1997). HIV-infected children with hemophilia: One- and two-year follow-up of neuropsychological functioning. *Pediatric AIDS HIV Infectious Disease, 8*, 91–97.

Hosek, S. G., Harper, G. W., & Domanico, R. (2005) Predictors of medication adherence among HIV-infected youth. *Psychology, Health & Medicine, 10*, 166–179.

Jeremy, R. J., Kim, S., Nozyce, M., Nachman, S., McIntosh, K., Pelton, S. I.,...Stanley, K.; Pediatric AIDS Clinical Trials Group (PACTG) 338 & 377 Study Teams. (2005). Neuropsychological functioning and viral load in stable antiretroviral therapy-experienced HIV-infected children. *Pediatrics, 115*, 380–387. doi: 10.1542/peds.2004-1108

Kammerer, B., Isquith, P., & Lundy, S. (in press). Approaches to assessment of very young children in Africa in the context of HIV. In M. Boivin & B. Giordani (Eds.). *Neuropsychology of children in Africa: Risk and resilience.* New York: Springer Publishing.

Keller, M. A., Venkatraman, T. N., Thomas, A., Deveikis, A., LoPresti, C., Hayes, J.,...Chang, L. (2004). Altered neurometabolite development in HIV-infected children: Correlation with neuropsychological tests. *Neurology, 62*, 1810–1817.

Koekkoek, S., de Sonneville, L. M., Wolfs, T. F., Licht, R., & Geelen, S. P. (2008). Neurocognitive function profile in HIV-infected school-age children. *European Journal Paediatric Neurology, 12*, 290–297.

Lentz, M. R., Kim, W., Kim, H., Soulas, C., Lee, V., Venna, N.,...González, R. G. (2011). Alterations in brain metabolism during the first year of HIV infection. *Journal of Neurovirology, 17*, 220–229. doi 10.1007/s13365–011–0030–9

Lesch, A., Swartz, L., Kagee, A., Moodley, K., Kafaar, Z., Myer, L., & Cotton, M. (2007). Paediatric HIV/AIDS disclosure: Towards a developmental and process-oriented approach. *AIDS Care, 19*, 811–816.

Letendre, S. (2011). Central nervous system complications in HIV disease: HIV-associated neurocognitive disorder. *Topics in Antiviral Medicine, 19*, 137–142.

Malda, M., Van De Vijver, F., Srinivasan, K., Transler, C., Sukumar, P., & Rao, P. (2008). Adapting a cognitive test for a different culture: An illustration of qualitative procedures. *Psychology Science Quarterly, 50*, 451–468.

Malee, K. M., Tassiopoulos, K., Huo, Y., Siberry, G., Williams, P. L., Hazra, R.,...Mellins, C. A. (2011). Mental health functioning among children and adolescents with perinatal HIV infection and perinatal HIV exposure. *AIDS Care.* doi: 10.1080/09540121.2011.575120

Malee, K., Williams, P., Montepiedra, G., McCabe, M., Nichols, S., Sirois, P. A.,...Kammerer, B. (2011). Medication adherence in children and adolescents with HIV infection: Associations with behavioral impairment. *AIDS Patient Care STDS, 25*, 191–200. doi: 10.1089/apc.2010.0181

Malee, K., Williams, P. L., Montepiedra, G., Nichols, S., Sirois, P. A., Storm, D.,...Kammerer, B. (2009). The role of cognitive functioning in medication adherence of children and adolescents with HIV infection. *Journal of Pediatric Psychology, 34*, 164–175. doi: 10.1093/jpepsy/jsn068

Marcotte, T. D., Heaton, R. K., Wolfson, T., Taylor, M. J., Alhassoon, O., Arfaa, K., Grant, I., & the HNRC Group. (1999). The impact of HIV-related neuropsychological dysfunction on driving behavior. *Journal of the International Neuropsychological Society, 7*, 579–592.

Martin, S., Elliott-DeSorbo, D. K., Wolters, P. L., Toledo-Tamula, M. A., Roby, G.,...Wood, L. V. (2007). Patient, caregiver and regimen characteristics associated with adherence to highly active antiretroviral therapy among HIV-infected children and adolescents. *Pediatric Infectious Disease Journal, 26*, 61–67.

Martin, S. C., Wolters, P. L., Toledo-Tamula, M. A., Zeichner, S. L., Hazra, R., & Civitello, L. (2006). Cognitive functioning in school-aged children with vertically acquired HIV infection being treated with highly active antiretroviral therapy (HAART). *Developmental Neuropsychology, 30*, 633–657. doi: 10.1207/s15326942dn3002_1

Marzolini, C., Telenti, A., Decosterd, L. A., Greub, G., Biollaz, J., & Buclin, T. (2001). Efavirenz plasma levels can predict treatment failure and central nervous system side effects in HIV-1 infected patients. *AIDS, 15*, 71–75.

McArthur, J. C., Steiner, J., Sacktor, N., & Nath, A. (2010). Human immunodeficiency virus-associated neurocognitive disorders: Mind the gap. *Annals of Neurology, 67*, 699–714.

McGrath, N., Fawzi, W. W., Bellinger, D., Robins, J., Msamanga, G. I., Manji, K., & Tronick, E. (2006). The timing of mother-to-child transmission of human immunodeficiency virus infection and the neurodevelopment of children in Tanzania. *Pediatric Infectious Disease Journal, 25*, 47–52.

Mellins, C. A., Brackis-Cott, E., Dolezal, C., & Abrams, E. J. (2006). Psychiatric disorders in youth with perinatally acquired Human Immunodeficiency Virus infection. *Pediatric Infectious Disease Journal, 25*, 432–437. doi: 10.1097/01.inf.0000217372.10385.2a

Mellins, C., Brackis-Cott, E., Dolezal, C., Richards, A., Nicholas, S., & Abrams, E. (2002) Patterns of status disclosure to perinatally HIV-infected children and subsequent mental health outcomes. *Clinical Child Psychology and Psychiatry. 7*, 101–114.

Mellins, C., Brackis-Cott, E., Leu, C., Elkington, K. S., Dolezal, C., Wiznia, A.,...Abrams, E. J. (2009). Rates and types of psychiatric disorders in perinatally human immunodeficiency virus-infected youth and seroreverters. *Journal of Child Psychology and Psychiatry, 50*, 1131–1138.

Mellins, C. A., Smith, R., O'Driscoll, P., Magder, L. S., Brouwers, P., Chase, C.,...Matzen, E. (2003). High rates of behavioral problems in perinatally HIV-infected children are not linked to HIV disease. *Pediatrics, 111*, 384–393.

Mialky, E., Vagnoni, J., & Rutstein, R. (2001). School-age children with perinatally acquired HIV infection: Medical and psychosocial issues in a Philadelphia cohort. *AIDS Patient Care and STDs, 15*, 575–579.

Moss, H. A., Wolters, P.L., Brouwers, P., Hendricks, M. L., & Pizzo, P. A. (1996). Impairment of expressive behavior in pediatric HIV-infected patients with evidence of CNS disease. *Journal of Pediatric Psychology, 21*, 379–400.

Nichols, S., Mahoney, E. M., Sirois, P. A., Bordeaux, J. D., Stehbens, J. A., Loveland, K. A., & Amodei, N. (2000). HIV-associated changes in adaptive, emotional, and behavioral functioning in children and adolescents with hemophilia: Results from the Hemophilia Growth and Development Study. *Journal of Pediatric Psychology, 25*, 545–556.

Paramesparan, Y., Garvey, L. J., Ashby, J., Foster, C. J., Fidler, S., & Winston, A. (2010). High rates of asymptomatic neurocognitive impairment in vertically acquired HIV-1-infected adolescents surviving to adulthood. *Journal of Acquired Immune Deficiency Syndrome, 55*, 134–136.

Patel, K., Ming, X., Williams, P. L., Robertson, K. R., Oleske, J. M., & Seage, G. R., 3rd. (2009). Impact of HAART and CNS-penetrating antiretroviral regimens on HIV encephalopathy among perinatally infected children and adolescents. *AIDS, 23*, 1893–1901. doi: 10.1097/QAD.0b013e32832dc041

Petersen, I., Bhana, A., Myeza, N., Alicea, S., John, S., Holst, H.,...Mellins, C. (2010). Psychosocial challenges and protective influences for socio-emotional coping of HIV+ adolescents in South Africa: A qualitative investigation. *AIDS Care, 1*, 1–9.

Pfefferbaum, A., Rosenbloom, M. J., Rohlfing, T., Kemper, C. A., Deresinski, S., & Sullivan, E. (2009). Frontostriatal fiber bundle compromise in HIV infection without dementia. *AIDS, 23*, 1977–1985.

Prado, P. T., Escorsi-Rosset, S., Cervi, M. C., & Santos, A. C. (2011). Image evaluation of HIV encephalopathy: A multimodal approach using quantitative MR techniques. *Neuroradiology*. doi: 10.1007/s00234-011-0869-8

Reger, M., Welsh, R., Razani, J., Martin, D. J., & Boone, K. B. (2002). A meta-analysis of the neuropsychological sequelae of HIV infection. *Journal of the International Neuropsychological Society, 8*, 410–424.

Rice, M. L., Buchanan, A. L., Siberry, G. K., Malee, K. M., Zeldow, B., Frederick, T.,...Williams, P. L. for the Pediatric HIV/AIDS Cohort Study (PHACS). (2012). Language impairment in perinatally HIV-infected children and HIV-exposed uninfected children. *Journal of Developmental and Behavioral Pediatrics, 33, 112–123.*

Scharko, A. M. (2006). DSM psychiatric disorders in the context of pediatric HIV/AIDS. *AIDS Care, 18,* 441–445.

Shanbhag, M. C., Rutstein, R. M., Zaoutis, T., Zhao, H., Chao, D., & Radcliffe, J. (2005). Neurocognitive functioning in pediatric human immunodeficiency virus infection: Effects of combined therapy. *Archives of Pediatric and Adolescent Medicine, 159,* 651–656. doi: 10.1001/archpedi.159.7.651

Sharer, L. R. (2005). Neuropathological aspects of HIV-1 infection in children. In H. E. Gendelman, I. Grant, I. P. Everall, S. A. Lipton, & S. Swindells (Eds.), *The neurology of AIDS: Second edition* (pp. 659–666). Oxford: Oxford University Press.

Sherr, L., Mueller, J., & Varrall, R. (2009). A systematic review of cognitive development and child human immunodeficiency virus infection. *Psychology, Health, and Medicine, 14,* 387–404.

Shonkoff, J. P., Garner, A. S., The Committee on Psychosocial Aspects of Child and Family Health, Committee on Early Childhood, Adoption, and Dependent Care, and Section on Developmental and Behavioral Pediatrics,…, Wood, D. L. (2012). The lifelong effects of early childhood adversity and toxic stress. *Pediatrics, 129,* e232. doi: 10.1542/peds.2011-2663

Smith, R., Malee, K., Leighty, R., Brouwers, P., Mellins, C., Hittelman, J.,…Blasini, I. (2006). Effects of perinatal HIV infection and associated risk factors on cognitive development among young children. *Pediatrics, 117,* 851–862. doi: 10.1542/peds.2005-0804

Smith, R., Chernoff, M., Rutstein, R., Malee, K., Garvie, P., Kammerer, B.,…Wilkins, M., for the Pediatric HIV/AIDS Cohort Study (PHACS). (2010). The long-term impact of HIV disease severity on cognitive and adaptive functioning during childhood and adolescence. 17th Conference on Retroviruses and Opportunistic Infections (CROI 2010), San Francisco, CA, February 16–19, 2010 (Abstract #861).

Souza, E., Santos, N., Valentini, S., Silva, G., & Falbo, A. (2010). Long-term follow-up outcomes of perinatally HIV-infected adolescents: Infection control but school failure. *Journal of Tropical Pediatrics, 56,* 421–426.

Steele, R. G., Nelson, T. D., & Cole, B. P. (2007). Psychosocial functioning of children with AIDS and HIV infection: Review of the literature from a socioecological framework. *Journal of Developmental and Behavioral Pediatrics, 28,* 58–69.

Sternberg, R. J. (2004). Culture and intelligence. *American Psychologist, 59,* 325–338.

Stiles, J. (2008). *The fundamentals of brain development: Integrating nature and nurture.* Cambridge, MA and London, England: Harvard University Press.

Tate, D. F., Conley, J. J., Meier, D. S., Navia, B. A., Cohen, R., & Guttmann, C. R. G. (2009). Neuroimaging among HIV-infected patients: Current knowledge and future directions. In R. H. Paul, N. Sacktor, V. Valcour, & K. T. Tashima (Eds.), *HIV and the brain: New challenges in the modern era* (pp. 187–211). New York: Humana Press.

Van Rie, A., Mupuala, A., & Dow, A. (2008). Impact of the HIV/AIDS epidemic on the neurodevelopment of preschool-aged children in Kinshasa, Democratic Republic of the Congo. *Pediatrics, 122,* e123–e128. doi: 10.1542/peds.2007-2558

Vaz, L. M., Maman, S., Eng, E., Barbarin, O. A., Tshikandu, T., & Behets, F. (2011). Patterns of disclosure of HIV status to infected children in sub-Sharan Africa. *Journal of Developmental and Behavioral Pediatrics, 32,* 307–315.

Watkins, J. M., Cool, V. A., Usner, D., Stehbens, J. A., Nichols, S., Loveland, K. A.,…Nuechterlein, K. H. (2000). Attention in HIV-infected children: Results from the Hemophilia Growth and Development Study. *Journal of the International Neuropsychological Society, 6,* 443–454.

Wiener, L., Kohrt, B., Battles, B., & Pao, M. (2011). The HIV experience: Youth identified barriers for transitioning from pediatric to adult care. *Journal of Pediatric Psychology, 36*, 141–154.

Wiener, L., Mellins, C., Marhefka, S., & Battles, H. B. (2007). Disclosure of an HIV diagnosis to children: History, current research, and future directions. *Journal of Developmental and Behavioral Pediatrics, 28*, 155–166.

Willen, E. J. (2006). Neurocognitive outcomes in pediatric HIV. *Mental Retardation and Developmental Disabilities Research Reviews, 12*, 223–228. doi: 10.1002/mrdd.20112

Williams, P. L., Marino, M., Malee, K., Brogly, S., Hughes, M. D., Mofenson, L. M.; PACTG 219C Team. (2010). Neurodevelopment and in utero antiretroviral exposure of HIV-exposed uninfected infants. *Pediatrics, 125*, e250–e260.

Williams, P. L., Storm, D., Montepiedra, G., Nichols, S., Kammerer, B., Sirois, P. A., . . . Malee, K. (2006). Predictors of adherence to antiretroviral medications in children and adolescents with HIV infection. *Pediatrics, 118*, e1745–e1757. doi: 10.1542/peds.2006-0493

Wilson, C. M., Wright, P. F., Safrit, J. T., & Rudy, B. (2010). Epidemiology of HIV infection and risk in adolescents and youth. *JAIDS Journal of Acquired Immune Deficiency Syndromes, 54*, S5–S6. doi: 10.1097/QAI.1090b1013e3181e1243a1091

Wolters, P. L., & Brouwers, P. (2005a). Neurobehavioral function and assessment of children and adolescents with HIV-1 infection. In S. L. Zeichner & J. S. Read (Eds.), *Textbook of pediatric HIV care* (pp. 269–286). Cambridge: Cambridge University Press.

Wolters, P. L., & Brouwers, P. (2005b). Evaluation of neurodevelopmental deficits in children with HIV-1 infection. In H. E. Gendelman, I. Grant, I. P. Everall, S. A. Lipton, & S. Swindells (Eds.), *The neurology of AIDS: Second edition* (pp. 667-682). Oxford: Oxford University Press.

Wolters, P. L., Brouwers, P., Civitello, L., & Moss, H. A. (1997). Receptive and expressive language function of children with symptomatic HIV infection and relationship with disease parameters: A longitudinal 24-month follow-up study. *AIDS, 11*, 1135–1144.

Wood, S. M., Shah, S. S., Steenhoff, A. P., & Rutstein, R. M. (2009). The impact of AIDS diagnosis on long-term neurocognitive and psychiatric outcomes of surviving adolescents with perinatally acquired HIV. *AIDS, 23*, 1859–1865.

World Health Organization. (2010). *Global report: UNAIDS report on the global AIDS epidemic, 2010.* Geneva, Switzerland: World Health Organization.

7 Neonatal Encephalopathy

Alex Kline, Katherine Ann Leonberger, and Ida Sue Baron

Neonatal hypoxic-ischemic encephalopathy (NE) is a significant cause of brain injury in term newborns, often resulting in serious cognitive and motor disabilities. It is a syndrome characterized by disturbed neurological functioning, beginning on the infant's first day of life, that is due to acute hypoxic-ischemic perinatal events (Parikh et al., 2009). This syndrome is typically exhibited by difficulty initiating and maintaining respiration, depression of tone and reflexes, a subnormal level of consciousness, and seizures during the infant's earliest days of life (Nelson & Leviton, 1991). As one of the leading causes of infant death in the developed world (Little et al., 2010), it is important to understand NE and to determine the most effective means of treatment.

EPIDEMIOLOGY

Hypoxic-ischemic disruptions are caused by lack of sufficient blood flow in combination with decreased oxygen content in the blood; this leads to an interruption in normal cerebral autoregulation and subsequent brain injury (Chao, Zaleski, & Patton, 2006). Because the brain has particularly high metabolic requirements, it is extremely susceptible to damage due to oxygen deprivation in the blood (Busl & Greer, 2010). The possible events leading up to such injury are diverse and can include uteroplacental insufficiency, infection, maternal hypotension, placental abruption, uterine rupture, maternal hemorrhage, cardiorespiratory arrest, severe fetal bradycardia, or prolonged labor, among others (Sarnat & Sarnat, 1976; Shankaran, 2009). When the neonate's blood is deprived of oxygen in such ways before or during birth, the risks of disrupted neurological and cognitive functioning become a serious concern.

It is estimated that NE affects approximately 1 to 6 of every 1000 newborns in the developed world (Parikh et al., 2009; Shankaran, 2009). Asphyxia accounts for approximately 23% of the 4 million global neonatal deaths annually (Lawn, Cousens, Zupan, & Lancet Neonatal Survival Steering, 2005). About 80% of survivors with severe NE go on to develop serious neurological impairments, and 30%–50% of survivors with moderate NE will develop long-term neurological difficulties. Currently, approximately 15%–20% of infants with NE die during infancy, and another 25% survive and develop neurosensory impairments and childhood disabilities (Shankaran, 2009). These impairments include cerebral palsy, mental retardation, epilepsy, deafness, and increased risk of infant death in severe cases (Robertson & Finer, 1988; Shankaran, Woldt, Koepke, Bedard, & Nandyal, 1991). Moderate cases of NE are correlated with motor deficits, memory impairment, visual motor/ visual perceptive difficulties, hyperactivity, and learning difficulties during childhood (Robertson & Finer, 1988; Shankaran et al., 1991; Vannucci & Perlman, 1997). These differences persist into adolescence. It has been found that adolescents with moderate neonatal encephalopathy display delayed recall for verbal and visual tasks, delayed perceptual–motor speed, impaired attention, and impaired executive functioning compared with controls and adolescents with mild NE (Maneru, Junque, Botet, Tallada, & Guardia, 2001). Fortunately, mild cases of NE do not tend to result in motor or cognitive impairments in childhood or adolescence (Shankaran, 2009; Maneru et al., 2001).

PATHOPHYSIOLOGY

There are several pathophysiologic mechanisms that cause brain injury in NE. It is now recognized that there are two distinct phases of injury. The primary phase occurs at the time of initial insult and as a result of the hypoxia and/or ischemia. Due to lack of blood flow and/or oxygenation, the body switches to anaerobic metabolism, which is a much less efficient method of adenosine triphosphate (ATP) synthesis. As a result, cellular membrane ion gradients that are ATP dependent cannot be maintained, resulting in cytotoxic edema, excessive intracellular accumulation of calcium, and increased extracellular excitatory amino acids, primarily glutamate (Lorek et al., 1994; Tan et al., 1996). Many infants with severe NE will show normal cerebral metabolism after birth (Azzopardi, 1999). Following resuscitation and restoration of cerebral blood flow and oxygenation, there is a latent phase, usually 6–15 hours later, that may extend for many days. The observation that the injury in NE is not limited to the primary insult, but is an evolving process, has transformed the investigation into treatments for NE. It is now known that although many neurons will die during the initial insult, many neurons will die hours or even days later. Roth and colleagues (1997) showed that the degree of secondary energy failure after the initial 24–48 hours is correlated with neurodevelopmental outcome at age 4 years. During the latent phase, infants often improve clinically, followed by the secondary phase of injury, which is clinically characterized by seizures, failure of cerebral mitochondrial function, and, ultimately, cell death (Beilharz, Williams, Dragunow, Sirimanne, & Gluckman, 1995; Gunn, Gunn, de Haan, Williams, & Gluckman, 1997). The mechanisms of delayed cell death, which are not completely understood, are likely multifactorial. Ultimately, cell death is likely due to a combination of both necrosis and apoptosis. It was the recognition of this delayed phase of injury that led to the possibility of further therapies extending past the time of initial injury.

CLINICAL MANIFESTATIONS

Although NE is an identifiable clinical syndrome in infancy, none of its potential manifestations are exclusive to this disorder, and there are multiple other etiologies for neonatal encephalopathy. These can include cerebrovascular accidents, seizures, respiratory etiologies, metabolic disturbances, and infectious causes (Nelson & Leviton, 1991), making diagnosis somewhat difficult. Early postnatal neurological abnormalities and other systemic abnormalities seen in the first days after birth must be considered when determining if a child has sustained NE (Sarnat & Sarnat, 1976; Perlman & Tack, 1988). Importantly, the most useful method of diagnosing NE in infancy is a neurological examination. It is recommended that all infants be given a detailed neurologic examination in the days after birth to identify even mild encephalopathy (Shankaran, 2009).

It has been suggested that diagnostic criteria for NE must include the following: early onset of encephalopathy (no more than a few days after birth); metabolic acidosis with an umbilical cord pH of <7 or a base deficit of 12 mmol/L at minimum; organ dysfunction in multiple systems; and, finally, exclusion of other causes such as trauma (external physical force damage to the brain), coagulation disorders, metabolic disorders, and genetic disorders (Shankaran, 2009). The first step in diagnosing NE is a detailed history of the pregnancy and birth, such that events that may have compromised blood and oxygen supply to the neonate can be identified and examined (Shankaran, 2009). Of particular importance is a history of maternal temperature elevation during pregnancy and labor; moderate gestational temperature elevation increases an infant's risk of developing neonatal encephalopathy (Shankaran, 2009). A history of fetal and maternal tachycardia should be taken, and laboratory examinations of placenta pathology and elevated biomarkers such as cytokines should be performed (Shankaran, 2009). Although there is no foolproof diagnostic test for NE, these steps can increase the probability of accurate diagnosis and effective treatment plans.

Recent neuroimaging and magnetic resonance imaging (MRI) studies have collectively demonstrated that perinatal asphyxia results in lesions in the basal ganglia, brain stem, thalamus, and hippocampus of term babies (Maneru et al., 2001). In particular, the hippocampus, the striatum, and the basal ganglia are at increased risk for hypoxic-ischemic injury in the neonatal brain (Armstrong-Wells, Bernard, Boada, & Manco-Johnson, 2010; Maneru et al., 2003). This may account for the deficits in memory, learning difficulties, and motor deficits frequently observed in survivors with moderate or severe injury. MRI studies have detected white matter lesions, often manifested as myelinization decay and corpus callosum thinning, in the brains of infants who suffered moderate or severe NE (Maneru et al., 2001). Studies using magnetic resonance spectroscopy (MRS) have also observed higher levels of lactate and reduced levels of N-acetylaspartate in neonatal brains following hypoxic ischemia, with more severe discrepancies correlating with later cognitive deficits in childhood (Little et al., 2010). Additionally, using MRI, it was found that adolescents who had suffered from moderate NE had smaller corpus callosums in comparison with controls and adolescents with mild NE (Maneru et al., 2001). This may contribute to the neuropsychological deficits observed in children with moderate and severe NE because the corpus callosum is implicated in executive functioning skills.

Whereas the predictive value of MRIs and other neuroimaging techniques is somewhat limited in the neonate's first days due to a lack of sensitivity to neuronal damage well suited to predicting very early abnormalities (Hallberg, Grossmann, Bartocci, & Blennow, 2010). Maynard, Prior and Scott (1969) developed amplitude-integrated EEG (aEEG) in the 1960s for use during anesthesia and in adult critical care; it was first used in newborns in the late 1970s and early 1980s (Viniker, Maynard, & Scott, 1984). The amplitude-integrated EEG tracing is generated from the raw EEG tracing that is amplified, filtered, rectified, and then smoothed. This makes for relative ease of interpretation and allows for evaluation of trends in background activity through pattern recognition. Ease of lead placement and observation of long-term trends make it an ideal bedside tool. Its use in neonatal intensive care units has increased over the last several years. Studies show that severity of injury can be predicted by amplitude-integrated EEG abnormalities, with more pronounced abnormalities correlating with more severe outcomes later in childhood (Hallberg et al., 2010). Additionally, the sooner these abnormalities subside during the infant's first 3 days of life, the better the outcome for the neonate with NE (Hallberg et al., 2010). The amplitude-integrated EEG is not meant to replace conventional EEG, which remains the gold standard, and its use is limited by the fact that it can miss both brief and localized seizures. Studies have also shown that the combination of amplitude-integrated EEG and early neurologic examination improves the ability to identify at-risk infants who may benefit from therapy (Shalak, Laptook, Velaphi, & Perlman, 2003). Sleep–wake cycling can be seen on EEG as early as 30 weeks gestation and is seen with advancing brain maturation. Studies have also shown that in term infants with suspected NE, time to recovery of sleep–wake cycling is predictive of ultimate neurodevelopmental outcome (Osredkar et al., 2005).

TRADITIONAL TREATMENT METHODS

In large part, the rehabilitative methods traditionally used to treat NE have been based upon treatment used for traumatic and other brain injuries (Arciniegas, 2010). This is due to a relative lack of research on neurorehabilitation for NE survivors (Arciniegas, 2010). Until recently, the primary treatment for NE included supportive intensive care, including correction of cardiopulmonary disturbances such as hypotension and hypoventilation. Many infants with moderate to severe NE have a decreased respiratory drive and will require mechanical ventilation. These infants are also at increased risk of pulmonary hypertension, at times due to meconium aspiration syndrome. Another important aspect of care is the correction of metabolic disturbances (particularly glucose, calcium, magnesium, and electrolytes). Fluid restriction is often necessary to help decrease cerebral edema and also as a result of decreased renal function. Detection and treatment of seizures is an extremely important part of the management of infants with NE. More than 50% of infants with moderate to severe NE will have seizures (Gluckman et al., 2005). Although these approaches help to manage symptoms and treat potential injuries resulting from NE, they do not target the pathophysiological events that lead to brain injury (Shankaran, 2009). Put differently, traditional treatment is aimed at rehabilitating, rather than preventing, cognitive and motor difficulties that result from NE.

CURRENT MEDICAL APPROACHES TO TREATMENT

As noted above, a key advance in the treatment of neonatal encephalopathy was the recognition that the injury that occurs in NE is not limited to a single point in time but rather is ongoing beyond the initial stage of insult. Clinical and experimental studies have shown that a secondary phase of energy failure occurs 8–48 hours later (Thoresen et al., 1995). These findings opened the door for further therapeutic interventions that would extend beyond the time of primary injury and ameliorate the effects of secondary injury.

There has been much interest in therapeutic modalities over the years due to the often unfavorable outcomes in infants with NE. Among diverse therapies investigated have been oxygen free radical inhibitors, endogenous scavengers, excitatory amino acid antagonists, calcium channel blockers, growth factors, Phenobarbital, and, more recently, hypothermia. Allopurinol is an oxygen free radical inhibitor that has been shown to reduce neuropathologic injury in animal models (Palmer, Vannucci, & Towfighi, 1990). A trial of allopurinol did not show improvement in newborns with NE compared with the control group, and the authors speculated that giving allopurinol postnatally might be too late to significantly decrease free radical levels (Benders et al., 2006). Magnesium sulfate is a glutamate receptor antagonist that has been shown in retrospective studies to decrease the risk of cerebral palsy in premature infants whose mothers were given magnesium for the treatment of preeclampsia (Nelson & Grether, 1995). In one study on the use of magnesium sulfate for the prevention of cerebral palsy in infants whose mothers were at imminent risk of delivery at 24–31 weeks' gestation, magnesium was shown to decrease the risk of moderate to severe cerebral palsy (Rouse et al., 2008). Phenobarbital, an anticonvulsant that increases gamma-aminobutyric acid (GABA) subtype A receptor activity, is frequently used to treat seizures in newborns. With high doses (40 mg/kg), it has been shown to significantly reduce seizures and improve neurologic outcomes at age 3 years when used in term infants with severe NE (Hall, Hall, & Daily, 1998). However, there are more recent concerns about the effect of GABAergic drugs, such as Phenobarbital, being associated with apoptotic neurodegeneration in the developing brains of animals (Bittigau, Sifringer, & Ikonomidou, 2003). Based on these and other studies, caution is needed when using these drugs in neonates. Although these and many other potential therapies showed initial promise in the laboratory, early results did not translate to the bedside or side effects made them prohibitive in newborns.

HYPOTHERMIA TREATMENT

Hypothermia as a treatment for NE was suggested as far back as 300 years ago by John Floyer (Floyer, 1722). Temple Fay performed studies in the 1930s and 1940s that showed successful resuscitation of hypothermic drowning victims. In the 1950s and 1960s animal studies by Westin and Miller showed improved survival and learning with rapid cooling after asphyxia (Westin, Miller, & Boles, 1963). Progress in the use of hypothermia in infants with NE was stalled when a paper published in 1958 showed decreased survival of premature infants when kept hypothermic (Silverman, Fertig, & Berger, 1958). These results, when extrapolated to term infants, were a serious setback in the use of hypothermia in newborns. Little progress was made over the next several decades in the use of hypothermia to treat NE.

In animal studies, hypothermia has been consistently found to be a safe and effective option for treating neonatal encephalopathy. Early studies of neonatal gerbils showed that NE results in functional abnormalities caused by hippocampal cell loss and that hypothermia applied for 2–6 hours following ischemic injury helps protect the hippocampus from cell damage (Carroll & Beek, 1992; Colbourne & Corbett, 1994). Gunn and colleagues (1997) examined the effects of hypothermia on neonatal lambs with hypoxic ischemic encephalopathy (HIE). Hypothermia decreased the extent of neuronal loss, reduced cortical infarction, and resulted in increased EEG activity (Gunn et al., 1997). These animal studies also showed that hypothermia was safe and that there were no significant side effects. O'Brien and colleagues (2006) found that hypothermia applied to newborn piglets with HIE decreased the severity of cerebral energy failure and that effects were similar whether the whole-body hypothermia was applied at 35°C or 33°C. Thoresen and colleagues (1996) examined the effects of cooling on neonatal rats with HIE and found that hypothermia significantly reduced brain damage in the cortex, hippocampus, basal ganglia, and thalamus of these rats compared with noncooled peers. In summary, neonatal animals with HIE appeared to benefit from hypothermia because it reduced brain damage, reduced neuronal loss, and decreased the severity of energy failure after hypoxia.

In human adults, hypothermia has been explored as a treatment for HIE caused by ventricular fibrillation cardiac arrest or ischemic stroke. In a retrospective study, Oddo and colleagues (2006) determined that adult patients who had been treated with hypothermia following cardiac arrest had better outcomes and lower rates of death compared with patients who had not undergone hypothermia treatment. A randomized, controlled multicenter study of adults following cardiac arrest similarly showed that patients who received brain hypothermia treatment had improved neurological outcomes and a decreased risk of death (Hypothermia after Cardiac Arrest Study, 2002). Additionally, Nagao and colleagues (2010) found that patients with cardiac arrest who attained a core temperature of 34°C for 3 days with hypothermia treatment showed improved neurological outcomes. Studies of hypothermia used for adult patients with stroke have not yet demonstrated such definitive neurological benefits but they have found that therapeutic hypothermia for stroke victims is a safe procedure that results in minimal discomfort or shivering (Guluma, Hemmen, Olsen, Rapp, & Lyden, 2006; Hemmen & Lyden, 2009; Kammersgaard et al., 2000).

Only recently has brain hypothermia in neonates emerged as a promising treatment for neuroprotection against the direct effects of NE. Although previous treatments for this disorder have been primarily supportive, recent studies show that reducing an infant's brain temperature by 2–5 degrees following perinatal hypoxic-ischemia for 24–72 hours can positively impact physical, functional, and neuropathological outcomes (Gluckman et al., 2005).

The mechanisms of action for hypothermia as a treatment for neonatal encephalopathy are not yet fully understood. It is unlikely that hypothermia improves outcomes due to a single mechanism of action; likely, it works at a variety of levels. A primary mode of action seems to be by reduction of cellular metabolic demands (Erecinska, Thoresen, & Silver, 2003). Hypothermia has been shown to decrease cerebral metabolism by 5% per degree of decrease in temperature (Laptook, Corbett, Sterett, Garcia, & Tollefsbol, 1995). However, hypothermia is also known to reduce neuronal death, reduce cerebral metabolism, inhibit the release of glutamate in the brain and spinal cord, inhibit platelet-activating factor, preserve endogenous antioxidants/decrease free radical activity, and reduce extent of brain injury in treated infants (Parikh et al.,

2009). One study found that infants treated with hypothermia following NE had significantly larger subcortical white matter volume after treatment compared with peers not treated with hypothermia (Parikh et al., 2009). This suggests that the treatment works primarily by preserving subcortical white matter, an area that is often injured in infants suffering from this disorder (Parikh et al., 2009). Other studies have suggested that hypothermia works primarily by protecting cortical gray matter and can lead to significant decreases in basal ganglia and thalamic lesions (Inder et al., 2004; Rutherford et al., 2005).

Hypothermia Clinical Trials

There have now been several multicenter, randomized, controlled clinical trials in the use of hypothermia for newborns with moderate to severe NE. The largest trials are discussed here, and each trial shares many similarities and some differences in recruitment, study design, and methodology. The CoolCap trial used selective head cooling (SHC) with mild systemic hypothermia; a cooling device was used to preferentially cool the infant's head while attempting to minimize systemic effects of hypothermia. Both the National Institute of Child Health and Development (NICHD)–sponsored trial and the Total Body Hypothermia for Neonatal Encephalopathy Trial (TOBY) trial used whole-body hypothermia, with the infants placed on a cooling mattress. The CoolCap and TOBY trials used amplitude-integrated EEG criteria in the recruitment of patients, while the NICHD trial did not. Each trial enrolled only infants ≥ 36 weeks gestation who were less than 6 hours of age at time of enrollment and cooled the infants for 72 hours before rewarming. The CoolCap trial cooled infants to a rectal temperature of 34°C–35°C, while the NICHD and TOBY trials cooled infants to a central temperature of 33.5°C. Importantly, each trial used the same primary outcome, which was a composite outcome of death or moderate to severe disability. Severe neurodevelopmental disability was defined as a score of <70 on the Mental Developmental Index (MDI) of the Bayley Scales of Infant Development–II, a score of 3–5 on the Gross Motor Function Classification System (GMFCS), with scores ranging from 1 to 5, and a higher score indicating more severe impairment or bilateral cortical visual impairment with no useful vision (Palisano et al., 2000).

In the multicenter CoolCap Study, which examined 243 term infants with moderate or severe encephalopathy, infants' brains were cooled to a rectal temperature of 34°C–35°C for 72 hours using SHC with mild systemic hypothermia (Gluckman et al., 2005). Primary outcome was defined as death or severe disability at 18 months. In the hypothermia group, 59/108 (55%) of infants died or survived with severe disability, while 73/110 (66%) of infants in the NE no hypothermia treatment control group had the same outcome. This was not statistically significant, with a p value = 0.10. In those infants with the most severe amplitude-integrated EEG changes, hypothermia was not found to be protective (odds ratio [OR] 1.8; 95% confidence interval [CI], 0.49–6.4; $p = 0.51$). In a prespecified secondary analysis, hypothermia seemed effective in those infants with less severe amplitude-integrated EEG changes (OR 0.47; 95% CI, 0.26–0.87; $p = 0.021$). Although hypothermia was not protective in the entire cohort studied, a significant protective effect was found for infants with less severe encephalopathy treated with hypothermia, with decreases in death as well as severe disability among this group (Gluckman et al., 2005). The authors speculated that improvement was not seen in the most severely affected group either because there was not enough time for the treatment to be effective prior to the secondary deterioration or because the injury was too severe for treatment to be effective.

Another randomized, controlled multicenter study examined infants with NE who underwent whole-body hypothermia at 33°C for 48 hours (Eicher et al., 2005). Although increased side effects were observed within the hypothermia group, it was found that 52% of the hypothermia infants suffered death or severe motor disability at 12 months compared with 84% of the nonhypothermia infants (Eicher et al., 2005).

The NICHD whole-body cooling (WBC) trial randomized 239 eligible infants: 102 to the hypothermia group and 106 to the control group. This study used whole-body hypothermia, with the infants placed on a cooling mattress to decrease the esophageal temperature to 33.5°C for 72 hours, followed by slow rewarming over 12 hours. Primary outcome was a combined endpoint of death or moderate to severe disability at age 18–22 months. The primary outcome occurred in 45 of 102 infants (44%) in the hypothermia group and 64 of 103 infants (62%) in the control group (risk ratio [RR] 0.72; 95% CI, 0.54–0.95; $p = 0.01$). Twenty-four infants (24%) in the hypothermia group died; 38 (37%) in the control group died (RR, 0.68; 95% CI, 0.44–1.05; $p = 0.08$). The authors concluded that whole-body hypothermia reduced the risk of the primary outcome in infants with moderate to severe NE (Shankaran et al., 2005).

The TOBY trial, published in 2009, enrolled 325 infants, with 163 undergoing cooling and 162 remaining in the control group with maintenance of normothermia. As in the NICHD trial, the TOBY trial used WBC. In the hypothermia group, 42 infants died and 32 survived but had severe neurodevelopmental disability; in the control group, 44 infants died and 42 had severe disability (RR for either outcome, 0.86; 95% CI, 0.68–1.07; $p = 0.17$). Importantly, infants in the cooled group had an increased rate of survival without neurologic abnormality (RR, 1.57; 95% CI, 1.16–2.12; $p = 0.003$). Cerebral palsy was also reduced in survivors who also had improved scores on the MDI and Psychomotor Developmental Index (PDI) of the Bayley Scales of Infant Development (Azzopardi et al., 2009). An important difference between the TOBY trial and other hypothermia trials is that the TOBY trial routinely sedated all infants undergoing hypothermia.

The three largest trials to date (CoolCap, NICHD, and TOBY) share many similarities in recruitment and study protocol. Each study also used the same primary outcome, which was a composite outcome of death or moderate to severe disability. This allows for comparison of outcomes between studies. Only the NICHD trial showed a significant reduction in the primary outcome; the TOBY trial was the only trial to show a reduction in specific neurologic outcomes, including a reduction in survival without neurologic impairment.

Unfortunately, hypothermia may not be equally beneficial for all infants with NE. The treatment becomes less protective as severity of cerebral damage increases. It is most beneficial for those with milder forms of the disorder (Bona, Hagberg, Loberg, Bagenholm, & Thoresen, 1998). Additionally, hypothermia becomes significantly less beneficial if it is started more than 6 hours after injury, and it has no protective effects if the infant has had seizures prior to initiating treatment (Gunn & Gunn, 1998). For these reasons, it is important to begin treatment as early as possible once cerebral insult is suspected.

Overall, therapeutic hypothermia is a safe and effective method of neuroprotection for those infants who meet eligibility criteria used in published studies. Side effects that have been consistently observed are usually mild and easily managed in an intensive care setting. In all of the cooling trials to date, meta-analysis has shown that physiological sinus bradycardia and thrombocytopenia are the only significant adverse effects (S. Jacobs, Hunt, Tarnow-Mordi, Inder, & Davis, 2007; Shah, 2010). Sinus bradycardia in hypothermia results from slowing of the atrial pacemaker as well as slowing intracardiac conduction (Gluckman et al., 2005; Shankaran et al., 2005). Meta-analysis has shown an increase in hypotension treated with inotropes (S. Jacobs et al., 2007). However, this was shown in another study to be more related to changes in physician management, with slower weaning of inotropes in those infants undergoing hypothermia (Battin et al., 2009). Although there is some concern over an increased risk of persistent pulmonary hypertension of the newborn (PPHN) in infants treated with hypothermia, the three largest cooling trials did not show an increased risk in cooled infants versus noncooled infants (Azzopardi et al., 2009; Gluckman et al., 2005; Shankaran et al., 2005). The same studies showed that despite an increased incidence of thrombocytopenia, this did not result in an increase in bleeding complications.

Hypothermia has been shown to have effects on several medications that are frequently used in infants with encephalopathy and those undergoing hypothermia. Certain anticonvulsants, neuromuscular paralysis agents, and sedatives have their metabolism affected by hypothermia. Clinicians caring for infants undergoing hypothermia must be aware of the potential for changes in drug levels. For drugs that are metabolized by the liver, the effect on drug metabolism is related to effects on the temperature-dependent cytochrome P450 enzyme system. Antibiotics such as gentamicin and inotropes such as dopamine, both of which are metabolized through the kidneys, do not seem to be affected by hypothermia. However, it is important to consider that many infants with NE have undergone some degree of renal impairment. Although studies in infants have not shown increased risk of infection, studies in adults have shown increased infection, in particular, pneumonia.

Clinicians caring for infants undergoing hypothermic therapy must also be aware of the potential for skin changes, including acrocyanosis, erythema, and sclerema. Subcutaneous fat necrosis is also a known complication of hypothermic therapy. Also, there must be diligence on the part of staff and frequent positioning changes. As discussed above, side effects of controlled hypothermia are mild and easily managed. However, more severe side effects are observed when the infant's temperature is not properly monitored during hypothermia therapy. More severe side effects include arrhythmias other than sinus bradycardia, hypotension, uncontrolled bleeding due to coagulopathy, pulmonary hemorrhage, renal failure, and acid–base and electrolyte disturbances (Laptook & Corbett, 2002).

To date, all published clinical trials have used similar entry criteria as well as duration and depth of cooling. Hypothermia for neonatal NE is now being used more frequently by NICUs worldwide outside of clinical trials; however, it is recommended that units adhere as closely as possible to guidelines established by the large trials that have been published. This includes not cooling infants <36 weeks gestation or infants who cannot begin hypothermia by 6 hours after birth. There is currently an NICHD-sponsored clinical trial of cooling infants who meet current clinical criteria and are up to 24 hours of age. It is also recommended that clinicians maintain the temperature guidelines, with a goal of 33.5°C, as used in the large published trials. The effects of deeper or more prolonged cooling on newborns are not known at this time. One study published in Italy in 2007 enrolled 39 term infants with asphyxia into three groups: a control group, a mild hypothermia groups (goal temperature 32°C–34°C), and a deep hypothermia group (goal temperature 30°C–33°C). There were no significant differences between the mild hypothermia and deep hypothermia groups with regard to safety and major clinical neurologic abnormalities (Compagnoni et al., 2008). Further studies are needed before changes are made to existing protocols.

It should also be noted that all outcomes published to date are relatively short term. All of the larger published cooling trials conducted follow-up at age 18–22 months. Further school-age follow-up at age 4–5 years is ongoing, but no additional follow-up studies have been published. It will be important to see if the neurologic improvements seen at 18–22 months persist into school age and beyond. To date there is also little published on the behavioral and subtle performance outcomes of infants who have undergone cooling. This will also be an important area for follow-up in the future.

There have now been several meta-analyses on the topic of hypothermia used to treat NE (Higgins, 2005; S. Jacobs et al., 2007; Shah, 2010; Speer & Perlman, 2006). The Cochrane review in 2003, which concluded that there was not enough evidence at that time to make a recommendation, was published prior to many of the larger, more recent trials. The most recent meta-analysis by Shah (2010) reviewed the results of 13 studies and included almost 1000 infants. Using a primary outcome of mortality or neurodevelopmental disability in childhood, there was found to be a significant reduction in the risk of mortality or of moderate to severe neurodevelopmental disability in infants who received hypothermia compared with control infants (pooled RR, 0.74; 95% CI, 0.65–0.83; RD: –0.15, 95% CI, –0.21, –0.09; NNTB: 795% CI 5–11) (Figure 7.1). Mortality was reduced in the hypothermia group (RR, 0.78 [95% CI, 0.65–0.92]; number needed to benefit, 15 [95% CI, 8–50]) (Figure 7.2). With regard to safety, the rates of bradycardia and thrombocytopenia were higher in the treatment group. Secondary outcomes measured included a subgroup analysis based on severity of encephalopathy (moderate or severe). There was a significant reduction in the risk of death or moderate to severe neurodevelopmental disability in infants with moderate NE. However, there was not a significant reduction in those infants with severe NE, although this consisted of a relatively small group of infants. In previous studies there was concern that infants with severe NE would be less likely to have support withdrawn and that the outcome of death would be replaced with an increased burden of severe disability. However, the studies have shown not only that the number of infants in both groups that had support withdrawn was similar but also that neurodevelopmental outcomes were improved in survivors (Shah, 2010).

Therapeutic hypothermia does have a statistically significant effect on the intermediate outcomes of term and near-term infants with NE; however, the improvement effect is modest overall and the rate of neurologic morbidity remains high. Recent work has begun to focus not only on maximizing results with hypothermia but also on looking for adjunctive treatments to be used in conjunction with hypothermia. Several promising treatments are being investigated. Recombinant erythropoietin (rEpo), which was approved by the US Food and Drug Administration in 1989 for anemia due to chronic renal disease, is now widely used to treat anemia of prematurity. In vitro studies have shown that rEpo activates anti-apoptotic pathways (Digicaylioglu & Lipton, 2001) and improves the viability of neurons cultured in conditions encountered in NE, including hypoxia-ischemia, glutamate toxicity, and nitric oxide toxicity (Morishita, Masuda, Nagao, Yasuda, & Sasaki, 1997). There is also evidence that rEpo improves later brain recovery because it promotes neurogenesis, angiogenesis, and migration of regenerating neurons (Tsai et al., 2006). Although rEpo does not

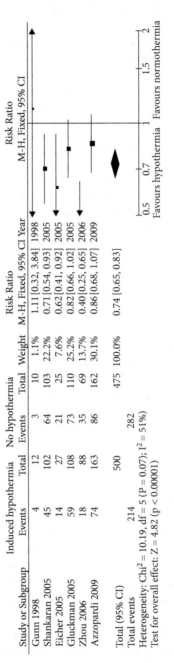

Study or Subgroup	Induced hypothermia		No hypothermia		Weight	Risk Ratio M-H, Fixed, 95% CI	Year	Risk Ratio M-H, Fixed, 95% CI
	Events	Total	Events	Total				
Gunn 1998	4	12	3	10	1.1%	1.11 [0.32, 3.84]	1998	
Shankaran 2005	45	102	64	103	22.2%	0.71 [0.54, 0.93]	2005	
Eicher 2005	14	27	21	25	7.6%	0.62 [0.41, 0.92]	2005	
Gluckman 2005	59	108	73	110	25.2%	0.82 [0.66, 1.02]	2005	
Zhou 2006	18	88	35	69	13.7%	0.40 [0.25, 0.65]	2006	
Azzopardi 2009	74	163	86	162	30.1%	0.86 [0.68, 1.07]	2009	
Total (95% CI)		500		475	100.0%	0.74 [0.65, 0.83]		
Total events	214		282					

Heterogeneity: Chi^2 = 10.19, df = 5 (P = 0.07); I^2 = 51%)
Test for overall effect: Z = 4.82 (p < 0.00001)

Favours hypothermia   Favours normothermia

FIGURE 7.1

Forest plot of primary outcome of death or moderate-to-severe neurodevelopmental disability in survivors.

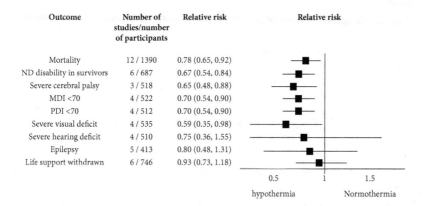

Outcome	Number of studies/number of participants	Relative risk
Mortality	12 / 1390	0.78 (0.65, 0.92)
ND disability in survivors	6 / 687	0.67 (0.54, 0.84)
Severe cerebral palsy	3 / 518	0.65 (0.48, 0.88)
MDI <70	4 / 522	0.70 (0.54, 0.90)
PDI <70	4 / 512	0.70 (0.54, 0.90)
Severe visual deficit	4 / 535	0.59 (0.35, 0.98)
Severe hearing deficit	4 / 510	0.75 (0.36, 1.55)
Epilepsy	5 / 413	0.80 (0.48, 1.31)
Life support withdrawn	6 / 746	0.93 (0.73, 1.18)

FIGURE 7.2

Efficacy outcomes. ND, neurodevelopmental; MDI, Mental Developmental Index; PDI, Psychomotor Developmental Index.

easily cross the blood–brain barrier, studies have used high-dose rEpo (5000 units/kg) and have shown neuroprotection in adult models (Brines et al., 2000). A randomized controlled trial published in 2009 in China enrolled 167 term infants with moderate to severe NE who received either rEpo or conventional treatment. The study showed that death or disability occurred in 44% of controls versus 24.6% of infants treated with rEpo at 18 months follow-up (Zhu et al., 2009). Though questions remain about potential adverse effects and optimal dosing, rEpo seems to be a promising treatment to be used adjunctively with hypothermia for neonatal NE (Juul, 2000).

Xenon, which is an anesthetic gas that is widely used in Europe, has also shown some promise in preliminary studies. Xenon is an antagonist of the N-methyl-D-aspartate subtype of the glutamate receptor, with an advantage in that it readily crosses the blood–brain barrier (Dworschak, 2008). Animal studies using subanesthetic doses of xenon in rats have shown global neuroprotection with reduced neurotransmitter release during ischemia and an improvement in neuronal injury and cell death (Carpentier, Mullins, Elkin, & Wolfe-Christensen, 2008). Other studies have shown a synergistic effect of xenon when combined with hypothermia in rat pups, as well as a greater improvement in histologic and functional outcome than either therapy alone (Hobbs et al., 2008). Although many questions still remain about the use of xenon for neonatal NE, it is a promising potential therapy, and early clinical trials are now underway.

NEUROPSYCHOLOGICAL OUTCOMES FOLLOWING ENCEPHALOPATHY

Because symptoms associated with more moderate NE are often subtle and occur distant from the original injury, cognitive impairment may initially go undetected as these infants mature (Armstrong-Wells et al., 2010). Neurodevelopmental and neuropsychological impairments may become evident among survivors of neonatal encephalopathy even in the absence of severe neuromotor deficits (Gonzalez & Miller, 2006; Marlow, Rose, Rands, & Draper, 2005; Moster, Lie, & Markestad, 2002). Such subtle problems may present as mild learning impairments or academic underachievement. However, relatively little is known about the milder neuropsychological problems in children who do not demonstrate major neurological deficits (van Handel, Swaab, de Vries, & Jongmans, 2007).

Cognitive and neuropsychological performances may vary based on severity of injury. For example, survivors of severe encephalopathy who had no neuromotor impairment had significantly lower general cognitive scores than controls on the British Ability Scales–Second Edition (BAS-II). Those who had moderate encephalopathy had cognitive scores that did not vary significantly from that of controls, but the scores were slightly lower. Children with severe injuries demonstrated impaired attention, memory, and executive functioning, whereas children with moderate injury scored lower on tasks of narrative memory and sentence repetition but otherwise demonstrated neuropsychological performances similar to that of controls (Marlow et al., 2005). These investigators also found that children with both severe and moderate neonatal encephalopathy demonstrated lower academic achievement than controls, with the severe group having the lowest scores and underachieving across all areas of academic achievement. It was found that the moderate group principally had spelling and reading problems. Children with severe encephalopathy also demonstrated more behavior problems than controls. Specifically, they were rated as more hyperactive, less prosocial, and as having more difficulty with daily functioning in the classroom setting (Marlow et al., 2005). Other studies have found that children who were exposed to moderate perinatal asphyxia demonstrated subtle neuropsychological deficits in comparison with controls, particularly in the areas of delayed recall for visual and verbal information, perceptual–motor speed, attention, and executive functioning (Maneru et al., 2001).

A history of neonatal encephalopathy but without major neurological impairment was associated with an increased need for resource assistance in kindergarten and elementary school and impaired performance in reading and mathematics compared with controls. Additionally, these children demonstrated problems with fine-motor skills and were at greater risk of minor motor impairments in childhood. Teachers also reported that these children were more likely to demonstrate such emotional problems as aggression, passivity, and anxiety than their peers (Moster et al., 2002).

Region of brain injury appears to influence the type of neuropsychological impairments observed. A watershed pattern of brain injury without consequent functional motor impairment following NE was associated with impaired language abilities (Steinman et al., 2009). As severity of injury with a watershed pattern increased, verbal scores decreased. In another study, those who sustained injuries restricted to the basal ganglia also demonstrated lower verbal scores, but not at a statistically significant level. Performance IQ was unaffected by severity of injury in either watershed or basal ganglia regions (Steinman et al., 2009). Memory disorders in childhood have been related to perinatal hypoxic ischemia and hippocampal involvement. In a study of developmentally amnesic patients who sustained hypoxic injury either perinatally or during early childhood, dissociation was found between episodic and semantic memory, with individuals who had hypoxic ischemic damage demonstrating impaired episodic memory but intact semantic memory. Additionally, dissociation between recall and recognition was found, with recall severely impaired but recognition intact (Vargha-Khadem, Gadian, & Mishkin, 2001). The impairments in episodic and recall memory were related to hippocampal damage during the hypoxic event; whether the dissociations resulted from structural reorganization of the brain or preservation of portions of the hippocampus after injury was not determined.

In summary, neuropsychological impairments may occur in the absence of major neurological impairments in children who have had encephalopathy. These may be most prominent in the domains of general cognition, academic achievement, attention, verbal skills, perceptual–motor skills, and memory and are most likely to occur after moderate or severe injury. Moreover, the type of impairment often is related to the location of injury. Therefore, it is important that infants experiencing NE be considered at elevated risk and undergo routine neuropsychological evaluation at an early age in order to maximize detection of any cognitive or behavioral deficits and to institute timely rehabilitation as symptoms arising from this disorder are detected.

NEUROPSYCHOLOGICAL OUTCOMES FOLLOWING COOLING

Hypothermia for infants who experience hypoxic ischemic encephalopathy has been associated with a reduction of later disability and learning difficulties. In a meta-analysis by Edwards and colleagues (2010), therapeutic hypothermia was found to lessen the likelihood of severe disability at age 18 months. Infants who had hypothermia treatment had a greater likelihood of survival without cerebral palsy and to have a Bayley MDI score of 84 or higher. In a study of infants aged 12 months who had been cooled for NE and compared with those who received no treatment, 64% of the normothermia patients had severely abnormal Bayley PDI scores (2 standard deviations below the mean) compared with 24% of those who had been treated with hypothermia. Additionally, 42% of the normothermia group had severely abnormal cognitive scores compared with only 24% of the hypothermia group (Eicher et al., 2005).

Shankaran and colleagues (2008) used similar methods to assess neurodevelopment in cooled infants. Severe disability was defined as an MDI score below 70, a GMFCS rating of 3–5, bilateral blindness, or deafness. Moderate disability was defined as an MDI score of 70–84, GMFCS rating of 2, hearing deficits, or seizure disorder requiring electroconvulsive therapy. At age 18 months, the hypothermia group had 24 deaths of 102 participants (23%), 19 severe disabilities, and 2 moderate disabilities. In contrast, infants who had not received hypothermia treatment had 38 deaths of 106 participants (36%), 25 severe disabilities, and 1 moderate disability.

Rutherford and colleagues (2005) examined whether hypothermia treatment results in different patterns of brain injury than does traditional normothermia treatment. They compared WBC and SHC methods and found that hypothermia treatment was associated with a decrease in basal ganglia and thalamic lesions, both of which have been related to abnormal neurodevelopmental outcomes later in life. Specifically, they found these lesions in 88.4% of noncooled infants, 50% of infants treated with SHC, and 75% of infants treated with WBC. SHC also resulted in a decrease in severe cortical lesions. Notably, infants with severe aEEG findings did not benefit from either hypothermia treatment, further evidence that this particular intervention may be most useful for infants whose injuries are less severe.

Other studies have also provided support for the findings that hypothermia treatment reduces the risk of neurodevelopmental disabilities. For example, Jacobs and colleagues (2011) found that 51.4% of infants in their hypothermia group had major sensorineural disabilities at age 2 years compared with 66.3% of control infants. Additionally, data from the NICHD study suggest that mild to moderate hypothermia may ameliorate brain damage caused by NE (Blackmon & Stark, 2006). Although more research is needed to determine the impact of hypothermia on the presence and severity of adverse neuropsychological outcomes after age 2 years, preliminary evidence suggests that hypothermia is a safe treatment that reduces the incidence of cognitive and neuromotor disability later in life.

FUTURE DIRECTIONS

Therapeutic hypothermia has emerged in recent years as a promising therapy for NE. There are now several large clinical trials supporting its use in a specified population of infants with NE. Several meta-analyses have also confirmed that hypothermia is safe and effective. Although all follow-up studies to date have been relatively short term, long-term studies are being completed. However, several questions remain unanswered by the current trials. For instance, the optimal depth and length of cooling are unknown, as are the possible benefits of hypothermia beyond the initial 6 hours after birth. Considering that neonatal NE is such a devastating illness with a large burden of long-term neurodevelopmental disability, the search is now underway for additional therapies that, when combined with hypothermia, may improve outcomes even further. Much additional research and follow-up must be conducted in order to improve the outcomes of these most vulnerable infants.

REFERENCES

Arciniegas, D. B. (2010). Hypoxic-ischemic brain injury: Addressing the disconnect between pathophysiology and public policy. *NeuroRehabilitation, 26*, 1–4. doi: 10.3233/ NRE-2010-0530

Armstrong-Wells, J., Bernard, T. J., Boada, R., & Manco-Johnson, M. (2010). Neurocognitive outcomes following neonatal encephalopathy. *NeuroRehabilitation, 26*, 27–33. doi: 10.3233/NRE-2010-0533

Azzopardi, D. V., Strohm, B., Edwards, A. D., Dyet, L., Halliday, H. L., Juszczak, E.,... Group, T. S. (2009). Moderate hypothermia to treat perinatal asphyxial encephalopathy. *The New England Journal of Medicine, 361*, 1349–1358. doi: 10.1056/NEJMoa0900854

Battin, M. R., Thoresen, M., Robinson, E., Polin, R. A., Edwards, A. D., Gunn, A. J., & Cool Cap Trial Group. (2009). Does head cooling with mild systemic hypothermia affect requirement for blood pressure support? *Pediatrics, 123*, 1031–1036. doi: 10.1542/ peds.2008-1610

Beilharz, E. J., Williams, C. E., Dragunow, M., Sirimanne, E. S., & Gluckman, P. D. (1995). Mechanisms of delayed cell death following hypoxic-ischemic injury in the immature rat: Evidence for apoptosis during selective neuronal loss. *Brain Research. Molecular Brain Research, 29*, 1–14.

Benders, M. J., Bos, A. F., Rademaker, C. M., Rijken, M., Torrance, H. L., Groenendaal, F., & van Bel, F. (2006). Early postnatal allopurinol does not improve short term outcome after severe birth asphyxia. *Archives of Disease in Childhood. Fetal and Neonatal Edition, 91*, F163–F165. doi: 10.1136/adc.2005.086652

Bittigau, P., Sifringer, M., & Ikonomidou, C. (2003). Antiepileptic drugs and apoptosis in the developing brain. *Annals of the New York Academy of Sciences, 993*, 103–114; discussion 123–104.

Blackmon, L. R., & Stark, A. R., American Academy of Pediatrics Committee on Fetus and Newborn. (2006). Hypothermia: A neuroprotective therapy for neonatal hypoxic-ischemic encephalopathy. *Pediatrics, 117,* 942–948. doi: 10.1542/peds.2005-2950

Bona, E., Hagberg, H., Loberg, E. M., Bagenholm, R., & Thoresen, M. (1998). Protective effects of moderate hypothermia after neonatal hypoxia-ischemia: Short- and long-term outcome. *Pediatric Research, 43,* 738–745.

Brines, M. L., Ghezzi, P., Keenan, S., Agnello, D., de Lanerolle, N. C., Cerami, C.,...Cerami, A. (2000). Erythropoietin crosses the blood-brain barrier to protect against experimental brain injury. *Proceedings of the National Academy of Sciences of the United States of America, 97,* 10526–10531.

Buol, K. M., & Greer, D. M. (2010). Hypoxic-ischemic brain injury: Pathophysiology, neuropathology and mechanisms. *NeuroRehabilitation, 26,* 5–13. doi: 10.3233/NRE-2010-0531

Carpentier, M. Y., Mullins, L. L., Elkin, T. D., & Wolfe-Christensen, C. (2008). Predictors of health-harming and health-protective behaviors in adolescents with cancer. *Pediatric Blood & Cancer, 51,* 525–530.

Carroll, M., & Beek, O. (1992). Protection against hippocampal CA1 cell loss by post-ischemic hypothermia is dependent on delay of initiation and duration. *Metabolic Brain Disease, 7,* 45–50.

Chao, C. P., Zaleski, C. G., & Patton, A. C. (2006). Neonatal hypoxic-ischemic encephalopathy: Multimodality imaging findings. *Radiographics, 26,* S159–S172. doi: 26/suppl_1/S159 [pii]10.1148/rg.26si065504

Colbourne, F., & Corbett, D. (1994). Delayed and prolonged post-ischemic hypothermia is neuroprotective in the gerbil. *Brain Research, 654,* 265–272.

Compagnoni, G., Bottura, C., Cavallaro, G., Cristofori, G., Lista, G., & Mosca, F. (2008). Safety of deep hypothermia in treating neonatal asphyxia. *Neonatology, 93,* 230–235. doi: 10.1159/111101

Digicaylioglu, M., & Lipton, S. A. (2001). Erythropoietin-mediated neuroprotection involves cross-talk between Jak2 and NF-kappaB signalling cascades. *Nature, 412,* 641–647. doi: 10.1038/35088074

Dworschak, M. (2008). Pharmacologic neuroprotection—is xenon the light at the end of the tunnel? *Critical Care Medicine, 36,* 2477–2479. doi: 10.1097/CCM.0b013e31818113d2

Edwards, A. D., Brocklehurst, P., Gunn, A. J., Halliday, H., Juszczak, E., Levene, M.,...Azzopardi, D. (2010). Neurological outcomes at 18 months of age after moderate hypothermia for perinatal hypoxic ischaemic encephalopathy: Synthesis and meta-analysis of trial data. *British Medical Journal, 340,* c363. doi: 10.1136/bmj.c363

Eicher, D. J., Wagner, C. L., Katikaneni, L. P., Hulsey, T. C., Bass, W. T., Kaufman, D. A.,...Yager, J. Y. (2005). Moderate hypothermia in neonatal encephalopathy: Efficacy outcomes. *Pediatric Neurology, 32,* 11–17. doi: 10.1016/j.pediatrneurol.2004.06.014

Erecinska, M., Thoresen, M., & Silver, I. A. (2003). Effects of hypothermia on energy metabolism in Mammalian central nervous system. *Journal of Cerebral Blood Flow and Metabolism, 23,* 513–530. doi: 10.1097/01.WCB.0000066287.21705.21

Gluckman, P. D., Wyatt, J. S., Azzopardi, D., Ballard, R., Edwards, A. D., Ferriero, D. M.,...Gunn, A. J. (2005). Selective head cooling with mild systemic hypothermia after neonatal encephalopathy: Multicentre randomised trial. *Lancet, 365,* 663–670. doi: 10.1016/S0140-6736(05)17946-X

Gonzalez, F. F., & Miller, S. P. (2006). Does perinatal asphyxia impair cognitive function without cerebral palsy? *Archives of Disease in Childhood. Fetal and Neonatal Edition, 91,* F454–F459. doi: 10.1136/adc.2005.092445

Guluma, K. Z., Hemmen, T. M., Olsen, S. E., Rapp, K. S., & Lyden, P. D. (2006). A trial of therapeutic hypothermia via endovascular approach in awake patients with acute ischemic stroke: Methodology. *Academic Emergency Medicine: Official Journal of the Society for Academic Emergency Medicine, 13*, 820–827. doi: 10.1197/j.aem.2006.03.559

Gunn, A. J., & Gunn, T. R. (1998). The "pharmacology" of neuronal rescue with cerebral hypothermia. *Early Human Development, 53*, 19–35. doi: S0378-3782(98)00033-4 [pii]

Gunn, A. J., Gunn, T. R., de Haan, H. H., Williams, C. E., & Gluckman, P. D. (1997). Dramatic neuronal rescue with prolonged selective head cooling after ischemia in fetal lambs. *The Journal of Clinical Investigation, 99*, 248–256. doi: 10.1172/JCI119153

Hall, R. T., Hall, F. K., & Daily, D. K. (1998). High-dose phenobarbital therapy in term newborn infants with severe perinatal asphyxia: A randomized, prospective study with three-year follow-up. *Journal of Pediatrics, 132*, 345–348.

Hallberg, B., Grossmann, K., Bartocci, M., & Blennow, M. (2010). The prognostic value of early aEEG in asphyxiated infants undergoing systemic hypothermia treatment. *Acta Paediatrica, 99*, 531–536. doi: 10.1111/j.1651-2227.2009.01653.x

Hemmen, T. M., & Lyden, P. D. (2009). Hypothermia after acute ischemic stroke. *Journal of Neurotrauma, 26*, 387–391. doi: 10.1089/neu.2008.0574

Higgins, R. D. (2005). Hypoxic ischemic encephalopathy and hypothermia: A critical look. *Obstetrics and Gynecology, 106*, 1385–1387. doi: 10.1097/01.AOG.0000190206. 70375.b4

Hobbs, C., Thoresen, M., Tucker, A., Aquilina, K., Chakkarapani, E., & Dingley, J. (2008). Xenon and hypothermia combine additively, offering long-term functional and histo-pathologic neuroprotection after neonatal hypoxia/ischemia. *Stroke, 39*, 1307–1313. doi: 10.1161/STROKEAHA.107.499822

Hypothermia after Cardiac Arrest Study Group. (2002). Mild therapeutic hypothermia to improve the neurologic outcome after cardiac arrest. *The New England Journal of Medicine, 346*, 549–556. doi: 10.1056/NEJMoa012689

Inder, T. E., Hunt, R. W., Morley, C. J., Coleman, L., Stewart, M., Doyle, L. W., & Jacobs, S. E. (2004). Randomized trial of systemic hypothermia selectively protects the cortex on MRI in term hypoxic-ischemic encephalopathy. *The Journal of Pediatrics, 145*, 835–837. doi: 10.1016/j.jpeds.2004.07.034

Jacobs, S., Hunt, R., Tarnow-Mordi, W., Inder, T., & Davis, P. (2007). Cooling for newborns with hypoxic ischaemic encephalopathy. *Cochrane Database of Systematic Reviews*(4), CD003311. doi: 10.1002/14651858.CD003311.pub2

Jacobs, S. E., Morley, C. J., Inder, T. E., Stewart, M. J., Smith, K. R., McNamara, P. J.,...Doyle, L. W. (2011). Whole-body hypothermia for term and near-term newborns with hypoxic-ischemic encephalopathy: A randomized controlled trial. *Archives of Pediatric and Adolescent Medicine, 165*, 692–700. doi: archpediatrics.2011.43 [pii]10.1001/archpediatrics.2011.43

Juul, S. E. (2000). Nonerythropoietic roles of erythropoietin in the fetus and neonate. *Clinics in Perinatology, 27*, 527–541.

Kammersgaard, L. P., Rasmussen, B. H., Jorgensen, H. S., Reith, J., Weber, U., & Olsen, T. S. (2000). Feasibility and safety of inducing modest hypothermia in awake patients with acute stroke through surface cooling: A case-control study: The Copenhagen Stroke Study. *Stroke, 31*, 2251–2256.

Laptook, A. R., & Corbett, R. J. (2002). The effects of temperature on hypoxic-ischemic brain injury. *Clinics in Perinatology, 29*, 623–649.

Laptook, A. R., Corbett, R. J., Sterett, R., Garcia, D., & Tollefsbol, G. (1995). Quantitative relationship between brain temperature and energy utilization rate measured in vivo using 31P and 1H magnetic resonance spectroscopy. *Pediatric Research, 38*, 919–925.

Lawn, J. E., Cousens, S., Zupan, J., & Lancet Neonatal Survival Steering, T. (2005). 4 million neonatal deaths: When? Where? Why? *Lancet, 365*, 891–900. doi: 10.1016/S0140-6736(05)71048-5

Little, D. M., Kraus, M. F., Jiam, C., Moynihan, M., Siroko, M., Schulze, F., & Geary, E. K. (2010). Neuroimaging of hypoxic-ischemic brain injury. *NeuroRehabilitation, 26*, 15–25. doi: 10.3233/NRE-2010-0532

Lorek, A., Takei, Y., Cady, E. B., Wyatt, J. S., Penrice, J., Edwards, A. D., . . . Reynolds, E. (1994). Delayed ("secondary") cerebral energy failure after acute hypoxia-ischemia in the newborn piglet: Continuous 48-hour studies by phosphorus magnetic resonance spectroscopy. *Pediatric Research, 36*, 699–706.

Maneru, C., Junque, C., Botet, F., Tallada, M., & Guardia, J. (2001). Neuropsychological long-term sequelae of perinatal asphyxia. *Brain Injury, 15*, 1029–1039. doi: 10.1080/02699050110074178

Maneru, C., Junque, C., Salgado-Pineda, P., Serra-Grabulosa, J. M., Bartres-Faz, D., Ramirez-Ruiz, B., . . . Botet, F. (2003). Corpus callosum atrophy in adolescents with antecedents of moderate perinatal asphyxia. *Brain Injury, 17*, 1003–1009.

Marlow, N., Rose, A. S., Rands, C. E., & Draper, E. S. (2005). Neuropsychological and educational problems at school age associated with neonatal encephalopathy. *Archives of Disease in Childhood. Fetal and Neonatal Edition, 90*, F380–F387. doi: 10.1136/adc.2004.067520

Morishita, E., Masuda, S., Nagao, M., Yasuda, Y., & Sasaki, R. (1997). Erythropoietin receptor is expressed in rat hippocampal and cerebral cortical neurons, and erythropoietin prevents in vitro glutamate-induced neuronal death. *Neuroscience, 76*, 105–116.

Moster, D., Lie, R. T., & Markestad, T. (2002). Joint association of Apgar scores and early neonatal symptoms with minor disabilities at school age. *Archives of Disease in Childhood: Fetal and Neonatal Edition, 86*, F16–F21.

Nagao, K., Kikushima, K., Watanabe, K., Tachibana, E., Tominaga, Y., Tada, K., . . . Yagi, T. (2010). Early induction of hypothermia during cardiac arrest improves neurological outcomes in patients with out-of-hospital cardiac arrest who undergo emergency cardiopulmonary bypass and percutaneous coronary intervention. *Circulation Journal: Official Journal of the Japanese Circulation Society, 74*, 77–85.

Nelson, K. B., & Grether, J. K. (1995). Can magnesium sulfate reduce the risk of cerebral palsy in very low birthweight infants? *Pediatrics, 95*, 263–269.

Nelson, K. B., & Leviton, A. (1991). How much of neonatal encephalopathy is due to birth asphyxia? *American Journal of Diseases in Children, 145*, 1325–1331.

O'Brien, F. E., Iwata, O., Thornton, J. S., De Vita, E., Sellwood, M. W., Iwata, S., . . . Robertson, N. J. (2006). Delayed whole-body cooling to 33 or 35 degrees C and the development of impaired energy generation consequential to transient cerebral hypoxia-ischemia in the newborn piglet. *Pediatrics, 117*, 1549–1559. doi: 117/5/1549 [pii]10.1542/peds.2005-1649

Oddo, M., Schaller, M. D., Feihl, F., Ribordy, V., & Liaudet, L. (2006). From evidence to clinical practice: Effective implementation of therapeutic hypothermia to improve patient outcome after cardiac arrest. *Critical Care Medicine, 34*, 1865–1873. doi: 10.1097/01.CCM.0000221922.08878.49

Osredkar, D., Toet, M. C., van Rooij, L. G., van Huffelen, A. C., Groenendaal, F., & de Vries, L. S. (2005). Sleep-wake cycling on amplitude-integrated electroencephalography in term newborns with hypoxic-ischemic encephalopathy. *Pediatrics, 115*, 327–332. doi: 10.1542/peds.2004-0863

Palisano, R. J., Hanna, S. E., Rosenbaum, P. L., Russell, D. J., Walter, S. D., Wood, E. P., . . . Galuppi, B. E. (2000). Validation of a model of gross motor function for children with cerebral palsy. *Physical Therapy, 80*, 974–985.

Palmer, C., Vannucci, R. C., & Towfighi, J. (1990). Reduction of perinatal hypoxic-ischemic brain damage with allopurinol. *Pediatric Research, 27*, 332–336.

Parikh, N. A., Lasky, R. E., Garza, C. N., Bonfante-Mejia, E., Shankaran, S., & Tyson, J. E. (2009). Volumetric and anatomical MRI for hypoxic-ischemic encephalopathy: Relationship to hypothermia therapy and neurosensory impairments. *Journal of Perinatology: Official Journal of the California Perinatal Association, 29,* 143–149. doi: 10.1038/jp.2008.184

Perlman, J. M., & Tack, E. D. (1988). Renal injury in the asphyxiated newborn infant: Relationship to neurologic outcome. *Journal of Pediatrics, 113,* 875–879.

Robertson, C. M., & Finer, N. N. (1988). Educational readiness of survivors of neonatal encephalopathy associated with birth asphyxia at term. *Journal of Developmental and Behavioral Pediatrics, 9,* 298–306.

Roth, S. C., Baudin, J., Cady, E., Johal, K., Townsend, J. P., Wyatt, J. S.,...Stewart, A. L. (1997). Relation of deranged neonatal cerebral oxidative metabolism with neurodevelopmental outcome and head circumference at 4 years. *Developmental Medicine and Child Neurology, 39,* 718–725.

Rouse, D. J., Hirtz, D. G., Thom, E., Varner, M. W., Spong, C. Y., Mercer, B. M.,...Eunice Kennedy Shriver, N. M.-F. M. U. N. (2008). A randomized, controlled trial of magnesium sulfate for the prevention of cerebral palsy. *The New England Journal of Medicine, 359,* 895–905. doi: 10.1056/NEJMoa0801187

Rutherford, M. A., Azzopardi, D., Whitelaw, A., Cowan, F., Renowden, S., Edwards, A. D., & Thoresen, M. (2005). Mild hypothermia and the distribution of cerebral lesions in neonates with hypoxic-ischemic encephalopathy. *Pediatrics, 116,* 1001–1006. doi: 10.1542/peds.2005-0328

Sarnat, H. B., & Sarnat, M. S. (1976). Neonatal encephalopathy following fetal distress. A clinical and electroencephalographic study. *Archives of Neurology, 33,* 696–705.

Shah, P. S. (2010). Hypothermia: A systematic review and meta-analysis of clinical trials. *Seminars in Fetal and Neonatal Medicine, 15,* 238–246. doi: 10.1016/j.siny.2010.02.003

Shalak, L. F., Laptook, A. R., Velaphi, S. C., & Perlman, J. M. (2003). Amplitude-integrated electroencephalography coupled with an early neurologic examination enhances prediction of term infants at risk for persistent encephalopathy. *Pediatrics, 111,* 351–357.

Shankaran, S. (2009). Neonatal encephalopathy: Treatment with hypothermia. *Journal of Neurotrauma, 26,* 437–443. doi: 10.1089/neu.2008.0678

Shankaran, S., Laptook, A. R., Ehrenkranz, R. A., Tyson, J. E., McDonald, S. A., Donovan, E. F.,...Human Development Neonatal Research, N. (2005). Whole-body hypothermia for neonates with hypoxic-ischemic encephalopathy. *The New England Journal of Medicine, 353,* 1574–1584. doi: 10.1056/NEJMcps050929

Shankaran, S., Pappas, A., Laptook, A. R., McDonald, S. A., Ehrenkranz, R. A., Tyson, J. E.,...Network, N. N. R. (2008). Outcomes of safety and effectiveness in a multicenter randomized, controlled trial of whole-body hypothermia for neonatal hypoxic-ischemic encephalopathy. *Pediatrics, 122,* e791–e798. doi: 10.1542/peds.2008-0456

Shankaran, S., Woldt, E., Koepke, T., Bedard, M. P., & Nandyal, R. (1991). Acute neonatal morbidity and long-term central nervous system sequelae of perinatal asphyxia in term infants. *Early Human Development, 25,* 135–148.

Silverman, W. A., Fertig, J. W., & Berger, A. P. (1958). The influence of the thermal environment upon the survival of newly born premature infants. *Pediatrics, 22,* 876–886.

Speer, M., & Perlman, J. M. (2006). Modest hypothermia as a neuroprotective strategy in high-risk term infants. *Clinics in Perinatology, 33,* 169–182, ix. doi: 10.1016/j.clp.2005.11.012

Steinman, K. J., Gorno-Tempini, M. L., Glidden, D. V., Kramer, J. H., Miller, S. P., Barkovich, A. J., & Ferriero, D. M. (2009). Neonatal watershed brain injury on magnetic resonance imaging correlates with verbal IQ at 4 years. *Pediatrics, 123,* 1025–1030. doi: 10.1542/peds.2008-1203

Tan, W. K., Williams, C. E., During, M. J., Mallard, C. F., Gunning, M. I., Gunn, A. J., & Gluckman, P. D. (1996). Accumulation of cytotoxins during the development of seizures and edema after hypoxic-ischemic injury in late gestation fetal sheep. *Pediatric Research, 39,* 791–797.

Thoresen, M., Bagenholm, R., Loberg, E. M., Apricena, F., & Kjellmer, I. (1996). Posthypoxic cooling of neonatal rats provides protection against brain injury. *Archives of Disease in Childhood. Fetal and Neonatal Edition, 74,* F3–F9.

Thoresen., M., Penrice, J., Lorek, A., Cady, E. B., Wylezinska, M., Kirkbride, V.,...Reynolds, E. (1995). Mild hypothermia after severe transient hypoxia-ischemia ameliorates delayed cerebral energy failure in the newborn piglet. *Pediatric Research, 37,* 667–670.

Tsai, P. T., Ohab, J. J., Kertesz, N., Groszer, M., Matter, C., Gao, J.,...Carmichael, S. T. (2006). A critical role of erythropoietin receptor in neurogenesis and post-stroke recovery. *The Journal of Neuroscience, 26,* 1269–1274. doi: 10.1523/JNEUROSCI.4480-05.2006

van Handel, M., Swaab, H., de Vries, L. S., & Jongmans, M. J. (2007). Long-term cognitive and behavioral consequences of neonatal encephalopathy following perinatal asphyxia: A review. *European Journal of Pediatrics, 166,* 645–654. doi: 10.1007/s00431-007-0437-8

Vannucci, R. C., & Perlman, J. M. (1997). Interventions for perinatal hypoxic-ischemic encephalopathy. *Pediatrics, 100,* 1004–1014.

Vargha-Khadem, F., Gadian, D. G., & Mishkin, M. (2001). Dissociations in cognitive memory: The syndrome of developmental amnesia. *Philosophical Transactions of the Royal Society of London. Series B, Biological Sciences, 356,* 1435–1440. doi: 10.1098/rstb.2001.0951

Viniker, D. A., Maynard, D. E., & Scott, D. F. (1984). Cerebral function monitor studies in neonates. *Clinical Electroencephalography, 15,* 185–192.

Westin, B., Miller, J. A., Jr., & Boles, A. (1963). Hypothermia induced during asphyxiation: Its effects on survival rate, learning and maintenance of the conditioned response in rats. *Acta Paediatrica, 52,* 49–60.

Zhu, C., Kang, W., Xu, F., Cheng, X., Zhang, Z., Jia, L.,...Wang, X. (2009). Erythropoietin improved neurologic outcomes in newborns with hypoxic-ischemic encephalopathy. *Pediatrics, 124,* e218–e226. doi: 10.1542/peds.2008-3553

8 Neuropsychological Functioning in Chronic Kidney Disease Across the Lifespan

Stephen R. Hooper and Arlene C. Gerson

The problem of kidney disease is so concerning that in 2000 the Healthy People Program established the reduction of chronic kidney disease (CKD) and its complications, disability, death, and economic costs as one of the program's main objectives. In order to achieve the targeted improvements, a multitiered approach was executed on local, state, and national levels. The approach included early identification of kidney disease, decreased prevalence, treatment of health conditions known to cause kidney damage, and implementation of rigorous evaluation of treatment of end-stage kidney disease (United States Department of Health and Human Services, 2000). These objectives were extended into Healthy People 2010 and provided support for kidney disease objectives to continue to be included in Healthy People 2020 (United States Department of Health and Human Services, 2011). The current Healthy People 2020 objectives include the following: (1) improvements in the early identification of kidney disease, (2) a slight decline in CKD prevalence, and (3) increased physician adherence with diabetes and hypertension evidence-based treatment protocols.

Further, there are health-related concerns for both children and adults with CKD. For example, the presence of pediatric CKD, particularly as it progresses toward the severe end of the spectrum where dialysis treatment is necessary, increases the death rate to between 30 and 150 times that of the general population of children and adolescents (USRDS, 2007). Moreover, once a child or young adolescent begins dialysis, the average length of life is only about 20 years (USRDS, 2007). In the adult arena, more than half of the individuals with severe kidney disease will experience some form of cerebrovascular accident. Given these sobering statistics, it is no wonder that kidney disease is a significant health concern that will manifest across the lifespan.

Given the national importance of CKD, this chapter focuses on what is currently known about the neuropsychological functioning of individuals with CKD across the lifespan. First, we provide an overview of CKD and its associated epidemiology. Next, we describe the available literature on the neuropsychological functioning of both children and adults with CKD, with a focus on potential underlying neurobiological mechanisms that contribute to the neurocognitive manifestations in individuals across the lifespan. Additionally, specific issues pertinent to individuals with CKD across the lifespan are addressed, including a list of clinical practice applications to assist neuropsychologists and other professionals working with this population.

OVERVIEW OF CHRONIC KIDNEY DISEASE

Definition

CKD manifests as deterioration of kidney functioning that typically progresses to the point of end-stage kidney disease (ESKD). For individuals aged 2 years and older, CKD is defined as kidney damage or estimated glomerular filtration rate (eGFR) <60 mL/min/1.73 m^2 for a time period of at least 3 months regardless of etiology. The eGFR can be estimated by using a number of different equations (Levey et al., 2005; Schwartz et al., 2010). For those younger than age 2 years, however, the above definition is not applicable because infants generally have a lower eGFR than older youth and because a CKD diagnosis is based on clinical symptoms.

Severity of Kidney Impairment

Kidney failure can produce a wide range of health-related concerns that can be transient and resolve or, more typically, are permanent and progressive. Generally speaking, the degree of impairment in kidney functioning is associated with disease severity. For kidney failure, disease severity provides a key strategy for determining the integrity of the filtration rate in the kidneys. As noted in the definition above, the eGFR is the primary method used to quantify the severity of kidney damage, with lower eGFR reflecting more severe kidney dysfunction. At present, kidney disease severity is classified into five stages according to the level of GFR (National Kidney Foundation, 2002). For example, severe kidney disease is defined as having an eGFR <30 mL/min/1.73 m^2 and described as a health state in which the kidneys are not adequately filtering toxins and waste products from the blood. In accordance with the National Kidney Foundation (2002), current severity stages include:

- Stage 1 – Kidney damage with normal or elevated GFR (GFR $\geq$ 90)
- Stage 2 – Kidney damage with mildly decreased GFR (GFR = 60–89)
- Stage 3 – Kidney damage with moderately decreased GFR (GFR = 30–59)
- Stage 4 – Severely decreased GFR (GFR = 15–29)
- Stage 5 – Kidney failure (GFR <15 or dialysis)

In addition to assisting with understanding the severity of the kidney disease, these stages also aid in making clinical determinations that pertain to patient management and treatments. Consequently, a variety of maintenance therapies are used for stages 1 through 3, while preparation and/or initiation of renal replacement therapies, including transplant, are involved at stages 4 and 5 (National Kidney Foundation, 2002).

Epidemiology

What is known about incidence and prevalence rates of CKD largely comes from the data relating to ESKD. This is not a scientific oversight but, rather, a function of the fact that many patients in the early stages of CKD present with few symptoms (Warady & Chadha, 2007). Coresh and colleagues (2003) estimated that the rates of patients with non–end-stage CKD may be 50 times more prevalent than those with ESKD. Overall, the number of patients with CKD has increased significantly, particularly in the adult population (Lysaght, 2002), with rates reflecting approximately 6%–16% of the population worldwide (Hallan et al., 2006; Warady & Chadha, 2007). This is a major factor that has contributed to an emphasis on CKD in Healthy People objectives.

Coresh and colleagues (2007) found that 50% of individuals aged 70 years or older meet the definition of CKD, with 38% of this age group having moderate to severe impairment when compared with a rate of 13% in the general United States population. Further, in a separate epidemiological study, Hailpern and colleagues (2007) estimated that approximately 1 million Americans between the ages of 20 and 59 years have CKD of a moderate nature, with the feeder system for this approximation coming from the child and adolescent populations.

To date, however, there are little comparable data of the incidence and prevalence of CKD in the pediatric population (Warady & Chadha, 2007). This is due, in part, to the different etiologies of CKD for children versus adults. The population-based data that do exist suggest a rate of approximately 74.7 cases per million in children younger than age 20 years (Ardissiono et al., 2003). Rates do seem to vary by age; the incidence rate for adolescents aged 15–19 years is about twice as high as that of children aged 10–14 years and nearly three times as high as that of children aged birth–4 years (USRDS, 2005). Additionally, it is important to note that CKD typically affects males more than females (NAPRTCS, 2005), perhaps secondary to the more frequent occurrence of congenital disorders in males (Warady & Chadha, 2007). Also, it tends to be seen more frequently in African Americans at a rate of two to three times that seen in Caucasian children (USRDS, 2001).

Etiology and Progression of Acute Kidney Injury and Chronic Kidney Disease

Acute kidney injury (AKI) can affect both children and adults and is characterized by a rapidly progressive loss of renal functioning. Unlike CKD, which results from congenital anomalies or from chronic health problems such as cardiovascular disease, diabetes, or obesity, this acute decline in renal functioning may be reversible. Temporary dialysis is often used early on in the treatment of AKI to treat the underlying cause of the kidney insult and to allow sufficient time for recovery of kidney functions (Pannu et al., 2008). In instances of AKI, there is a more heightened level of uremia than in those with CKD and, subsequently, greater vulnerability to encephalopathy secondary to changes in sodium–water balance, uremic toxins, and associated inflammatory effects on the brain (Arieff & Massry, 1974; De Deyn et al., 2003; Nguyen et al., 2006).

When this occurs, the individual may evidence a number of immediate and significant neurocognitive difficulties including poor attention, motor clumsiness, cognitive fatigue, and seizures.

Similar to AKI, CKD affects children and adults of all ages. In contrast to AKI, CKD encompasses patients with kidney function below approximately 75% of normal and extends downward to include those with no native function and who are dependent on dialysis or have received a kidney transplant. With progressively less kidney function, the body begins to accumulate waste products that the kidney fails to clear. The individual is at risk for an ever-increasing number and variety of complications related to kidney failure including neuropsychological deficits and dysfunction. In general, CKD is characterized by a slow onset and gradual increase in symptoms, eventually resulting in irreversible kidney damage. In both children and adults, the rate of kidney decline is not easily predicted for individual patients. However, in epidemiological studies it has been noted to take up to 10 years to progress to a severe enough stage that dialysis or transplantation is required (Hemmelgarn et al., 2006).

With respect to the etiology of CKD, data from the North American Pediatric Renal Transplant Cooperative Study (El Nahas et al., 2005) showed that about 50% of the patients experienced CKD secondary to obstructive uropathy (22%), aplasia/hypoplasia/dysplasia (18%), and reflux nephropathy (8%). In general, etiologies related to structural causes were more prevalent in patients younger than age 12 years, while cases of CKD secondary to glomerulonephritis appear more frequently in children older than age 12 years. In the latter cases, focal segmental glomerulosclerosis accounted for about 8.7% of the patients; however, when combined, all of the other glomerulonephrities account for <10% of the etiological agents in pediatric CKD.

In adult-onset CKD, etiology is generally described as being a consequence of genetic factors, lifestyle factors, and age. Genetic factors frequently implicated in adult-onset CKD include hypertension, dyslipidemia, and diabetes mellitus (Coresh et al., 2007). Lifestyle factors commonly associated with adult-onset CKD include smoking, sedentary lifestyle, and obesity (Lash et al., 2009). Age-related anatomic and physiologic renal changes include decreased renal mass, reduced tubular mass, and increased renal vascular resistance (Abdelhafiz et al., 2011).

NEUROIMAGING FINDINGS IN CHRONIC KIDNEY DISEASE

Across both child and adult populations, there have been approximately 24 structural and functional imaging studies conducted on various populations of individuals with CKD over the past 30 years. Within the adult population, earlier structural imaging studies using computer axial tomography (CT) scans revealed the presence of intracranial arachnoid cysts (Schievink et al., 1995), as well as changes in white and gray matter density, following hemodialysis in adults with acute renal failure (Ronco et al., 1999). Subsequent structural scans using magnetic resonance imaging (MRI) showed the presence of silent cerebral infarctions (Bouchi et al., 2010), deep white matter hyperintensities (Ishikawa et al., 2009), and cerebral micro-bleeds (Shima et al., 2010) in a wide range of individuals with CKD.

For the pediatric population, a similar set of findings has begun to emerge. Specifically, earlier studies using CT scans showed cerebral atrophy in severe CKD (Papageorgiou et al., 1982; Steinberg et al., 1985), while later studies that employed MRI evidenced cerebral atrophy and concerns for ischemic lesions in the vasculature region in the brain (Valanne et al., 2004). A recent functional brain scan using transcranial ultrasound Doppler in a pediatric sample with essential hypertension, ages 7–20 years, showed abnormal vasodilatory reactivity (Wong et al., 2011). Although children with CKD were excluded from this study, the findings hold significance for studying children with CKD given that a large percentage of pediatric patients with CKD have diagnosed hypertension.

NEUROPSYCHOLOGICAL FINDINGS IN CHRONIC KIDNEY DISEASE

Findings in Children

Although clinical research efforts over the past 50 years have examined the neuropsychological functioning of children with CKD, many of the pre-1990 findings likely were contaminated by a variety of factors including uncontrolled anemia and aluminum exposure secondary to many of the renal replacement therapies of that time period. The improvement of these therapies since that time has ushered in a new era of research in the neuropsychological functioning of children with CKD. However, even with these changes in treatment, a variety of neurocognitive dysfunctions and impairments continue to surface.

In this regard, a number of researchers have examined the neuropsychological functioning of children with CKD (Gerson et al., 2006; Gipson et al., 2004; Gipson, Hooper et al., 2006; Gipson & Hooper, 2012; Icard et al., 2010), with several of these reviews highlighting various neuropsychological assessment strategies in the evaluation of children and adolescents with CKD (Gipson & Hooper, 2009). Taken together, these reviews have documented a long-standing history of neurocognitive difficulties being present across the age range of infancy through late adolescence. They also have documented a wide range of difficulties ranging from general to specific, with severity of the cognitive impairments ranging from mild to severe.

Infants, Toddlers, and Preschoolers. For the youngest children, few efforts have been made to document neurocognitive concerns. Earlier studies certainly evidenced a number of concerns for infants and preschoolers with kidney disease, with significant developmental delays being noted in approximately a quarter of the patients (Hulstijn-Dirkmaat et al., 1995; Ledermann et al., 2000; Warady et al., 1999). For example, Ledermann and colleagues (2000) showed general developmental delays in dialysis-dependent infants when compared with children with renal insufficiency or typically developing infants. Further, in one of the few long-term follow-up studies, Warady and colleagues (1999) reported a low average range of intellectual functioning for about 21% of the sample who experience ESKD from infancy, with nonverbal abilities being lower than verbal abilities for about 44% of the sample.

More recently, Duquette and colleagues (2009) examined the early neurodevelopmental and adaptive behavior functions of infants and preschool children who had CKD. The sample included 16 patients with mild, moderate, severe, and end-stage CKD and 16 healthy matched controls. Findings revealed significant differences between the CKD and control groups on both developmental level and adaptive behavior, with the CKD group obtaining lower scores on both indices. For this young sample, the overall developmental level fell within the borderline range, while the overall adaptive behavior was rated as within the low-average range for chronological age. In addition, approximately 28% of the sample with CKD evidenced significant cognitive delays, as defined by scores falling at least 2 standard deviations below the average score. Disease severity also was strongly correlated to cognitive and adaptive functioning such that lower scores were associated with more impaired renal function. These findings serve to demonstrate that infants and preschoolers with CKD are at increased risk for early neurodevelopmental and adaptive behavior delays, with the magnitude of the delay correlating with the severity of the disease. In addition, these findings hold strong implications for the deployment of early intervention and special education services to facilitate overall development.

Children and Adolescents. Compared with the infants, toddlers, and preschool ers, there are significantly more empirical studies examining various neurocognitive aspects of CKD in children and adolescents. In general, the overall level of intellectual functioning for school-aged children with CKD is within the low-average range, with there being some sense that the more severe the kidney disease (e.g., ESKD), the lower the overall intellectual capabilities (Duquette et al., 2007; Hooper et al., 2011). Additionally, Lande and colleagues (2011) showed that children with CKD and elevated blood pressure evidence lower IQ. Specifically, in a cross-sectional analysis of the relation between blood pressure and IQ in 383 children aged 6–18 years, findings revealed that children with elevated blood pressure manifested lower IQ scores. In particular, Lande and colleagues (2011) noted that the blood pressure index correlated inversely with nonverbal IQ, and this relationship was maintained even after controlling for demographic and disease-related variables.

In addition to the intellectual findings, children and adolescents with CKD have shown a number of specific neuropsychological difficulties. Most notable among these are attention and executive function problems. Using a sample of children who received kidney transplants, Qvist and colleagues (2002) found no group differences on measures of attention regulation; however, 24% of the sample was experiencing a significant attention problem. In their CKD sample, Gipson, Duquette, and colleagues (2006) also showed the presence of difficulties with the executive functions of initiation and sustaining; these findings remained even after adjusting for IQ. In contrast, the executive functions of set-shifting and inhibitory control appeared to be uninvolved.

Similarly, concerns have been raised with respect to the presence of problems with the neuropsychological functions of memory (Fennell et al., 1990), with close to 20% of children with CKD showing significant generalized memory impairment (Qvist et al., 2002). Gipson, Duquette, and colleagues (2006) also documented that different kinds of memory can be impaired in children with CKD. Less empirical work has been done in the neurocognitive areas of sensory–motor, language, and visual–spatial abilities in children with CKD, but the data that are available suggest significant concerns for deficits in these neurocognitive domains as well (Bawden et al., 2004; Fennell et al., 1990; Groothoff et al., 2002; Qvist et al., 2002).

In one of the largest studies following children with CKD, Hooper and colleagues (2011) examined the neurocognitive difficulties in children with mild to moderate CKD and the relationship of targeted disease-related variables to neurocognitive outcomes. The sample comprised 368 children and adolescents, aged 6–16 years (mean = 13.0 years) enrolled in the National Institute of Diabetes and Digestive and Kidney Diseases funded Chronic Kidney Disease in Children Prospective Cohort Study

(CKiD). Measures included tests of intelligence, academic achievement, attention regulation, and parental ratings of executive functions. Results from this cross-sectional analysis of data, which were obtained shortly after the children entered the study, indicated that the median cognitive functioning for the sample fell within the average range, although 21%–40% of participants scored at least 1 standard deviation below the mean on IQ, achievement, attention, and/or executive functioning tests. At this baseline assessment, relatively few CKD-related variables were predictive of overall performance or risk status on the cognitive variables. In terms of overall performance, participants having elevated proteinuria scored modestly, but significantly lower, on IQ and attention variability than those without elevated proteinuria. Further, participants with elevated proteinuria were about 2.5 times more likely to be at risk for having low IQ; those having a glomerular diagnosis as their cause for CKD were 2.5 times more likely to be at risk for inattention; and those with a higher glomerular filtration rate (i.e., better kidney function) had less risk for overall executive dysfunction. Findings from this study are important in that they show that the majority of children with mild to moderate CKD do not manifest major neurocognitive deficits. Despite these relatively encouraging group findings, the study also showed that a substantial number of children with mild to moderate CKD do evidence cognitive dysfunction and that several disease-related variables do have modest relationships with cognitive risk status at this early stage of the disease process.

Finally, it is important to understand how renal replacement therapies such as dialysis and renal transplant can affect a child's neuropsychological functioning. A number of studies have examined the impact of transplant on subsequent neurocognitive capabilities. For example, transplant recipients have been described as having higher intellectual levels when compared with pretransplant levels, as well as when compared with children receiving dialysis (Fennell et al., 1990; Lawry et al., 1994), although the latter finding has been debated in the literature (Brouhard et al., 2000). Significant improvements in sustained attention and processing speed have also been documented to occur after transplant (Mendley & Zelko, 1999). In contrast to the above-noted positive associations between transplantation and neurocognitive functioning, Fennell and colleagues (1990) found memory functions deteriorated over a 1-year period regardless of the treatments utilized. In addition, Qvist and colleagues (2002) documented ongoing memory problems (20%) and attention/executive function problems (24%) in their posttransplant sample.

Findings in Adults

For adults who had childhood-onset CKD, research suggests that neuropsychological challenges apparent in childhood may impact educational and vocational outcomes in adulthood. Research evaluating adult survivors of childhood-onset ESKD has shown that verbal and nonverbal IQ is about 10 points lower than in uninvolved peers and that many achieve lower educational and poorer vocational outcomes (Bartosh et al., 2003; Groothoff et al., 2002). Findings that point out the difficulty in reversing ESKD-associated neuropsychological challenges and the negative long-term impact of these challenges have led to the increased emphasis on preemptive transplantation for children with non–end-stage CKD. In addition, these findings have been used to inform transition programs for young adults (Icard et al., 2008).

The prevalence of cognitive dysfunction in adult-onset CKD appears to be elevated across the spectrum of kidney disease severity. A sizeable amount of cross-sectional and longitudinal data have portrayed an increased risk of neuropsychological problems in adults with ESKD requiring dialysis. For example, the prevalence of severe cognitive impairment in patients receiving hemodialysis and peritoneal dialysis has been reported to be significantly higher than the prevalence of dementia in community-based population studies (Kalirao et al., 2011). Even after adjusting for the confounders of age, sex, race, education, depression, diabetes, hypertension, and stroke, Kalirao and colleagues (2011) and Murray and colleagues (2006) reported that the prevalence of severe cognitive impairment in their samples was much higher than the 5%–10% estimated prevalence of dementia in community-based non-ESKD population studies involving individuals aged 65 years and older.

Murray and colleagues (2006) measured cognitive function in 338 patients receiving hemodialysis, aged 55–89 years (mean = 71.2, standard deviation [SD] = 9.5), with the goal of comparing their neurocognitive function to a non-ill control group. They found that 70% of the cohort had moderate to severe cognitive impairment. In addition, it was observed that the hemodialysis group was 3.5 times more likely to have severe cognitive impairment relative to the non-ill comparison group, even after adjusting for age, sex, race, education, depression, diabetes, hypertension, and stroke (Murray et al., 2006). Kalirao and colleagues (2011) studied 51 patients undergoing peritoneal dialysis, with the goal of comparing their neurocognitive functioning to that of patients on hemodialysis and a non-ill control group. Findings revealed that approximately 75% of the peritoneal dialysis cohort had moderate to severe cognitive impairment, with about one-third of the group demonstrating severe cognitive impairment. Furthermore, the peritoneal dialysis group was >2.5 times more likely than the non-CKD participants to develop moderate to severe cognitive impairment. In addition to the observation of a high prevalence of global cognitive functioning impairments in adults with kidney disease receiving dialysis treatment, neuropsychological dysfunction in executive function, verbal fluency, attention, and perceptual–motor skills has been observed (Fazekas et al., 1996; Kurella et al., 2004; Pereira et al., 2007; Post et al., 2010).

Of critical importance in adult CKD, a number of studies have sought to determine whether the disproportionate prevalence of moderate to severe cognitive dysfunction is attributable to dialysis treatment, renal failure itself, or differences in demographic factors and comorbid conditions. When adjusting for these confounding factors, a number of studies have provided support for the likelihood that dialysis treatment may independently have a negative impact on both short-term and long-term neurocognitive functioning (Kalirao et al., 2011; Kurella et al, 2010a; Murray et al., 2006). Specifically, Murray and colleagues (2006) found that undergoing dialysis treatment for a duration longer than 24 months is associated with a 1.6-fold increased risk for an individual to show severe cognitive impairment. Consequently, although dialysis treatment is necessary to support an individual's kidney functioning, these findings do implicate the negative effects that can occur in the area of neuropsychological functioning. Possible explanatory mechanisms for this relationship include the following: (1) the process of hemodialysis can induce recurrent episodes of acute cerebral ischemia that, in turn, may contribute to acute decline in cognitive function during dialysis (Kobayashi et al., 2010; Murray et al., 2006; Post et al., 2010); and (2) the process of hemodialysis can contribute to metabolic dysregulation that, in turn, may reduce cognitive performance, especially in tasks that require attention, concentration, organization, and planning (Murray et al., 2006).

Similar to the observations of study cohorts with ESKD receiving dialysis, cohorts that are primarily comprised of adults with moderate to severe CKD who are not receiving dialysis also have higher rates of severe cognitive dysfunction compared with healthy patient groups. For example, analysis of data from the Cardiovascular Health Cognition Study revealed that among study participants with nonelevated creatinine and reporting good to excellent health at baseline (N = 2557), moderate kidney damage at follow-up (reflected by an increase in serum creatinine from 1.0 mg/DL to 2.0 mg/DL) was independently associated with a 37% increase in risk of a new diagnosis of vascular-type dementia (Seliger et al., 2004). In addition, recent analyses of data from the Chronic Renal Insufficiency Cohort Study show a 2-fold higher prevalence of severe cognitive dysfunction in participants with advanced CKD who are not on dialysis (eGFR <30 mL/min/1.73 m^2) compared with participants with mild to moderate CKD (Yaffe et al., 2010). In addition to findings regarding associations between CKD and global cognitive impairment, a number of studies have replicated this association between moderate reductions in eGFR and/or moderate elevations in creatinine and lower levels of performance on neurocognitive measures of perceptual–motor, attention, language, and higher-order executive functions (Elias et al., 2009; Jassal et al., 2008; Seliger et al., 2004; Yaffe et al., 2010).

Cognitive dysfunction has also been observed in adults with mild and moderate kidney disease. In a landmark study using computerized cognitive function tests obtained as part of the National Health and Nutrition Examination Survey, it was observed that moderate CKD was independently associated with poorer learning/concentration and a nearly 3-fold increased risk of visual attention impairment (Hailpern et al., 2007). In addition, analysis of data from a multisite prospective observational cohort study of 5529 community-dwelling men who were enrolled in the Osteoporotic Fractures in Men Study found evidence of an independent association between mild to moderate reductions in kidney function and poorer executive function (Slinin et al., 2008).

Finally, a number of studies have sought to determine whether this increased rate of neurocognitive dysfunction and dementia in the adult population is attributable to renal failure, differences in sociodemographic factors, and/or comorbid conditions. In sum, after adjusting for confounding variables, findings generally provide support for the likelihood that mild to moderate kidney disease may independently have a harmful impact on both short-term and long-term neurocognitive functioning (Elias et al., 2009; Etgen et al., 2009; Seliger et al., 2004; Slinin et al., 2008).

Factors Affecting Neuropsychological Impairment Across the Lifespan

What CKD-related factors can affect the neuropsychological functioning of both children and adults? The available research supports the likelihood that multiple pathogenetic processes contribute to the development of kidney disease, the rate of kidney deterioration, the occurrence of neurocognitive dysfunction, and the tempo of neuropsychological deterioration. There are several biologically plausible mechanisms through which impairment of renal function could result in an increased risk for neurocognitive declines or, in the adult population, dementia. All of these factors need to be taken into account when examining the neurocognitive functioning of children and adults with CKD.

First, there is a significant body of evidence regarding the bidirectional association between cardiovascular integrity and renal function (i.e., cardio–renal association), indicating that CKD is a risk factor for cardiac disease and, conversely, that cardiac disease is a risk factor for the development of kidney disease (Hailpern et al., 2007; Seliger et al., 2004). Notable among these variables is hypertension. What is known is that more than 50% of children with CKD have hypertension (Flynn et al., 2008; Mitsnefes et al., 2003) and that many adults with hypertension evidence a variety of neurocognitive difficulties when compared with nonhypertensive peers (Lande et al., 2003; Waldstein et al., 2001). In addition to the efforts by Lande and colleagues (2011), the field is striving toward increasing our understanding of this relationship in children, particularly in children with milder variants of CKD (Mitsnefes et al., 2010).

Second, there is mounting evidence of a cerebrorenal association demonstrating that poor kidney function is associated with increased risk of cerebrovascular problems and, conversely, that cerebrovascular disease predicts kidney function outcomes (Elias et al., 2009; Kobayashi et al., 2010; Kurella et al, 2011). Neuropathological changes brought about by atherosclerosis, microvascular disease, clinical stroke, silent stroke, oxidative stress, and white matter lesions have been found to be associated with incremental changes in cognitive functioning in both community-based healthy cohorts and CKD cohorts (Fazekas et al., 1996; Jassal et al., 2008; Jassal et al., 2010; Kurella et al., 2004; Kobayashi et al., 2010; Murray et al., 2006; Pereira et al., 2004; Seliger et al., 2004; Tryc et al., 2011; Ikram et al., 2008). For example, in a community-based cross-sectional study of 923 individuals, Elias and colleagues (2009) found that for participants with eGFR <60 (mean = 49.7, SD = 10.7) there was a 2-fold increased risk of having cognitive impairment compared with those with eGFR ≥ 60. More specifically, they found that after adjusting for numerous covariates (i.e., age, sex, education, race, diabetes, blood pressure, body mass index, lipid levels, stroke), higher levels of serum creatinine (2 mg/dL versus 1 mg/dL) were associated with worse performance on neurocognitive assessments of executive functioning. From a developmental perspective, how the vascular system changes across the lifespan in individuals with CKD, such that there is an increase in neurological manifestations in adulthood, remains to be determined. Further, continued efforts to uncover childhood vascular precursors may serve to facilitate earlier intervention and ameliorate the manifestation of adult neurological problems.

A third factor, anemia, has been tagged as another common consequence of kidney disease. Anemia has been associated with both cognitive functioning problems and clinical dementia in adults with ESKD (Kurella et al., 2010b). These findings have led to the establishment of clinical practice guidelines that prioritize the treatment of anemia in adults with deteriorating kidney function. Moreover, the efficacy of treating anemia has been established through the observation that increases in hemoglobin can result in improvements in patient perceptions of quality of life (Foley et al., 2009).

Finally, a number of other mechanistic factors have been implicated in the relationship between CKD and neurocognitive impairment. For example, the relationship between depression and cognitive dysfunction has been well described in both nonclinical and health-impaired groups. Within adult kidney disease cohorts, depression prevalence rates have ranged from 11% to 29%, with the highest rates of depression occurring in patients who were receiving dialysis (Elias et al., 2009; Etgen et al., 2009;

Jassal et al., 2008; Kalirao et al., 2011; Murray et al., 2006). It is important to point out that the relationship between depression and cognitive dysfunction is well recognized in adult patients with CKD and is routinely addressed using statistical procedures that identify and mediate its influence so that the unique contributions of kidney disease to neurocognitive functioning can be ascertained (Elias et al., 2009; Etgen et al., 2009; Jassal et al., 2008; Kalirao et al., 2011; Murray et al., 2006). It is important to note, however, that this is less well understood in the child CKD population (Hooper et al., 2009).

Metabolic dysregulation, which is characterized by inflammation and oxidative stress, has also been found to be associated with both kidney failure and the pathogenesis of dementia. Similarly, malnutrition, weight loss, and sarcopenia are common clinical consequences of kidney deterioration and have been shown to increase the risk of both cognitive dysfunction and physical difficulties (Seliger et al., 2004).

RELATED ISSUES IN THE NEUROPSYCHOLOGICAL FUNCTIONING OF INDIVIDUALS WITH CKD

Adherence to Medical Procedures

Cognitive impairment in adults with CKD has been associated with a variety of adverse outcomes with respect to kidney disease progression and treatment costs. For example, the integrity of cognitive functioning has been shown to influence medication adherence (Stilley et al., 2010) and, when impaired, may impede compliance with dialysis schedules, fluid restrictions, and dietary recommendations (Kalirao et al., 2011; Murray et al., 2006; Sehgal et al., 1997). Furthermore, cognitive impairment and dementia among patients undergoing hemodialysis appear to increase the risk of hospitalization, annual Medicare costs for adults, and mortality (USRDS, 2011). Sehgal and colleagues (1997) sought to evaluate the implications of cognitive impairment among 336 patients receiving hemodialysis and found that cognitive impairment was independently associated with increased technician time caring for patients after dialysis and with increased hospital days.

Adolescent and Adult Transition

Adolescent and adult transition issues have become a national focus. Indeed, for children with CKD, this is the natural pathway into adulthood, and the associated burden of CKD will be an unfortunate partner in this process. Children with CKD face many barriers during their transition through adolescence into adulthood, and these barriers undoubtedly will have an impact on how an individual manages his or her CKD. Childhood-onset CKD and the associated medical complications can prevent many adolescents from making this transition and facing these developmental challenges successfully.

Icard and colleagues (2008) discussed a number of key transition issues (e.g., vocational rehabilitation services, mental health) and emphasized the need for more evidence-based transition programs that would facilitate the movement from late adolescence into adulthood. Further, it is essential that the healthcare needs of individuals with CKD be taken into account in this process. Bell and colleagues (2011) noted that the design of healthcare transition services for adolescents and emerging adults with

CKD needs to take into account a variety of issues (e.g., family factors, healthcare resources), including the individual's neurocognitive capabilities. These latter functions and dysfunctions undoubtedly can have a positive or negative impact on the individual's compliance with medical procedures, understanding of their medical care, and ability to engage in preventative actions with respect to this illness.

Clinical Applications

Despite what appears to be a fair amount of literature on the neurocognitive functioning of individuals with CKD across the lifespan, we are only beginning to provide an evidence base to this field and to our understanding of the neurocognitive presentation of children and adults with CKD. Nonetheless, there are a number of clinical applications of the available empirical literature about what is known that can be asserted. These include the following:

- Recognizing the potential symptoms of kidney disease so that you can be aware of physical symptoms that your patients might experience. Biochemical symptoms of kidney disease vary from person to person and can include the following: (1) high levels or urea in the blood that may result in appetite loss, nausea, vomiting, diarrhea, weight loss, and/or changes in frequency, amount, or color of urine; (2) a build-up of phosphates in the blood that may result in itching and muscle cramps and/or sleep problems; (3) a build-up of potassium in the blood that may result in abnormal heart rhythms and/or muscle paralysis; (4) fluid retention that may result in shortness of breath due to extra fluid on the lungs and swelling of the legs, ankles, feet, face, and/or hands; and (5) decreased production of the hormone erythropoietin, which may result in fatigue, feeling weak, dizziness, difficulty concentrating, and/or low blood pressure (Murtagh et al., 2007).
- Developing prevention strategies that target modification of vascular risk factors. Increased physical and cognitive activities have shown some promise in influencing cognitive outcomes in adults with CKD (Tamura & Yafee, 2011; Middleton et al., 2011; Geda et al., 2011; Geda et al., 2010). In addition, interventions targeting improved sleep, along with improved medication adherence, may serve to improve cognitive functioning in adults and children with CKD (Pace-Schott & Spencer, 2011).
- Given the progressive nature of CKD, a baseline assessment of neuropsychological functioning is recommended before the initiation of any renal replacement therapies (i.e., dialysis, transplant). Findings should be communicated in a manner such that healthcare providers understand the implications of the testing results. This type of pre–post assessment strategy also will be useful when evaluating the benefit versus risk of receiving dialysis (Murray et al., 2006).
- Although much remains to be learned about the pathophysiology of cognitive impairment in kidney disease, its prevalence indicates an imperative for serial assessment of neurocognitive functioning prior to ESKD to characterize neurocognitive deficits across the lifespan.
- With respect to CKD management, it is important for the service provider to be keenly aware of aspects of a patient's cognitive functioning that remain intact, are deteriorating, or have deteriorated to a point where self-care and/or medical decision making are compromised. Although applicable to all patients with CKD,

this is particularly important for the aging CKD population. In this population, it becomes even more important to guide treatment and establish safeguards if cognitive deterioration prevents a patient from being able to manage his or her healthcare independently or to take on the independent management of healthcare during the transition from a pediatric to adult medical practice.

- If possible, avoid engaging your patient in important conversations during dialysis treatments. Due to the prevalence of acute neurocognitive functioning deficits observed during hemodialysis treatment, efforts should be made to communicate information of import prior to or after dialysis treatment. Further, information concerning healthcare regimen changes or new medical recommendations should be provided in writing to the patient or the patient's healthcare representative, and efforts to ensure that they have understood the instructions should be made.
- CKD is a complex disease that appears to involve a number of bodily systems and can have an impact on a wide range of life events. In this regard, it is important to implement an interdisciplinary management team model that is employed when working with this patient population across the lifespan.

CONCLUSIONS AND DIRECTIONS

This chapter has focused on what is currently known about the neuropsychological functioning of individuals with CKD across the lifespan. In addition to an overview of CKD, we described what is known about the neuropsychological functioning of both children and adults with CKD, and we provided a discussion of several key CKD-related factors that could affect neurocognitive outcomes. In sum, it is clear that CKD is not just a medical illness but, rather, a complex problem that can affect neurocognitive abilities, learning, adaptive functions, child–adult transition challenges, and long-standing medical care issues. At present, it appears that a number of neurocognitive abilities can be affected, with the preponderance of available evidence on both children and adults pointing to vulnerable attention/executive functions and memory capabilities. However, little is known about other major neurocognitive domains such as language or sensory-motor functions.

Similarly, there appears to be multiple underlying neurological mechanisms that contribute to these difficulties, with available evidence, largely from the literature on adults, directing efforts to vascular abnormalities and dysfunction. The linkage of these adult-related findings may have a pathway via hypertension because this may provide an avenue for developmental continuity of vascular problems into adulthood. The role of the neuropsychologist appears to be important not only for understanding the impact of CKD on brain-related functions but also for assisting in the management of individuals with CKD in the family, medical, school, and other community settings.

Finally, it will be important for professionals in the fields of nephrology and neuropsychology to continue to work in a collaborative fashion in both the adult and pediatric realms. The intersection of these fields is critical to improving our understanding of the neurocognitive issues presented by individuals with CKD at all ages. Such a collaboration should contribute to improvement in our understanding of the underlying mechanisms that contribute to the neurocognitive functioning of pediatric and adult patients with mild, moderate, severe, and end-stage kidney disease. Ongoing dialogues about clinical observations and research findings will be critical to facilitation of professional partnerships aimed at improving the well-being of children and adults with CKD.

ACKNOWLEDGEMENTS

This chapter was completed with support from the Maternal Child Health Bureau (#MCJ379154A); the Administration on Developmental Disabilities (#90DD043003); and the National Institute of Diabetes and Digestive and Kidney Diseases, the National Institute of Neurological Disorders and Stroke, the National Institute of Child Health and Human Development, and the National Heart, Lung, and Blood Institute (U01-DK-66143, U01-DK-66174, U01-DK-66116, U01-DK-082194).

REFERENCES

Abdelhafiz, A. H., Ahmed, S., Flint, K., & El-Nahas, M. (2011). Is chronic kidney disease in older people a new geriatric giant? *Aging Health, 7*, 749–762.

Ardissino, G., Dacco, V., Testa, S., Bonaudo, R., Claris-Appiani, A., Taioli, E.,...Sereni, F. (2003). Epidemiology of chronic renal failure in children: Data from the ItalKid project. *Pediatrics, 111*, e382–387.

Arieff, A. I., & Massry, S. G. (1974). Calcium metabolism of brain in acute renal failure. Effects of uremia, hemodialysis, and parathyroid hormone. *Journal of Clinical Investigation, 53*, 387–392.

Bartosh, S. M., Leverson, G., Robillard, D., & Sollinger, H.W. (2003). Long-term outcomes in pediatric renal transplant recipients who survive into adulthood. *Transplantation, 76*, 1195–1200.

Bawden, H. N., Acott, P., Carter, J., Lirenman, D., MacDonald, G. W., McAllister, M.,...Crocker, J. (2004). Neuropsychological functioning in end-stage renal disease. *Archives of the Diseases of Childhood, 89*, 644–647.

Bell, L. E., Ferris, M. E., Fenton, N., & Hooper, S. R. (2011). Health care transition in pediatric CKD. *Advances in Chronic Kidney Disease, 18*, 384–390.

Bouchi, R., Babazono, T., Yoshida, N., Nyumura, I., Toya, K., Hayashi, T.,...Iwamoto, Y. (2010). Relationship between chronic kidney disease and silent cerebral infarction in patients with Type 2 diabetes. *Diabetic Medicine, 27*, 538–543.

Brouhard, B. H., Donaldson, L. A., Lawry, K. W., McGowan, K. R., Drotar, D., Davis, I.,...Tejani, A. (2000). Cognitive functioning in children on dialysis and post-transplantation. *Pediatric Transplantation, 4*, 261–267.

Coresh, J., Astor, B. C., Greene, T., Eknoyan, G., & Levey, A. S. (2003). Prevalence of chronic kidney disease and decreased kidney function in the adult US population: Third National Health and Nutrition Examination Survey. *American Journal of Kidney Diseases, 41*, 1–12.

Coresh, J., Selvin, E., Stevens, L. A., Manzi, J., Kusek, J. W., Eggers, P., ... & Levey, A. S. (2007). Prevalence of chronic kidney disease in the United States. *Journal of the American Medical Association, 298*, 2038–2047.

DeDeyn, P. P., Vanholder, R., & DHooge, R. (2003). Nitric oxide in uremia: Effects of several potentially toxic guanidine compounds. *Kidney International Supplement, 84*, S25–S28.

Duquette, P. J., Hooper, S. R., Icard, P. F., Mamak, E. G., Wetherington, C. E., & Gipson, D. S. (2009). Early neurodevelopment in children with chronic kidney disease. *Journal of Special Education, 43*, 45–51.

Duquette, P. J., Hooper, S. R., Wetherington, C. E., Jenkins, T. L., & Gipson, D. S. (2007). Brief Report: Intellectual and academic functioning in pediatric chronic kidney disease. *Journal of Pediatric Psychology, 32,* 1011–1017.

Elias, M. F., Elias, P. K., Seliger, S. L., Narsipur, S. S., Dore, G. A., & Robbins, M. A. (2009). Chronic kidney disease, creatinine, and cognitive functioning. *Nephrology, Dialysis, and Transplant, 24,* 2446–2452.

El Nahas, A. M., & Bello, A. K. (2005). Chronic kidney disease: The global challenge. *Lancet, 365,* 31–40.

Etgen, T., Sander, D., Chonchol, M., Briesenick, C., Poppert, H., Forstl, H., & Bicket, H. (2009). Chronic kidney disease is associated with incident cognitive impairment in the elderly: The INVADE study. *Nephrology, Dialysis, and Transplant, 24,* 3144–3150.

Fazekas, G., Fazekas, F., Schmidt, R., Flooh, E., Valetitsch, H., Kapeller, P., & Krejs, G. J. (1996). Pattern of cerebral blood flow in cognition in patients undergoing chronic haemodialysis treatment. *Nuclear Medicine Communications, 17,* 603–608.

Fennell, R. S., Fennell, E. B., Carter, R. L., Mings, E. L., Klausner, A. B., & Hurst, J. R. (1990). A longitudinal study of the cognitive function of children with renal failure. *Pediatric Nephrology, 4,* 11–15.

Flynn, J. T., Mitsnefes, M., Pierce, C., Cole, S. R., Parekh, R. S., Furth, S. L.,...Chronic Kidney Disease in Children Study Group. (2008). Blood pressure in children with chronic kidney disease: A report from the chronic kidney disease in children study. *Hypertension, 52,* 631–637.

Foley, R. N., Curtis, B. M., & Parfrey, P. S. (2009). Erythropoietin therapy, hemoglobin targets, and quality of life in healthy hemodialysis patients: A randomized trial. *Clinical Journal of the American Society of Nephrology, 4,* 726–733.

Geda, Y. E., Topazian, H. M., Lewis, R. A., Robers, R. O., Knopman, D. S., Pankratz, V. S.,...Petersen, R. C. (2011). Engaging in cognitive activities, aging, and mild cognitive impairment: A population-based study. *Journal of Neuropsychiatry and Clinical Neuroscience, 23,* 149–154.

Geda, Y. E., Roberts, R. O., Knopman, D. S., Christianson, T. J. H., Pankratz, V. S., Ivnik, R. J.,...Rocca, W. H. (2010). Physical exercise, aging, and mild cognitive impairment: A population-based study. *Archives of Neurology, 67,* 80–86.

Gerson, A. C., Butler, R., Moxy-Mims, M., Wentz, A., Shinnar, S., Lande, M.,...Hooper, S. R. (2006). Neurocognitive outcomes in children with chronic kidney disease: Current findings and contemporary endeavors. *Mental Retardation and Developmental Disabilities Research Reviews, 12,* 208–215.

Gipson, D. S., Duquette, P. J., Icard, P. F., & Hooper, S. R. (2006). The central nervous system in childhood chronic kidney disease. *Pediatric Nephrology, 22,* 1703–1710.

Gipson, D. S., & Hooper, S. R. (2009). Neurodevelopmental issues in chronic renal disease. In D. F. Geary, & F. Schaefer (Eds.), *Comprehensive pediatric nephrology* (pp. 733–742). Cambridge, MA: Elsevier.

Gipson, D. S., & Hooper, S. R. (2012). Neurocognitive complications and management in pediatric kidney disease. In B. A. Warady, F. Schaefer, & S. R. Alexander (Eds.), *Pediatric dialysis* (2nd ed., pp. 581–592). New York: Springer.

Gipson, D. S., Hooper, S. R., Duquette, P. J., Wetherington, C. E., Stellwagen, K. K., Jenkins, T. L, & Ferris, M. E. (2006). Memory and executive functions in pediatric chronic kidney disease. *Child Neuropsychology, 12,* 1–15.

Gipson, D. S, Wetherington, C. E., Duquette, P. J., & Hooper, S. R. (2004). The nervous system and chronic kidney disease in children. *Pediatric Nephrology, 19,* 832–839.

Groothoff, J. W., Grootenhuis, M., Dommerholt, A., Gruppen, M. P., Offringa, M., & Heymans, H. S. (2002). Impaired cognition and schooling in adults with end stage renal disease since childhood. *Archives of the Diseases of Childhood, 87,* 380–385.

Hailpern, S. M., Melamed, M. L., Cohen, H. W., & Hostetter, T. H. (2007). Moderate chronic kidney disease and cognitive function in adults 20–59 years of age: Third National Health and Nutrition Examination Survey (NHANES III). *Journal of the American Society of Nephrology, 18*, 2205–2213.

Hallan, S. I., Coresh, J., Astor, B. C., Asberg, A., Powe, N. R., Romundstad, S., . . . Holmen, J. (2006). International comparison of the relationship of chronic kidney disease prevalence and ESRD risk. *Journal of the American Society of Nephrology, 17*, 2275–2284.

Hemmelgarn , B. R., Zhang, J., Manns, B. J., Tonelli, M., Larsen, E., Ghali, W. A., . . . Culleton, B. F. (2006). Progression of kidney dysfunction in the community-dwelling elderly. *Kidney International, 69*, 2155–2161.

Hooper, S. R., Duquette, P. J., Icard, P., Wetherington, C. E., Harrell, W, & Gipson, D. S. (2009). Social-behavioral functioning in pediatric chronic kidney disease. *Child: Care, Health & Development, 35*, 832–840.

Hooper, S. R., Gerson, A. C., Wentz, A., Abraham, A., Mendley, S., Butler, R., . . . Furth, S. (2011). Neurocognitive functioning of children and adolescents with mild to moderate chronic kidney disease: Baseline findings. *Clinical Journal of the American Society of Nephrology, 6*, 1824–1830.

Hulstijn-Dirkmaat, G. M., Damhuis, I. H., Jetten, M. L., Koster, A. M., & Schroder, C. H. (1995). The cognitive development of pre-school children treated for chronic renal failure. *Pediatric Nephrology, 9*, 464–469.

Icard, P., Hooper, S. R., & Gipson, D. S. (2010). Cognitive improvement in children with CKD after transplant. *Pediatric Transplantation, 14*, 887–890.

Icard, P. F., Hower, S. J., Kuchenreuther, A. R., Hooper, S. R., & Gipson, D. S. (2008). The transition from childhood to adulthood with ESRD: Educational and social challenges. *Clinical Nephrology, 69*, 1–7.

Ishikawa, K., Ikeda, M., Hamasaki, Y., Hataya, H., Shishido, S., Asanuma, H., . . . Honda, M. (2009). Posterior reversible encephaolopathy syndrome in children: Its high prevalence and more extensive imaging findings. *American Journal of Kidney Diseases, 48*, 231–238.

Ikram, M. A., Vernooij, M. W., Hofman, A., Neissen, W. J., van der Lugt, A., & Breteler, M. M. B. (2008). Kidney function is related to cerebral small vessel disease. *Stroke, 39*, 55–61.

Jassal, S. K., Kritz-Silverstein, D., & Barrett-Connor, E. (2010). A prospective study of albuminuria and cognitive function in older adults: The Rancho Bernardo Study. *American Journal of Epidemiology, 171*, 277–286.

Jassal, S., Roscoe, J., LeBlanc, D., Devins, G. M., & Rourke, S. (2008). Differential impairment of psychomotor efficiency and processing speed in patients with chronic kidney disease. *International Urology and Nephrology, 40*, 849–854.

Kalirao, P., Pederson, S., Foley, R. N., Kolste, A., Tupper, D., Zaun, D., . . . & Murray, A. M. (2011). Cognitive impairment in peritoneal dialysis patients. *American Journal of Kidney Disease, 57*, 612–620.

Kobayashi, M., Hirawa, N., Morita, S., Yatsu, K., Kobayashi, Y., Yamamoto, Y., . . . Umemura, S. (2010). Silent brain infarction and rapid decline in kidney function in patients with CKD: A prospective cohort study. *American Journal of Kidney Disease, 56*, 468–476.

Kurella, M., Chertow, G. M., Luan, J., & Yaffe, K. (2004). Cognitive impairment in chronic kidney disease. *Journal of the American Geriatrics Society, 52*, 1863–1869.

Kurella, T. M., Larive, B., Unruh, M. L., Stokes, J. B., Nissenson, A., Mehta, R.L., & Chertow, G.M. (2010a). Frequent Hemodialysis Network Trial Group. Prevalence and correlates of cognitive impairment in hemodialysis patients: The Frequent Hemodialysis Network trials. *Clinical Journal of the American Society of Nephrology, 5*, 1429–1438.

Kurella, T. M., Wadley, V. G., Newsome, B. B., Zakai, N.A., McClure, L. A., Howard, G., . . . McClellan, W. (2010b). Hemoglobin concentration and cognitive impairment in the renal REasons for Geographic And Racial Differences in Stroke (REGARDS) Study. *Journal of Gerontology, 65,* 1380–1386.

Kurella, T. M., Xie, D., Yaffe, K., Cohen, D. L., Teal, V., Kasner, S. E.,...Go, A. S. (2011). Vascular risk factors and cognitive impairment in chronic kidney disease: The Chronic Renal Insufficiency Cohort (CRIC) study. *Clinical Journal of the American Society of Nephrology, 6,* 248–256.

Kuyer, J. M., Hulstihn-Dirkmaat, G. M., & van Aken, M. A. (1990). Effects of kidney transplantation on cognitive functioning in children. *Tiffschr Kindergeneeskd, 58,* 83–89.

Lande, M. B., Gerson, A., Hooper, S. R., Cox, C., Matheson, M., Mendley, S.,...Flynn, J. (2011). Blood pressure and neurocognitive function in children with chronic kidney disease: A report of the Children with Chronic Kidney Disease Cohort Study. *Clinical Journal of the American Society of Nephrology, 6,* 1831–1837.

Lande, M. B., Kaczorowski, J. M., Auinger, P., Schwartz, G. J., & Weitzman, M. (2003). Elevated blood pressure and decreased cognitive function among school-age children and adolescents in the United States. *Journal of Pediatrics, 143,* 720–724.

Lash, J. P., Go, A. S., Appel, L. J., He, J., Ojo, A., Rahman, M.,...Feldman H. I. (2009). Chronic Renal Insufficiency Cohort (CRIC) Study: Baseline characteristics and associations with kidney function. *Clinical Journal of the American Society of Nephrology, 4,* 1302–1311.

Lawry, K. W., Brouhard, B. H., & Cunningham, R. J. (1994). Cognitive functioning and school performance in children with renal failure. *Pediatric Nephrology, 8,* 326–329.

Ledermann, S. E., Scanes, M. E., Fernando, O. N., Duffy, P. G., Madden, S. J., & Trompeter, R. S. (2000) Long-term outcome of peritoneal dialysis in infants. *Journal of Pediatrics, 136,* 24–29.

Levey, A. S., Eckardt, K. U., Tsukamoto, Y., Levin, A., Coresh, J., Rossert, J.,...Eknoyan, G. (2005). Definition and classification of chronic kidney disease: A position statement from Kidney Disease: Improving global outcomes (KDIGO). *Kidney International, 67,* 2089–2100.

Lysaght, M. J. (2002). Maintenance dialysis population dynamics: Current trends and long-term implications. *Journal of the American Society of Nephrology, 13,* 37–40.

Mendley, S. R., & Zelko, F. A. (1999). Improvement in specific aspects of neurocognitive performance in children after renal transplantation. *Kidney International, 56,* 318–323.

Middleton, L. E., Manini, T. M., Simonsick, E. M., Harris, T. B., Barnes, D. E., Tylavsky, F.,...Yaffe, K. (2011). Activity energy expenditure and incident cognitive impairment in older adults. *Archives of Internal Medicine, 171,* 1251–1257.

Murtagh, F. E., Addington-Hall, J., & Higginson, I. J. (2007). The prevalence of symptoms in end-stage renal disease: A systematic review. *Advances in Chronic Kidney Disease, 14,* 82–99.

Mitsnefes, M., Flynn, J., Cohn, S., Samuels, J., Blydt-Hansen, T., Saland, J.,...CKiD Study Group (2010). Masked hypertension associates with left ventricular hypertrophy in children with CKD. *Journal of the American Society of Nephrology, 21,* 137–144.

Mitsnefes, M., Ho, P. L., & McEnery, P. T. (2003). Hypertension and progression of chronic renal insufficiency in children: A report of the North American Pediatric Renal Transplant Cooperative Study (NAPRTCS). *Journal of the American Society of Nephrology, 14,* 2618–2622.

Murray, A. M., Tupper, D. E., Knopman, D. S., Gilbertson, D. T., Pederson, S. L., Li, S.,...Kane, R. L. (2006). Cognitive impairment in hemodialysis patients is common. *Neurology, 67,* 216–223.

National Kidney Foundation. (2002). K/DOQI clinical practice guidelines for chronic kidney disease: Evaluation, classification, and stratification. *American Journal of Kidney Disease, 39,* S1-S266.

Nguyen, D. N., Spopen, H., Su, F., Schiettecatte, J., Shi, L., Hachimi-Idrissi, S., & Huyghens, I. (2006). Elevated levels of S-100 beta protein and neuron-specific enolase associated with brain injury in patients with severe sepsis and septic shock. *Critical Care Medicine*, *34*, 1967–1974.

North American Pediatric Renal Transplant Cooperative Study (NAPRTCS). (2005). *2005 Annual Report*. Rockville, MD: The EMMES Corporation.

Pace-Schott, E. F., & Spencer, R. M. (2011). Age-related changes in the cognitive function of sleep. *Progress in Brain Research*, *191*, 75–89.

Pannu, N., Klarenbach, S., Wiebe, N., Manns, B., & Tonelli, M. (2008). Renal replacement therapy in patients with acute renal failure: A systematic review. *Journal of the American Medical Association*, *299*, 793–805.

Papageorgiou, C., Ziroyannis, P., Vathylakis, J., Grigoriadis, A., Hatzikonstantinou, V., & Capsalakis, Z. (1982). A comparative study of brain atrophy by computerized tomography in chronic renal failure and chronic hemodialysis. *Acta Neurologica Scandinavica*, *66*, 378.

Pereira, A. A., Weiner, D. E., Scott, T., Chandra, P., Bluestein, R., Griffith, J., & Sarnak, M. J. (2007). Subcortical cognitive impairment in dialysis patients. *Hemodialysis International*, *11*, 309–314.

Post, J. B., Jegede, A. B., Morin, K., Spungen, A. M., Langhoff, E., & Sano, M. (2010). Cognitive profile of chronic kidney disease and hemodialysis patients without dementia. *Nephron Clinical Practice*, *116*, 247–255.

Qvist, E., Pihko, H., Fagerudd, P.L., Valanne, L., Lamminranta, S., Karikoski, J.,…Holmberg, C. (2002). Neurodevelopmental outcome in high-risk patients after renal transplantation in early childhood. *Pediatric Transplantation*, *6*, 53–62.

Ronco, C., Bellomo, R., Brendolan, A., Pinna, V., & La Greca, G. (1999). Brain density changes during renal replacement in critically ill patients with acute renal failure. Continuous hemofiltration versus intermittent hemodialysis. *Journal of Nephrology*, *12*, 173–178.

Schievink, W. I., Huston, J., Torres, V. E., & Marsh, W. R. (1995). Intracranial cysts in autosomal dominant polycystic kidney disease. *Journal of Neurosurgery*, *83*, 1004–1007.

Schwartz, G. J., Abraham, A. G., Furth, S. L., Warady, B. A., & Munoz, A. (2010). Optimizing iohexol plasma disappearance curves to measure the glomerular filtration rate in children with chronic kidney disease. *Kidney International*, *77*, 65–71.

Sehgal, A. R., Grey, S. F., DeOreo, P. B., & Whitehouse, P. J. (1997). Prevalence, recognition, and its implications of mental impairment among hemodialysis patients. *American Journal of Kidney Disease*, *30*, 41–49.

Seliger, S. L., Siscovick, D. S., Stehman-Breen, C. O., Gillen, D. L., Fitzpatrick, A., Bleyer, A., & Kuller, L. H. (2004). Moderate renal impairment and risk of dementia among older adults: The Cardiovascular Health Cognition Study. *Journal of the American Society of Nephrology*, *15*, 1904–1911.

Shima, H., Ishimura, E., Naganuma, T., Yamazaki, T., Kobayashi, I., Shidara, K.,…Nishizawa, Y. (2010). Cerebral microbleeds in predialysis patients with chronic kidney disease. *Nephrology, Dialysis, Transplantation*, *25*, 1554–1559.

Slinin, Y., Paudel, M. L., Ishani, A., Taylor, B. C., Yaffe, K., Murray, A. M.,…Ensrud, K. E. (2008). Osteoporotic Fractures in Men Study Group. Kidney function and cognitive performance and decline in older men. *Journal of the American Geriatric Society*, *56*, 2082–2088.

Steinberg, A., Efrat, R., Pomeranz, A., & Drukker, A. (1985). Computerized tomography of the brain in children with chronic renal failure. *The International Journal of Pediatric Nephrology*, *6*, 121–126.

Stilley, C. S., Bender, C. M., Dunbar-Jacob, J., Sereika, S., & Ryan, C. M. (2010). The impact of cognitive function on medication management: Three studies. *Health Psychology, 29,* 50–55.

Tamura, M. K., & Yafee, K. (2011). Dementia and cognitive impairment in ESRD: Diagnostic and therapeutic strategies. *Kidney International, 79,* 14–22.

Tryc, A. B., Alwan, G., Bokemeyer, M., Goldbecker, A., Hecker, H., Haubitz, M., & Weissenborn, K. (2011). Cerebral metabolic alterations and cognitive dysfunction in chronic kidney disease. *Nephrology, Dialysis, and Transplant, 26,* 2635–2641.

United States Department of Health and Human Services (2000). *Healthy People 2010* (2nd ed.). With Understanding and Improving Health and Objectives for Improving Health. Washington, DC: Author.

United States Department of Health and Human Services (2011). *Office of Disease Prevention and Health Promotion. Healthy People 2020.* Washington, DC: Author.

United States Renal Data System (2001). *USRDS 2001 Annual Data Report: Atlas of Chronic Kidney Disease and End-Stage Renal Disease in the United States.* Bethesda, MD: National Institutes of Health, National Institute of Diabetes and Digestive and Kidney Diseases.

United States Renal Data System (2005). *USRDS 2005 Annual Data Report: Atlas of Chronic Kidney Disease and End-Stage Renal Disease in the United States.* Bethesda, MD: National Institutes of Health, National Institute of Diabetes and Digestive and Kidney Diseases.

United States Renal Data System (2007). USRDS 2007 Annual Data Report: Atlas of Chronic Kideny Disease and End-Stage Renal Disease in the United States. Bethesda, MD. National Institues of Health, National Institue of Diabes and Digestive and Kidney Disease.

Valanne, L., Qvist, E., Jalanko, H., Holmberg, C., & Pihko, H. (2004). Neuroradiologic findings in children with renal transplantation under 5 years of age. *Pediatric Transplantation, 8,* 44–51.

Waldstein, S. R., Snow, J., Muldoon, M. F., & Katzel, L. I. (2001). Neuropsychological consequences of cardiovascular disease. In R. E. Tarter, M. Butters, & S. R. Beers (Eds.), *Medical Neuropsychology* (2nd ed., pp. 51–83). New York: Kluwer Academic/Plenum Publishers.

Warady, B. A., & Chadha, V. (2007). Chronic kidney disease in children: The global perspective. *Pediatric Nephrology, 22,* 1999–2009.

Warady, B. A., Belden, B., & Kohaut, E. (1999). Neurodevelopmental outcome of children initiating peritoneal dialysis in early infancy. *Pediatric Nephrology 13,* 759–765.

Wong, L. J., Kupferman, J. C., Prohovnik, I., Kirkham, F. J., Goodman, S., Paterno, K.,...Pavlakis, S. G. (2011). Hypertension impairs vascular reactivity in the pediatric brain. *Stroke, 42,* 1834–1838.

Yaffe, K., Ackerson, L., Kurella Tamura, M., Le Blanc, P., Kusek, J. W., Sehgal, A. R.,...Go, A. S. (2010). Chronic kidney disease and cognitive function in older adults: Findings from the chronic renal insufficiency cohort cognitive study. *Journal of the American Geriatric Society, 58,* 338–345.

9 Neuropsychological Outcomes in Pediatric Liver Disease and Transplantation

Lisa G. Sorensen

HISTORICAL MEDICAL PERSPECTIVE

Advances in the diagnosis and treatment of pediatric liver disease have dramatically reduced morbidity and mortality in this population. The advent of liver transplantation (LT) in 1967 revolutionized the treatment of liver disease (Jonas & Perez-Atayde, 2003; Lorincz, 2010). Since 1988, the first year for which the United Organ Sharing Organization (UNOS) provides data, the number of liver transplants performed in the United States has nearly quadrupled. In 2011, the figure reached 6341 (536 in those <18 years) based on Organ Procurement and Transplantation Network data as of April 6, 2012.[1] Current survival rates for pediatric LT are 85%–93% at 1 year and 76%–86% at 5 years. The majority of pediatric LT patients are <6 years (Figure 9.1).

Development of living donor LT in 1989 (Everson & Trotter, 2003) significantly reduced the wait time for patients with end-stage liver disease (ESLD) and allowed for LT to be performed when patients are more medically stable. Survival rates in pediatric acute liver failure (ALF) have increased from about one-third to three-quarters since the availability of LT (Arya, Gulati, & Deopujari, 2010). Policy changes have also helped reduce the incidence of ALF (e.g., avoidance of aspirin in children, shift to

[1] This work was supported, in part, by Health Resources and Services Administration contract 234–2005–37011C. The content is the sole responsibility of the authors alone and does not necessarily reflect the views or policies of the US Department of Health and Human Services, nor does mention of the trade names, commercial products, or organizations imply endorsement by the US government.

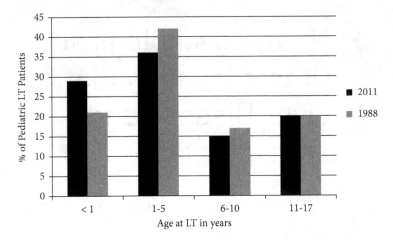

FIGURE 9.1

The distribution of age at liver transplantation (LT) in years for pediatric patients in the U.S. The pattern is similar for 1988 (the first year these data were available) and 2011. Most pediatric patients are transplanted under age 6, with nearly a third currently transplanted in the first year of life. Based on Organ Procurement and Transplantation Network (OPTN) data as of March 23, 2012

uniform acetaminophen dosing) (Jonas & Perez-Atayde, 2003; US Food and Drug Administration, 2011).

Due to the small number of pediatric patients with liver disease, resources such as The Studies in Pediatric Liver Transplantation (SPLIT) registry database (The SPLIT Research Group, 2001), Pediatric Acute Liver Failure (PALF) group (Squires et al., 2006), and Biliary Atresia Research Consortium (Goldman & Pranikoff, 2011) have formed over the last 15 years to provide the necessary infrastructure for a more sophisticated understanding of pediatric liver disease and transplant, including neuropsychological outcomes.

CURRENT MEDICAL FACTORS AND TREATMENT AND INTERVENTION UPDATE

Liver Disease

The liver is the largest organ in the body. Among its most critical functions are clearing toxins from the body; aiding digestion, absorption of nutrients, and metabolism; and fighting infection. Liver disease in children differs in epidemiology, etiology, disease course, and clinical manifestations compared with adults (Jonas & Perez-Atayde, 2003). Several factors make the infant and young child with liver disease particularly vulnerable. For example, they are less able to avoid perinatal infection, they experience nutritional deficiencies at a crucial time in brain development, and central nervous system (CNS) involvement in some diseases (e.g., metabolic syndromes) may lead to devastating brain damage (Leonis & Balistreri, 2008). Common etiologies of pediatric ESLD include biliary atresia (BA), progressive familial intrahepatic cholestasis (PFIC), Alagille syndrome, metabolic syndromes, neonatal and autoimmune hepatitis, α_1-antitrypsin deficiency (AATD), cirrhosis, primary sclerosing cholangitis, and Wilson's disease (WD). A few of the most common pediatric liver diseases and conditions are briefly reviewed, with special attention to those in which neuropsychological outcomes have been examined.

Biliary Atresia

Among pediatric patients, BA is the primary cause of death from liver failure and the most common reason for LT (Goldman & Pranikoff, 2011). This disorder involves obstruction of bile transfer from the liver (resulting in malnutrition) and occurs in 1 in 10,000 to 1 in 15,000 live births. The most common type (affecting 80%–90%) develops perinatally (Goldman & Pranikoff, 2011; Jonas & Perez-Atayde, 2003). Early surgical intervention using the Kasai procedure (prior to 3 months of age) is critical to survival (Goldman & Pranikoff, 2011; Jonas & Perez-Atayde, 2003). Even so, many patients with BA ultimately require LT.

α_1-Antitrypsin Deficiency

AATD is the most common genetic cause of pediatric liver disease, with an incidence of 1 in 1600 to 1 in 2000 live births (Perlmutter, 2003). Persistent jaundice may lead to diagnosis in the early neonatal period, although many patients are not symptomatic until early adolescence or even adulthood. In this disease, the liver cannot produce enough α_1-antitrypsin, which protects the liver and lungs, and liver disease and emphysema result. Liver, and sometimes lung, transplantation are required in severe cases (Perlmutter, 2003).

Metabolic Liver Disease

Various inherited metabolic syndromes involve liver dysfunction. For example, maple syrup urine disease (MSUD) is characterized by periodic metabolic crises and propionic acidemia involves episodic hyperammonemia, both of which can result in profound brain damage (Jonas & Perez-Atayde, 2003).

Acute Liver Failure

Pediatric ALF, or fulminant hepatic failure, is quite rare; it has been estimated at 50–100 cases per year in the United States (Alonso, Squires, & Whitington, 2007) and involves acute liver injury with no known evidence of chronic liver disease (Squires et al., 2006). Etiology is unknown in about half of pediatric patients (Narkewicz et al., 2009; Squires et al., 2006). When identified, etiologies include infectious, toxin/drug, metabolic, and autoimmune processes (Alonso et al., 2007). Outcomes are difficult to predict. The best prognosis is when there has been accidental acetaminophen overdose (more than 90% spontaneously recover); the worst prognosis is for patients <3 years (53% spontaneously recover, 19% die, 28% undergo LT); and in those who develop hepatic encephalopathy (HE) grade III–IV, only 33% and 22% spontaneously recover, respectively (Squires et al., 2006).

Hepatic Encephalopathy

HE may accompany both chronic and acute liver disease and is an important marker of disease severity as well as of CNS involvement. Particularly in children, the causes of HE are not well understood, but failure of the liver to eliminate neurotoxins (e.g., ammonia) is considered central (Alonso et al., 2007; Bismuth, Funakoshi, Cadranel, & Blanc, 2011). Associated cerebral edema becomes more pronounced with HE severity and subsides after LT or with improved liver function (Bismuth et al., 2011). Drugs such as Rifaximin and Lactulose can help reduce ammonia production (Arya et al., 2010). In chronic liver disease, encephalopathy may be episodic, persistent, or minimal (MHE); whereas in ALF, deterioration in mental status may lead to coma within hours of onset.

A staging system designed for HE in adults has been adapted for older children but it is less useful in young children and infants due to limited language skills (Alonso et al., 2007) (Table 9.1). The PALF study group operationally defined HE in young children in an attempt to better characterize this important condition (Squires et al., 2006) (Table 9.1).

Portal hypertension refers to increased pressure in the portal vein carrying blood to the liver from the digestive organs and may result from intrinsic liver disease or extrahepatic portal vein obstruction. A major complication of portal hypertension is HE (Bosch, D'Amico, & Garcia-Pagan, 2003).

Reye Syndrome

Reye syndrome, characterized by hyperammonemia and ALF, was most prevalent in the 1960s and 1970s, with only rare cases reported since the mid-1980s due to reduced aspirin use in young children. Treatment primarily focuses on maintaining metabolic homeostasis and limiting increased intracranial pressure associated with HE (Jonas & Perez-Atayde, 2003).

Wilson's Disease

WD often presents as ALF, although it is arguably better characterized as a chronic liver disease because the underlying problem is an inherited defect in copper metabolism (Alonso et al., 2007; Kodama, Fujisawa, & Bhadhprasit, 2011). The prevalence of WD is approximately 1 in 30,000 (Kodama et al., 2011). It accounts for only 3% of pediatric ALF patients (Squires et al., 2006) because it is typically diagnosed in adolescents and adults. However, copper is accumulating in the liver throughout early childhood and eventually is deposited in various tissues, including the brain.

The primary clinical manifestations are hepatic, neurologic, and psychiatric (Kodama et al., 2011; Lorincz, 2010). Those with primarily hepatic presentation are typically diagnosed earlier than those with a neurological presentation (Lorincz, 2010), and psychiatric symptoms (e.g., personality change) can lead to misdiagnosis (Lorincz, 2010). The most common neurological symptoms include dysarthria (58%) and dystonia (42%) (Lorincz, 2010).

Abnormal signal on magnetic resonance imaging (MRI) has been found in lentiform and caudate nuclei, thalamus, brainstem, and white matter (Kodama et al., 2011). Treatment involves use of chelating agents (e.g., penicillamine) and sometimes LT. Optimal outcomes are dependent on early treatment prior to significant progression of neurological symptoms (Kodama et al., 2011).

Liver Transplant

In a cohort of 461 5-year survivors in the SPLIT registry, BA accounted for 48%, metabolic liver disease 13%, ALF 11%, other cholestatic conditions 15%, other conditions 9%, and tumor 4% (Ng et al., 2008). More than 99% still had calcineurin inhibitor (CI)–based immunosuppression (74% tacrolimus and 24% cyclosporine), with one-fourth prescribed prednisone. Height was strongly correlated with continued steroid use and fell below the 10th percentile in one-third of this cohort.

Table 9.1 Stages of Hepatic Encephalopathy, by Age

Stage	Clinical Manifestation	
	Age 0–3 years[a]	Older Children and Adolescents[b]
I	• Inconsolable crying • Sleep reversal • Inattention to task • Unreliable hand-flapping tremor	• Mildly slowed thinking • Disturbed sleep–wake cycle • Slight hand-flapping tremor • Minimal EEG abnormalities
II	• Normal or hyperreflexia • Untestable neurological signs	• Drowsiness • Confusion • Inappropriate behavior • Disorientation • Mood swings • Definite hand-flapping tremor • Usually generalized slowing on EEG
III (stupor)	• Somnolence • Stupor • Combativeness • Hyperreflexia • Unreliable hand-flapping tremor • Most likely untestable neurological signs	• Very sleepy but arousable • Unresponsive to verbal commands • Marked confusion • Delirium • Hyperreflexia • Hand-flapping tremor present if patient cooperative • Positive Babinski sign • Grossly abnormal slowing on EEG
IV (coma)	• Unconscious • Decerebrate or decorticate • Response to pain present (IV A) or absent (IV B)	• Unconscious • Decerebrate or decorticate • Response to pain present (IV A) or absent (IV B) • Appearance of delta waves on EEG

Abbreviation: EEG, electroencephalogram.

[a]Adapted from Squires et al. (2006).

[b]Adapted from Alonso, Squires, & Whitington (2007).

LT clearly saves lives. Patient health may be negatively impacted by aspects of the peri- and post-LT treatment regimen. Hearing loss has been documented in 12%–15% of pediatric LT patients, associated with cumulative dose of amikacin (Deutsch et al., 1998), hepatoblastoma, and length of hospital stay post-LT (Bucuvalas et al., 2003). Other potential complications include acute or chronic rejection, hemorrhage, CI neurotoxicity, and infections such as cytomegalovirus (Everson & Trotter, 2003).

EARLY PSYCHOLOGICAL AND NEUROPSYCHOLOGICAL FINDINGS

The study of neuropsychological outcomes in children and adolescents with liver disease is relatively young. The shift from research focused on reducing mortality and medical morbidity to neuropsychological function did not occur until the mid-1980s, once survival rates improved. Research has also been limited because of the overall rarity of patients and resulting small numbers of potential participants at individual medical centers. Most data are published in case reports and studies with small, heterogeneous, single-center samples, often with broad age ranges. Interpretation of findings is made difficult by the necessity of administering multiple measures to individuals of different ages within the same sample (e.g., Bayley and Wechsler scales). Because the majority of children receiving LT are young, different measures are also needed when comparing patients' pre-LT versus post-LT functioning, resulting in limited utility of this type of data.

Liver Disease

Reye Syndrome

Early data on Reye syndrome survivors pointed to deficits primarily in motoric aspects of speech (Kotagal, Rolfe, & Escobar, 1984). However, more comprehensive assessment (N = 18; mean = 11.8 years) revealed that Reye syndrome may also impact intelligence (IQ) (Meekin, Glasgow, McCusker, & Rooney, 1999). Patients with disease onset in the first year of life had lower IQ compared with those with later onset (mean = 85.3 versus 109) and sibling controls (mean = 96.5). Further, patients with more severe disease (stages III–V) had significantly lower Verbal IQ (VIQ) than those with less severe disease (mean = 81 versus 98) and siblings (mean = 98.2). Similarly, speech defects were associated with more severe disease (initial and worst stage of illness stages III–V, ammonia levels >300 μg/dL, >24 hours altered consciousness) in a review of 43 patients (Reitman et al., 1984).

A study examining 26 patients with a history of Reye syndrome incidentally found higher levels than expected (27%) of premorbid learning disability (LD) by parent report at follow-up (Quart, Cruickshank, & Sarnaik, 1985). The significance of this finding is unclear; small sample size and use of retrospective report warrant cautious interpretation.

Wilson's Disease

WD can present with progressively worsening symptoms, which are not diagnosed for months or years, or with acute decompensation of neurological, psychiatric, and/or liver functioning. Thus, outcomes can be quite variable, in part, related to the progression of the disease prior to treatment initiation and the stage of treatment.

A large retrospective review of WD patients (N = 129) described clinical findings at the index admission (mean = 1.5 years of treatment; mean = 18.8 years of age) and two subsequent follow-ups (mean = 5.0 and 11.8 years of treatment; mean = 22.3 and 29.1 years of age) (Meekin et al., 1999). Results suggested a pattern of early improvement in hepatic, neurological, and psychiatric symptoms; cognitive impairment; dysarthria; and copper metabolism, with a subsequent plateau in these symptoms. However, a much smaller study (N = 7) assessed initial and long-term outcomes (21–34 years later) in WD patients (age 8–35 years at initial evaluation; IQ = 86–117) and did not find differences in IQ over time (Medalia & Scheinberg, 1991).

Biliary Atresia and End-Stage Liver Disease

A series of early studies conducted by the Stewart group at the University of Texas examined ESLD and end-stage BA, finding IQ/developmental functioning ranging from borderline to average. Early disease onset, liver function, and growth parameters (especially in younger children) were highlighted as important correlates of intellectual deficits. Younger patients (0.5–5 years) fared worse; overall cognitive functioning on the Bayley Scales of Infant Development (BSID) or Stanford-Binet L-M fell in the borderline range (infants, mean = 79.5; children, mean = 76.1) with extremely low motor skills (infants, mean = 69.7; children, mean = 56.9). Infants' mental and motor development were associated with growth parameters, whereas children's development was associated with liver function (Stewart, Uauy, Waller, Kennard, & Andrews, 1987).

Neuropsychological functioning was not as depressed in older, more heterogeneous ESLD samples, but patients with early disease onset (<1 year) had lower IQs than those with later onset (early onset, mean = 85.0 versus late onset, mean = 99.5) (Stewart et al., 1988). Worse outcomes were related to longer illness duration, poorer nutritional status, and vitamin E deficiency. In a subsequent study (Stewart, Campbell, McCallon, Waller, & Andrews, 1992), lower IQ was found in early versus late-onset patients and compared with controls with cystic fibrosis (CF). On the Wechsler Intelligence Scale for Children–Revised (WISC–R), late-onset patients scored lower than test norms only on VIQ. IQ was best predicted by liver function and duration of disease, suggesting that patients with the highest risk for poor cognitive outcomes are those with onset of liver disease in the first year of life.

Liver Transplantation

Post-Liver Transplant Neurological Outcomes

An early retrospective review of post-LT (Rothfus, Hirsch, Latchaw, & Starzl, 1988) reported neurological problems in 48% (N = 71; aged 0.6–18 years). Seizures were most common (24%), followed by major mental status change and coma (14%), prolonged HE (3%), and brain death (3%). Computed tomography scans revealed significant intracerebral hemorrhage in three of four comatose patients. About one-third of patients with neurological problems had prominent sulci and ventricles, but this was not associated with symptoms or steroid dose.

Post-Liver Transplant Neuropsychological Functioning

The Stewart group conducted two small studies to examine neuropsychological outcomes in pediatric LT patients compared with controls with CF; their studies reinforced and expanded on earlier findings in ESLD patients (Stewart, Hiltebeitel, et al., 1991; Stewart, Silver, et al., 1991). VIQ (91.5–92.0) and Performance IQ (PIQ; 89.0–89.1) on the Wechsler Scales were consistent with prior studies. PIQ differed from controls in both studies, but VIQ only differed in one study (Stewart, Silver, et al., 1991). Neuropsychological testing with Reitan-Indiana and Halstead-Reitan tests indicated somewhat different areas of deficit in the two studies: in visuospatial and abstraction/reasoning abilities but not in attention, motor, or sensory–perceptual processing (Stewart, Silver, et al., 1991), as well as a similar pattern with the addition of deficits in learning/memory and motor skills in the other. Academic achievement was also lower for LT patients versus controls, with mean scores in the low 80s on the Wide Range Achievement Test–Revised (WRAT–R) (Stewart, Hiltebeitel, et al., 1991).

Pre- Versus Post-Liver Transplant Neuropsychological Functioning

A handful of studies compared pre- and post-LT neuropsychological functioning, often finding no significant change over time (despite heterogeneous ages and measures within samples) and support for early age of disease onset/LT, growth deficits, and liver function as important predictors (Beath et al., 1997; Kennard et al., 1999; Stewart et al., 1989; Wayman, Cox, & Esquival, 1997; Zitelli et al., 1988). Two studies specifically examined very young children, similarly finding an initial dip followed by return to pre-LT levels. Wayman and colleagues (1997) found that BA patients (N = 40; aged <2 years at LT) declined at 3 months post-LT but returned to pre-LT levels at 12 months on the BSID (Mental Development Index = 92.7, Psychomotor Development Index = 80.9). Delays at 12 months post-LT were associated with growth delay (weight deficit), abnormal liver function (albumen), disease severity (length of hospital stay), and age at LT. Beath and colleagues (1997) (N = 19; aged <1 year at LT) found declines in social skills and eye–hand coordination 1 year post-LT on the Griffiths Mental Development Scales (GMDS), but recovery to pre-LT levels by 4 years post-LT. No changes were seen for motor skills and problem solving.

In a prospective study, no differences were found in IQ from pre-LT to 1 year post-LT (N = 29; aged 0–15 years pre-LT) (Stewart et al., 1989). Patients with mental and motor delays post-LT had earlier disease onset than those without delays. However, because the younger and older groups were administered different measures (BSID or Stanford-Binet L-M vs. WISC), interpretation must be cautious. In a retrospective review of LT patients (N = 50; aged 6–23 years) (Kennard et al., 1999), the same group found no IQ differences pre-LT and 3–9 years post-LT. Post-LT, IQ and achievement fell below norms for all composite scores. A quarter of the sample (26%) showed a pattern suggesting learning disability (IQ–achievement discrepancy), but only 10% had received special education services. A large proportion (18%) had an IQ <70 compared with 2.3% in the normative population. In a relatively large sample (N = 65; aged 3–21 years), which also examined long-term outcomes post-LT (2–5 years), 9% were receiving special education and 12% were described as 2 years behind grade level (Zitelli et al., 1988). A subgroup (n = 29) was examined both pre- and post-LT using the BSID, Merrill-Palmer, Stanford-Binet-LM, WPPSI, or WISC-R; no changes were found over time (post-LT IQ = 93.3).

In some disorders, LT appears to halt inevitable decline due to liver disease or perhaps even result in slight improvement. For example, a case report of a patient with citrullinemia (a urea cycle disorder associated with episodes of hyperammonemia, increased intracranial pressure, and progressive decline) found the child's IQ scores declining from "normal" to low average to borderline between ages 5 and 13 years (Fletcher, Couper, Moore, Coxon, & Dorney, 1999). At age 15, 1 year post-LT, Full-Scale IQ (FSIQ) remained in the borderline range, with some improvement in PIQ. In a survey of medical centers treating urea cycle disorders, qualitative reports by transplant physicians suggested mostly stable or slightly improved neurological and cognitive functioning following LT (Whitington et al., 1998).

Liver Disease

In the past decade, several studies have been conducted to examine neuropsychological outcomes in children with liver disease. Methodological concerns persist because most of these studies have been single-center, small samples, or case reports, with limited information beyond IQ. However, some gains have been made in elucidating the impact of liver disease on the brain.

Wilson's Disease

WD appears to primarily involve the basal ganglia, although widespread brain atrophy can occur (Lorincz, 2010). Broad neuropsychological deficits are also reported. A study of WD patients undergoing treatment (N = 20; aged 14–46 years) (Xu et al., 2010) reported basal ganglia lesions in 95%. Some patients also had abnormalities in the thalamus, brain stem, and frontal lobes. A subset (n = 8) that completed categorical and perceptual learning was deficient in both relative to healthy controls. Similarly, a small study (N = 12; aged 18–32 years) (Hegde, Sinha, Rao, Taly, & Vasudev, 2010) found 75% had MRI abnormalities: basal ganglia (75%), brainstem (42%), and cerebral atrophy (25%). All but one participant who had a normal MRI had neuropsychological deficits. These were found in motor speed, working memory/attention, learning/memory, visuo-constructive ability, mental speed, verbal fluency, and set-shifting.

Additional evidence supports potential improvement in neuropsychological function when WD is treated. A patient who was referred for learning problems at age 8 years was found to have below-average "cognitive functions," including language comprehension (Gronlund et al., 2006). The patient subsequently developed epigastric pain and periventricular white matter changes on MRI, leading to a diagnosis of WD. After two years of treatment with penicillamine, neuropsychological functioning improved and MRI returned to normal. By age 18 years he was reportedly functioning above average, as was his 16-year-old sister who was treated for WD while still asymptomatic.

Progressive Familial Intrahepatic Cholestasis

A case report describing a 16-year-old girl with progressive familial intrahepatic cholestasis (PFIC) type 1 (Byler's disease) presented as the first case of pediatric acquired chronic hepatocerebral degeneration due to ESLD (Papapetropoulos et al., 2008). Symptoms of this disorder resemble those of WD and include neuropsychiatric symptoms (e.g., apathy, cognitive impairment) and extrapyramidal syndrome.

Biliary Atresia

Few additional studies have been published about BA, although it is the largest single disease leading to pediatric LT. A small study (N = 15; aged 4–20 months) (Caudle, Katzenstein, Karpen, & McLin, 2010) mirrored earlier findings of very significant delays, particularly in very young patients. All composites on the Mullen Scales of Early Learning were below norms, with the weakest performance apparent on the Gross Motor (mean = 71.8) and Expressive Language (mean = 79.9) Scales. Modest associations were found with liver function, growth parameters, and age at Kasai procedure (the earlier the better). Of note, because nearly half of the sample was primarily Spanish speaking and required an interpreter for testing, the language results should be interpreted cautiously.

Minimal Hepatic Encephalopathy

An area that has received much attention in recent years with exciting results is MHE. Several studies in the United States (Foerster, Conklin, Petrou, Barker, & Schwarz, 2009) and India (Srivastava et al., 2011; Yadav, Saksena, et al., 2010; Yadav, Srivastava, et al., 2010) have examined MHE in children using magnetic resonance spectroscopy, finding significant correlations between brain metabolites and biochemical markers of encephalopathy (plasma ammonia levels and the ratio of branched-chain to aromatic amino acids). In addition, correlations between mean diffusivity on diffusion tensor imaging, plasma ammonia, and brain glutamine/glutamate suggest that ammonia may play a causal role in the development of low-grade cerebral edema in MHE in children, as in adults (Srivastava et al., 2011; Yadav, Saksena, et al., 2010; Yadav, Srivastava, et al., 2010). One study (Srivastava et al., 2011) also found increased pro-inflammatory cytokines in patients with MHE relative to controls, suggesting that both hyperammonemia and pro-inflammatory cytokines play a role in the development of cerebral edema associated with MHE. These studies, conducted in both patients with chronic liver disease and those with extrahepatic portal vein obstruction with portal systemic shunts (PSS), provide important clues regarding the mechanism for development of HE and a role for imaging in diagnosis of MHE in children. Also, greater deficits in visuomotor coordination, short-term memory, and visual perception were seen in patients with MHE, and these were associated with increased mean diffusivity (indicating edema) (Yadav, Srivastava, et al., 2010).

A handful of small studies suggested that MHE-related neuropsychological impairment may improve, especially in fluid abilities, with treatment of portal hypertension (Eroglu et al., 2004; Lautz, Tantemsapya, Rowell, & Superina, 2011; Mack et al., 2006). Two patients with surgical repair of congenital PSS (age 17 years and 4 years) showed improvement in learning/memory, stamina/energy, mood, fine motor speed, reading, and IQ (Eroglu et al., 2004). Improvement was reported in all 4 patients who had neuropsychological deficits in a retrospective review of 10 patients who had surgical repair of congenital PSS, (Lautz et al., 2011). A prospective study of 12 patients who had extrahepatic portal vein thrombosis and no overt HE found improvement in fluid abilities (attention, mental speed, and verbal memory) and motor speed/dexterity following surgical repair (Mack et al., 2006). Further evidence of disruption in fluid abilities was seen in a multisite, longitudinal study of children with hepatitis C virus (N = 114; aged 5–18 years) (Rodrigue et al., 2011; Rodrigue et al., 2009). Patients showed worse executive function on a parental questionnaire compared with norms, but function was not worse than in those diagnosed as having attention-deficit/hyperactivity disorder. Executive deficits did not improve after 24 weeks of pharmacological treatment.

Neurological Outcomes

A small retrospective review (Nachulewicz et al., 2006) found a prevalence of neurological complications in only 20% (N = 20) of children transplanted for ALF. As in the earlier, larger study of neurological outcomes following LT (Rothfus et al., 1988), severity/duration of pre-LT HE (grades III–IV) correlated with incidence of neurological complications. An unfortunate and serious complication of LT is immunosuppressant neurotoxicity. This has been documented in adults taking cyclosporine, tacrolimus, and prednisone (Everson & Trotter, 2003) but has only been recently reported in children. Two case reports (ALF and BA) describe the development of akinetic mutism, speech apraxia, dysfluency, and dysarthria with abnormally high tacrolimus levels in the context of relatively preserved comprehension (Matoth, Jurim, Lotem, & Granot, 2000; Sokol, Molleston, Filo, Van Valer, & Edwards-Brown, 2003). Speech abnormalities partially recovered over a period of 6 months to 1 year. In the first case, brain imaging was normal (Matoth et al., 2000); in the second case, imaging indicated cerebellar lesions consistent with drug-induced edema and scattered lesions in gray and white matter consistent with hypertension (Sokol et al., 2003).

Post-Liver Transplant Neuropsychological Functioning

Studies examining post-LT functioning over the past decade have mostly reinforced earlier findings. IQ has nearly universally fallen below published norms (Adeback, Nemeth, & Fischler, 2003; Kaller et al., 2010; Kaller et al., 2005; Schulz, Wein, Boeck, Rogiers, & Burdelski, 2003; Sorensen et al., 2011). Pediatric LT patients clearly have a downward shift in IQ, with mean IQ scores typically in the mid-80s to low-90s, with an increased prevalence (up to 27% versus 2% expected) of scores falling below 70 (Adeback et al., 2003; Gilmour, Adkins, Liddell, Jhangri, & Robertson, 2009; Krull, Fuchs, Yurk, Boone, & Alonso, 2003; Sorensen et al., 2011). Of note, the only multicenter study to examine IQ in pediatric LT patients, which had the largest sample (N = 144; aged 5–6), found the smallest proportion of patients functioning at or below 70 (4%), although FSIQ, VIQ, and PIQ were all significantly below norms (FSIQ = 94.7, VIQ = 95.0, PIQ = 94.9) and twice as many as expected (26% versus 14% expected) had mild to moderate IQ delays (IQ = 71–85) (Sorensen et al., 2011).

As in prior studies using CF controls, recent efforts using healthy (Gritti et al., 2001) and CF (Krull et al., 2003) controls are inconsistent, with lower IQ for LT patients in the former, but only a trend toward weaker VIQ in the latter. Interpretation of these contradictory findings remains hampered by small, single-center samples (both studies N <20). Furthermore, at least one study has documented cognitive concerns in CF patients (Wray & Radley-Smith, 2010), suggesting they are not ideal controls.

The broader pattern of neuropsychological functioning in pediatric LT patients is less clear because few studies have comprehensively assessed domains other than IQ. As in prior studies, verbal and nonverbal IQs are typically similarly delayed (Adeback et al., 2003; Gilmour et al., 2009; Sorensen et al., 2011). However, Krull and colleagues (2003) found significantly weaker language processing on the Clinical Evaluation of Language Fundamentals–Preschool or Revised compared with CF controls but not weaker visual perception on the Developmental Test of Visual Perception, 2nd edition. Only two other studies of children with liver disease have suggested a relative weakness in language: in children aged <2 years with a large proportion of non-English speakers (Caudle et al., 2010) and in a retrospective review (Stewart et al., 1992).

In contrast, Haavisto and colleagues (2011) (N = 18; aged 7–16 years) reported poorer PIQ (mean = 88.9), but not VIQ (mean = 99.6) or FSIQ (mean = 94.0), compared with WISC–III norms. This study also found poorer performance on visuospatial, visuoconstructive, and social perception tasks on the NEPSY: A Developmental Neuropsychological Assessment, second edition (NEPSY–II) but not in language, attention/executive function, or memory and learning. Other studies have reported deficits in visuomotor skills (mean = 82) (Gilmour et al., 2009) as well as lower PIQ (mean = 84.5) than VIQ (mean = 90.6) in 30% of patients on the Wechsler scales (Adeback et al., 2003). Such findings are in line with the prior report by the Stewart group (Stewart, Hiltebeitel, et al., 1991) and a recent report of MHE outcome (Yadav, Srivastava, et al., 2010).

The few pediatric studies of attention and executive functioning post-LT have typically found deficits. Several studies using the Kaufman Assessment Battery for Children have found deficits in both Sequential and Simultaneous Scale performance relative to norms (Kaller, Boeck, et al., 2010; Kaller et al., 2005; Schulz et al., 2003). Performance on the Sequential Scale, which taps working memory, ranged from 90.8 to 92.3, while performance on the Simultaneous Scale, which more closely aligns with nonverbal reasoning and problem solving, ranged from 93.9 to 95.5. It should be noted that these studies a priori excluded patients with IQ <70. In a recent study by the same group (N = 137; aged 6–18 years), LT patients demonstrated poorer performance compared with norms in alertness, working memory, sustained attention, and divided attention on the Test of Attentional Performance and the children's version of that test (Kaller, Langguth, Ganschow, Nashan, & Schulz, 2010). A large multicenter study (Sorensen et al., 2011) reported significant executive deficits relative to norms on the Behavior Rating Inventory of Executive Function, particularly by teacher report (Global Executive Composite = 58). The one study that did not find specific deficits in attention/executive function had a small sample and used the NEPSY–II (Haavisto et al., 2011).

Consistent with earlier findings by Stewart and colleagues, recent studies have documented significant problems with learning and school functioning. Achievement was found to be below norms in medium to large studies (Schulz et al., 2003; Sorensen et al., 2011) and in a smaller study (Gilmour et al., 2009) but not compared with CF controls (Krull et al., 2003). In a large multicenter study (Sorensen et al., 2011), young LT patients demonstrated school readiness concepts consistent with peers on the Bracken Basic Concepts Scale, Revised, but differed from norms in both word reading (mean = 92.7) and math (mean = 93.1) on the WRAT–4.

In the largest study of academic outcomes to date in pediatric LT patients (N = 823; aged 6–18 years) (Gilmour et al., 2010), 34% of patients were receiving special education services, 11% had received accommodations, and 20% had repeated a grade, by parent report. Diagnosis of learning disability was reported in 17.4% and mental retardation in 5.2%. The other large multicenter study of pediatric LT patients (Sorensen et al., 2011) similarly reported that 31% had received special education in the past year and 25% had profiles suggesting learning disability. These results are consistent with earlier findings (Kennard et al., 1999).

Although recent studies have examined predictors of neuropsychological and academic functioning after LT in children, results remain mixed. Younger age at LT was found to be an important factor leading to poorer outcomes in one study (Krull et al., 2003) but not in another (Schulz et al., 2003). A retrospective review (N = 40; aged <6 months at LT) found "long-term" outcomes of "regular mental development" in only 28% of participants (Grabhorn, Ganschow, Helmke, Rogiers, & Burdelski, 2002). In contrast, another study reported that younger age at transplant predicted "better" performance, but only for simultaneous processing and achievement, not for sequential processing (Kaller et al., 2005).

Although one study did not find a significant effect of diagnosis or time since transplant (Adeback et al., 2003), LT patients with BA performed better than those with other diagnoses in another study (Gilmour et al., 2009). A large study (Kaller, Langguth, et al., 2010) found worse attention/executive function in patients with "diagnoses affecting the brain" (Crigler-Najjar syndrome, citrullinemia, Alagille syndrome, metabolic disorders, WD, tyrosinemia) compared with those who had diagnoses that presumably do not directly affect the brain (BA, AATD, oxalosis, cholestasis, ALF, autoimmune hepatitis, liver tumor). It should be noted that this distinction is debatable.

In a moderately large sample (N = 44), longer duration of illness and deficient height at LT predicted Simultaneous Processing and Achievement (Kaller et al., 2005). Another small to moderate sized study (Gilmour et al., 2009) found that 45% of variance in PIQ was explained by growth deficits pre-LT and elevated serum ammonia, while 23% of variance in VIQ was due to elevated CI levels. In another study (Krull et al., 2003), language deficits were associated with disease severity and peri-/post-LT complications, as reflected by more days in intensive care, more days in the hospital post-LT, and elevated bilirubin pre-LT. In a large multicenter school outcomes study (Gilmour et al., 2010), special education was predicted by type of immunosuppression (cyclosporine or other immunosuppressant being worse than tacrolimus), cytomegalovirus post-LT, and pre-LT special education (odds ratio: 22.5), pointing to the importance of pretransplant factors in neuropsychological and academic outcomes. In contrast, a smaller study found that age (younger being better) and height (closer to normal being better) at LT explained 66% of variance in achievement (Schulz et al., 2003). In one study (Kaller, Langguth, et al., 2010), slow reaction time and poor sustained attention were predicted by type of LT (deceased donor), longer duration of disease, older age at LT, and gender, although the amount of variance explained was modest (14%–25%).

Pre- Versus Post-Liver Transplant Neuropsychological Functioning

Consistent with older studies, recent evidence suggests that progressive cognitive decline may be halted or even reversed. A case series of patients with Crigler-Najjar syndrome type 1 (a genetic disorder involving hyperbilirubinemia from birth and high risk for brain damage) suggested that earlier LT (i.e., prior to brain injury) results in better outcome (Schauer et al., 2003). A 4-year-old without brain injury remained cognitively intact post-LT, whereas children aged 7 years and 12 years who had mild to moderate deficits pre-LT improved incompletely following LT. Similarly, a small series (N = 14) of patients with MSUD showed stable IQ in 57% and improved IQ in 36% post-LT (Shellmer et al., 2011). Neuropsychological function due to another metabolic disorder, propionic acidemia, also stabilized or improved post-LT according to a retrospective review (N = 12) (Barshes et al., 2006). Another study (Yoshitoshi et al., 2009) reported stable or improved functioning up to 15 years post-LT in WD patients (N = 32; aged 6–40 years).

Other ESLD and BA groups were found to demonstrate stable functioning post-LT versus pre-LT. A follow-up to an earlier report (Beath et al., 1997) on infants (<1 year) undergoing LT found a slight dip in some areas of cognitive function on the GMDS initially but then a return to pre-LT levels by 4 years post-LT (N = 25) (van Mourik et al., 2000). One case report suggested improved cognitive and/or academic functioning post-LT in a child with BA (Ikegami et al., 2000). The child's school functioning was reduced relative to her healthy identical twin by the second year of school. However, following LT in middle school, her performance steadily and dramatically improved until she was performing at the level of her twin in the third year of high school.

INTERVENTION AND TREATMENT GAINS

Unfortunately, because the full scope and nature of neuropsychological deficits in pediatric liver disease are not yet well defined, we are not able to determine appropriate interventions, apart from the medical treatments described above (e.g., LT, copper chelation for WD). Although Lactulose and Rifaximin are sometimes given to pediatric patients with suspected MHE, their effectiveness in children has not been examined using neuropsychological measures, as they have in adults (Prasad et al., 2007). It is unclear whether psychostimulants might have the same benefits in pediatric patients with liver disease/LT who evidence attention/executive deficits as in other brain injury populations (Butler & Mulhern, 2005). Currently, standard of care dictates developmental or neuropsychological evaluation as soon as concerns arise, in addition to advocacy for needed school services.

CURRENT RESOURCES

To date, there is no established set of guidelines for assessing and managing neuropsychological outcomes in pediatric patients with liver disease/LT. With appropriate documentation via neuropsychological evaluation or school-based testing, patients can receive special education services. Even if school performance is adequate in the early grades, parents should be vigilant for signs of increased difficulty keeping pace with academic demands and seek evaluation and/or services in a timely manner when such concerns arise. Because LT most commonly occurs prior to the start of formal education, teachers may not be aware of the child's history and the extent to which it may impact neuropsychological and academic functioning.

Several Web sites provide information and resources regarding liver function and disorders in children. The Children's Liver Disease Foundation (www.childrensliverdisease.org), the American Liver Foundation (www.liverfoundation.org), and Children's Liver Association for Support Services (CLASS; www.classkids.org) provide informational handouts and resources. The Children's Liver Disease Foundation has appealing and kid-friendly animations explaining normal and abnormal liver functioning. The CLASS Web site provides numerous links to additional support organizations. UNOS (www.unos.org) provides statistics on LT and information for patients and families. The Childhood Liver Disease Research and Education Network (ChiLDREN) is a collaborative network of medical centers and patient support organizations designed to encourage and facilitate participation in research studies (http://childrennetwork.org).

FUTURE AIMS AND RESEARCH OPPORTUNITIES

As data accumulate and as some clarity is provided about these populations, many questions with regard to neuropsychological function in pediatric liver disease/LT remain unanswered. There are several priorities for the next generation of research. Pediatric patients with liver disease clearly demonstrate deficits in IQ that typically persist after LT. However, the longitudinal course of these deficits over the lifespan and in terms of time since LT is not well described. It is not clear which patients will improve after LT and which will remain stable. IQ deficits are expected; however, more data are needed regarding the pattern of functioning across neuropsychological domains. Few studies have examined areas other than IQ, and these have provided mixed results. Attention/executive function is an area of particular interest given the potential for intervention and relation to HE.

Most research has been conducted on chronic liver disease and specific disorders that present acutely, such as WD and Reye syndrome. Larger, more heterogeneous studies targeting pediatric ALF are needed to clarify neuropsychological issues in this group pre- and post-LT. A particularly exciting avenue of research is examination of brain correlates of neuropsychological deficits. Intriguing data have emerged using diffusion tensor imaging and magnetic resonance spectroscopy in pediatric patients with MHE. Additional imaging studies are needed to clarify the impact of liver disease on the brain. An important goal is to better delineate predictors of neuropsychological outcomes in this population. Inconsistent findings to date are likely related to methodological issues such as small, single-center samples. The final model is likely multilayered, with a combination of pre-, peri-, and post-LT factors contributing to neuropsychological outcomes with both permanent and reversible effects (Figure 9.2).

Once the scope and nature of the problems have been clarified, potential changes in policy (e.g., age at LT listing) and standard of care (e.g., use of post-LT medications, surgical interventions) can be proposed to promote optimal outcomes.

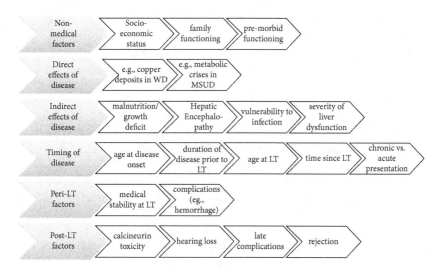

FIGURE 9.2

This model proposes several factors that may act in conjunction to determine neuropsychological outcomes in pediatric patients with liver disease. LT, liver transplantation; MSUD, Maple syrup urine disease; WD, Wilson's disease.

Finally, when all modifiable medical variables contributing to neuropsychological outcomes have been addressed, research must pursue additional means for improving outcomes by assessing the efficacy of targeted interventions (e.g., medications for HE, psychostimulants for inattention). These goals can only be accomplished with more multicenter collaboration and efforts to carefully design prospective studies with large, representative samples. Use of different tests based on age in the same sample should be minimized, or at least standardized, since this practice introduces a confound with age at disease onset and LT and makes interpretation more challenging. Neuropsychological outcomes in children with liver disease and LT represent an exciting "new frontier" whose exploration will hopefully lead to a better understanding and more effective prevention and management of deficits in the coming years.

REFERENCES

Adeback, P., Nemeth, A., & Fischler, B. (2003). Cognitive and emotional outcome after pediatric liver transplantation. *Pediatric Transplantation, 7,* 385–389.

Alonso, E. M., Squires, R. H., & Whitington, P. F. (2007). Acute liver failure in children. In F. J. Suchy, R. J. Sokol & W. F. Balistreri (Eds.), *Liver disease in children, third edition* (pp. 71–96). Cambridge, UK: Cambridge University Press.

Arya, R., Gulati, S., & Deopujari, S. (2010). Management of hepatic encephalopathy in children. *Postgraduate Medical Journal, 86,* 34–41.

Barshes, N. R., Vanatta, J. M., Patel, A. J., Carter, B. A., O'Mahony, C. A., Karpen, S. J., & Goss, J. A. (2006). Evaluation and management of patients with propionic acidemia undergoing liver transplantation: A comprehensive review. *Pediatric Transplantation, 10,* 773–781.

Beath, S. V., Cash, A. J., Brook, G. A., Mayer, A. D., Buckels, J. A. C., & Kelly, D. A. (1997). Long term outcome of liver transplantation (LTx) in babies aged less than 12 months. *Journal of Pediatric Gastroenterology and Nutrition, 24,* 485.

Bismuth, M., Funakoshi, N., Cadranel, J. -F., & Blanc, P. (2011). Hepatic encephalopathy: From pathophysiology to therapeutic management. *European Journal of Gastroenterology & Hepatology, 23,* 8–22.

Bosch, J., D'Amico, G., & Garcia-Pagan, J. C. (2003). Portal Hypertension. In E. R. Schiff, M. F. Sorrell & W. C. Maddrey (Eds.), *Schiff's Diseases of the Liver* (9th ed., Vol. 1, pp. 430–485). Philadelphia: Lippincott Williams & Wilkins.

Bucuvalas, J. C., O'Connor, A., Buschle, K., Krug, S., Ryckman, F. C., Atherton, H., ... Balistreri, W. F. (2003). Risk of hearing impairment in pediatric liver transplant recipients: A single center study. *Pediatric Transplantation, 7,* 265–269.

Butler, R. W., & Mulhern, R. K. (2005). Neurocognitive interventions for children and adolescents surviving cancer. *Journal of Pediatric Psychology, 30,* 65–78.

Caudle, S. E., Katzenstein, J. M., Karpen, S. J., & McLin, V. A. (2010). Language and motor skills are impaired in infants with biliary atresia before transplantation. *Journal of Pediatrics, 156,* 936–940.

Deutsch, E. S., Bartling, V., Lawenda, B., Schwegler, J., Falkenstein, K., & Dunn, S. (1998). Sensorineural hearing loss in children after liver transplantation. *Archives of Otolaryngology—Head & Neck Surgery, 124,* 529–533.

Eroglu, Y., Donaldson, J., Sorensen, L. G., Vogelzang, R. L., Melin-Aldana, H., Andersen, J., & Whitington, P. F. (2004). Improved neurocognitive function after radiologic closure of congenital portosystemic shunts. *Journal of Pediatric Gastroenterology and Nutrition, 39,* 410–417.

Everson, G. T., & Trotter, J. F. (2003). Transplantation of the liver. In E. R. Schiff, M. F. Sorrell & W. C. Maddrey (Eds.), *Schiff's Diseases of the Liver* (9th ed., Vol. 2, pp. 1585–1614) Philadelphia: Lippincott Williams & Wilkins.

Fletcher, J. M., Couper, R., Moore, D., Coxon, R., & Dorney, S. (1999). Liver transplantation for citrullinaemia improves intellectual function. *Journal of Inherited Metabolic Disease*, *22*, 581–586.

Foerster, B. R., Conklin, L. S., Petrou, M., Barker, P. B., & Schwarz, K. B. (2009). Minimal hepatic encephalopathy in children: Evaluation with proton MR spectroscopy. *American Journal of Neuroradiology*, *30*, 1610–1613.

Gilmour, S., Adkins, R., Liddell, G. A., Jhangri, G., & Robertson, C. M. (2009). Assessment of psychoeducational outcomes after pediatric liver transplant. *American Journal of Transplantation*, *9*, 294–300.

Gilmour, S., Sorensen, L. G., Anand, R., Yin, W., Alonso, E. M., on behalf of the SPLIT Research Consortium (2010). School outcomes in children registered in the Studies for Pediatric Liver Transplant (SPLIT) Consortium. *Liver Transplantation*, *16*, 1041–1048.

Goldman, M., & Pranikoff, T. (2011). Biliary disease in children. *Current Gastroenterology Reports*, *13*, 193–201.

Grabhorn, E., Ganschow, R., Helmke, K., Rogiers, X., & Burdelski, M. (2002). Liver transplantation in infants younger than 6 months old. *Transplantation Proceedings*, *34*, 1964–1965.

Gritti, A., Di Sarno, A. M., Comito, M., De Vincenzo, A., De Paola, P., & Vajro, P. (2001). Psychological impact of liver transplantation on children's inner worlds. *Pediatric Transplantation*, *5*, 37–43.

Gronlund, J., Nanto-Salonen, K., Venetoklis, J., Holmberg, R.-L., Heinonen, A., & Stahlberg, M.-R . (2006). Poor cognitive development and abdominal pain: Wilson's disease. *Scandinavian Journal of Gastroenterology*, *41*, 361–364.

Haavisto, A., Korkman, M., Tormanen, J., Holmberg, C., Jalanko, H., & Qvist, E. (2011). Visuospatial impairment in children and adolescents after liver transplantation. *Pediatric Transplantation*, *15*, 184–192.

Hegde, S., Sinha, S., Rao, S. L., Taly, A. B., & Vasudev, M. K. (2010). Cognitive profile and structural findings in Wilson's disease: A neuropsychological and MRI-based study. *Neurology India*, *58*, 708–713.

Ikegami, T., Nishizaki, T., Hiroshige, S., Hashimoto, K., Yanaga, K., & Sugimachi, K. (2000). Effect of liver transplantation in a twin for biliary atresia on physical development and intellectual performance: Report of a case. *Surgery Today*, *30*, 841–843.

Jonas, M. M., & Perez-Atayde, A. R. (2003). Liver disease in infancy and childhood. In E. R. Schiff, M. F. Sorrell & W. C. Maddrey (Eds.), *Schiff's Diseases of the Liver* (Ninth ed., Vol. 2, pp. 1459–1496). Philadelphia: Lippincott Williams and Wilkins.

Kaller, T., Boeck, A., Sander, K., Richterich, A., Burdelski, M., Ganschow, R., & Schulz, K.-H. (2010). Cognitive abilities, behaviour, and quality of life in children after liver transplantation. *Pediatric Transplantation*, *14*, 496–503.

Kaller, T., Langguth, N., Ganschow, R., Nashan, B., & Schulz, K.-H. (2010). Attention and executive functioning deficits in liver transplanted children. *Clinical and Translational Research*, *90*, 1567–1573.

Kaller, T., Schulz, K.-H., Sander, K., Boeck, A., Rogiers, X., & Burdelski, M. (2005). Cognitive abilities in children after liver transplantation. *Transplantation*, *79*, 1252–1256.

Kennard, B. D., Stewart, S. M., Phelan-McAuliffe, D., Waller, D. A., Bannister, M., Fioravani, V., & Andrews, W. S. (1999). Academic outcome in long-term survivors of pediatric liver transplantation. *Developmental and Behavioral Pediatrics*, *20*, 17–23.

Kodama, H., Fujisawa, C., & Bhadhprasit, W. (2011). Pathology, clinical features and treatments of congenital copper metabolic disorders—Focus on neurologic aspects. *Brain and Development*, *33*, 243–251.

Kotagal, S., Rolfe, U., Schwarz, K. B., & Escober, W. (1984). "Locked-in" state following Reye's syndrome. *Annals of Neurology, 15,* 599–601.

Krull, K., Fuchs, C., Yurk, H., Boone, P., & Alonso, E. (2003). Neurocognitive outcome in pediatric liver transplant recipients. *Pediatric Transplantation, 7,* 111–118.

Lautz, T. B., Tantemsapya, N., Rowell, E., & Superina, R. A. (2011). Management and classification of type II congenital portosystemic shunts. *Journal of Pediatric Surgery, 46,* 308–314.

Leonis, M. A., & Balistreri, W. F. (2008). Evaluation and management of end-stage liver disease in children. *Gastroenterology, 134,* 1741–1751.

Lorincz, M. T. (2010). Neurologic Wilson's disease. *Annals of the New York Academy of Sciences, 1184,* 173–187.

Mack, C. L., Zelko, F. A., Lokar, J., Superina, R., Alonso, E. M., Blei, A. T., & Whitington, P. F. (2006). Surgically restoring portal blood flow to the liver in children with primary extrahepatic portal vein thrombosis improves fluid neurocognitive ability. *Pediatrics, 117,* e405-e412.

Matoth, I., Jurim, O., Lotem, S., & Granot, E. (2000). Speech disturbances in a child after living related liver transplant. *Transplantation Proceedings, 32,* 699–700.

Medalia, A., & Scheinberg, H. (1991). Intellectual functioning in treated Wilson's disease. *Annals of Neurology, 29,* 573–574.

Meekin, S. L., Glasgow, J. F. T., McCusker, C. G., & Rooney, N. (1999). A long-term follow-up of cognitive, emotional, and behavioural sequelae to Reye syndrome. *Developmental Medicine and Child Neurology, 41,* 549–553.

Nachulewicz, P., Kaminski, A., Kalicinski, P., Kmiec, T., Szaplyko, W., Teisseyre, J., & Kowalski, A. (2006). Analysis of neurological complications in children transplanted due to fulminant liver failure. *Transplantation Proceedings, 38,* 253–254.

Narkewicz, M. R., Olio, D. D., Karpen, S. J., Murray, K. F., Schwarz, K., Yazigi, N.,... Pediatric Acute Liver Failure Study Group. (2009). Pattern of diagnostic evaluation for the causes of pediatric acute liver failure: An opportunity for quality improvement. *Journal of Pediatrics, 155,* 801–806.

Ng, V. L., Fecteau, A., Shepherd, R., Magee, J., Bucuvalas, J., Alonso, E.,... Anand, R. (2008). Outcomes of 5-year survivors of pediatric liver transplantation: Report on 461 children from a North American multicenter registry. *Pediatrics, 122,* e1128-e1135.

Papapetropoulos, S., Tzakis, A., Sengun, C., Reddy, C., Boukas, K., Zitser, J., & Singer, C. (2008). Case of pediatric acquired chronic hepatocerebral degeneration. *Pediatric Neurology, 38,* 67–70.

Perlmutter, D. H. (2003). α1-Antitrypsin deficiency In E. R. Schiff, M. F. Sorrell & W. C. Maddrey (Eds.), *Schiff's diseases of the liver* (9th ed., Vol. 2, pp. 1207–1229). Philadelphia: Lippincott Williams & Wilkins.

Prasad, S., Dhiman, R. K., Duseja, A., Chawla, Y. K., Sharma, A., & Agarwal, R. (2007). Lactulose improves cognitive functions and health-related quality of life in patients with cirrhosis who have minimal hepatic encephalopathy. *Hepatology, 45,* 549–559.

Quart, E. J., Cruickshank, W. M., & Sarnaik, A. (1985). Prior history of learning disabilities in Reye's syndrome survivors. *Journal of Learning Disabilities, 18,* 345–349.

Reitman, M. A., Casper, J., Coplan, J., Weiner, L. B., Kellman, R. M., & Kanter, R. K. (1984). Motor disorders of voice and speech in Reye's syndrome survivors. *American Journal of Diseases of Children, 138,* 1129–1131.

Rodrigue, J. R., Balistreri, W., Haber, B., Jonas, M. M., Mohan, P., Molleston, J. P.,... Gonzalez-Peralta, R. P. (2011). Peginterferon with or without ribavirin has minimal effect on quality of life, behavioral/emotional, and cognitive outcomes in children. *Hepatology, 53,* 1468–1475.

Rodrigue, J. R., Balistreri, W., Haber, B., Jonas, M. M., Mohan, P., Molleston, J. P.,... Gonzalez-Peralta, R. P. (2009). Impact of Hepatitis C virus infection on children and their caregivers: Quality of life, cognitive, and emotional outcomes. *Journal of Pediatric Gastroenterology and Nutrition, 48,* 341–337

Rothfus, W. E., Hirsch, W. L., Latchaw, R. E., & Starzl, T. E. (1988). Neuroradiologic aspects of pediatric orthotopic liver transplantation. *American Journal of Neuroradiology, 9,* 303–306.

Schauer, R., Strangl, M., Lang, T., Zimmermann, A., Chouker, A., Gerbes, A. L.,...Rau, H. G. (2003). Treatment of Crigler-Nijjar type I disease: Relevance of early liver transplantation. *Journal of Pediatric Surgery, 38,* 1227–1231.

Schulz, K.-H., Wein, C., Boeck, A., Rogiers, X., & Burdelski, M. (2003). Cognitive performance of children who have undergone liver transplantation. *Transplantation, 75,* 1236–1240.

Shellmer, D. A., DeVito Dabbs, A., Dew, M. A., Noll, R. B., Feldman, H., Strauss, K. A.,...Mazariegos, G. V. (2011). Cognitive and adaptive functioning after liver transplantation for maple syrup urine disease: A case series. *Pediatric Transplantation, 15,* 58–64.

Sokol, D. K., Molleston, J. P., Filo, R. S., Van Valer, J., & Edwards-Brown, M. (2003). Tacrolimus(FK506)-induced mutism after liver transplant. *Pediatric Neurology, 28,* 156–158.

Sorensen, L. G., Neighbors, K., Martz, K., Zelko, F., Bucuvalas, J. C., Alonso, E. M.,..., F. O. G. (2011). Cognitive and academic outcomes after pediatric liver transplantation: Functional Outcomes Group (FOG) results. *American Journal of Transplantation, 11,* 303–311.

The SPLIT Research Group. (2001). Studies of Pediatric Liver Transplantation (SPLIT): Year 2000 outcomes. *Transplantation, 72,* 463–476.

Squires, R. H., Shneider, B. L., Bucuvalas, J., Alonso, E., Sokol, R. J., Narkewicz, M. R.,...Hynan, L. S. (2006). Acute liver failure in children: The first 348 patients in the Pediatric Acute Liver Failure Study Group. *Journal of Pediatrics, 148,* 652–658.

Srivastava, A., Yadav, S. K., Yachha, S. K., Thomas, M. A., Saraswat, V. A., & Gupta, R. K. (2011). Pro-inflammatory cytokines are raised in extrahepatic portal venous obstruction, with minimal hepatic encephalopathy. *Journal of Gastroenterology and Hepatology, 26,* 979–986.

Stewart, S. M., Campbell, R. A., McCallon, D., Waller, D. A., & Andrews, W. S. (1992). Cognitive patterns in school-age children with end-stage liver disease. *Developmental and Behavioral Pediatrics, 13,* 331–338.

Stewart, S. M., Hiltebeitel, C., Nici, J., Waller, D. A., Uauy, R., & Andrews, W. S. (1991). Neuropsychological outcome of pediatric liver transplantation. *Pediatrics, 87,* 367–376.

Stewart, S. M., Silver, C. H., Nici, J., Waller, D., Campbell, R., Uauy, R., & Andrews, W. S. (1991). Neuropsychological function in young children who have undergone liver transplantation. *Journal of Pediatric Psychology, 16,* 569–583.

Stewart, S. M., Uauy, R., Kennard, B. D., Waller, D. A., Benser, M., & Andrews, W. S. (1988). Mental development and growth in children with chronic liver disease of early and late onset. *Pediatrics, 82,* 167–172.

Stewart, S. M., Uauy, R., Waller, D. A., Kennard, B. D., & Andrews, W. S. (1987). Mental and motor development correlates in patients with end-stage biliary atresia. *Pediatrics, 79,* 882–888.

Stewart, S. M., Uauy, R., Waller, D. A., Kennard, B. D., Benser, M., & Andrews, W. S. (1989). Mental and motor development, social competence, and growth one year after successful pediatric liver transplantation. *Journal of Pediatrics, 114,* 574–581.

U.S. Food and Drug Administration. (2011). Reducing fever in children: Safe use of acetaminophen, from www.fda.gov/consumer

van Mourik, I. D. M., Beath, S. V., Brook, G. A., Cash, A. J., Mayer, A. D., Buckels, J. A. C., & Kelly, D. A. (2000). Long-term nutritional and neurodevelopmental outcome of liver transplantation in infants aged less than 12 months. *Journal of Pediatric Gastroenterology and Nutrition, 30,* 269–275.

Wayman, K. I., Cox, K. L., & Esquival, C. O. (1997). Neurodevelopmental outcome of young children with extrahepatic biliary atresia 1 year after liver transplantation. *Journal of Pediatrics, 131,* 894–898.

Whitington, P. F., Alonso, E. M., Boyle, J. T., Molleston, J. P., Rosenthal, P., Edmond, J. C., & Millis, J. M. (1998). Liver transplantation for the treatment of urea cycle disorders. *Journal of Inherited Metabolic Disease, 21*(Suppl. 1), 112–118.

Wray, J., & Radley-Smith, R. (2010). Cognitive and behavioral functioning of children listed for heart and/or lung transplantation. *American Journal of Transplantation, 10,* 2527–2535.

Xu, P., Lu, Z.-L., Wang, X., Dosher, B., Zhou, J., Zhang, D., & Zhou, Y. (2010). Category and perceptual learning in subjects with treated Wilson's disease. *PLoS ONE, 5.* e9635. doi:10.1371/journal.pone.0009635.

Yadav, S. K., Saksena, S., Srivastava, A., Srivastava, A., Saraswat, V. A., Thomas, M. A.,…Gupta, R. K. (2010). Brain MR imaging and 1H-MR spectroscopy changes in patients with extrahepatic portal vein obstruction from early childhood to adulthood. *American Journal of Neuroradiology, 31,* 1337–1342.

Yadav, S. K., Srivastava, A., Srivastava, A., Thomas, M. A., Agarwal, J., Pandey, C. M.,…Gupta, R. K. (2010). Encephalopathy assessment in children with extra-hepatic portal vein obstruction with MR, psychometry, and critical flicker frequency. *Journal of Hepatology, 52,* 348–354.

Yoshitoshi, E. Y., Takada, Y., Oike, F., Sakamoto, S., Ogawa, K., Kanazawa, H.,…Uemoto, S. (2009). Long-term outcomes for 32 cases of Wilson's disease after living-related donor liver transplantation. *Transplantation, 87,* 261–267.

Zitelli, B. J., Miller, J. W., Gartner, J. C., Jr., Malatack, J. J., Urbach, A. H., Belle, S. H.,…Starzl, T. E. (1988). Changes in life-style after liver transplantation. *Pediatrics, 82,* 173–180.

10 Multiple Sclerosis

William S. MacAllister and Lana Harder

HISTORICAL MEDICAL PERSPECTIVE

The understanding of multiple sclerosis (MS) diagnosis and management has undergone a dramatic transformation in the past two decades. Not long ago, MS was considered essentially untreatable, and physicians of the day could offer little in the way of disease modification or symptom management. Fortunately, a surge of research and clinical efforts changed the landscape of MS management since those early years. Not only do we have a greater understanding of the underlying pathophysiology of the disease, we also have a better understanding of disease presentation and progression. More importantly, we also have gained a small arsenal of disease-modifying therapies (DMTs) to slow the overall progression of the disease, as well as a host of symptomatic treatments to allay the effects of specific symptoms of MS.

Symptoms suggestive of what is now known as multiple sclerosis have been documented as early as the fourteenth century when the case of St. Ludwina of Schiedam was described (Murray, 2009). Her symptoms included weakness in her legs, loss of balance, and visual disturbance. Symptoms presented and were followed by remission; her condition slowly progressed across decades. Her case is believed to be one of the earliest documented accounts of a patient with MS. In 1822, based on his personal diary spanning 26 years, Sir Augustus d'Este, the grandson of King George III, documented his own medical course, which began at age 28 years (Landtblom, Fazio, Fredrikson, & Granieri, 2010). Initial symptoms were consistent with optic neuritis followed by intermittent central nervous system (CNS) symptoms, eventually reaching a secondary progressive form including paraparesis, urinary problems, and impotence. Approximately two decades following Augustus's death, Jean Marie Charcot formally defined MS in 1868, putting forth diagnostic criteria that would later undergo several revisions (Landtblom et al., 2010).

Despite progress toward identification and classification of MS, researchers have struggled to identify its underlying pathophysiology. Many ideas have emerged regarding the pathogenesis of MS and, as the notion of mechanisms underlying MS have changed, so too have treatment approaches, evolving considerably over the decades to follow. For example, in the early nineteenth century, CNS disorders were thought to be the result of a buildup of toxins and were treated with purgatives (Murray, 2011). Another theory was related to over- or understimulation of the nerves, and treatment included nerve stimulation through chemical, herbal, electric, or physical means. By 1935, a review on the treatment of MS identified more than 150 treatments including anticoagulants, antibiotics, diet modification, vaccines, and agents used to treat cancer (Murray, 2009). Research methods improved considerably, particularly after the 1960s, and studies focused on the pathophysiology of MS, exploring biochemical, immunological, genetic, geographical, and environmental features of the disease (Murray, 2011).

The advent of magnetic resonance imaging (MRI) technology in the early 1980s had a profound impact on the understanding of the MS disease process because it allowed for observation of the active disease across time. Lesions associated with MS and related diseases are visualized on MRI of the brain and spinal cord, and such technology is now central to the diagnostic and disease monitoring process. MRI technology has revealed that disease activity may be ongoing despite clinically silent periods, demonstrating the progressive, rather than episodic, nature of MS (Murray, 2009). MRI research has also promoted understanding of the link between brain-based changes associated with MS and cognitive functioning. For example, research examining the adult MS population has revealed both gray and white brain matter atrophy associated with neuropsychological deficits (Sanfilipo, Benedict, Weinstock-Guttman, & Bakshi, 2006).

Currently, MS is conceptualized as an inflammatory autoimmune disease of the CNS with onset in a predisposed individual related to an unknown event, likely an exposure to an environmental pathogen many years prior to the disease manifestation. In MS, the immune system response involves an attack on myelin, resulting in axonal damage. Underlying the onset of MS is thought to be a multifactorial process that includes a genetic susceptibility, environmental factors, immunology, and infectious agents. Research has shown a higher degree of MS among family members, with concordance rates of 30% in homozygous twins and 5%–7% in heterogenous twins (Ebers, Sadovnick, & Risch, 1995). Additionally, epidemiology studies have indicated that the risk of developing MS may be influenced by one's geographical location prior to age 15 years, with an increased risk associated with greater distance from the equator (Kurtzke, Beebe, & Norman, 1985). Currently, this is thought to be related to vitamin D deficiency but may also reflect a genetic distribution of predisposed individuals in particular regions. Research has investigated infectious agents, with particular focus on the Epstein-Barr virus (Murray, 2009), and their relation to MS, though no single agent has been identified. As stated by Landtblom and colleagues (2010), "...the search for the code revealing the secret of MS goes on."

Although a full understanding of the underlying mechanisms associated with MS has yet to be reached, significant strides have been made in the last several decades, leading to the current therapeutic era of MS (Murray, 2011). Again, whereas MS was previously thought to be an untreatable disease, it is now considered to be a disease responsive to pharmacotherapies (Stuve et al., 2010). In the 1990s, the first US Food and Drug Administration (FDA)–approved treatment for MS was introduced, altering the disease course; this treatment is believed to improve long-term outcomes for patients. Current treatment aims to reduce MS exacerbations, delaying the disease progression and the patient's subsequent level of disability, and is described below. This idea emphasizes the importance of early diagnosis and initiation of treatment.

Diagnostic criteria for MS have certainly evolved since Charcot's initial descriptions. The most recent revision of diagnostic criteria, known as the McDonald Criteria, occurred in 2010 and is expected to allow for more rapid diagnosis while simplifying the overall process (Polman et al., 2011). The diagnosis of MS requires evidence of dissemination of CNS lesions across space and time. The patient must have two or more objective clinical attacks or a clinical attack(s) with positive MRI findings. Previously, events had to be separated in time by at least 30 days. However, this is no longer the case, and a new lesion may establish dissemination across time regardless of the number of days from the baseline MRI. Dissemination of lesions in space can be demonstrated in at least one T2 lesion in two of the following four areas in the CNS: periventricular, juxtacortical, infratentorial, and/or spinal cord. The clinical manifestations of MS are numerous, but the most common symptoms seen in acute MS relapses include optic neuritis, paresthesias (i.e., sensation of numbness and tingling), weakness, ataxia, speech problems (e.g., dysarthria), diplopia, fatigue, urinary incontinence, and cognitive loss.

There are four distinct clinical courses that MS may follow, known as relapsing-remitting, primary progressive, secondary progressive, and progressive relapsing (Vollmer, 2007). Relapsing-remitting MS is the most common form, accounting for approximately 85% of adult MS cases. It is marked by relapses, also known as exacerbations or attacks, followed by periods of recovery. The primary progressive form accounts for 10%–15% of MS cases and continues to progress steadily from the time of onset. This form tends to impact older individuals, and though it accounts for fewer MS cases, those with this form of the disease may have a shorter lifespan in comparison with those with other forms of the disease (Grytten Torkildsen, Lie, Aarseth, Nyland, & Myhr, 2008). Secondary progressive MS begins with a relapsing-remitting course and transitions to a progressive form, which may or may not involve relapses. Approximately half of patients with the relapsing-remitting form will progress to this form. Finally, the progressive relapsing form constitutes approximately 5% of MS patients and presents as the progressive form from onset with relapses superimposed with or without periods of remission.

To be sure, MS, with an average age of onset of about 30 years, is usually thought of as a disease of young adulthood. However, in the last two decades, there has been an increasing awareness that MS can occur in children and adolescents. Moreover, there has been a significant increase in the understanding of pediatric MS in the last 5 years (Chitnis et al., 2011). Estimates indicate that 2.7%–5% of MS cases emerge prior to age 18 years, though onset prior to the start of puberty is far less common (Boiko et al., 2002; Duquette et al., 1987). As such, research has increasingly begun to focus on children and adolescents diagnosed with MS and related demyelinating diseases. Though MS in childhood is in many ways quite similar to MS of adulthood, there are some noteworthy differences. For example, relapsing-remitting MS is by far the most common form of MS observed in pediatric patients, accounting for more than 96% of cases (Dale, Brilot, & Banwell, 2009). Further, though MS is more common in females across the age range, the disparities between females and males appears to be more extreme in the teenage years. Of note, however, in prepubescent children and among late-onset MS populations (i.e., onset after age of menopause), the gender ratios are more or less equal (Banwell, Ghezzi, Bar-Or, Mikaeloff, & Tardieu, 2007; Renoux et al., 2007).

Diagnosing MS in childhood presents some unique challenges because several conditions that children experience share many similarities with the initial presentations of MS. For example, conditions such as acute disseminated encephalomyelitis (ADEM) and transverse myelitis (TM) are CNS demyelinating diseases that are more commonly seen in childhood. These conditions present with similar sensory disturbances such as optic neuritis and limb weakness/numbness. Symptoms associated with ADEM, a demyelinating disease that is more common in children and adolescents than in adults, are preceded by a viral or bacterial infection or routine immunization in about 75% of cases (Tenembaum, Chitnis, Ness, Hahn, & International Pediatric MS Study Group, 2007). ADEM is typically monophasic but may be recurring. Importantly, some clinicians believe that recurrent ADEM represents a childhood form of MS (Belman, Chitnis, Renoux, Waubant, & International Pediatric MS Study Group, 2007) and it is also important to note that as many as 29% of children presenting with ADEM will go on to have MS (Mar, Lenox, Benzinger, Brown, & Noetzel, 2010). An ADEM event may last for up to 3 months and often includes evidence of encephalopathy and a polysymptomatic presentation. TM is a CNS demyelinating disease that produces lesions in the spinal cord only. Approximately 20% of TM cases occur prior to age 18 years. In the largest single case series of pediatric TM, Pidcock and colleagues (2007) reviewed 47 pediatric patients. They found that age of onset ranged from 0 to 17 years. Febrile illness and vaccination occurred in 47% and 28% of cases, respectively. The risk of reaching a subsequent MS diagnosis following a diagnosis of TM was quite low. Functional impairment was severe; 89% of patients were nonambulatory and/or required assistance with ventilation. At approximately 3 years follow-up, approximately half of the patients had difficulty with ambulation and required bladder catheterization. Younger age at onset, larger MRI lesions, and cervical lesions were associated with the poorest outcomes.

CURRENT MEDICAL FACTORS AND TREATMENT AND INTERVENTION UPDATE

The treatment of MS in both adults and their younger counterparts involves several tiers, including managing (and reducing the severity of) acute relapse, the use of DMTs to slow the overall disease progression, and adjunctive therapies to manage specific MS symptoms. Treatment for acute relapses involves the use of corticosteroids, which are typically administered intravenously once per day for a period of 3–5 days. In many cases, this is followed by an oral prednisone taper. Alternatively, high-dose oral prednisone may be administered to adults. Those working with younger MS patients should be aware that the high oral dose has not been tested for use in children and adolescents (Barnes et al., 1997; Martinelli et al., 2009; Morrow, Stoian, Dmitrovic, Chan, & Metz, 2004). For neuropsychologists evaluating individuals with MS, it is important to recognize that steroid treatments are often associated with significant side effects; these often include insomnia and irritability and, less commonly, psychosis, hyperglycemia, and hypertension. Steroids may adversely impact attention and memory as a result of these side effects. As such, it may be wise for neuropsychologists to delay evaluation of these individuals until after steroid treatments and related side effects have resolved. For those in whom steroid treatment proves ineffective in managing severe relapses, plasmapheresis or intravenous immunoglobulin may be considered by the treating neurologist. Importantly, these therapies have shown effectiveness in pediatric-onset MS cases (Duzova & Bakkaloglu, 2008; Weinshenker et al., 1999).

Whereas the above treatments are used primarily to quell acute relapses, they do not directly affect the disease course. Medications used to alter the overall progression of the disease are typically referred to as disease-modifying therapies. The first DMT arrived on the scene in the1990s, and there is now a small arsenal of medications used in this pursuit. For example, there are several formulations of injectable interferon drugs (IFNs), including several formulations of IFN beta 1a (brand names include Avonex and Rebif), several formulations of IFN 1b (brand names include Betaseron and Extavia), and glatiramer acetate for injection (brand name Copaxone). The purpose of these drugs is to delay relapses and slow the overall progression of the disease. All of these medications are approved for use in adults with MS and have also been used successfully in children (Banwell et al., 2006; Banwell, Bar-Or, Giovannoni, Dale, & Tardieu, 2011; Banwell et al., 2007; Chitnis et al., 2012; Krupp & MacAllister, 2005; Pohl et al., 2007). Of note, in retrospective studies comparing the relative efficacy of three interferon preparations, there were no noteworthy differences in effectiveness (Limmroth, Putzki, & Kachuck, 2011).

For individuals with particularly active disease (i.e., that is disease resistant to the first-line treatments described above), the drug mitoxantrone (brand name Novantrone) is sometimes utilized. Mitoxantrone is a synthetic anthracenedione derivative. This medication is classified as an immunosuppressant, historically used in the treatment of certain cancers, and is administered as an intravenous infusion. Studies have shown that treatment with mitoxantrone may improve disability and delay further progression of MS in patients with the relapsing-remitting form of the disease. Further, this medication shows some promise in those with progressive forms of MS, the forms with fewer available effective treatment options (Scott & Figgitt, 2004).

The drug natilizumab (brand name Tysabri), another medication administered by monthly infusion, has recently gained substantial attention. Natilizumab is a recombinant, humanized monoclonal antibody. As with all DMTs, this drug was developed for use with adults but has been used in children who are experiencing breakthrough disease; this treatment was well tolerated and appeared effective in reducing relapse rate in younger MS patients (Ghezzi et al., 2010). Natilizumab received unfortunate press early on due to the fact that several individuals using the medication in combination with other DMTs experienced an extremely rare complication, that is, the development of progressive multifocal leukoencephalopathy (PML). Thereafter, the medication was briefly removed from the market but was later reestablished for use as a monotherapy. Unfortunately, several more cases of PML have since come to light, and therefore it does not appear that natalizumab-associated PML is restricted to combination therapies (Warnke et al., 2010). Fortunately, this complication remains rare.

A drawback of all of the above-mentioned DMTs is the fact that they require either injection or infusions, making their use somewhat onerous for the patient. This, no doubt, adversely impacts treatment compliance in some, especially considering the injection site reactions experienced by many on these medications. Fortunately, FDA approval has recently been obtained for the first oral disease-modification medication for the treatment of MS. Fingolimod (brand name Gilenya), a sphingosine 1-phosphate receptor modulator, has a unique mechanism of action—it works by inhibiting the departure of lymphocytes from the lymph nodes. Recent 2-year phase 3 clinical trials of fingolimod showed that not only did this agent improve annualized relapse rate in comparison with placebo (Kappos et al., 2010) as well as IFN beta 1a (Cohen et al., 2010), it also prevented progression of disability and improved several

MRI parameters, including reducing gadolinium-enhancing lesions and brain volume loss. Despite the apparent effectiveness of this medication, there are some significant risks associated with it that may limit its use. In clinical trials, risks included two fatal herpes infections, and there is a suggestion of an increased risk of cancers. As such, this medication is currently considered a second-line agent reserved for use in those without adequate disease control on the IFNs or glatiramer acetate (see Yadav & Bourdette, 2010).

EARLY PSYCHOLOGICAL AND NEUROPSYCHOLOGICAL FINDINGS

Cognitive dysfunction/neuropsychological impairment in MS has been well described in the literature. Several prominent working groups throughout the United States, Canada, and Europe have defined the major areas of deficits and risks for more severe deficits. Though there is some variability across studies, the larger investigations of cognitive dysfunction generally suggest that about 43%–56% of adults with MS will show noteworthy cognitive deficits (see Heaton, Nelson, Thompson, Burks, & Franklin, 1985; Rao, Leo, Bernardin, & Unverzagt, 1991). In terms of MS subtype, most cognitive impairments are generally seen in the progressive forms of the disease (i.e., secondary progressive and primary progressive). Unfortunately, cognitive dysfunction can be seen very early in the disease course (Achiron & Barak, 2006) and even in very mild forms of the disease (Rovaris et al., 2008).

In terms of domains affected, the now classic study by Rao and colleagues (1991) of adults with MS demonstrated that the most frequently affected neuropsychological functions are those of memory, information processing, executive functions such as problem solving, as well as visuospatial functions. Language skills are less frequently impaired, though some may show subtle difficulties in naming and verbal fluency. In terms of predictors of cognitive dysfunction, in addition to progressive disease courses, men with MS appear to have more cognitive difficulties than do their female counterparts (Savettieri et al., 2004). Though some studies have suggested that African Americans with MS may show a greater degree of cognitive deficit, these differences may merely reflect socioeconomic factors.

Although cognitive impairment in adult patients with MS has been investigated extensively, less is known about cognitive functioning in individuals with pediatric-onset MS. Research has indicated that approximately one-third of pediatric patients with MS experience cognitive impairment (Amato et al., 2008; MacAllister et al., 2005). It has been suggested that youth with MS experience greater cognitive impairment given the impact of the disease process on the developing CNS (Amato et al., 2008). Consistent with this idea, younger age at onset has emerged as a risk factor for adverse cognitive outcomes (Amato, Zipoli, & Portaccio, 2008; Banwell & Anderson, 2005). Previous studies have also identified disease duration and relapse rate as risk factors associated with cognitive impairment (Banwell & Anderson, 2005; MacAllister et al., 2005). Indeed, a longitudinal study of a cohort including 56 pediatric MS patients and 50 healthy controls revealed cognitive impairment (defined as failure on at least three tests) in 70% of patients and deteriorating cognitive performance in 75% of patients. Cognitive deficits have been reported in the areas of verbal and visual memory, complex attention, verbal fluency, receptive language, visuomotor integration, and global IQ (Amato et al., 2008; Amato et al., 2010; Banwell & Anderson, 2005; MacAllister et al., 2005). Such cognitive impairment associated with pediatric MS has been linked to adverse academic outcomes (MacAllister et al., 2005). Compared with adult studies, findings suggest that although pediatric MS patients may have some overlap in deficits, they may show additional problems with language. Despite significant contributions toward the understanding of the cognitive sequelae associated with pediatric MS, consensus regarding a neuropsychological profile associated with pediatric MS has yet to be reached.

Although limited, existing research on psychological and neuropsychological outcomes in pediatric demyelinating disorders has focused largely on MS. However, given brain involvement of the disease process in ADEM, some research has focused on cognitive outcomes in this population. Deery and colleagues (2010) compared nine patients with MS and nine patients with ADEM, aged 7–18 years. Results showed that patients with ADEM demonstrated subtle cognitive problems while those with MS experienced greater impairment. Another study of six children diagnosed with ADEM revealed that, as a group, performance was in the average range; however, a review of individual patient profiles exposed mild cognitive deficits in each subject (Hahn et al., 2003). Conclusions of both studies indicated that, in general, cognitive problems are present but are less severe in pediatric ADEM patients as compared with pediatric MS patients.

Psychological problems associated with MS in adulthood have been well documented in the literature. Unfortunately, depression among adults with MS is extremely common with a lifetime prevalence of 40%–60%. Research suggests that the rate of depression in MS is greater than that in any other chronic illness group (Pucak, Carroll, Kerr, & Kaplin, 2007). Depression has been linked to poor cognitive functioning, suicide or suicidal intent, poor compliance with DMTs, and reduced quality of life (Feinstein, 2011). It is important to note that symptoms of depression are believed to be immune mediated, occurring secondary to inflammation, rather than stemming from the psychological stress associated with living with a chronic and often unpredictable disease alone (Pucak et al., 2007). It has also been suggested that brain lesion location and lesion volume may be associated with symptoms of depression (Feinstein et al., 2004; Feinstein, 2011; Pujol, Bello, Deus, Marti-Vilalta, & Capdevila, 1997).

Not surprisingly, less is known about psychological functioning in the pediatric MS population. Research examining pediatric patients with chronic illness has established that, in general, patients are at risk for the development of psychiatric problems (Weisbrot et al., 2010). Studies of pediatric MS patients have revealed estimates of affective disorders ranging from 30% to almost 50%. One study of 23 pediatric patients with CNS demyelinating diseases, ranging from age 6 years to 17 years, showed that almost half of the participants met criteria for psychiatric diagnoses, including 27% with depressive disorders and 64% with anxiety disorders (Weisbrot et al., 2010). In another study of 39 children diagnosed with MS, approximately one-third of these patients presented with an affective disorder, with the majority meeting criteria for depression (Goretti et al., 2010). MacAllister and colleagues (2005) found that 46% of pediatric MS patients met criteria for a diagnosis of an affective disorder. Follow-up studies have shown poorer quality of life, including sleep disturbance, academic difficulties, and poorer emotional functioning, more generally in children and adolescents with MS (MacAllister et al., 2009). Taken together, the existing literature clearly indicates that pediatric patients with MS are at risk for the development of psychiatric disorders, particularly internalizing disorders such as anxiety and depression.

Qualitative study of the experience of living with MS described by pediatric patients has yielded important insights for those working with these individuals (Boyd & MacMillan, 2005). Twelve pediatric patients diagnosed with MS participated in a semistructured interview. Themes emerged in the data including lack of knowledge about MS, feelings of distress at the time of diagnosis, and concerns over activity limitations. Stressors related to treatment, unpredictability of the disease, and school absences were identified. Both positive coping strategies (e.g., distraction, deriving support from others) and negative coping strategies (e.g., denial, avoidance) were identified.

In discussing the ramifications of MS, one must carefully consider the symptom of fatigue, especially considering the dramatic effect that this one symptom may have on an individual's life. The pathophysiology of MS-related fatigue is quite complex and multifactorial in nature. Though a comprehensive review of these factors is outside the scope of this chapter, fatigue is related to dysregulation of the immune system and changes in the nervous system related to the disease process (e.g., demyelination results in increased energy expenditure during neuronal transmission). For a more comprehensive review of these factors, see MacAllister and Krupp (2005).

Unfortunately, fatigue is the most commonly reported symptom in adults with MS (Freal, Kraft, & Coryell, 1984; Krupp, Alvarez, LaRocca, & Scheinberg, 1988; Minden et al., 2006). The symptom of fatigue often adversely impacts physical functioning, may be present even without significant exertion, and is often exacerbated by heat. Not surprisingly, fatigue is often perceived to be the most disruptive and disabling symptom of the disease. The impact of fatigue in MS is widespread. Not only does it prevent individuals with MS from participating in life activities and adversely affects quality of life (Benedict et al., 2005; Lobentanz et al., 2004), MS often results in lost time at work and the need to reduce work hours (Edgley, Sullivan, & Dehoux, 1991; Smith & Arnett, 2005).

Fatigue not only affects adults with MS; recent investigations have assessed fatigue in children and adolescents with the disease. For example, an Italian group of children and adolescents with MS were assessed via the Fatigue Severity Scale. Surprisingly, only 9% of this sample reported significant fatigue on this measure when the adult-derived cutoffs were applied (Amato et al., 2008), suggesting that this adult-oriented scale, which is not normed on children and adolescents, may be inappropriate for use in younger populations. In the United States, a group of children and adolescents with MS were studied via the PedsQL Multidimensional Fatigue Scale (MacAllister et al., 2009). In this sample, a quarter of the sample had mild fatigue and a third reported severe fatigue. It is also important to recognize that fatigue was not related to use of DMTs, nor was level of fatigue correlated with clinical factors such as age of onset, disease duration, relapse rate, or number of relapses. Though fatigue rates may be slightly lower in children and adolescents with MS as compared with adults, this is still an important aspect of the disease in this subpopulation because more than half reported at least mild fatigue.

Fatigue in MS is often thought of as a "hidden disability" given the fact that, unlike mobility impairment, it cannot easily be seen by coworkers, friends, or family. In pediatric samples, this has led to noteworthy psychosocial ramifications (MacAllister et al., 2009). Those working with teens with MS should seek to educate school personnel about these issues and document the special considerations that must be made for such individuals in a formal individualized education plan. Considerations may include being excused from strenuous gym activities, having classmates carry the student's books between classes, and being excused for tardiness.

RECENT PSYCHOLOGICAL AND NEUROPSYCHOLOGICAL FINDINGS

Whereas early research on neuropsychological functioning in individuals with MS has focused on outlining areas of dysfunction and progression, more recent work has focused on defining the best assessment tools for examining cognitive loss in MS and the relations between neuropsychological functioning, clinical factors, and neuroimaging parameters that predict cognitive loss.

As indicated previously, depression is quite common among individuals with MS. Unfortunately, those with MS and depression tend to show more cognitive deficits than nondepressed patients with MS, particularly processing speed and working memory deficits (see Arnett, Higginson, Voss, Bender et al., 1999; Arnett, Higginson, Voss, Wright et al., 1999). Interestingly, the relations between fatigue and cognitive functioning, despite the intuitive link, have been quite difficult to elucidate. Though it has long been known that individuals with MS tend to self-report that fatigue impairs their cognition (Krupp et al., 1988), showing this empirically has been challenging. For example, some studies have demonstrated significant relations between fatigue and processing speed deficits (Andreasen, Spliid, Andersen, & Jakobsen, 2010), but others have failed to find such relations (Parmenter, Denney, & Lynch, 2003).

It is also important to note that though earlier studies have shown that cognitive dysfunction and physical disability are only weakly associated, more recent work suggests that these variables are more strongly related than previously thought (Lynch, Parmenter, & Denney, 2005). Genetic markers for cognitive loss have also been explored, but results remain inconclusive. For example, the apolipoprotein E-4 (ApoE-4) polymorphism has been implicated in other disorders, but recent data suggest that there is no association between ApoE-4 and neuropsychological impairment in MS (Carmona et al., 2011).

With respect to neuroimaging, studies have demonstrated that central atrophy is a strong predictor of neuropsychological dysfunction in individuals with MS (Christodoulou et al., 2003). The relations between atrophy and neuropsychological dysfunction have even been seen in pediatric samples. For example, a recent study showed strong relations between both global brain volume and thalamic atrophy and cognition in a sample of young subjects (Till et al., 2011). Overall lesion load also correlates modestly with neuropsychological dysfunction (Calabrese et al., 2009; Christodoulou et al., 2003).

Interesting studies utilizing fMRI have shown evidence for the functional reorganization of cognitive processes in individuals with MS. For example, in a study comparing those with clinically isolated syndromes, relapsing-remitting MS, and secondary progressive MS with healthy controls, evidence for the recruitment of wider neural networks was seen. Specifically, those with relapsing-remitting MS showed greater activation in the precuneous, parietal lobes, and right fusiform gyrus, as well as hippocampi during a go/no-go task. Moreover, those with secondary progressive disease additionally recruited superior and inferior parietal lobes, dorsolateral prefrontal regions, right precentral regions, postcentral regions, and right temporal brain areas bilaterally. Thus, MS patients compensate for cognitive loss, at least to some degree, by recruiting additional brain regions to perform cognitive tasks (Loitfelder et al., 2011).

Two recent studies have examined the role of cognitive reserve in MS. The cognitive reserve model holds that neuropsychological deficits are lessened for individuals with higher education and/or greater premorbid intelligence. One study showed that processing speed declines were moderated by high cognitive reserve (Benedict, Morrow, Weinstock Guttman, Cookfair, & Schretlen, 2010), and another study demonstrated that the impact of brain atrophy on cognitive loss was moderated by higher cognitive reserve (Sumowski, Chiaravalloti, Wylie, & Deluca, 2009). Specifically, individuals with MS and greater cognitive reserve were able to withstand greater neuropathology (as measured by atrophy inferred from third ventricle width) without showing greater deficits in information processing speed.

Cognitive screening tools have been validated and are widely used as a cost-effective tool for evaluating adults with MS. In 2001, a panel of neuropsychologists and psychologists with specialization in MS met to develop a minimal neuropsychological examination for clinical monitoring and research purposes (Benedict et al., 2006). This meeting resulted in the compilation of a 90-minute battery called the Minimal Assessment of Cognitive Function in MS (MACFIMS). This battery includes the following seven subtests targeting areas most commonly impacted in MS: Controlled Oral Word Association Test; Judgment of Line Orientation Test; California Verbal Learning Test, Second Edition; Brief Visuospatial Memory Test–Revised; Symbol Digit Modalities Test; Paced Auditory Serial Addition Test; and Delis-Kaplan Executive Function System Sorting Test. Additionally, the Brief Repeatable Battery of Neuropsychological Tests (BRB) was developed as a 40-minute battery administered to screen for cognitive dysfunction (Bever, Grattan, Panitch, & Johnson, 1995). A short version of the BRB has been validated and includes the following three tests: Selective Reminding Test, Paced Auditory Serial Addition Test–3, and Symbol Digit Modalities Test (Portaccio et al., 2009). In comparing these screening batteries, it was determined that both the MACFIMS and the BRB have similar sensitivity in detecting cognitive impairment in adult MS patients in general. However, the Brief Visuospatial Memory Test of the MACFIMS may be more sensitive in detecting visual memory impairment in comparison with the 10/36 Spatial Memory Task of the BRB (Strober et al., 2009). A formal battery for clinical monitoring and research has not yet been developed for a pediatric population.

INTERVENTION AND TREATMENT GAINS

In addition to the DMTs described previously, there are many symptomatic treatments used to improve the quality of life of individuals with MS that target specific symptoms of the disease. Though a survey of all symptomatic treatments is outside the scope of this chapter, what follows is a brief survey of interventions that have been used to improve major symptoms of the disease, including treatments to improve mood and psychological function more generally, as well as fatigue and cognition, which are of particular interest to neuropsychologists.

The most obvious symptom of MS that is most easily observed by others is mobility impairment. Above and beyond the use of canes, walkers, and wheelchairs, numerous treatments have been employed to improve mobility in individuals with MS. For example, recent work has shown the utility of functional electrical stimulators in improving factors such as toe drag, circumduction, and overall energy expenditure during walking (Barrett, Mann, Taylor, & Strike, 2009). Further, such interventions have been shown to improve walking speed and overall scores on the Expanded Disability Status Scale (Ratchford et al., 2010). In 2010, the FDA approved the drug dalfampridine for use in individuals with MS. Dalfampridine is a potassium channel blocker that increases the duration of action potentials, thereby exerting an excitatory effect. Recent phase 3 clinical trials have shown that this medication can improve walking speed in those with mobility impairment (Goodman et al., 2009). Exercise programs have also shown promise in increasing strength (de Souza-Teixeira et al., 2009).

Given the importance of sleep to cognition, it is important to note that sleep disruption is frequently seen in individuals with MS. Neuropsychologists assessing these patients should routinely assess for sleep problems and possibly refer to a sleep specialist when appropriate. Sleep disorders commonly seen in MS patients include insomnia, disordered breathing, and restless leg syndrome, all of which typically respond to standard treatments (Brass, Duquette, Proulx-Therrien, & Auerbach, 2010). With respect to mood, pharmacologic agents are commonly used to treat depression, though few studies have evaluated the efficacy of such medications in individuals with MS. The Cochrane Collaboration, which was established to evaluate pharmacologic treatment of depression in MS, included two randomized studies, one controlled and the other blinded, that both showed a trend toward effectiveness of pharmacologic treatment (for desipramine and paroxetine), but both failed to reach statistical significance (Koch, Glazenborg, Uyttenboogaart, Mostert, & De Keyser, 2011).

Literature on nonpharmacological intervention has shown promise for MS patients. For example, cognitive-behavioral therapy (CBT) has been found to be just as effective as medication (i.e., selective serotonin reuptake inhibitors [SSRIs]) in patients with MS (Mohr, Boudewyn, Goodkin, Bostrom, & Epstein, 2001). CBT conducted via telephone has also shown efficacy among MS patients. Allowing access to therapeutic treatment from home is especially appealing for MS patients, many of whom have mobility impairments that make attending regular sessions outside the home very challenging (Feinstein, 2011). Psychopharmacological therapy and CBT for depression in children have been studied extensively, and each has been established as effective treatment modalities. However, little is known about the efficacy of these treatments in the pediatric MS population.

Support groups have also been shown to be an effective treatment strategy because patients with a relatively rare medical condition have the opportunity to connect with other patients coping with the same problem. This type of intervention has been provided through a camp for pediatric patients with MS (MacAllister, Boyd, Holland, Milazzo, & Krupp, 2007). Such an opportunity allows patients to connect with others with MS, receive education, and discuss a variety of topics with their peers. Feedback from interviews following camp suggests a positive response (Block et al., 2011).

The presentation of fatigue is multifactorial in nature. As such, its management can be quite complex. Clinicians must recognize that there are both primary factors in the manifestation of fatigue (i.e., related to demyelination, neurological factors, etc.) as well as secondary factors (e.g., secondary to sleep disturbance, depression, physical deconditioning, medication side effects) (MacAllister & Krupp, 2005). Accordingly, the effective management of fatigue should seek to first reduce or eliminate factors that may contribute to it, such as depression, sleep problems, or medications with side effects of fatigue. Again, individuals with MS often respond positively to cognitive behavioral psychotherapy. When necessary, pharmacological interventions, such as SSRIs, may prove helpful. When fatigue persists after eliminating these factors, alternate approaches, including nonpharmacological approaches, should be sought. For example, formal exercise programs are helpful in reducing physical deconditioning that may occur when fatigued individuals avoid tasks, resulting in lost muscle mass and increasing weakness, which is part of a vicious cycle. Further, energy conservation programs and cooling programs (for individuals whose fatigue is exacerbated by heat) may prove helpful. Given these, referral to an occupational therapist with expertise in fatigue in MS is often invaluable. For those with treatment-resistant fatigue, several medications have proven effective. First-line agents for the treatment of fatigue in MS include amantadine for mild fatigue and modafinil for more severe fatigue. Interestingly, a recent study showed that modafinil (in comparison with placebo) may not only improve fatigue in select individuals with MS but may also improve focused attention and manual dexterity (Lange, Volkmer, Heesen, & Liepert, 2009). An earlier study that examined the effects of amantadine and pemoline failed to show differences in attention, memory, or motor speed in comparison with placebo (Geisler et al., 1996).

Though it was known that individuals with MS did show some cognitive improvement on first-line DMTs (see Barak & Achiron, 2002; Fischer et al., 2000; Pliskin et al., 1996), it has been clear that cognitive deficits continue to affect many. As such, investigators began to seek agents to improve cognition in this group. Given that acetylcholine is plentiful throughout the basal forebrain and cortex and that MS often affects the periventricular regions containing pathways that serve these regions, the use of acetylcholinesterase inhibitors, such as donepezil, seemed like a viable option. Early investigations on the effectiveness of this agent, including a single-center randomized placebo-controlled study of 69 patients with MS (Krupp et al., 2004), are promising. In this study, those treated with donepezil showed significant improvement in verbal memory (as measured by the Selective Reminding Test) in comparison with those receiving placebo. This effect remained significant even after controlling for age, level of disability, reading ability, MS subtype, and gender. Unfortunately, this study proved difficult to replicate. A follow-up to this initial study, a larger multicenter investigation that used a randomized placebo-controlled study of donepezil, failed to show any treatment effect on the primary outcome measures, improvement in selective reminding test scores, and patient subjective report of improved memory (Krupp et al., 2011). As such, donepezil is not presently considered to be a viable treatment option for memory dysfunction in individuals with MS. Interestingly, however, the medication rivastigmine, another cholinergic agent, may show promise in improving cognitive processing speed in patients with MS (Huolman et al., 2011). As such, it seems that the use of cholinergic agents in those with MS may warrant further study. It is worth noting that there has been no demonstrated efficacy for natural substances, such as *Ginkgo biloba*, in improving memory in MS (Lovera et al., 2007).

As indicated above, some improvements in attention and motor speed have been seen with medications such as modafinil (Lange et al., 2009). Recent work has also examined the effects of stimulant medications to improve cognition. Again, though no effect in comparison with placebo was seen for stimulants such as pemoline (Geisler et al., 1996), a more recent study of l-amphetamine sulfate did show some preliminary support. In a within-subjects counterbalanced study of this agent at 15-mg, 30-mg, and

45-mg doses versus placebo, improvement on tests of processing speed (e.g., Symbol Digit Modalities Test) was seen for the highest dosage (Benedict et al., 2008).

The issue of cognitive rehabilitation in neurologic illness has become a hot topic in recent years. Unfortunately, empirical support for such interventions remains elusive. Generally speaking, interventions involve either cognitive retraining (e.g., Mattioli et al., 2010) or the learning of compensatory strategies (e.g., Mattioli et al., 2010; Tesar, Bandion, & Baumhackl, 2005). A recent Cochrane Review of cognitive rehabilitation studies in MS considered 14 studies that met their criteria in terms of study design. Unfortunately, the main conclusion of the review was that, overall, there was "low evidence" that cognitive rehabilitation improved neuropsychological functioning in MS. That said, they noted that the majority of these studies (12 of 14), when considered individually, did provide at least some evidence for a positive effect for aspects of learning and memory as well as working memory. The review concluded by noting the sample size limitations and methodological issues that characterized many of the studies and discussed the need for better research designs on larger patient populations before firm conclusions can be drawn (Rosti-Otajarvi & Hamalainen, 2011). It is important to note that, to date, there have been no formal studies of cognitive remediation in younger MS patients. This is an area in desperate need of future research.

CURRENT RESOURCES

Fortunately for those with MS and the clinicians treating them, there are numerous resources that are geared toward patient education and support. Those working with individuals with MS should provide references whereby patients can gain further information about the disease in layman's terms, as well as seek support. These information sources also provide educational materials appropriate for clinicians in all disciplines, including physicians, nurses, physical therapists, occupational therapists, and psychologists, who may be involved in the care of persons with MS. Though not an exhaustive list, below are some good resources with which one may wish to become familiar.

The National MS Society (NMSS) is the first place to start in terms of resources (www.nationalmssociety.org). The society provides education, outreach, and support to patients with MS and the family members who may be involved in their care. Further, the NMSS supports research to pursue prevention, treatment, and cure. The foundation also has a significant advocacy role, working with politicians and legislatures to address the needs of people with MS. The national society has state-level chapters that provide fund-raising and outreach activities. A list of local chapters can be found on the national Web site.

Similar to the NMSS of the United States (described above), the Multiple Sclerosis Society of Canada provides similar support. Their Web site is available in both French (http://mssociety.ca/fr/) and English (http://mssociety.ca/en/). In Europe, the MS Society in the United Kingdom performs a similar role (http://www.mssociety.org.uk/).

Several smaller organizations also provide support. For example, the Multiple Sclerosis Association of America (www.msaa.com) is a nonprofit organization with a mission to enrich the quality of life for individuals affected by MS. The Accelerated Cure Project (www.acceleratedcure.org) is a national nonprofit organization dedicated to curing MS by determining its causes.

Given the recent surge in interest of pediatric MS, it is not surprising that there are now numerous support services available for this unique population. In the United States, there are several centers dedicated to the coordinated study of children and adolescents with MS that began with generous startup funding support from the NMSS. These centers are located in California, Alabama, Minnesota, Massachusetts, and New York. The Web sites and contact information for these centers can be found at: http://www.nationalmssociety.org/about-multiple-sclerosis/pediatric-ms/pediatric-ms-centers-of-excellence/index.aspx. Beyond these coordinated research centers, there are a number of US and international pediatric MS programs. In Canada, for example, the Hospital for Sick Kids is a well-established center with expertise in the diagnosis and management of MS in children and adolescents. Centers with expertise in MS as it pertains to children are also available throughout Europe and Australia. Moreover, several recent publications from the NMSS offer information and support for children and teens with MS. These include *Students with MS & the Academic Setting: A Handbook for School Personnel* and *Managing School-Related Issues: A Guide for Parents with a Child or Teen Living with MS*. The book, *Kids get MS too: A Guide for Parents Whose Child or Teen has MS* is available online at: http://mssociety.ca/en/pdf/kidsgetmstoo.pdf.

It is also important to note that several MS centers that work with children and teens have established structured camp experiences for these individuals. The first such camp was offered through the National Pediatric MS Center at Stony Brook University in New York (http://www.pediatricmscenter.org/camp.aspx). Other camps as well as teen support networks (e.g., telephone chat groups) are available on the NMSS Web site. For camps in Canada, see http://mssociety.ca/en/help/camp.htm.

FUTURE AIMS AND RESEARCH OPPORTUNITIES

Many significant gains have been made in the past 10 years with respect to our knowledge of the pathophysiology of MS, the manifestation of the disease, its clinical course, and the associated neuropsychological deficits. Given the advances made in the last decade that have led to earlier diagnosis, more prompt initiation of treatment, as well as a wider array of treatment options to choose from (in terms of both DMTs and symptomatic treatments), the future for MS patients looks considerably brighter than it did just a few short decades ago. That said, there remain several avenues to explore, and neuropsychologists are uniquely qualified and positioned to make a significant impact.

As indicated throughout this chapter, less is known about neuropsychological and psychosocial outcomes for pediatric patients with MS. Further longitudinal study with larger cohorts is warranted in order to better understand developmental trajectories of these patients in the context of this chronic brain-based disease. An understanding of the relation of clinical variables (i.e., age at onset, disease duration, relapse rate) on outcomes will deepen our knowledge of the impact of the disease process on the developing brain. Additionally, as has been established for the adult MS population, a brief neuropsychological screening battery should be validated in pediatric MS patients to provide a timely and cost-effective way to identify cognitive problems and provide intervention for patients who are likely to benefit from such services.

Again, prior research has demonstrated that use of the first DMTs has led to improved cognition in many. Since the time of these early studies, several new medications have been offered, including the first oral medication (i.e., fingolimod). It remains to be seen if patients treated with this novel medication fare better cognitively than do patients treated with standard interferon treatment and/or glatiramer acetate.

Unfortunately, the use of medications such as acetylcholinesterase inhibitors to improve memory function in those with MS has resulted in mixed results, with the consensus being that these medications are not ready for "prime time" in this population. However, as newer cognitive-enhancing medications become available, it is incumbent on the profession to carefully consider the utility of the agents in the MS population, especially considering the potential success seen with medications such as the l-amphetamines. To date, no systematic studies have examined the efficacy of these medications in younger samples (i.e., pediatric MS). This is an area worthy of consideration.

Perhaps the area of greatest need is that of cognitive rehabilitation. As indicated above, there are but a handful of well-designed studies regarding cognitive rehabilitation in MS that employ meaningful outcome measures that are ecologically valid. Further, there are no studies at all on cognitive rehabilitation in pediatric MS samples. It is anticipated that these shortcomings will be addressed in the next few years. It is also worth noting that there have been some meaningful advances in the area of working memory rehabilitation in recent years. Specifically, a computer-based working memory rehabilitation program has shown preliminary empirical support (Klingberg, 2010). This program has shown some effectiveness in conditions such as developmental attention-deficit/hyperactivity disorder (Holmes et al., 2009) and stroke (Westerberg et al., 2007). The generalizability of these findings to other populations that present with working memory deficits, such as MS, remains largely unknown.

Considering pediatric MS more specifically, there remains several "treatment gaps" between this group and their older counterparts. For example, there are currently no clinical trials of symptomatic therapy in children with MS. Likewise, treatment of mood disturbance in adults with MS has been studied, but the effectiveness of treatments in children with the disease remains unexamined. Likewise, there is no data regarding the treatment of bladder dysfunction, bowel dysfunction, or mobility impairment in this young group.

In sum, though significant advances have been made, much work remains to be done. That said, this is an exciting time in MS research and clinical work. Neuropsychologists should be proud of the contributions they have made to the understanding of this disease, which have no doubt led to substantial improvement in the lives of many afflicted with this illness. Personally, we are quite excited to see what lies ahead.

REFERENCES

Achiron, A., & Barak, Y. (2006). Cognitive changes in early MS: A call for a common framework. *Journal of the Neurological Sciences, 245,* 47–51. doi: 10.1016/j.jns.2005.05.019

Amato, M. P., Goretti, B., Ghezzi, A., Lori, S., Zipoli, V., Moiola, L.,... Multiple Sclerosis Study Group of the Italian Neurological Society. (2010). Cognitive and psychosocial features in childhood and juvenile MS: Two-year follow-up. *Neurology, 75,* 1134–1140. doi: 10.1212/WNL.0b013e3181f4d821

Amato, M. P., Goretti, B., Ghezzi, A., Lori, S., Zipoli, V., Portaccio, E.,... Multiple Sclerosis Study Group of the Italian Neurological Society. (2008). Cognitive and psychosocial features of childhood and juvenile MS. *Neurology, 70,* 1891–1897. doi: 10.1212/01. wnl.0000312276.23177.fa

Amato, M. P., Zipoli, V., & Portaccio, E. (2008). Cognitive changes in multiple sclerosis. *Expert Review of Neurotherapeutics, 8,* 1585–1596. doi: 10.1586/14737175.8.10.1585

Andreasen, A. K., Spliid, P. E., Andersen, H., & Jakobsen, J. (2010). Fatigue and processing speed are related in multiple sclerosis. *European Journal of Neurology : The Official Journal of the European Federation of Neurological Societies, 17,* 212–218. doi: 10.1111/j.1468-1331.2009.02776.x

Arnett, P. A., Higginson, C. I., Voss, W. D., Bender, W. I., Wurst, J. M., & Tippin, J. M. (1999). Depression in multiple sclerosis: Relationship to working memory capacity. *Neuropsychology, 13,* 546–556.

Arnett, P. A., Higginson, C. I., Voss, W. D., Wright, B., Bender, W. I., Wurst, J. M., & Tippin, J. M. (1999). Depressed mood in multiple sclerosis: Relationship to capacity-demanding memory and attentional functioning. *Neuropsychology, 13,* 434–446.

Banwell, B., Bar-Or, A., Giovannoni, G., Dale, R. C., & Tardieu, M. (2011). Therapies for multiple sclerosis: Considerations in the pediatric patient. *Nature Reviews. Neurology, 7,* 109–122. doi: 10.1038/nrneurol.2010.198

Banwell, B., Reder, A. T., Krupp, L., Tenembaum, S., Eraksoy, M., Alexey, B.,...Antonijevic, I. (2006). Safety and tolerability of interferon beta-1b in pediatric multiple sclerosis. *Neurology, 66,* 472–476.

Banwell, B. L., & Anderson, P. E. (2005). The cognitive burden of multiple sclerosis in children. *Neurology, 64,* 891–894. doi: 10.1212/01.WNL.0000152896.35341.51

Banwell, B., Ghezzi, A., Bar-Or, A., Mikaeloff, Y., & Tardieu, M. (2007). Multiple sclerosis in children: Clinical diagnosis, therapeutic strategies, and future directions. *Lancet Neurology, 6,* 887–902.

Barak, Y., & Achiron, A. (2002). Effect of interferon-beta-1b on cognitive functions in multiple sclerosis. *European Neurology, 47,* 11–14.

Barnes, D., Hughes, R. A., Morris, R. W., Wade-Jones, O., Brown, P., Britton, T.,...Frankel, J. (1997). Randomised trial of oral and intravenous methylprednisolone in acute relapses of multiple sclerosis. *Lancet, 349,* 902–906.

Barrett, C. L., Mann, G. E., Taylor, P. N., & Strike, P. (2009). A randomized trial to investigate the effects of functional electrical stimulation and therapeutic exercise on walking performance for people with multiple sclerosis. *Multiple Sclerosis, 15,* 493–504. doi: 10.1177/1352458508101320

Belman, A. L., Chitnis, T., Renoux, C., Waubant, E., & International Pediatric MS Study Group. (2007). Challenges in the classification of pediatric multiple sclerosis and future directions. *Neurology, 68,* S70–S74. doi: 10.1212/01.wnl.0000259421.40556.76

Benedict, R. H., Cookfair, D., Gavett, R., Gunther, M., Munschauer, F., Garg, N., & Weinstock-Guttman, B. (2006). Validity of the minimal assessment of cognitive function in multiple sclerosis (MACFIMS). *Journal of the International Neuropsychological Society, 12,* 549–558.

Benedict, R. H., Morrow, S. A., Weinstock Guttman, B., Cookfair, D., & Schretlen, D. J. (2010). Cognitive reserve moderates decline in information processing speed in multiple sclerosis patients. *Journal of the International Neuropsychological Society, 16,* 829–835. doi: 10.1017/S1355617710000688

Benedict, R. H., Munschauer, F., Zarevics, P., Erlanger, D., Rowe, V., Feaster, T., & Carpenter, R. L. (2008). Effects of l-amphetamine sulfate on cognitive function in multiple sclerosis patients. *Journal of Neurology, 255,* 848–852. doi: 10.1007/s00415-008-0760-7

Benedict, R. H., Wahlig, E., Bakshi, R., Fishman, I., Munschauer, F., Zivadinov, R., & Weinstock-Guttman, B. (2005). Predicting quality of life in multiple sclerosis: Accounting for physical disability, fatigue, cognition, mood disorder, personality, and behavior change. *Journal of the Neurological Sciences, 231,* 29–34. doi: 10.1016/j.jns.2004.12.009

Bever, C. T., Grattan, L., Panitch, H. S., & Johnson, K. P. (1995). The brief repeatable battery of neuropsychological tests for multiple sclerosis: A preliminary serial study. *Multiple Sclerosis, 1,* 165–169.

Block, P., Rodriguez, E. L., Milazzo, M. C., MacAllister, W. S., Krupp, L. B., Nishida, A.,... Keys, C. B. (2011). Building pediatric multiple sclerosis community using a disability studies framework of empowerment. *Disability and Community, 6,* 85–112.

Boyd, J. R., & MacMillan, L. J. (2005). Experiences of children and adolescents living with multiple sclerosis. *The Journal of Neuroscience Nursing, 37,* 334–342.

Brass, S. D., Duquette, P., Proulx-Therrien, J., & Auerbach, S. (2010). Sleep disorders in patients with multiple sclerosis. *Sleep Medicine Reviews, 14,* 121–129. doi: 10.1016/j. smrv.2009.07.005

Calabrese, M., Agosta, F., Rinaldi, F., Mattisi, I., Grossi, P., Favaretto, A.,... Filippi, M. (2009). Cortical lesions and atrophy associated with cognitive impairment in relapsing-remitting multiple sclerosis. *Archives of Neurology, 66,* 1144–1150. doi: 10.1001/archneurol.2009.174

Carmona, O., Masuet, C., Santiago, O., Alia, P., Moral, E., Alonso-Magdalena, L.,... Arbizu, T. (2011). Multiple sclerosis and cognitive decline: Is ApoE-4 a surrogate marker? *Acta Neurologica Scandinavica, 124,* 258–263. doi: 10.1111/j.1600-0404.2010.01473.x; 10.1111/j.1600-0404.2010.01473.x

Chitnis, T., Krupp, L., Yeh, A., Rubin, J., Kuntz, N., Strober, J. B.,... Waubant, E. (2011). Pediatric multiple sclerosis. *Neurologic Clinics, 29,* 481–505. doi: 10.1016/j. ncl.2011.01.004

Chitnis, T., Tenembaum, S., Banwell, B., Krupp, L., Pohl, D., Rostasy, K.,... and the International Pediatric Multiple Sclerosis Study Group. (2012). Consensus statement: Evaluation of new and existing therapeutics for pediatric multiple sclerosis. *Multiple Sclerosis, 18,* 116–127. doi: 10.1177/1352458511430704

Christodoulou, C., Krupp, L. B., Liang, Z., Huang, W., Melville, P., Roque, C.,... Peyster, R. (2003). Cognitive performance and MR markers of cerebral injury in cognitively impaired MS patients. *Neurology, 60,* 1793–1798.

Cohen, J. A., Barkhof, F., Comi, G., Hartung, H. P., Khatri, B. O., Montalban, X.,... TRANSFORMS Study Group. (2010). Oral fingolimod or intramuscular interferon for relapsing multiple sclerosis. *The New England Journal of Medicine, 362,* 402–415. doi: 10.1056/NEJMoa0907839

Dale, R. C., Brilot, F., & Banwell, B. (2009). Pediatric central nervous system inflammatory demyelination: Acute disseminated encephalomyelitis, clinically isolated syndromes, neuromyelitis optica, and multiple sclerosis. *Current Opinion in Neurology, 22,* 233–240.

de Souza-Teixeira, F., Costilla, S., Ayan, C., Garcia-Lopez, D., Gonzalez-Gallego, J., & de Paz, J. A. (2009). Effects of resistance training in multiple sclerosis. *International Journal of Sports Medicine, 30,* 245–250. doi: 10.1055/s-0028-1105944

Deery, B., Anderson, V., Jacobs, R., Neale, J., & Kornberg, A. (2010). Childhood MS and ADEM: Investigation and comparison of neurocognitive features in children. *Developmental Neuropsychology, 35,* 506–521. doi: 10.1080/87565641.2010.494921

Duquette, P., Murray, T. J., Pleines, J., Ebers, G. C., Sadovnick, D., Weldon, P.,... Hader, W. (1987). Multiple sclerosis in childhood: Clinical profile in 125 patients. *The Journal of Pediatrics, 111,* 359–363.

Duzova, A., & Bakkaloglu, A. (2008). Central nervous system involvement in pediatric rheumatic diseases: Current concepts in treatment. *Current Pharmaceutical Design, 14,* 1295–1301.

Ebers, G. C., Sadovnick, A. D., & Risch, N. J. (1995). A genetic basis for familial aggregation in multiple sclerosis. canadian collaborative study group. *Nature, 377,* 150–151. doi: 10.1038/377150a0

Edgley, K., Sullivan, M. J. L., & Dehoux, E. (1991). A survey of multiple sclerosis: Part 2. determinants of employment status. *Canadian Journal of Rehabilitation, 4*, 127–132.

Feinstein, A. (2011). Multiple sclerosis and depression. *Multiple Sclerosis, 17*, 1276–1281. doi: 10.1177/1352458511417835

Feinstein, A., Roy, P., Lobaugh, N., Feinstein, K., O'Connor, P., & Black, S. (2004). Structural brain abnormalities in multiple sclerosis patients with major depression. *Neurology, 62*, 586–590.

Fischer, J. S., Priore, R. L., Jacobs, L. D., Cookfair, D. L., Rudick, R. A., Herndon, R. M.,...Kooijmans-Coutinho, M. F. (2000). Neuropsychological effects of interferon beta-1a in relapsing multiple sclerosis. multiple sclerosis collaborative research group. *Annals of Neurology, 48*, 885–892.

Freal, J. E., Kraft, G. H., & Coryell, J. K. (1984). Symptomatic fatigue in multiple sclerosis. *Archives of Physical Medicine and Rehabilitation, 65*, 135–138.

Geisler, M. W., Sliwinski, M., Coyle, P. K., Masur, D. M., Doscher, C., & Krupp, L. B. (1996). The effects of amantadine and pemoline on cognitive functioning in multiple sclerosis. *Archives of Neurology, 53*, 185–188.

Ghezzi, A., Pozzilli, C., Grimaldi, L. M., Brescia Morra, V., Bortolon, F., Capra, R.,...Comi, G. (2010). Safety and efficacy of natalizumab in children with multiple sclerosis. *Neurology, 75*, 912–917. doi: 10.1212/WNL.0b013e3181f11daf

Goodman, A. D., Brown, T. R., Krupp, L. B., Schapiro, R. T., Schwid, S. R., Cohen, R.,...Fampridine MS-F203 Investigators. (2009). Sustained-release oral fampridine in multiple sclerosis: A randomised, double-blind, controlled trial. *Lancet, 373*, 732–738. doi: 10.1016/S0140-6736(09)60442-6

Goretti, B., Ghezzi, A., Portaccio, E., Lori, S., Zipoli, V., Razzolini, L.,...Study Group of the Italian Neurological Society. (2010). Psychosocial issue in children and adolescents with multiple sclerosis. *Neurological Sciences, 31*, 467–470. doi: 10.1007/s10072-010-0281-x

Grytten Torkildsen, N., Lie, S., Aarseth, J., Nyland, H., & Myhr, K. (2008). Survival and cause of death in multiple sclerosis: Results from a 50-year follow-up in western Norway. *Multiple Sclerosis, 14*, 1191–1198. doi: 10.1177/1352458508093890

Hahn, C. D., Miles, B. S., MacGregor, D. L., Blaser, S. I., Banwell, B. L., & Hetherington, C. R. (2003). Neurocognitive outcome after acute disseminated encephalomyelitis. *Pediatric Neurology, 29*, 117–123.

Heaton, R. K., Nelson, L. M., Thompson, D. S., Burks, J. S., & Franklin, G. M. (1985). Neuropsychological findings in relapsing-remitting and chronic-progressive multiple sclerosis. *Journal of Consulting and Clinical Psychology, 53*, 103–110.

Holmes, J., Gathercole, S. E., Place, M., Dunning, D. L., Hilton, K. A., & Elliot, J. G. (2009). Working memory deficits can be overcome: Impacts of training and medication on working memory in children with ADHD. *Applied Cognitive Psychology, 24*, 827–836.

Huolman, S., Hamalainen, P., Vorobyev, V., Ruutiainen, J., Parkkola, R., Laine, T., & Hamalainen, H. (2011). The effects of rivastigmine on processing speed and brain activation in patients with multiple sclerosis and subjective cognitive fatigue. *Multiple Sclerosis, 17*, 1351–1361. doi: 10.1177/1352458511412061

Kappos, L., Radue, E. W., O'Connor, P., Polman, C., Hohlfeld, R., Calabresi, P.,...FREEDOMS Study Group. (2010). A placebo-controlled trial of oral fingolimod in relapsing multiple sclerosis. *The New England Journal of Medicine, 362*, 387–401. doi: 10.1056/NEJMoa0909494

Klingberg, T. (2010). Training and plasticity of working memory. *Trends in Cognitive Sciences, 14*, 317–324. doi: 10.1016/j.tics.2010.05.002

Koch, M. W., Glazenborg, A., Uyttenboogaart, M., Mostert, J., & De Keyser, J. (2011). Pharmacologic treatment of depression in multiple sclerosis. *Cochrane Database of Systematic Reviews*, CD007295. doi: 10.1002/14651858.CD007295.pub2

Krupp, L. B., Alvarez, L. A., LaRocca, N. G., & Scheinberg, L. C. (1988). Fatigue in multiple sclerosis. *Archives of Neurology, 45*, 435–437.

Krupp, L. B., Christodoulou, C., Melville, P., Scherl, W. F., MacAllister, W. S., & Elkins, L. E. (2004). Donepezil improved memory in multiple sclerosis in a randomized clinical trial. *Neurology, 63*, 1579–1585.

Krupp, L. B., Christodoulou, C., Melville, P., Scherl, W. F., Pai, L. Y., Muenz, L. R.,...Wishart, H. (2011). Multicenter randomized clinical trial of donepezil for memory impairment in multiple sclerosis. *Neurology, 76*, 1500–1507. doi: 10.1212/WNL.0b013e318218107a

Krupp, L. B., & MacAllister, W. S. (2005). Treatment of pediatric multiple sclerosis. *Current Treatment Options in Neurology, 7*, 191–199.

Kurtzke, J. F., Beebe, G. W., & Norman, J. E. (1985). Epidemiology of multiple sclerosis in US veterans: III. migration and the risk of MS. *Neurology, 35*, 672–678.

Landtblom, A. M., Fazio, P., Fredrikson, S., & Granieri, E. (2010). The first case history of multiple sclerosis: Augustus d'este (1794–1848). *Neurological Sciences, 31*, 29–33. doi: 10.1007/s10072-009-0161-4

Lange, R., Volkmer, M., Heesen, C., & Liepert, J. (2009). Modafinil effects in multiple sclerosis patients with fatigue. *Journal of Neurology, 256*, 645–650. doi: 10.1007/s00415-009-0152-7

Limmroth, V., Putzki, N., & Kachuck, N. J. (2011). The interferon beta therapies for treatment of relapsing-remitting multiple sclerosis: Are they equally efficacious? A comparative review of open-label studies evaluating the efficacy, safety, or dosing of different interferon beta formulations alone or in combination. *Therapeutic Advances in Neurological Disorders, 4*, 281–296. doi: 10.1177/1756285611413825

Lobentanz, I. S., Asenbaum, S., Vass, K., Sauter, C., Klosch, G., Kollegger, H.,...Zeitlhofer, J. (2004). Factors influencing quality of life in multiple sclerosis patients: Disability, depressive mood, fatigue and sleep quality. *Acta Neurologica Scandinavica, 110*, 6–13. doi: 10.1111/j.1600-0404.2004.00257.x

Loitfelder, M., Fazekas, F., Petrovic, K., Fuchs, S., Ropele, S., Wallner-Blazek, M.,...Enzinger, C. (2011). Reorganization in cognitive networks with progression of multiple sclerosis: Insights from fMRI. *Neurology, 76*, 526–533. doi: 10.1212/WNL.0b013e31820b75cf

Lovera, J., Bagert, B., Smoot, K., Morris, C. D., Frank, R., Bogardus, K.,...Bourdette, D. (2007). Ginkgo biloba for the improvement of cognitive performance in multiple sclerosis: A randomized, placebo-controlled trial. *Multiple Sclerosis, 13*, 376–385. doi: 10.1177/1352458506071213

Lynch, S. G., Parmenter, B. A., & Denney, D. R. (2005). The association between cognitive impairment and physical disability in multiple sclerosis. *Multiple Sclerosis, 11*, 469–476.

MacAllister, W. S., Belman, A. L., Milazzo, M., Weisbrot, D. M., Christodoulou, C., Scherl, W. F.,...Krupp, L. B. (2005). Cognitive functioning in children and adolescents with multiple sclerosis. *Neurology, 64*, 1422–1425.

MacAllister, W. S., Boyd, J. R., Holland, N. J., Milazzo, M. C., & Krupp, L. B. (2007). The psychosocial consequences of pediatric multiple sclerosis. *Neurology, 68*, S66–S69.

MacAllister, W. S., Christodoulou, C., Troxell, R., Milazzo, M., Block, P., Preston, T. E.,...Krupp, L. B. (2009). Fatigue and quality of life in pediatric multiple sclerosis. *Multiple Sclerosis, 15*, 1502–1508. doi: 10.1177/1352458509345902

MacAllister, W. S., & Krupp, L. B. (2005). Multiple sclerosis-related fatigue. *Physical Medicine and Rehabilitation Clinics of North America, 16*, 483–502.

Mar, S., Lenox, J., Benzinger, T., Brown, S., & Noetzel, M. (2010). Long-term prognosis of pediatric patients with relapsing acute disseminated encephalomyelitis. *Journal of Child Neurology, 25*, 681–688. doi: 10.1177/0883073809343320

Martinelli, V., Rocca, M. A., Annovazzi, P., Pulizzi, A., Rodegher, M., Boneschi, F. M.,...Filippi, M. (2009). A short-term randomized MRI study of high-dose oral vs intravenous methylprednisolone in MS. *Neurology, 73,* 1842–1848. doi: 10.1212/WNL.0b013e3181c3fd5b

Mattioli, F., Stampatori, C., Bellomi, F., Capra, R., Rocca, M., & Filippi, M. (2010). Neuropsychological rehabilitation in adult multiple sclerosis. *Neurological Sciences, 31*(Suppl 2), S271–S274. doi: 10.1007/s10072-010-0373-7

Minden, S. L., Frankel, D., Hadden, L., Perloffp, J., Srinath, K. P., & Hoaglin, D. C. (2006). The Sonya Slifka longitudinal multiple sclerosis study: Methods and sample characteristics. *Multiple Sclerosis, 12,* 24–38.

Mohr, D. C., Boudewyn, A. C., Goodkin, D. E., Bostrom, A., & Epstein, L. (2001). Comparative outcomes for individual cognitive-behavior therapy, supportive-expressive group psychotherapy, and sertraline for the treatment of depression in multiple sclerosis. *Journal of Consulting and Clinical Psychology, 69,* 942–949.

Morrow, S. A., Stoian, C. A., Dmitrovic, J., Chan, S. C., & Metz, L. M. (2004). The bioavailability of IV methylprednisolone and oral prednisone in multiple sclerosis. *Neurology, 63,* 1079–1080.

Murray, T. J. (2011). The history of multiple sclerosis: From the age of description to the age of therapy. In B. Giesser (Ed.), *Primer of Multiple Sclerosis,* Oxford University Press, New York, NY.

Murray, T. J. (2009). The history of multiple sclerosis: The changing frame of the disease over the centuries. *Journal of the Neurological Sciences, 277* Suppl 1, S3–S8. doi: 10.1016/S0022-510X(09)70003-6

Parmenter, B. A., Denney, D. R., & Lynch, S. G. (2003). The cognitive performance of patients with multiple sclerosis during periods of high and low fatigue. *Multiple Sclerosis, 9,* 111–118.

Pidcock, F. S., Krishnan, C., Crawford, T. O., Salorio, C. F., Trovato, M., & Kerr, D. A. (2007). Acute transverse myelitis in childhood: Center-based analysis of 47 cases. *Neurology, 68,* 1474–1480. doi: 10.1212/01.wnl.0000260609.11357.6f

Pliskin, N. H., Hamer, D. P., Goldstein, D. S., Towle, V. L., Reder, A. T., Noronha, A., & Arnason, B. G. (1996). Improved delayed visual reproduction test performance in multiple sclerosis patients receiving interferon beta-1b. *Neurology, 47,* 1463–1468.

Pohl, D., Waubant, E., Banwell, B., Chabas, D., Chitnis, T., Weinstock-Guttman, B., & Tenembaum, S. (2007). Treatment of pediatric multiple sclerosis and variants. *Neurology, 68,* S54–S65.

Polman, C. H., Reingold, S. C., Banwell, B., Clanet, M., Cohen, J. A., Filippi, M.,...Wolinsky, J. S. (2011). Diagnostic criteria for multiple sclerosis: 2010 revisions to the McDonald criteria. *Annals of Neurology, 69,* 292–302. doi: 10.1002/ana.22366; 10.1002/ana.22366

Portaccio, E., Goretti, B., Zipoli, V., Siracusa, G., Sorbi, S., & Amato, M. P. (2009). A short version of Rao's brief repeatable battery as a screening tool for cognitive impairment in multiple sclerosis. *The Clinical Neuropsychologist, 23,* 268–275. doi: 10.1080/13854040801992815

Pucak, M. L., Carroll, K. A., Kerr, D. A., & Kaplin, A. I. (2007). Neuropsychiatric manifestations of depression in multiple sclerosis: Neuroinflammatory, neuroendocrine, and neurotrophic mechanisms in the pathogenesis of immune-mediated depression. *Dialogues in Clinical Neuroscience, 9,* 125–139.

Pujol, J., Bello, J., Deus, J., Marti-Vilalta, J. L., & Capdevila, A. (1997). Lesions in the left arcuate fasciculus region and depressive symptoms in multiple sclerosis. *Neurology, 49,* 1105–1110.

Rao, S. M., Leo, G. J., Bernardin, L., & Unverzagt, F. (1991). Cognitive dysfunction in multiple sclerosis. I. frequency, patterns, and prediction *Neurology, 41,* 685–691.

Ratchford, J. N., Shore, W., Hammond, E. R., Rose, J. G., Rifkin, R., Nie, P., … Kerr, D. A. (2010). A pilot study of functional electrical stimulation cycling in progressive multiple sclerosis. *NeuroRehabilitation, 27,* 121–128. doi: 10.3233/NRE-2010-0588

Renoux, C., Vukusic, S., Mikaeloff, Y., Edan, G., Clanet, M., Dubois, B., … Adult Neurology Departments KIDMUS Study Group. (2007). Natural history of multiple sclerosis with childhood onset. *The New England Journal of Medicine, 356,* 2603–2613. doi: 10.1056/NEJMoa067597

Rosti-Otajarvi, E. M., & Hamalainen, P. I. (2011). Neuropsychological rehabilitation for multiple sclerosis. *Cochrane Database of Systematic Reviews, 11,* CD009131. doi: 10.1002/14651858.CD009131.pub2

Rovaris, M., Riccitelli, G., Judica, E., Possa, F., Caputo, D., Ghezzi, A., … Filippi, M. (2008). Cognitive impairment and structural brain damage in benign multiple sclerosis. *Neurology, 71,* 1521–1526. doi: 10.1212/01.wnl.0000319694.14251.95

Sanfilipo, M. P., Benedict, R. H., Weinstock-Guttman, B., & Bakshi, R. (2006). Gray and white matter brain atrophy and neuropsychological impairment in multiple sclerosis. *Neurology, 66,* 685–692. doi: 10.1212/01.wnl.0000201238.93586.d9

Savettieri, G., Messina, D., Andreoli, V., Bonavita, S., Caltagirone, C., Cittadella, R., … Quattrone, A. (2004). Gender-related effect of clinical and genetic variables on the cognitive impairment in multiple sclerosis. *Journal of Neurology, 251,* 1208–1214. doi: 10.1007/s00415-004-0508-y

Scott, L. J., & Figgitt, D. P. (2004). Mitoxantrone: A review of its use in multiple sclerosis. *CNS Drugs, 18,* 379–396.

Smith, M. M., & Arnett, P. A. (2005). Factors related to employment status changes in individuals with multiple sclerosis. *Multiple Sclerosis, 11,* 602–609.

Strober, L., Englert, J., Munschauer, F., Weinstock-Guttman, B., Rao, S., & Benedict, R. H. (2009). Sensitivity of conventional memory tests in multiple sclerosis: Comparing the rao brief repeatable neuropsychological battery and the minimal assessment of cognitive function in MS. *Multiple Sclerosis, 15,* 1077–1084. doi: 10.1177/1352458509106615

Stuve, O., Kieseier, B. C., Hemmer, B., Hartung, H. P., Awad, A., Frohman, E. M., … Eagar, T. N. (2010). Translational research in neurology and neuroscience 2010: Multiple sclerosis. *Archives of Neurology, 67,* 1307–1315. doi: 10.1001/archneurol.2010.158

Sumowski, J. F., Chiaravalloti, N., Wylie, G., & Deluca, J. (2009). Cognitive reserve moderates the negative effect of brain atrophy on cognitive efficiency in multiple sclerosis. *Journal of the International Neuropsychological Society, 15,* 606–612. doi: 10.1017/S1355617709090912

Tenembaum, S., Chitnis, T., Ness, J., Hahn, J. S., & International Pediatric MS Study Group. (2007). Acute disseminated encephalomyelitis. *Neurology, 68,* S23–S36. doi: 10.1212/01.wnl.0000259404.51352.7f

Tesar, N., Bandion, K., & Baumhackl, U. (2005). Efficacy of a neuropsychological training programme for patients with multiple sclerosis – a randomised controlled trial. *Wiener Klinische Wochenschrift, 117,* 747–754. doi: 10.1007/s00508-005-0470-4

Till, C., Ghassemi, R., Aubert-Broche, B., Kerbrat, A., Collins, D. L., Narayanan, S., … Banwell, B. L. (2011). MRI correlates of cognitive impairment in childhood-onset multiple sclerosis. *Neuropsychology, 25,* 319–332. doi: 10.1037/a0022051

Vollmer, T. (2007). The natural history of relapses in multiple sclerosis. *Journal of the Neurological Sciences, 256* Suppl 1, S5–S13. doi: 10.1016/j.jns.2007.01.065

Warnke, C., Menge, T., Hartung, H. P., Racke, M. K., Cravens, P. D., Bennett, J. L., … Stuve, O. (2010). Natalizumab and progressive multifocal leukoencephalopathy: What are the causal factors and can it be avoided? *Archives of Neurology, 67*, 923–930. doi: 10.1001/archneurol.2010.161

Weinshenker, B. G., O'Brien, P. C., Petterson, T. M., Noseworthy, J. H., Lucchinetti, C. F., Dodick, D. W.,...Rodriguez, M. (1999). A randomized trial of plasma exchange in acute central nervous system inflammatory demyelinating disease. *Annals of Neurology, 46*, 878–886.

Weisbrot, D. M., Ettinger, A. B., Gadow, K. D., Belman, A. L., MacAllister, W. S., Milazzo, M.,...Krupp, L. B. (2010). Psychiatric comorbidity in pediatric patients with demyelinating disorders. *Journal of Child Neurology, 25*, 192–202. doi: 10.1177/0883073809338519

Westerberg, H., Jacobaeus, H., Hirvikoski, T., Clevberger, P., Ostensson, M. L., Bartfai, A., & Klingberg, T. (2007). Computerized working memory training after stroke – a pilot study. *Brain Injury, 21*, 21–29. doi: 10.1080/02699050601148726

Yadav, V., & Bourdette, D. (2010). Oral disease-modifying therapies for multiple sclerosis: Are we there yet? *Current Neurology and Neuroscience Reports, 10*, 333–335. doi: 10.1007/s11910-010-0126-2

11 Phenylketonuria

Susan E. Waisbren and Kevin M. Antshel

The warning label on diet soda cans that contain the artificial sweetener aspartame reads, "Phenylketonurics: contains phenylalanine." This warning has greatly increased the public's awareness of phenylketonuria (PKU), which is caused by a genetic mutation that leads to a defect in the metabolism of phenylalanine, an essential amino acid. The mutated PKU gene results in a defect in the liver enzyme phenylalanine hydroxylase, resulting in a block in the conversion of phenylalanine to tyrosine.

An autosomal recessive disorder, PKU is inherited from each parent and affects males and females at an equal rate. When both the mother and father are carriers, the chance of a child inheriting PKU is 1 in 4. (in the United States, 1 in 50 people are carriers.) PKU is almost unknown among individuals of African descent but fairly common among those of European decent, with prevalence rates ranging from 1 in 5400 in Ireland, to 1 in 11,000 in the United States, to 1 in 16,000 in Switzerland (Woo, Lidsky, Guttler, Chandra, & Robson, 1983).

Treatment for PKU consists of a phenylalanine-restricted diet, including a special formula and foods low in phenylalanine. Until recently, the only formula option was amino acid–based formulas that contain all of the necessary nutrients (amino acids) in protein, apart from phenylalanine. Currently, PKU can be cured only by liver transplantation (Vajro et al., 1993). However, liver transplantation is not without significant risks; thus, the "cure" is generally not considered to be a treatment option.

HISTORICAL MEDICAL PERSPECTIVE

PKU is likely to have originated more than 300 years ago in an isolated community in San'a, the capital of Yemen (Wright, 1990). At the time, the Jews of Yemen were not permitted to marry outside of their faith. Thus, the gene for PKU spread only within this community. Different mutations for PKU have been traced to the Vikings and to gene bearers in Japan, Italy, Denmark, Scotland, Ireland, Kuwait, South America, and South Africa.

Asbjorn Følling, a Norwegian physician, discovered PKU in 1934 when a mother with two children with mental retardation came to see him after consulting many other doctors. The mother insisted that both her children had a similar degree of mental retardation and both excreted urine with a unique odor. Følling discovered that the children's urine contained a large amount of phenylpyruvic acid, a metabolite of phenylalanine (Folling, 1994). Følling concluded that the children's condition was caused by a defect in phenylalaine metabolism and termed the children's condition "oligophrenia phenylpyrouvica."

Twenty years later, a treatment for the condition (now termed PKU) was discovered by Horst Bickel after he was consulted about a 17-month-old child who had the typical features of PKU: mental retardation, eczema, awkward gait, spastic reflexes, and no language abilities. Bickel hypothesized that if the child's phenylalanine intake were limited, the buildup of the toxic amino acid could be prevented. With Louis Woolf, Bickel created an amino acid mixture that contained all the necessary parts of protein except for phenylalanine (Bickel, Gerrard, & Hickmans, 1954). Through a series of case study experiments, Bickel demonstrated that excessive phenylalanine was responsible for neurological problems and that dietary treatment was helpful.

Nearly 10 years later, two fathers of children with mental retardation, Robert Guthrie and Robert MacCready, advanced the field by developing a screening test for PKU. Guthrie, a microbiologist, developed a bacterial assay for the filter paper blood test (Guthrie & Susi, 1963). With only a drop of blood obtained from the heel of a newborn infant, PKU could be identified within the first few days of life and treatment could be initiated. MacCready, the director of the Diagnostic Division of the Massachusetts Public Health Laboratories in Boston, was so impressed by this new technology that he started the first newborn screening program for PKU in Massachusetts in 1964 (MacCready, 1963). By 1975, the majority of US states had enacted a newborn screening law (Paul, 1999). Currently, laws mandating newborn screening for PKU exist throughout North America and most of Europe.

CURRENT MEDICAL FACTORS AND TREATMENT AND INTERVENTION UPDATE

The precise reason why PKU causes neurological dysfunction remains elusive. Nonetheless, several hypotheses have been forwarded, all of which suggest that the accumulation of phenylalanine metabolites in blood is not directly related to neurological and neuropsychological deficits in PKU. Rather, excess blood phenylalanine is indirectly linked to aberrations in myelin, competition across the blood brain barrier (BBB), and reductions in neurotransmitters (Surtees & Blau, 2000). These three hypotheses are described below.

Myelin Synthesis and Turnover. Large quantities of phenylalanine or its metabolites may be toxic to the brain by inhibiting myelin development (Scriver & Kaufman, 2001). For example, magnetic resonance imaging (MRI) studies suggest that when phenylalanine levels are elevated, myelination in the brain is reduced (Scarabino et al., 2009). Moreover, in untreated or poorly treated children with PKU, myelination is delayed; in adults who discontinue the PKU diet, demyelination occurs (Huttenlocher, 2000).

Competition for Transport. Phenylalanine competes with several other essential amino acids (large neutral amino acids, or LNAAs) for transport across the BBB. In the presence of elevated levels of phenylalanine, more phenylalanine is transported across the BBB than other LNAAs. When this occurs, other amino acids such as tyrosine and tryptophan fail to reach the brain (Miller, Pardridge, Braun, & Oldendorf, 1985). Tyrosine and tryptophan are precursors of neurotransmitters dopamine and serotonin, respectively. When precursors are reduced, lower levels of the neurotransmitter typically result (Guttler & Lou, 1986). Additionally, reduction of important amino acids inhibits protein synthesis in the brain, which is critical for cognitive functioning (Hoeksma et al., 2009).

Dopamine Reduction. When phenylalanine cannot be metabolized to tyrosine in PKU, tyrosine and the metabolites of tyrosine are reduced. One of these metabolites is the neurotransmitter dopamine; as expected, dopamine levels are reduced in the cerebrospinal fluid of individuals with PKU (Burlina et al., 2000). Treatment with large doses of tyrosine, however, does not prevent the neurological effects of PKU (Batshaw, Valle, & Bessman, 1981; Pietz et al., 1995). Thus, high phenylalanine levels, and not low tyrosine levels, are still considered the most likely pathological agent in PKU. The prefrontal cortex is highly sensitive to even modest dopamine reductions and this explains why specific cognitive functions related to the prefrontal cortex are selectively impaired in individuals with PKU (Diamond, Ciaramitaro, Donner, Djali, & Robinson, 1994).

Genetics

Very soon after the discovery of PKU, physicians and parents noted that not all children with PKU had the same phenylalanine levels when off the diet nor did they have the same tolerance for phenylalanine before their blood levels rose. In 1983, the gene for phenylalanine hydroxylase, the enzyme responsible for the conversion of phenylalanine to tyrosine, was cloned (Woo et al., 1983). Following cloning, it became evident that many mutations exist in the phenylalanine hydroxylase gene. Mapped to chromosome 12, the phenylalanine hydroxylase gene is 90 kb in length (q22–q24.2; 13 exons) (Scriver & Kaufman, 2001). More than 500 mutations have been identified in the phenylalanine hydroxylase gene (www.PAHdb.mcgill.ca).

As a function of the heterogeneity of mutations, the following three categories have been artificially defined: *classic PKU,* individuals who have blood phenylalanine levels >20 mg/dL while on a normal diet and with no activity of the phenylalanine hydroxylase enzyme; *mild PKU,* individuals with blood phenylalanine levels of 10–20 mg/dL and 5%–15% residual activity of the enzyme; and *non-PKU hyperphenylalaninemia,* individuals with blood phenylalanine levels of 2–10 mg/dL and an estimated 25% residual activity of phenylalanine hydroxylase).

Genotype-to-phenotype correlations, however, depend primarily on the particular combination of genes inherited from the mother and father. For example, a patient with the genotype of R408W/IVS-12 will have a more severe biochemical defect than a patient with the genotype R408W/Y414C, even though the two patients share the R408W gene. The reason is that although the R408W mutation confers no phenylalanine hydroxylase enzyme activity, the Y414C allows for enough enzyme activity to produce mild PKU, while the IVS-12 mutation also confers no phenylalanine hydroxylase activity and thus results in classic PKU. In addition to the genetic factors related to the phenylalanine hydroxylase genotype, other physiological and genetic factors affect the PKU phenotype (Lichter-Konecki et al., 1989).

Treatment

Standard Treatment. Until the 1980s, most clinics in North America and Europe recommended diet discontinuation during middle childhood (Schuett & Brown, 1984). Thus, at about age 5 or 6 years, most children with PKU were suddenly allowed to eat as much protein (phenylalanine) as they desired. Although it was known that their blood phenylalanine levels would rise, it was thought that their cognitive abilities would be unaffected.

Despite the appeal of considering PKU a disease of early childhood, evidence suggesting that diet discontinuation resulted in diminished IQ in a large percentage of children with PKU began to mount (Waisbren, Schnell, & Levy, 1980). For example, the age at which blood phenylalanine levels consistently exceeded 15 mg/dL was the best predictor of IQ and school achievement at ages 8 and 10 years (Holtzman, Kronmal, van Doorninck, Azen, & Koch, 1986).

In 2000, a National Institutes of Health Consensus Conference convened in Washington, DC, to prepare guidelines for the treatment of PKU. At that time, continuation of the PKU diet throughout the lifespan was recommended, with the understanding that the diet may be relaxed in adults depending on individual needs (NIH, 2000). Women with PKU who consider getting pregnant were advised to maintain blood phenylalanine levels at 2–6 mg/dL beginning 3 months before pregnancy and continuing throughout pregnancy (NIH, 2000).

Recommendations from the various PKU clinics vary with regard to what constitutes metabolic control in children. Nevertheless, the recommendation from most clinics is now 2–6 mg/dL. However, due to the restrictiveness of the diet, few teenagers are able to maintain levels within this range (Walter et al., 2002). For example, in a study of children in the United Kingdom, only 12% were following a strict diet by age 14 years, and only 4% were following a strict diet by age 18 years (Beasley, Costello, & Smith, 1994). It is largely for these reasons that new and emerging treatments for PKU continue to be developed.

New and Emerging Treatments. In 2007, oral administration of sapropterin dihydrochloride (BH4) received approval from the US Federal Drug Administration (FDA) for the treatment of PKU. A cofactor of phenylalanine-hydroxylase, BH4 is the enzyme responsible for converting phenylalanine to tyrosine. BH4 boosts the activity of this enzyme in individuals with PKU who have residual enzyme activity. Sapropterin dihydrochloride appears to be more effective in individuals with mild PKU; approximately 80% of individuals with mild PKU and about 10% of those with classic PKU who take sapropterin dihydrochloride respond with lowered phenylalanine levels and increased tolerance of phenylalanine (protein) (Blau et al., 2009; Levy et al., 2007).

LNAA therapy is another supplemental therapy. In large quantity, LNAAs can compete with phenylalanine at the BBB so that less phenylalanine and more LNAAs cross into the brain (Matalon et al., 2007; Matalon et al., 2003; Schindeler et al., 2007). Unlike BH4, however, LNNA therapy does not reduce the blood phenylalanine level, although LNAA therapy may lower brain phenylalanine concentrations (Matalon et al., 2007).

A phenylalanine-free source of protein has also been recently identified. This protein, glycomacropeptide (GMP), is produced during cheese-making and, when isolated from cheese whey, contains virtually no phenylalanine (Ney et al., 2009). Some evidence suggests that GMP improves protein retention and phenylalanine utilization and also lowers phenylalanine levels in the brain (van Calcar et al., 2009). GMP may emerge as an alternative to the current amino acid formulas, especially if a GMP formula with a more palatable taste and odor than the amino acid formula can be developed (Laclair, Ney, MacLeod, & Etzel, 2009).

In current clinical trials, an investigational enzyme substitution therapy termed "pegylated recombinant phenylalanine ammonia lyase" has been shown theoretically to reduce blood phenylalanine levels in all individuals with PKU (Bélange-Quintana et al., 2011). This potential therapy involves weekly or more frequent subcutaneous injections. Animal model research suggests that phenylalanine levels could be controlled without diet by using this therapy (Sarkissian et al., 2008).

At this time, gene therapy research for PKU is being performed in animal models. The results are mixed (Lavri & Lorberboum-Galski, 2007; Eisensmith & Woo, 1994; Jung et al., 2008) and suggest that gene therapy will not be a viable treatment option any time in the near future.

EARLY PSYCHOLOGICAL AND NEUROPSYCHOLOGICAL FINDINGS

Intelligence

If untreated, children with classic PKU have severe intellectual disabilities, eczema, seizures, ataxia, motor deficits, and behavioral problems such as self-mutilation, aggression, impulsivity, and psychosis (Partington, 1978; Partington & Laverty, 1978; Pitt, 1971). Because the early identification of individuals with PKU was not standard practice until after 1964, there is a cohort of adults with PKU who have intellectual disability. The introduction of a phenylalanine-restricted diet to adults with untreated PKU results in little or no improvement in cognitive function. However, case reports suggest moderate and sometimes even dramatic improvement in behavior if metabolic control is achieved and maintained on a long-term basis (Harper & Reid, 1987; Yannicelli & Ryan, 1995).

Until the 1980s, diet restriction recommendations did not extend beyond middle childhood (Schuett & Brown, 1984). Subsequently, studies demonstrated diminished IQ associated with diet discontinuation (Waisbren et al., 1980); discontinuation of treatment predicted IQ and school achievement in middle childhood (Holtzman et al., 1986). Even with continued treatment, children with PKU usually attained IQ scores that were 6–9 points lower than those of their siblings and parents (Fishler, Azen, Henderson, Friedman, & Koch, 1987) and IQ scores dropped following diet discontinuation (Seashore, Friedman, Novelly, & Bapat, 1985).

Other cognitive domains

In addition to IQ effects, visual–motor deficits (Koff, Boyle, & Pueschel, 1977), global processing problems including impaired reaction times (Waisbren, Brown, de Sonneville, & Levy, 1994), and executive functioning deficits (Pennington, van Doorninck, McCabe, & McCabe, 1985) are some of the earliest reported findings.

Diamond and colleagues were one of the first groups to study PKU systematically as an exemplar disorder of executive functioning (Diamond, Prevor, Callender, & Druin, 1997). They reported that children with blood phenylalanine levels >360 μmol/L (6 mg/dL) performed less well on tasks of executive function (working memory and inhibitory control) than on nonexecutive function tasks. Others have similarly reported negative correlations between blood phenylalanine levels and performance of laboratory measures of executive functioning (Weglage, Pietsch, Funders, Koch, & Ullrich, 1996; Welsh, Pennington, Ozonoff, Rouse, & McCabe, 1990).

Using early and continuously treated sample of individuals with PKU, multiple research groups reported that individuals with PKU perform less well relative to age-matched peers on executive tasks designed to assess attention, problem-solving abilities, impulsivity, planning, and organization (Huijbregts, de Sonneville, van Spronsen, Licht, & Sergeant, 2002; Ris, Williams, Hunt, Berry, & Leslie, 1994; Stemerdink et al., 1995).

Academic functioning

Relative to discrete cognitive domains, academic functioning and achievement have been less well studied. Nonetheless, several trends emerged in early PKU research. Math difficulties were some of the most commonly reported school struggles in children and adolescents with PKU, regardless of dietary control (Azen, Koch, & Gross-Friedman, 1991; Fishler, Azen, Friedman, & Koch, 1989; Weglage, Funders, Wilken, Schubert, & Ullrich, 1993). Although reading decoding generally is an area of strength for children and adolescents with PKU, reading comprehension difficulties are more common (Fishler et al., 1989; Fishler et al., 1987; Koch, Azen, Friedman, & Williamson, 1984).

Phenylalanine: cognition associations

In addition to describing the cognitive domains affected by elevated levels of phenylalanine, early research also considered dose–response relationships. Concurrent blood phenylalanine levels in individuals with PKU have been negatively correlated with reaction time (Clarke, Gates, Hogan, Barrett, & MacDonald, 1987; Huijbregts, de Sonneville, Licht, van Spronsen, & Sergeant, 2002; Schmidt et al., 1994). Nonetheless, most neuropsychological test results in adults with PKU, both on and off diet, correlated with phenylalanine levels during childhood but not with concurrent levels in adulthood (Brumm et al., 2004).

Behavioral/Psychiatric manifestations

In addition to cognition, the behavioral manifestations of PKU have received research attention. For example, researchers and clinicians alike have alluded to an increased prevalence of attentional problems and attention-deficit/hyperactivity disorder (ADHD) diagnoses in PKU (Antshel & Waisbren, 2003; Burgard, Rey, Rupp, Abadie, & Rey, 1997; Lou, 1994). Some data suggest that 25% children with early-treated PKU receive stimulant medication for ADHD compared with 7% of children with diabetes (Arnold, Vladutiu, Orlowski, Blakely, & DeLuca, 2004).

Anxiety, including panic disorder and agoraphobia, has also been reported as a complication of elevated phenylalanine levels (Rothenberg & Sills, 1968; Smith, Beasley, Wolff, & Ades, 1988; Sullivan & Chang, 1999; Waisbren & Levy, 1991; Waisbren & Zaff, 1994). Reductions in phenylalanine levels generally result in reductions in anxiety symptoms (Pietz et al., 1997; Sullivan & Chang, 1999).

In addition to ADHD and anxiety, the effects of PKU on personality and tempera-ment, including lower levels of "persistence," "intensity," and "rhythmicity," were noted by early researchers (Fisch, Sines, & Chang, 1981; Schor, 1983) as well as higher levels of hypersensitivity and talkativeness (Siegel, Balow, Fisch, & Anderson, 1968). Parents noted unfavorable changes in the child's personality as a function of increased pheny-lalanine levels (Schuett, 1997). Finally, lower levels of social maturity and functional independence in young adults with PKU were also reported by earlier research groups (Waisbren, Hamilton, St James, Shiloh, & Levy, 1995; Weglage et al., 1992).

Maternal PKU

With the progress made in newborn screening and more effective interventions, most young adult women with PKU did not have intellectual disability by the early 1980s. Given the improvements in functioning, many adult women with PKU were marry-ing and having children. However, as these women became pregnant, it became clear that elevated levels of phenylalanine were not only detrimental to the woman with PKU but also to the developing fetus (Levy & Waisbren, 1983). The phrase "maternal PKU" was coined in the early 1980s to refer to the risks to the fetus when the mother has PKU.

The risks in maternal PKU occur secondary to the teratogenic effect of elevated levels of phenylalanine in the intrauterine environment because the fetus relies on the mother to metabolize phenylalanine (Ghavami, Levy, & Erbe, 1986). If untreated, con-genital birth defects including intellectual disability (95%), microcephaly (90%), and congenital heart disease (17%) (Lenke & Levy, 1980) occur in the offspring of women with maternal PKU. These outcomes are very similar to those noted in the fetal alcohol syndrome population (Levy & Waisbren, 1983). The risks to the developing fetus are reduced significantly if the mother with PKU initiates strict dietary treatment prior to pregnancy and maintains metabolic control throughout pregnancy (Hanley, Clarke, & Schoonheyt, 1987; Koch et al., 1990).

To better understand the processes and outcomes associated with maternal PKU, the International Collaborative Study of Maternal Phenylketonuria, which is a lon-gitudinal, prospective study of the effects of dietary treatment during pregnancy in women with PKU in the United States, Canada, and Germany, was conducted (Koch et al., 1993). Results indicated a dose–response relationship between the number of gestational weeks at which the mother reduced her blood phenylalanine level and the child's neonatal course, birth head circumference, infant developmental quotient (DQ), and childhood IQ (Hanley et al., 1996; Rouse et al., 1997; Waisbren et al., 1998). For example, the DQ at age 6–12 months in maternal PKU offspring whose mothers attained metabolic control by 20 weeks gestation was within the average range, whereas the DQ of offspring whose mothers were not in metabolic control until after 20 weeks gestation was <85 (Hanley et al., 1996). Similar results were reported in childhood; the mean IQ of offspring whose mothers attained metabolic control by 10 weeks was 93, 88 for those whose mothers attained metabolic control between 10 and 20 weeks, and 73 for those whose mothers were not in control until after 20 weeks (Hanley et al., 1996).

The Maternal PKU Collaborative Study data also suggest that despite treatment, offspring from maternal PKU pregnancies often function developmentally and cog-nitively below average levels (Koch et al., 1990). This is possibly secondary to the fact that >60% of women with PKU who become pregnant do so unintentionally and are not in metabolic control at the time of conception (Waisbren et al., 1995). In the 1990s and continuing forward, efforts to improve treatment adherence have focused on adolescents and include social support designed to improve attitudes about the efficacy and acceptability of treatment (Waisbren et al., 1995; Waisbren, Shiloh, St James, & Levy, 1991).

RECENT PSYCHOLOGICAL AND NEUROPSYCHOLOGICAL FINDINGS

PKU

Neurological. With the tremendous advances in technology, it has become easier to identify specific neurological anomalies and associations with elevated levels of phenylalanine. The myelin aberrations have become easier to identify with protocols such as diffusion tensor imaging and magnetic resonance spectroscopy. In general, imaging studies have demonstrated that PKU is associated with diffuse white matter pathology in both treated and untreated individuals (Anderson & Leuzzi, 2010). In those untreated for PKU, hypomyelination (lack of myelin formation) occurs, while in individuals with PKU who are treated early intramyelinic edema occurs in a fashion that is negatively associated with the level of metabolic control (Anderson & Leuzzi, 2010). This pathology can be reversed, however, with adherence to a strict low-phenylalanine diet for at least 2 months (Anderson & Leuzzi, 2010).

A recent diffusion tensor imaging study examined the development of the microstructural integrity of white matter across six regions of the corpus callosum in 34 children (aged 7–18 years) with early-treated and continuously treated PKU and in 61 age- and gender-matched controls (White et al., 2010). Results demonstrated that relative anisotropy was comparable to that of controls across all six regions of the corpus callosum. However, mean diffusivity was restricted in children with PKU in anterior yet not posterior corpus callosum regions (White et al., 2010). Moreover, the mean diffusivity was more restricted in older adolescents with PKU (White et al., 2010).

Studies using functional magnetic resonance imaging (fMRI) protocols have also recently emerged in the PKU literature. For example, Christ and colleagues (2010) recently compared six individuals with early-treated PKU (age range 11–27 years) during performance of an *n*-back working memory task and compared results with those of six age- and gender-matched neurologically intact individuals. fMRI results revealed that individuals with PKU demonstrated atypical neural activation within the prefrontal cortex and decreased neural synchronization between regions during working memory task performance (Christ, Moffitt, et al., 2010).

A recent study examined event-related potential (ERP) components elicited during a selective processing task (de Sonneville et al., 2010). Results indicated that children with PKU differed from controls on task performance accuracy. Performance accuracy was associated with both lifetime and concurrent phenylalanine levels, yet with a stronger association with lifetime phenylalanine levels. The researchers concluded that children with PKU differed from age-matched controls on selective attention tasks, observed in ERP components associated with relatively late attentional processing (de Sonneville et al., 2010).

Neuropsychological. A meta-analysis that focused on overall intelligence in children and adults with PKU confirmed the previously established relationship between blood phenylalanine levels and IQ. The combined results of 40 studies showed that in children with PKU, mean lifetime blood phenylalanine levels were significantly correlated with Full Scale IQ ($r = -0.34$). A similar correlation ($r = -0.35$) was noted between IQ and blood phenylalanine levels during the "critical period" (ages 0–12 years) and with the concurrent blood phenylalanine level ($r = -0.31$) (Waisbren et al., 2007).

Attempts to explain the variability in neuropsychological performance have also become more common. One novel approach to explaining variability in neuropsychological functioning among individuals with PKU posits an association between the stability of blood phenylalanine levels and functioning. In a retrospective study of 45 early-treated and continuously treated children with PKU, the stability of blood phenylalanine level was a better predictor of IQ ($r = -0.37$; $p = .06$) than lifetime mean blood phenylalanine level ($r = -0.18$; $p = .34$) (Anastasoaie, Kurzius, Forbes, & Waisbren, 2008).

Within the past 10 years, there has also been a push in the field to expand the neuropsychological focus beyond simply assessing IQ as an outcome variable (Brumm & Grant, 2010). For example, the assessment of specific executive functions such as working memory, inhibitory control, and set shifting has been emphasized. Although some discrepancies exist, many studies suggest that individuals with PKU have difficulties on executive tasks assessing working memory and response inhibition yet perform relatively better on tasks of set shifting (Christ, Huijbregts, de Sonneville, & White, 2010).

Findings using executive-function laboratory tasks designed to measure planning and organization are less consistent across studies and may be related to cohort differences (e.g., age, phenylalanine levels), variability in the extent to which tasks placed demands on executive working memory and/or response inhibition, and variability in the sensitivity of the tasks to detect subtle performance differences (Christ, Huijbregts, et al., 2010). Scores on questionnaires designed to assess day-to-day executive functioning are only weakly related to laboratory-based performance on tasks of executive functioning (Christ, Huijbregts, et al., 2010; Sharman, Sullivan, Young, & McGill, 2009). Despite the great interest and focus on executive functioning, a meta-analytic review (Moyle, Fox, Arthur, Bynevelt, & Burnett, 2007) documented that the largest effect sizes between individuals with PKU and typically developing control participants were on measures of processing speed.

More recent research has also considered the impact of novel treatments in improving neuropsychological outcomes in PKU. Gassio and colleagues (2010) assessed domains of cognition in nine children with PKU who had been treated for >5 years with 5–9 mg/kg/day of BH4. The authors compared the results of the current sample of children with their previous samples of children who were treated with diet. No statistically significant differences emerged on any of the cognitive domains (Gassio et al., 2010).

Psychological. Although very few studies have investigated the prevalence of ADHD, clinical focus has shifted toward improving the assessment and diagnostic validity of ADHD within the PKU population (Antshel & Waisbren, 2003; Arnold et al., 2004). Similar to ADHD, very few studies have assessed the prevalence of other psychiatric disorders in PKU. Nonetheless, elevated rates of psychiatric symptoms, especially anxiety and depression, are common in individuals with PKU, and symptom severity of anxiety and depressive features is positively associated with phenylalanine levels (Brumm, Bilder, & Waisbren, 2010).

Maternal PKU

Maternal PKU populations have also received considerable research attention in the past 10 years. Going beyond birth outcomes, most recent research has considered cognitive and psychiatric outcomes in children born to mothers with PKU. For example, in a study that included some offspring through 10 years of age, 44% were noted to exhibit significant behavioral problems (Ng, Rae, Wright, Gurry, & Wray, 2003). Likewise, a large longitudinal maternal PKU study (Maillot, Lilburn, Baudin, Morley, & Lee, 2008) followed 105 children born to 67 mothers with PKU, the majority of whom were in relatively good metabolic control of their condition during pregnancy. The mothers with PKU were divided into the following two groups: those who received a low phenylalanine diet prior to pregnancy and those who initiated the diet after they became pregnant, usually within the first trimester. At age 8 years, children born to mothers who received the diet prior to pregnancy had higher IQ scores than those whose mothers initiated the diet after they became pregnant (111 and 91, respectively) (Maillot et al., 2008). Blood phenylalanine variability during pregnancy correlated negatively with children's IQ scores, even when the blood phenylalanine level was within the recommended range, with correlations as high at –0.71 at age 14 years (Maillot et al., 2008).

Not surprisingly, much of the recent clinical research has considered how best to optimize the management of maternal PKU. Presently, a comprehensive approach that addresses all stages of the maternal PKU life cycle (prevention of unplanned pregnancy, reproductive decision making, treatment initiation before pregnancy begins, and treatment continuation) is recommended (Koch, Trefz, & Waisbren, 2010). The use of pharmaceutical therapies such as sapropterin may also help to improve metabolic control during pregnancy (Koch et al., 2010).

CURRENT RESOURCES

Considerable progress in understanding and treating PKU has been made over the last 80 years. Nonetheless, very early on in the history of PKU, it became apparent that the biggest challenge may be adherence to treatment. The PKU diet is one of the more difficult, if not the most difficult, medical diet to maintain. Every social gathering, school lunch period, travel plan, summer activity, and nightly meal must be carefully planned. Moreover, poor adherence will set off a cascade of events that makes it even more difficult to adhere to the diet. For example, the hyperactive or impulsive behavior common in children with PKU may lead to poor self-control with the diet. This produces an anxious or overly controlling response from parents, which may lead to an increase in poor dietary adherence and oppositional behavior in the child (Hendrikx, van der Schot, Slijper, Huisman, & Kalverboer, 1994).

In addition to improvements in the taste and flavor of medical foods such as formula and low-protein foods, recent advances in treatments may also improve adherence rates. For example BH4, LNAA therapy, a phenylalanine-free source of protein (GMP), and pegylated recombinant phenylalanine ammonia lyase all appear to have some promise in improving treatment adherence rates.

In addition to improving treatment adherence (and related to treatment adherence), the current focus is on improving the transition from pediatric care to adult care. Possibly owing to the once prevalent notion that PKU was a disease of childhood, most PKU clinics are housed within pediatric departments. As with other medical conditions (Lotstein, McPherson, Strickland, & Newacheck, 2005), an emphasis has been placed on providing adult care in adult settings. This makes intuitive sense because the concerns and issues for adults with PKU, including vitamin deficiencies, osteoporosis, and maternal PKU, are different from those of children (Hoeks, den Heijer, & Janssen, 2009).

The following issues, which are not necessarily specific to PKU, need to be addressed in order to best facilitate the transition from pediatric to adult care providers: patients should have an identified healthcare professional to oversee their individual transition; patients and providers need to identify the knowledge and skills required for developmentally appropriate care; an up-to-date and portable medical record (personal health summary) should be kept by patients; healthcare providers need to assist patients in writing a healthcare transition plan by the time the patient is aged 14 years; all patients should receive the necessary care to protect and optimize their health; and continuous and affordable health insurance should be guaranteed to ensure that all costs of the transition planning and care are covered (American Academy of Pediatrics, 2002). Although these steps seem reasonable, many families with a special needs child are not prepared to make the transition to adult healthcare (Reiss, Gibson, & Walker, 2005).

FUTURE AIMS AND RESEARCH OPPORTUNITIES

The ability to predict neuropsychological phenotype from genotype has presented significant challenges in PKU because there can be great differences in IQ among individuals with the same genotype. Likewise, despite evidence of myelin abnormalities in early-treated and untreated individuals, neuroimaging studies to date have not found a correlation between MRI abnormalities and neuropsychological performance. Future research, using continually advancing technology, should attempt to further clarify these relationships. Similarly, physiological factors beyond phenylalanine levels remain to be investigated, including variations in the BBB, the influence of other genes, and neurotransmitter regulation during standard treatments as well as with new alternative treatments.

Prospective studies should also extend research on the relationship between neuropsychological outcomes and psychosocial functioning in individuals with PKU across the lifespan. To date, far more research has considered the neuropsychology of individuals with PKU, and far less has considered the psychology of this population. Likewise, in the maternal PKU population, very little research has focused on parenting styles of continuously treated and untreated mothers, yet research in this area could be very significant toward understanding the psychosocial outcomes of maternal PKU offspring.

Finally, much of what we know about PKU in adulthood relates to young adults. There is less information on middle-aged adults and far less data on PKU in geriatric populations. Given our aging population, more research should focus on PKU in the context of middle and old age. Are treatments as efficacious? What types of psychiatric comorbidity exist? What is the relationship between PKU and cognitive decline/dementia? These are questions that presently have no real answers.

REFERENCES

American Academy of Pediatrics. (2002). A consensus statement on health care transitions for young adults with special health care needs. *Pediatrics, 110*, 1304–1306.

Anastasoaie, V., Kurzius, L., Forbes, P., & Waisbren, S. (2008). Stability of blood phenylalanine levels and IQ in children with phenylketonuria. *Molecular Genetics and Metabolism, 95*, 17–20.

Anderson, P. J., & Leuzzi, V. (2010). White matter pathology in phenylketonuria. *Molecular Genetics and Metabolism, 99* (Supplement 1), S3–S9.

Antshel, K. M., & Waisbren, S. E. (2003). Developmental timing of exposure to elevated levels of phenylalanine is associated with ADHD symptom expression. *Journal of Abnormal Child Psychology, 31*, 565–574.

Arnold, G. L., Vladutiu, C. J., Orlowski, C. C., Blakely, E. M., & DeLuca, J. (2004). Prevalence of stimulant use for attentional dysfunction in children with phenylketonuria. *Journal of Inherited Metabolic Disease, 27*, 137–143.

Azen, C. G., Koch, R., & Gross-Friedman, E. (1991). Intellectual development in 12-year-old children with phenylketonuria. *American Journal of Diseases of Children, 145*, 35–39.

Batshaw, M. L., Valle, D., & Bessman, S. P. (1981). Unsuccessful treatment of phenylketonuria with tyrosine. *Journal of Pediatrics, 99*, 159–160.

Beasley, M. G., Costello, P. M., & Smith, I. (1994). Outcome of treatment in young adults with phenylketonuria detected by routine neonatal screening between 1964 and 1971. *Quarterly Journal of Medicine, 87*, 155–160.

Bélanger -Quintana, A., Burlina, A., Harding, C. O., & Muntau, A. C. (2011). Up to date knowledge on different treatment strategies for phenylketonuria. *Molecular genetics and metabolism, 104* Suppl, S19–25. doi: 10.1016/j.ymgme.2011.08.009

Bickel, H., Gerrard, J., & Hickmans, E. M. (1954). The influence of phenylalanine intake on the chemistry and behaviour of a phenyl-ketonuric child. *Acta Paediatrica, 43*, 64–77.

Blau , N., Belanger-Quintana, A., Demirkol, M., Feillet, F., Giovannini, M., MacDonald, A., & van Spronsen, F. J. (2009). Optimizing the use of sapropterin (BH(4)) in the management of phenylketonuria. *Molecular Genetics and Metabolism, 96*, 158–163.

Brumm, V. L., Azen, C., Moats, R. A., Stern, A. M., Broomand, C., Nelson, M. D., & Koch, R. (2004). Neuropsychological outcome of subjects participating in the PKU adult collaborative study: A preliminary review. *Journal of Inherited Metabolic Disease, 27*, 549–566.

Brumm, V. L., Bilder, D., & Waisbren, S. E. (2010). Psychiatric symptoms and disorders in phenylketonuria. *Molecular Genetics and Metabolism, 99*, S59–S63.

Brumm, V. L., & Grant, M. L. (2010). The role of intelligence in phenylketonuria: A review of research and management. *Molecular Genetics and Metabolism, 99* (Supplement 1), S18–S21.

Burgard, P., Rey, F., Rupp, A., Abadie, V., & Rey, J. (1997). Neuropsychologic functions of early treated patients with phenylketonuria, on and off diet: Results of a cross-national and cross-sectional study. *Pediatric Research, 41*, 368–374.

Burlina, A. B., Bonafe, L., Ferrari, V., Suppiej, A., Zacchello, F., & Burlina, A. P. (2000). Measurement of neurotransmitter metabolites in the cerebrospinal fluid of phenylketonuric patients under dietary treatment. *Journal of Inherited Metabolic Disease, 23*, 313–316.

Christ, S. E., Huijbregts, S. C., de Sonneville, L. M., & White, D. A. (2010). Executive function in early-treated phenylketonuria: Profile and underlying mechanisms. *Molecular Genetics and Metabolism, 99*, S22–S32.

Christ, S. E., Moffitt, A. J., & Peck, D. (2010). Disruption of prefrontal function and connectivity in individuals with phenylketonuria. *Molecular Genetics and Metabolism, 99*, S33–S40.

Clarke, J. T., Gates, R. D., Hogan, S. E., Barrett, M., & MacDonald, G. W. (1987). Neuropsychological studies on adolescents with phenylketonuria returned to phenylalanine-restricted diets. *American Journal of Mental Retardation, 92,* 255–262.

de Sonneville, L. M., Huijbregts, S. C., van Spronsen, F. J., Verkerk, P. H., Sergeant, J. A., & Licht, R. (2010). Event-related potential correlates of selective processing in early- and continuously-treated children with phenylketonuria: Effects of concurrent phenylalanine level and dietary control. *Molecular Genetics and Metabolism, 99,* S10–S17.

Diamond, A., Ciaramitaro, V., Donner, E., Djali, S., & Robinson, M. B. (1994). An animal model of early-treated PKU. *Journal of Neuroscience, 14,* 3072–3082.

Diamond, A., Prevor, M. B., Callender, G., & Druin, D. P. (1997). Prefrontal cortex cognitive deficits in children treated early and continuously for PKU. *Monographs of the Society for Research in Child Development, 62,* 1–208.

Eavri, R., & Lorberboum-Galski, H. (2007). A novel approach for enzyme replacement therapy. The use of phenylalanine hydroxylase-based fusion proteins for the treatment of phenylketonuria. *Journal of Biological Chemistry, 282,* 23402–23409.

Eisensmith, R. C., & Woo, S. L. (1994). Gene therapy for phenylketonuria. *Acta Paediatrica, 407,* 124–129.

Fisch, R. O., Sines, L. K., & Chang, P. (1981). Personality characteristics of nonretarded phenylketonurics and their family members. *Journal of Clinical Psychiatry, 42,* 106–113.

Fishler, K., Azen, C. G., Friedman, E. G., & Koch, R. (1989). School achievement in treated PKU children. *Journal of Mental Deficiency Research, 33,* 493–498.

Fishler, K., Azen, C. G., Henderson, R., Friedman, E. G., & Koch, R. (1987). Psychoeducational findings among children treated for phenylketonuria. *American Journal of Mental Deficiency, 92,* 65–73.

Folling, I. (1994). The discovery of phenylketonuria. *Acta Paediatrica, 407,* 4–10.

Gassio, R., Vilaseca, M. A., Lambruschini, N., Boix, C., Fuste, M. E., & Campistol, J. (2010). Cognitive functions in patients with phenylketonuria in long-term treatment with tetrahydrobiopterin. *Molecular Genetics and Metabolism, 99,* S75–S78.

Ghavami, M., Levy, H. L., & Erbe, R. W. (1986). Prevention of fetal damage through dietary control of maternal hyperphenylalaninemia. *Clinical Obstetrics and Gynecology, 29,* 580–585.

Guthrie, R., & Susi, A. (1963). A simple phenylalanine method for detecting phenylketonuria in large populations of newborn infants. *Pediatrics, 32,* 338–343.

Guttler, F., & Lou, H. (1986). Dietary problems of phenylketonuria: Effect on CNS transmitters and their possible role in behaviour and neuropsychological function. *Journal of Inherited Metabolic Disease, 9,* 169–177.

Hanley, W. B., Clarke, J. T., & Schoonheyt, W. (1987). Maternal phenylketonuria (PKU)—a review. *Clinical Biochemistry, 20,* 149–156.

Hanley, W. B., Koch, R., Levy, H. L., Matalon, R., Rouse, B., Azen, C., & de la Cruz, F. (1996). The North American Maternal Phenylketonuria Collaborative Study, developmental assessment of the offspring: Preliminary report. *European Journal of Pediatrics, 155,* S169–S172.

Harper, M., & Reid, A. H. (1987). Use of a restricted protein diet in the treatment of behaviour disorder in a severely mentally retarded adult female phenylketonuric patient. *Journal of Mental Deficiency Research, 31,* 209–212.

Hendrikx, M. M., van der Schot, L. W., Slijper, F. M., Huisman, J., & Kalverboer, A. F. (1994). Phenylketonuria and some aspects of emotional development. *European Journal of Pediatrics, 153,* 832–835.

Hoeks, M. P., den Heijer, M., & Janssen, M. C. (2009). Adult issues in phenylketonuria. *Netherlands Journal of Medicine, 67,* 2–7.

Hoeksma, M., Reijngoud, D. J., Pruim, J., de Valk, H. W., Paans, A. M., & van Spronsen, F. J. (2009). Phenylketonuria: High plasma phenylalanine decreases cerebral protein synthesis. *Molecular Genetics and Metabolism, 96,* 177–182.

Holtzman, N. A., Kronmal, R. A., van Doorninck, W., Azen, C., & Koch, R. (1986). Effect of age at loss of dietary control on intellectual performance and behavior of children with phenylketonuria. *New England Journal of Medicine, 314,* 593–598.

Huijbregts, S. C., de Sonneville, L. M., Licht, R., van Spronsen, F. J., & Sergeant, J. A. (2002). Short-term dietary interventions in children and adolescents with treated phenylketonuria: Effects on neuropsychological outcome of a well-controlled population. *Journal of Inherited Metabolic Disease, 25,* 419–430.

Huijbregts, S. C., de Sonneville, L. M., van Spronsen, F. J., Licht, R., & Sergeant, J. A. (2002). The neuropsychological profile of early and continuously treated phenylketonuria: Orienting, vigilance, and maintenance versus manipulation-functions of working memory. *Neuroscience and Biobehavioral Reviews, 26,* 697–712.

Huttenlocher, P. R. (2000). The neuropathology of phenylketonuria: Human and animal studies. *European Journal of Pediatrics, 159,* S102–S106.

Jung, S. C., Park, J. W., Oh, H. J., Choi, J. O., Seo, K. I., Park, E. S., & Park, H. Y. (2008). Protective effect of recombinant adeno-associated virus 2/8-mediated gene therapy from the maternal hyperphenylalaninemia in offsprings of a mouse model of phenylketonuria. *Journal of Korean Medical Science, 23,* 877–883.

Koch, R., Azen, C., Friedman, E. G., & Williamson, M. L. (1984). Paired comparisons between early treated PKU children and their matched sibling controls on intelligence and school achievement test results at eight years of age. *Journal of Inherited Metabolic Disease, 7,* 86–90.

Koch, R., Hanley, W., Levy, H., Matalon, R., Rouse, B., Dela Cruz, F., & Gross Friedman, E. (1990). A preliminary report of the collaborative study of maternal phenylketonuria in the United States and Canada. *Journal of Inherited Metabolic Disease, 13,* 641–650.

Koch, R., Levy, H. L., Matalon, R., Rouse, B., Hanley, W., & Azen, C. (1993). The North American Collaborative Study of Maternal Phenylketonuria. Status report 1993. *American Journal of Diseases of Children, 147,* 1224–1230.

Koch, R., Trefz, F., & Waisbren, S. (2010). Psychosocial issues and outcomes in maternal PKU. *Molecular Genetics and Metabolism, 99,* S68–S74.

Koff, E., Boyle, P., & Pueschel, S. M. (1977). Perceptual-motor functioning in children with phenylketonuria. *American Journal of Diseases of Children, 131,* 1084–1087.

Laclair, C. E., Ney, D. M., MacLeod, E. L., & Etzel, M. R. (2009). Purification and use of glycomacropeptide for nutritional management of phenylketonuria. *Journal of Food Science, 74,* E199–E206.

Lenke, R. R., & Levy, H. L. (1980). Maternal phenylketonuria and hyperphenylalaninemia. An international survey of the outcome of untreated and treated pregnancies. *New England Journal of Medicine, 303,* 1202–1208.

Levy, H. L., Milanowski, A., Chakrapani, A., Cleary, M., Lee, P., Trefz, F. K., & Dorenbaum, A. (2007). Efficacy of sapropterin dihydrochloride (tetrahydrobiopterin, 6R-BH4) for reduction of phenylalanine concentration in patients with phenylketonuria: A phase III randomised placebo-controlled study. *Lancet, 370,* 504–510.

Levy, H. L., & Waisbren, S. E. (1983). Effects of untreated maternal phenylketonuria and hyperphenylalaninemia on the fetus. *New England Journal of Medicine, 309,* 1269–1274.

Lichter-Konecki, U., Schlotter, M., Yaylak, C., Ozguc, M., Coskun, T., Ozalp, I., & Konecki, D. (1989). DNA haplotype analysis at the phenylalanine hydroxylase locus in the Turkish population. *Human Genetics, 81,* 373–376.

Lotstein, D. S., McPherson, M., Strickland, B., & Newacheck, P. W. (2005). Transition planning for youth with special health care needs: Results from the National Survey of Children with Special Health Care Needs. *Pediatrics, 115,* 1562–1568.

Lou, H. C. (1994). Dopamine precursors and brain function in phenylalanine hydroxylase deficiency. *Acta Paediatrica, 407*(Supplement), 86–88.

MacCready, R. A. (1963). Phenylketonuria screeing programs. *New England Journal of Medicine, 269,* 52.

Maillot, F., Lilburn, M., Baudin, J., Morley, D. W., & Lee, P. J. (2008). Factors influencing outcomes in the offspring of mothers with phenylketonuria during pregnancy: The importance of variation in maternal blood phenylalanine. *American Journal of Clinical Nutrition, 88,* 700–705.

Matalon, R., Michals-Matalon, K., Bhatia, G., Burlina, A. B., Burlina, A. P., Braga, C., & Guttler, F. (2007). Double blind placebo control trial of large neutral amino acids in treatment of PKU: Effect on blood phenylalanine. *Journal of Inherited Metabolic Disease, 30,* 153–158.

Matalon, R., Surendran, S., Matalon, K. M., Tyring, S., Quast, M., Jinga, W., & Szucs, S. (2003). Future role of large neutral amino acids in transport of phenylalanine into the brain. *Pediatrics, 112,* 1570–1574.

Miller, L. P., Pardridge, W. M., Braun, L. D., & Oldendorf, W. H. (1985). Kinetic constants for blood-brain barrier amino acid transport in conscious rats. *Journal of Neurochemistry, 45,* 1427–1432.

Moyle, J. J., Fox, A. M., Arthur, M., Bynevelt, M., & Burnett, J. R. (2007). Meta-analysis of neuropsychological symptoms of adolescents and adults with PKU. *Neuropsychology Review, 17,* 91–101.

Ney, D. M., Gleason, S. T., van Calcar, S. C., MacLeod, E. L., Nelson, K. L., Etzel, M. R., & Wolff, J. A. (2009). Nutritional management of PKU with glycomacropeptide from cheese whey. *Journal of Inherited Metabolic Disease, 32,* 32–39.

Ng, T. W., Rae, A., Wright, H., Gurry, D., & Wray, J. (2003). Maternal phenylketonuria in Western Australia: Pregnancy outcomes and developmental outcomes in offspring. *Journal of Paediatrics and Child Health, 39,* 358–363.

NIH. (2000). Phenylketonuria (PKU): Screening and management. *NIH Consensus Statement, 17,* 1–33.

Partington, M. W. (1978). Long term studies of untreated phenylketonuria II: The plasma phenylalanine level. *Neuropadiatrie, 9,* 255–267.

Partington, M. W., & Laverty, T. (1978). Long term studies of untreated phenylketonuria I: Intelligence or mental ability. *Neuropadiatrie, 9,* 245–254.

Paul, D. (1999). Contesting consent: The challenge to compulsory neonatal screening for PKU. *Perspectives in Biology and Medicine, 42,* 207–219.

Pennington, B. F., van Doorninck, W. J., McCabe, L. L., & McCabe, E. R. (1985). Neuropsychological deficits in early treated phenylketonuric children. *American Journal of Mental Deficiency, 89,* 467–474.

Pietz, J., Fatkenheuer, B., Burgard, P., Armbruster, M., Esser, G., & Schmidt, H. (1997). Psychiatric disorders in adult patients with early-treated phenylketonuria. *Pediatrics, 99,* 345–350.

Pietz, J., Landwehr, R., Kutscha, A., Schmidt, H., de Sonneville, L., & Trefz, F. K. (1995). Effect of high-dose tyrosine supplementation on brain function in adults with phenylketonuria. *J Pediatr, 127,* 936–943.

Pitt, D. (1971). The natural history of untreated phenylketonuria. *Medical Journal of Australia, 1,* 378–383.

Reiss, J. G., Gibson, R. W., & Walker, L. R. (2005). Health care transition: Youth, family, and provider perspectives. *Pediatrics, 115,* 112–120.

Ris, M. D., Williams, S. E., Hunt, M. M., Berry, H. K., & Leslie, N. (1994). Early-treated phenylketonuria: Adult neuropsychologic outcome. *Journal of Pediatrics, 124,* 388–392.

Rothenberg, M. B., & Sills, E. M. (1968). Iatrogenesis: The PKU anxiety syndrome. *Journal of the American Academy of Child and Adolescent Psychiatry, 7,* 689–692.

Rouse, B., Azen, C., Koch, R., Matalon, R., Hanley, W., de la Cruz, F., & Shifrin, H. (1997). Maternal Phenylketonuria Collaborative Study (MPKUCS) offspring: Facial anomalies, malformations, and early neurological sequelae. *American Journal of Medical Genetics, 69,* 89–95.

Sarkissian, C. N., Gamez, A., Wang, L., Charbonneau, M., Fitzpatrick, P., Lemontt, J. F., & Scriver, C. R. (2008). Preclinical evaluation of multiple species of PEGylated recombinant phenylalanine ammonia lyase for the treatment of phenylketonuria. *Proceedings of the National Academy of Sciences 105,* 20894–20899.

Scarabino, T., Popolizio, T., Tosetti, M., Montanaro, D., Giannatempo, G. M., Terlizzi, R., Salvolini, U. (2009). Phenylketonuria: White-matter changes assessed by 3.0-T magnetic resonance (MR) imaging, MR spectroscopy and MR diffusion. *Radiological Medicine, 114,* 461–474.

Schindeler, S., Ghosh-Jerath, S., Thompson, S., Rocca, A., Joy, P., Kemp, A., ... Christodoulou, J. (2007). The effects of large neutral amino acid supplements in PKU: An MRS and neuropsychological study. *Molecular Genetics and Metabolism, 91,* 48–54. doi: 10.1016/j.ymgme.2007.02.002

Schmidt, E., Rupp, A., Burgard, P., Pietz, J., Weglage, J., & de Sonneville, L. (1994). Sustained attention in adult phenylketonuria: The influence of the concurrent phenylalanine-blood-level. *Journal of Clinical and Experimental Neuropsyhology, 16,* 681–688.

Schor, D. P. (1983). PKU and temperament. Rating children three through seven years old in PKU families. *Clinical Pediatrics, 22,* 807–811.

Schuett, V. E. (1997). Off-diet young adults with PKU: Lives in danger. *National PKU News, 8,* 1–5.

Schuett, V. E., & Brown, E. S. (1984). Diet policies of PKU clinics in the United States. *American Journal of Public Health, 74,* 501–503.

Scriver, C. R., & Kaufman, S. (2001). Hyperphenylalaninemias: Phenylalanine hydroxylase deficiency. In C. R. Scriver, A. L. Baudet, W. S. Sly & D. Valle (Eds.), *The Metabolic and Molecular Bases of Inherited Disease* (8th ed., pp. 1667–1724). New York: McGraw-Hill.

Seashore, M. R., Friedman, E., Novelly, R. A., & Bapat, V. (1985). Loss of intellectual function in children with phenylketonuria after relaxation of dietary phenylalanine restriction. *Pediatrics, 75,* 226–232.

Sharman, R., Sullivan, K., Young, R., & McGill, J. (2009). Biochemical markers associated with executive function in adolescents with early and continuously treated phenylketonuria. *Clinical Genetics, 75,* 169–174.

Siegel, F. S., Balow, B., Fisch, R. O., & Anderson, V. E. (1968). School behavior profile ratings of phenylketonuric children. *American Journal of Mental Deficiency, 72,* 937–943.

Smith, I., Beasley, M. G., Wolff, O. H., & Ades, A. E. (1988). Behavior disturbance in 8-year-old children with early treated phenylketonuria. Report from the MRC/DHSS Phenylketonuria Register. *Journal of Pediatrics, 112,* 403–408.

Stemerdink, B. A., van der Meere, J. J., van der Molen, M. W., Kalverboer, A. F., Hendrikx, M. M., Huisman, J., & Verkerk, P. H. (1995). Information processing in patients with early and continuously-treated phenylketonuria. *European Journal of Pediatrics, 154,* 739–746.

Sullivan, J. E., & Chang, P. (1999). Review: Emotional and behavioral functioning in phenylketonuria. *Journal of Pediatric Psychology, 24,* 281–299.

Surtees, R., & Blau, N. (2000). The neurochemistry of phenylketonuria. *European Journal of Pediatrics, 159*, S109–S113.

Vajro, P., Strisciuglio, P., Houssin, D., Huault, G., Laurent, J., Alvarez, F., & Bernard, O. (1993). Correction of phenylketonuria after liver transplantation in a child with cirrhosis. *New England Journal of Medicine, 329*, 363.

van Calcar, S. C., MacLeod, E. L., Gleason, S. T., Etzel, M. R., Clayton, M. K., Wolff, J. A., & Ney, D. M. (2009). Improved nutritional management of phenylketonuria by using a diet containing glycomacropeptide compared with amino acids. *American Journal of Clinical Nutrition, 89*, 1068–1077.

Waisbren, S. E., Brown, M. J., de Sonneville, L. M., & Levy, H. L. (1994). Review of neuropsychological functioning in treated phenylketonuria: An information processing approach. *Acta Paediatrica, 407*, 98–103.

Waisbren, S. E., Chang, P., Levy, H. L., Shifrin, H., Allred, E., Azen, C., & Rouse, B. (1998). Neonatal neurological assessment of offspring in maternal phenylketonuria. *Journal of Inherited Metabolic Disease, 21*, 39–48.

Waisbren, S. E., Hamilton, B. D., St James, P. J., Shiloh, S., & Levy, H. L. (1995). Psychosocial factors in maternal phenylketonuria: Women's adherence to medical recommendations. *American Journal of Public Health, 85*, 1636–1641.

Waisbren, S. E., & Levy, H. L. (1991). Agoraphobia in phenylketonuria. *Journal of Inherited Metabolic Disease, 14*, 755–764.

Waisbren, S. E., Noel, K., Fahrbach, K., Cella, C., Frame, D., Dorenbaum, A., & Levy, H. (2007). Phenylalanine blood levels and clinical outcomes in phenylketonuria: A systematic literature review and meta-analysis. *Molecular Genetics and Metabolism, 92*, 63–70.

Waisbren, S. E., Schnell, R. R., & Levy, H. L. (1980). Diet termination in children with phenylketonuria: A review of psychological assessments used to determine outcome. *Journal of Inherited Metabolic Disease, 3*, 149–153.

Waisbren, S. E., Shiloh, S., St James, P., & Levy, H. L. (1991). Psychosocial factors in maternal phenylketonuria: Prevention of unplanned pregnancies. *American Journal of Public Health, 81*, 299–304.

Waisbren, S. E., & Zaff, J. (1994). Personality disorder in young women with treated phenylketonuria. *Journal of Inherited Metabolic Disease, 17*, 584–592.

Walter, J. H., White, F. J., Hall, S. K., MacDonald, A., Rylance, G., Boneh, A., & Vail, A. (2002). How practical are recommendations for dietary control in phenylketonuria? *Lancet, 360*, 55–57.

Weglage, J., Funders, B., Wilken, B., Schubert, D., Schmidt, E., Burgard, P., & Ullrich, K. (1992). Psychological and social findings in adolescents with phenylketonuria. *European Journal of Pediatrics, 151*, 522–525.

Weglage, J., Funders, B., Wilken, B., Schubert, D., & Ullrich, K. (1993). School performance and intellectual outcome in adolescents with phenylketonuria. *Acta Paediatrica, 82*, 582–586.

Weglage, J., Pietsch, M., Funders, B., Koch, H. G., & Ullrich, K. (1996). Deficits in selective and sustained attention processes in early treated children with phenylketonuria—result of impaired frontal lobe functions? *European Journal of Pediatrics, 155*, 200–204.

Welsh, M. C., Pennington, B. F., Ozonoff, S., Rouse, B., & McCabe, E. R. (1990). Neuropsychology of early-treated phenylketonuria: Specific executive function deficits. *Child Development, 61*, 1697–1713.

White, D. A., Connor, L. T., Nardos, B., Shimony, J. S., Archer, R., Snyder, A. Z., & McKinstry, S. C. (2010). Age-related decline in the microstructural integrity of white matter in children with early- and continuously-treated PKU: A DTI study of the corpus callosum. *Molecular Genetics and Metabolism, 99*, S41–S46.

Woo, S. L., Lidsky, A. S., Guttler, F., Chandra, T., & Robson, K. J. (1983). Cloned human phenylalanine hydroxylase gene allows prenatal diagnosis and carrier detection of classical phenylketonuria. *Nature, 306,* 151–155.

Wright, K. (1990). *Cradle of mutation. Discover,* 22–23.

Yannicelli, S., & Ryan, A. (1995). Improvements in behaviour and physical manifestations in previously untreated adults with phenylketonuria using a phenylalanine-restricted diet: A national survey. *Journal of Inherited Metabolic Disease, 18,* 131–134.

12 Preterm Birth Outcomes in Adolescence and Young Adulthood

Ida Sue Baron, Katherine Ann Leonberger, and Margot D. Ahronovich

Preterm birth interrupts the continuum of normal fetal development and results in the final stages of gestation occurring in an ex utero rather than in utero environment. Early birth is consequential for the individual and is a major public health concern worldwide. In the United States alone, more than a half-million infants are born preterm at a cost of more than $26 billion annually (March of Dimes, 2011), making preterm birth a high-priority condition. An infant born preterm today benefits from substantial advances in obstetric and neonatal care that have accrued over decades. Therefore, survival into adulthood is more assured for a larger number of early-birth survivors than ever before. However, despite considerable gains in neonatal intensive care, survival often is associated with a significant personal as well as societal cost.

A newborn is defined by gestational age or completed weeks of gestation at the time of delivery, based upon the onset of the mother's last menstrual period. Using gestational age, a baby delivered at 37–41 weeks has completed a full-term gestation, and birth at >41 weeks is referred to as "post-term." Delivery at <37 weeks meets criteria for preterm birth. Birth at 34–36 weeks is designated as "late preterm" (LPT), at 32–33 weeks birth as "moderate preterm," at <32 weeks as "very preterm," and at <28 weeks as "extremely preterm." Data showing differential outcome even within the term range has resulted in the use of the phrase "early term" for those born at 37–38 weeks.

Infant survival and outcome are affected by both gestational age and weight at birth. Thus, there is a stratification based upon birth weight as well. Birth weight of <2500 grams is considered low birth weight (LBW), <1500 grams as very low birth weight (VLBW), and <1000 grams as extremely low birth weight (ELBW). Additionally, the term "small for gestational age" is used if the newborn's birth weight falls below the 10th percentile for gestational age, and the term "intrauterine growth retardation" is used if there has been fetal growth restriction. Importantly, although both gestational age and birth weight are influential outcome factors, neither descriptor alone is sufficiently predictive of later neuropsychological functioning. Outcome varies in response to a wide and complex range of mediating and moderating medical, psychological, and socioenvironmental variables. Notably, the high incidence of neurodevelopmental impairment in preterm children is not fully explained by our current understanding of associated brain abnormalities (Counsell et al., 2008). In this chapter, the term "preterm" will be used generically to refer to either gestational age or birth weight descriptors.

This chapter summarizes current knowledge about the outcomes of individuals born at <37 weeks gestation, with particular focus on adolescents and young adults who were born ELBW or VLBW. A historical medical perspective is provided to assist the reader in appreciating the medical complications and treatment advances associated with premature birth over several decades. Second, psychological findings reported about those individuals who were born in the 1970s and 1980s are summarized. Discussion continues with a summary of psychological outcomes reported in adolescents and adults born post-1990. Finally, we summarize and conclude with proposed future directions.

HISTORICAL MEDICAL PERSPECTIVE

In 1990, the incidence of preterm birth in the United States was 10.6% of live births; this increased to a maximum of 12.8% by 2006 (Kirby & Wingate, 2010; Martin et al., 2008). Subsequently, there has been a decline over consecutive years, lowering the rate to 12.2% of live births in 2009 (Martin et al., 2011). Factors that contributed to the rate increase include more advanced interventions for maternal and fetal complications, higher rates of spontaneous delivery, medical complications associated with fertility assistance, and an increased incidence of elective delivery near term (Martin, Kirmeyer, Osterman, & Shepherd, 2009). The decrease in the preterm birth rate appears attributable to improved medical interventions as well as to educational outreach regarding elective early delivery and its potential adverse effects on the newborn. Although reduction in the preterm live birth rate is encouraging, preterm birth continues to be a significant public health issue and is associated with a considerable number of adverse early and late effects on the functioning of these individuals and their families well into adolescence and adulthood. It is difficult to identify the most critical etiological factors that affect long-term outcome and to accurately predict long-term consequences for an individual child.

Until recently, elective delivery at the late preterm stage was considered a safe option without short- or long-term risk to the newborn. However, the development of a fetus is incomplete at the moderately preterm (32–33 weeks) or even late preterm (34–36 weeks) stage. Interruption of the fetal maturational experience raises the risk of mortality and, for survivors, of immediate- or later-appearing medical complications that affect multiple body systems. These, in turn, may affect later neuropsychological functioning. The evidence is convincing that elective delivery prior to 39 weeks gestation in the absence of precipitating medical complications is an unnecessary risk (Ashton, 2010). In response to promulgated evidence-based education to this effect, fewer elective births are taking place in the absence of maternal or fetal complications, and the preterm birth rate has been reduced accordingly.

Many medical advances, which have been refined over several decades, are responsible for the improved preterm survival rate and decreased incidence of severe complications such as intraventricular hemorrhage, cerebral palsy (CP), neurosensory impairment, and mental retardation. The initiation of neonatal intensive care units in the 1970s, concerted societal efforts to expand access to prenatal maternal and fetal healthcare, and the introduction of specialized high-risk pregnancy units within medical centers have improved prenatal care and postnatal outcomes. These developments have also extended the lifespan and improved the quality of life for survivors. Ideally, neonatal care today includes systematic protocols in the critical first hours of life that are coordinated among multiple care providers committed to ensuring the neonate's optimal outcome. The introduction of antenatal corticosteroids, surfactant to improve lung function, improved modes of ventilator support, reduction and early treatment of infection, scheduling of at-risk infants for inborn delivery at a hospital with a neonatal intensive care unit, cesarean section for the smallest and highest-risk fetus, nutritional best practices that support neonatal growth and brain development, and overall rigorous evidence-based treatment protocols have all contributed to better outcomes for today's newborn. These have been important stimuli for the systematic study of early neurodevelopmental and long-term psychological effects.

Better medical management of early birth has lowered the limits of viability. Whereas 750 grams birth weight or birth at 28 weeks were the lower limits of viability in the 1980s, contemporary experience is that birth weight just over 400 grams or birth at 23–24 weeks are considered the cusp of viability. Rarely will the fragile neonate born at 22 weeks survive to hospital discharge, and profound medical complications are likely should such an infant survive. Not all physicians endorse aggressive resuscitation of these infants; some have reservations about whether survival will result in a sufficiently optimal quality of life to merit the extreme life-saving measures necessary at such an immature stage of development. Thus, aggressive life-support measures for those born at the lowest end of the preterm spectrum are not endorsed universally. However, some tertiary care centers find that a representative sample of their earliest-born neonates who might not have been resuscitated by others due to their extreme immaturity function within an average to above-average range in fundamental psychological domains (Baron, Erickson, Ahronovich, Baker, & Litman, 2011a).

In addition to gestational age and birth weight, knowledge of the individual's birth year is an additional essential reference characteristic. The outcomes of those born in earlier years of neonatal and obstetric intensive care continue to be reported contemporaneously, including as these individuals mature into adolescence and young adulthood. As noted above, individuals born in an era of nascent intensive medical care standards are at greater overall risk compared with those born preterm today. Thus, regardless of the year in which results are published, the data presented should be considered in context with what is known about neonatal medical procedures and treatments applicable during the birth era. For example, when surfactant therapy was introduced as a treatment for immature lung development in the mid-1980s, a dramatic reduction in the incidence and severity of lung disease resulted, and negative effects on general cognitive efficiency were reduced in survivors. In general, the outcomes of premature infants born prior to the 1980s are not comparable to outcomes of today's newborns who are cared for with current advanced treatment regimens. Until cohorts born after 2000 are studied into adolescence, some skepticism is warranted concerning expectations and generalizability of findings reported today about adolescents born preterm years ago.

Varied methodological choices further complicate cross-study comparisons. Highly variable sociodemographic characteristics across centers, inconsistent participant inclusion and exclusion characteristics, varied subgroup composition, disparate center treatment protocols, and a lack of systematic uniformity in their application both within and across centers are some of the inconsistencies across studies. In addition, because we are now seeing infants survive at earlier gestational ages than in prior decades, we now have an entirely new data set to analyze as these children reach adolescence.

Survival of extremely preterm infants has been a source of controversy related to the likelihood that these individuals will demonstrate later disability (Lorenz, Wooliever, Jetton, & Paneth, 1998). Reports of a worsened neurodevelopmental profile in recent birth cohorts that include a greater number of infants born prior to 26 weeks contribute to the opinion that there has been no substantial improvement in neurodevelopmental outcome in preterm children relative to those born in earlier years. Such data have been cited as evidence that decades of intensive preterm care have had only a minimal effect on the prevalence of disabilities. These reports have had the untoward effect of restricting some centers' endorsement of aggressive resuscitation efforts for those born at 23–25 weeks. However, others endorse aggressive life-saving efforts and find that a large percentage of these neonates do survive with average mean general intellectual level and less severe neuromotor compromise than did earlier cohorts. They have also found that intellectual, neuropsychological, and behavioral outcomes for those born at 23–25 weeks do not differ compared with those born at 26–28 weeks (Ahronovich, Baron, & Litman, 2007). Additionally, findings of group stability over birth epochs by several centers suggest that the many medical advances introduced have offset negative effects that might have been expected with inclusion of the earliest-born survivors. A consideration that adds to the controversy is that outcomes reported by large, multi-center national studies have inherent methodological variance related to the protocols of the individual care centers. Therefore, outcome may contrast greatly with that of a single center that provides more systematic and uniformly controlled neonatal services to newborns.

EARLY PSYCHOLOGICAL AND NEUROPSYCHOLOGICAL OUTCOMES

Preterm delivery's effect on psychological performance over the lifespan has been studied for decades. Before 1980, investigational emphases were justly placed on ways to extend the fetal period, increase neonatal survival, and decrease the debilitating medical complications associated with preterm birth, rather than on psychological outcome. Short- and long-term effects on general cognition became a more concerted focus of study in the 1980s, commensurate with improving preterm survival rates. In the earliest years of study, psychological data were principally obtained through qualitative impressions and nonstandardized observational methods. Additionally, standardized infant neurodevelopmental scales that provided summary mental and motor development scores were administered. Overall, longitudinal study was rare. Rather, data were principally obtained through cross-sectional study of new cohorts born in later birth years.

Beginning around the mid- to late-1980s, more rigorous retrospective cross-sectional studies were conducted, principally for those at school age and often employing broad measures of general intelligence. Those born in the presurfactant era, and thus at greater risk, were the source of most published data. Not surprisingly, the lowered infant development scale and IQ scores that were reported reflected the biological and physiological effects of preterm birth as well as the quality and impact of that era's medical care in the presurfactant era. For example, VLBW adolescents born between 1977 and 1979 (mean birth weight = 1179 grams; mean gestational age = 29.7 weeks) were studied at age 20 with regard to level of education, cognitive and academic achievement, and rates of chronic illness and risk-taking behavior. Compared with a normal birth weight group, VLBW adolescents were less likely to have graduated from high school, had a lower mean IQ (87 versus 92), and had higher rates of neurosensory impairment, additionally, males were less likely to be enrolled in postsecondary education. These individuals were at an educational disadvantage, had subnormal height, reported less substance abuse, and had lower rates of pregnancy than their peers born at normal birth weights (Hack et al., 2002). A large proportion of those born at this center between 1982 and 1986 (presurfactant) at a weight of <750 grams required physical and occupational therapy, special education services, and individualized educational plans as adolescents (Hack et al., 2000).

Studies of intelligence following preterm birth provide especially consistent findings. Intelligence level often is inversely related to birth weight or gestational age, and mean scores of preterm groups fall below those of term controls (for reviews see Baron & Rey-Casserly, 2010; Bhutta, Cleves, Casey, Cradock, & Anand, 2002). Thus, the mean IQ of children decreases as the gestational age at birth is lower compared with term populations (Moster, Lie, & Markestad, 2008).

Whereas IQ scores often fell below average limits in preterm cohorts born in the 1970s to early 1990s, cohorts born in the late 1990s to 2000s have more often demonstrated average IQ. The many studies of pre-1990 ELBW and VLBW cohorts have provided important insights into the diverse risk factors associated with preterm birth that influence cognitive functioning. However, these studies relied on single or general psychological instruments and often failed to explain these children's poor early academic performances and special educational needs. The introduction of comprehensive neuropsychological protocols has enabled a better appreciation of domain-specific influences and etiological factors. Notably, cognitive and neuropsychological development was rarely assessed during the critical preschool period (age 3–5 years), even in the most at-risk survivors. This gap has only recently begun to be bridged (Baron, Erickson, Ahronovich, Baker, & Litman, 2011a). Additionally, data regarding adolescent outcomes have been limited until individuals began to be studied retrospectively in the 1990s.

Neuropsychology was a rapidly growing area of specialty practice in the 1980s (Baron, Wills, Rey-Casserly, Armstrong, & Westerveld, 2011), providing both a theoretical and pragmatic basis for examining the effects of diverse neurological, systemic, and nonmedical insults in children, adolescents, and adults. Neuropsychological measures were introduced in preterm studies beginning around 1990 to better understand more discrete behavioral effects of disruption to the underlying brain substrate. Also, these measures aid in our ability to better address the substantial interaction of disorder, brain systems integrity, and consequent neuropsychological performance in this high-risk population. Overall, a lower incidence of mortality and of severely disabling complications began to be reported in this era. Reductions were seen in the rates of several conditions that severely impact neuropsychological functioning including sensorineural (hearing and vision) impairment, CP, mental retardation, hydrocephalus, intraventricular hemorrhage, and periventricular leukomalacia. Periventricular leukomalacia is the most common etiology of CP in premature infants (Kinney, 2006), and CP is a significant risk when there is hemorrhage of the medial portion of the cerebellum (Zayek, Benjamin, et al., 2011a).

In addition to low general intelligence and poor neuromotor function, the inclusion of neuropsychological measures in preterm studies showed that these survivors commonly experience diverse neuropsychological impairments including attentional, executive function, visuomotor, visuospatial, and processing speed deficits (Aarnoudse-Moens, Weisglas-Kuperus, van Goudoever, & Oosterlaan, 2009; Baron et al., 2009; Mulder, Pitchford, Hagger, & Marlow, 2009; Mulder, Pitchford, & Marlow, 2010). A review of attention development in preterm children concluded that attentional problems in infancy become more apparent by toddlerhood and that individual differences in early orienting and sustained attention are predictive of later attentional, cognitive, and behavioral functioning (van de Weijer-Bergsma, Wijnroks, & Jongmans, 2008). A particular vulnerability to experiencing nonverbal deficit has also been reported (Caldu et al., 2006; Lohaugen et al., 2010; Rickards, Kelly, Doyle, & Callanan, 2001), including in those born late preterm who were admitted to a neonatal intensive care unit (Baron, Erickson, et al., 2009). Nonverbal dysfunction has been found with some consistency in the preterm population. Also, the significant contribution of early white matter dysfunction to these persisting deficits, impairment of the cortical dorsal stream network, and its connections to parietal, frontal, and hippocampal regions may be explanatory (Atkinson & Braddick, 2007).

Language deficits were either not often examined or characterized as subtle and of less consequence in preterm children relative to their other areas of deficit. However, as shown in a meta-analysis review, preterm children often performed below term children on both simple (receptive vocabulary) and complex language tasks (van Noort-van der Spek, Franken, & Weisglas-Kuperus, 2012). The latter review found preterm and term group differences for complex, but not simple, language as the children's age increased from 3 years to 12 years. In individual studies, preterm adolescents who achieved average verbal IQ and verbal memory scores performed below term controls (Caldu et al., 2006). In a longitudinal study of children with birth weight of 1250 g or less tested at ages 8 years, 12 years, and 16 years, poorer general cognition and higher-order language skills (phonological awareness and phonemic decoding) were found in the teenagers compared with term controls. However the between-group difference in cognitive scores remained stable from age 8 years to 16 years, and catch-up gains in receptive vocabulary were found by age 16 years. These data suggest that this cohort's absence of neurosensory impairment and favorable socioeconomic variables (higher maternal education, ethnic nonminority) supported their more optimal developmental trajectories (Luu, Vohr, Allan, Schneider, & Ment, 2011).

Some negative effects attributed to preterm birth may have their etiology in socioenvironmental factors or genetic predisposition. These effects, which have been understudied in many early preterm studies, are more of a focus in recent investigations. Their influence may become especially apparent in case studies or in reports of outcomes of a single care center, especially when there is application of systematic treatment protocols for the newborn endorsed by all treating physicians. For example, a remarkable divergence in neuropsychological outcome characterized the early school age outcomes of triplets, including one born weighing 780 grams (1.7 pounds) (Baron, Litman, Ahronovich, & Gidley Larson, 2007). Comprehensive neuropsychological data obtained from each triplet when considered in context with their medical and family histories highlighted that individual outcome was not reliably predicted solely by birth weight. Rather, family factors and genetic predisposition were strong explanatory influences for the resultant neuropsychological profiles . Further, a review of studies that examined cognitive functioning in children born at term indicated that parental social class accounted for a larger proportion of the variance in intelligence than birth weight and that these two variables were largely independent (Shenkin, Starr, & Deary, 2004), findings that are relevant for the preterm population as well.

RECENT PSYCHOLOGICAL AND NEUROPSYCHOLOGICAL OUTCOMES

Differences of opinion exist regarding the course and functional outcomes of recent preterm newborns relative to those born in past years. As noted previously, some maintain that recent births at <29 gestational weeks have not shown gains, although they have been advantaged by contemporary medical care and despite reductions in the severity of illness and mortality. Yet, other reports provide a more optimistic outlook regarding a medical course that has been enhanced by improved screening, diagnosis, and treatment in those born since the early 1990s (Bode et al., 2009; Donohue, Boss, Shepard, Graham, & Allen, 2009; Wilson-Costello, Friedman, Minich, Fanaroff, & Hack, 2005; Zayek, Trimm, et al., 2011b), including for those born at <26 gestational weeks (Ahronovich et al., 2007).

Within-Center Comparisons

To address contradictory opinions, preterm cohorts born in different care eras at a single center should provide important indices of meaningful change over the decades of improving neonatal care. Several centers have reported such data. A comparison of children born at 22–24 weeks in 1993–1995 with those born in 2000–2003 found the latter to be advantaged by advanced care, sonographic surveillance, greater use of antenatal steroids, and more frequent life-sustaining interventions in the neonatal intensive care unit, without a change in the mortality rate (Donohue et al., 2009). At another center, live births at ≤30 weeks increased 35% from 1985–1986 to 2005–2006 and were accompanied by an 11% increase in survival, 25% greater survival of those born at <27 weeks, 10% decline in significant ultrasound abnormalities, and 19% increase in survival without severe neurodevelopmental impairment at age 24 months (Bode et al., 2009). At 18–24 months' corrected age, ELBW infants born at 22–26 weeks between January 1998 and June 2003 and compared with those born between July 2003 and December 2008 showed that survival rate increased from 20% to 40% in those born at 22 weeks, a neurodevelopmental impairment reduction from 54% to 28%, and severe neurodevelopmental impairment reduction from 35% to 8% in infants born at 23–24 weeks (Zayek et al., 2011b).

In another single-center comparison, the ELBW survival rate increased from 49% in a 1980s cohort to 68% in a 1990s cohort. In addition, there was a larger absolute number of developmentally normal children and fewer medical complications including sepsis, periventricular leukomalacia, and chronic lung disease. The higher rates of neurologic abnormality found in the 1990s cohort, including CP (16%–25%), deafness (3%–7%), and neurodevelopmental impairment (26%–36%), were attributed to greater survival of infants born at earlier gestational ages (Wilson-Costello et al., 2005). Their follow-up study of a cohort born since 2000 documented increased antenatal steroid use and cesarean section and decreased postnatal steroid treatment, resulting in lowered rates of sepsis, severe intraventricular hemorrhage, CP, and neurodevelopmental impairment (Wilson-Costello et al., 2007). Additional evidence that the incidence of childhood disabilities in ELBW children remains stable despite an increase in survival rate., and that the severity of neurodevelopmental disabilities has decreased was reported in a comparison of two cohorts of ELBW children born 10 years apart (1991–1995, 2001–2005). At age 5 years, 52% of 67 children born in 1991–1995 had survived compared with 63% of 49 children born in 2001–2005. Six children in the 1991–1995 cohort (17%) had disabilities, three with major neurodevelopmental disabilities compared with 19% born in 2001–2005, and one with severe disabilities (Jonsdottir et al., 2012). Such large changes across single centers emphasize that beneficial effects have indeed occurred over time.

Insights from Neuroimaging

Infants born more recently also benefit from advances in neuroimaging techniques that have improved surveillance at very young ages. These have also clarified the types of structural brain abnormalities commonly associated with preterm birth that are prominent etiologies of persistent long-term neuropsychological compromise. Such abnormalities are especially prevalent in VLBW and ELBW adolescents and generally absent in those born late preterm. Preterm birth has a negative effect on the development of cortical thickness (Nagy, Lagercrantz, & Hutton, 2011) and has been associated with decreased volumes of total brain, cortical gray matter, and right and left hippocampus in very preterm adolescents born in 1979–1980, as well as an association of increase in lateral ventricle size (Nosarti et al., 2002). A reduction in cerebellar volume was found in adolescence and young adulthood in a 1982–1984 cohort whose participants self-reported poor well-being (Parker et al., 2008).

Regional cerebral growth impairment following preterm birth may result from interruption of cerebellocerebral connectivity and loss of necessary neuronal activation (Limperopoulos, Chilingaryan, Guizard, Robertson, & Du Plessis, 2010). Cerebellar growth was found to be normal in the absence of supratentorial injury (Jaeger, Silveira, & Procianoy, 2011) (commonly found in infants born at early gestational ages). Cerebral white matter damage sustained by the immature preterm brain is a significant neuropathology that underlies the poor neuromotor outcomes associated with preterm birth (Volpe, 2003) as well as impairment of vulnerable major motor pathways, such as the corticospinal tract, which may occur prenatally (Deng, 2010). White matter microstructure appears to be compromised in a regionally specific pattern, and these abnormalities persist into childhood and adolescence, potentially affecting a wide range of neuropsychological functions. For example, in a VLBW cohort, attentional deficits observed in the presence of white matter disturbances in the posterior corpus callosum and internal capsules were not compensated for or improved by age 11 years (Nagy et al., 2003). Corpus callosum thinning was associated with abnormal language lateralization in preterm adolescents (Rushe et al., 2001), as were deficits in verbal fluency, executive function, everyday memory, and vocabulary (Narberhaus et al., 2008). Associations between anterior corpus callosum (genu) and prefrontal functioning and between posterior corpus callosum (splenium) and vocabulary in the latter study were related to respective connections to prefrontal and posterior parietal cortex. In a study of adolescents born very preterm between 1983 and 1994, reduced corpus callosum size was positively correlated with gestational age as well as Wechsler Performance IQ and the Working Memory Index, suggesting that corpus callosum thinning is a permanent consequence of premature birth and that myelinated fiber damage contributes significantly to these poor performances (Caldu et al., 2006).

Several studies utilizing advanced imaging techniques found evidence that supported hypotheses of neural compensation by preterm children and adolescents following perinatal brain injury. On a visual-association task that requires encoding, recognition, and same/different discrimination, functional magnetic resonance imaging (fMRI) showed that the preterm group relied on neural networks to process visual–perceptual material that were different from those used by control participants. Increased activity was found in the left caudate nucleus, right cuneus, and left superior parietal lobule during encoding, and decreased activity was found in the right inferior frontal gyrus during encoding. In addition, there was increased activity in the right cerebellum and anterior cingulate gyrus bilaterally during recognition, as well as smaller absolute gray matter (Narberhaus et al., 2009). Evidence of neuronal reorganization after early brain injury was also found in a study of verbal paired-associate learning in which young adults born very preterm had increased left parahippocampal and precentral gyri activity during encoding. These young adults also had increased precentral gyrus activity during recall, a pattern that differed from controls. Activity in the left parahippocampal gyrus during encoding was positively correlated with increased gray matter volume in this region, and those born at <28 weeks had the most activity and gray matter in this region (Lawrence et al., 2010).

Memory tasks have been administered to further address the issue of neural compensation. An fMRI study of explicit memory, spatial memory, and perceptuomotor function in preterm and term adolescents found no between-group differences in hippocampal activation. However, greater activation change was found on a perceptuomotor task in both the left and right caudate nucleus for the preterm participants, with significant activation change in the right caudate. The preterm group had greater activation change in the right caudate nucleus during spatial task encoding and less activation in both the right and left caudate during the test phase, whereas the term group's greater activation change occurred during the test phase. Although no observable performance differences were found and accuracy and reaction time were comparable between the groups, these results suggest that the observed activation of different brain regions on the memory task indicate compensation for earlier insult (Curtis, 2006). In another study, increased right hippocampal activation in preterm adolescents during an encoding memory task suggested contralateral reorganization to compensate for an impaired left hippocampus (Gimenez et al., 2005).

Adolescent Outcomes of Preterm Birth in the 1970s and 1980s

Adolescence is a time of continuing neurological, psychological, and social maturation. Longitudinal neuroimaging studies confirm that the adolescent brain continues to mature beyond the teen years (S. B. Johnson, Blum, & Giedd, 2009). Gender differences in the timing of adolescent brain development and resultant brain volume have been reported. These include the findings that females reach peak values of brain volumes earlier than males, males have a 9%–12% larger brain size than females, and male–female regional developmental differences occur in such regions as the basal ganglia, hippocampus, amygdala, and white matter (Lenroot & Giedd, 2010). Developmental delay or deficit associated with preterm delivery is likely to persist across the lifespan. As preterm individuals mature into adolescence and an extended range of outcomes is studied more rigorously, the extent and duration of functional impairment are increasingly understood.

.Yet, caution is advised when interpreting much of the published data about adolescent outcomes. Most contemporary reports are about individuals born in the 1970s and 1980s, an era of high mortality rates and viability boundaries that were of later gestational ages and heavier birth weights than for today's newborn. For example, 27% of those born at <37 weeks in 1977–1978 and hospitalized in a neonatal unit in the Netherlands did not survive (Schothorst, Swaab-Barneveld, & van Engeland, 2007). As noted above, individuals born in earlier eras of less advanced medical care carry a high risk of severe medical and intracerebral complications, sensorineural impairment, mental retardation, CP, and less adaptive functional outcomes. Moreover, those born at <26 weeks, who have survived in greater numbers since the 1990s, are only just beginning to enter adolescence and thus have not yet been thoroughly studied.

Intelligence and academic proficiency have been primary outcome measures in many preterm adolescent studies. In one early-born cohort, 53% of VLBW participants had an IQ >1 standard deviation below the comparison mean, none obtained an IQ >1 standard deviation above the mean, and specific problems were reported in arithmetic and visual perception (Lohaugen et al., 2010). Birth between 1979 and 1983 was associated with worse IQ and poorer phonological verbal fluency than in a control group at ages 15 years and 19 years. Interestingly, the term group showed improved semantic verbal fluency over time, but the preterm adolescents failed to show similar gain by age 19 years (Allin et al., 2006).

Psychological, psychiatric, and economic implications of preterm birth have been studied in early adolescent cohorts. Eight percent of those in a 1977–1978 cohort were physically or mentally disabled as adolescents, and 70% had persistent mild neurological abnormalities (gross and fine motor deficits) that, together with reduced verbal abilities and family adversity, likely mediated the development of psychopathology and internalizing disorder. Of the 8%, 16.3% had depressive disorder, 23.3% had anxiety disorder, and parental report indicated social problems (Schothorst et al., 2007). In another study of adolesents at age 19 years, more than 12% of those born in 1983 showed moderate to severe problems in cognitive or neurosensory functioning; 31.7% had ≥1 or more moderate or severe cognitive, neuromotor, academic, occupational, or neuroscensory problems; 24% required special education or a lesser level of academic services; and 7.6% had no paid employment nor had they continued their education. Compared with the general population on health status, perceived health, education, and occupation, twice as many preterm participants were poorly educated, three times as many were neither employed nor in school, and nearly one-third had moderate to severe limitations in their activities and participation in society (Hille et al., 2007). Twenty-one percent of a 1979–1980 ELBW cohort had neurosensory impairments, 46% had below-average IQ scores, 14% were severely disabled, 15% were moderately disabled, and 25% were mildly disabled at age 14 years (Doyle & Casalaz, in 1980–1982 who had no CP showed reduced IQ, visual processing, visual memory, problem-solving, and arithmetic achievement. Parental and teacher ratings indicated a higher likelihood of peer rejection and more learning problems requiring remedial education or special school services, and adolescent self-report indicated lower self-esteem (Rickards et al., 2001). An adolescent ELBW cohort born weighing equal to or less than 800 grams and at 23–29 weeks between 1981 and 1986 who had no physical handicaps and an IQ of at least 70 had poorer vocabulary, block design, digit span, reading, and arithmetic performances compared with controls. However, there was no difference in sustained attention. Self-reports indicated poor academic achievement and job competence, athletic inadequacy, and low confidence in establishing romantic relationships. Their parents reported clinically significant internalizing and externalizing behavioral problems, especially in males (Grunau, Whitfield, & Fay, 2004).

A series of Canadian studies of adolescents born preterm in 1977–1982 found that 28% had neurosensory impairment compared with only 1% of controls. Comparing ELBW, VLBW, and term groups, reading scores >2 standard deviations below the mean were found in 38%, 18%, and 2.5%, respectively. IQ scores <70 were found in 48% of ELBW and 24% of VLBW participants. Of those born ELBW, 25% repeated a grade and 50% required special education. Only 43% of ELBW and VLBW were mainstreamed into general education classrooms, and 72% of ELBW and 53% of VLBW reported academic difficulty in their mainstream setting (Saigal, Hoult, Streiner, Stoskopf, & Rosenbaum, 2000; Saigal et al., 2007). Additionally, those born ELBW also had more emotional problems, developmental delays, learning disorders, and hyperactivity compared with controls, and they required more healthcare services (Saigal, Stoskopf, Streiner, & Burrows, 2001). ELBW survivors were found to be less productive as adults compared with controls. In accordance with other studies, however, the productivity and adaptability of these ELBW subjects was evident (Goddeeris et al., 2010; Saigal et al., 2007; Saigal et al., 2006). Although these data are encouraging regarding functional adequacy in adolescence, the neurocognitive tasks administered to these participants at younger ages were often not readministered, leaving the extent and duration of cognitive weaknesses that had been documented in their childhood unresolved.

National registry records in Norway of those born at 23–36 weeks between 1967 and 1983 were reviewed in order to determine the incidence of medical and social disabilities in those aged 19–35 years. It was found that those born at 23–27 weeks were most disadvantaged; their survival rate of 17.8% contrasted with a term rate of 96.5%. In addition, they were at a greater risk of CP, mental retardation, blindness, hearing loss, sensorineural impairment, epilepsy, and behavioral and socioemotional disorders. Approximately one in nine in this group received a disability pension. For the entire sample, the percentage receiving disability support was inversely related to gestational age: 1 of 12 at 28–30 weeks, 1 of 24 at 31–33 weeks, 1 of 42 at 34–36 weeks, and 1 of 59 for term controls. Their preterm birth was also associated with lower levels of high school, college, and postgraduate education; lower income; and lower incidence of marrying and having a family, even in the absence of medical disability (Moster et al., 2008).

Perinatal brain damage and white matter abnormalities appear to be mediating factors of long-term psychiatric health and cognitive difficulties in preterm adolescents. A diffusion tensor imaging study found VLBW adolescents had poorer visual–motor skill, manual dexterity, visual perception, IQ, and attention compared with controls.

Greater white matter disruption in the internal and external capsule and in the inferior and middle superior fasciculus was associated with lower IQ and worse fine-motor, attentional, and social functioning (Skranes et al., 2007). Ventricular dilation, white matter reduction, and corpus callosum thinning were associated with symptoms of attention-deficit/hyperactivity disorder (ADHD), anxiety disorder, and Asperger syndrome in VLBW adolescents (Indredavik et al., 2005). In a 1986–1988 cohort, lower birth weight was associated with inattention, psychiatric diagnosis, and reduced psychosocial function, with the presence of intraventricular hemorrhage increasing the risk of inattention and a lower Apgar score increasing the risk of autism spectrum disorder symptoms and internalizing symptoms (Indredavik et al., 2010).

Behavioral outcomes of VLBW young adults born in 1977–1979 were assessed using parental- and self-report questionnaires. Males were less likely to engage in delinquent behavior and alcohol use but more likely to exhibit withdrawal and thought-disordered behaviors than controls, with no differences related to the quality of their interpersonal relationships. Females reported more withdrawal and internalizing behaviors, poorer interpersonal relationships, and less excessive alcohol use or delinquent behavior; their parents reported more anxious, depressed, and withdrawn symptoms; attentional problems; and internalizing behaviors. Singletons exhibited more anxious and depressed symptoms and fewer overall behavioral problems than did twins (Hack et al., 2004).

Adolescents and their parents, general practitioners, and teachers completed health and school performance questionnaires for an extremely preterm cohort born in 1983–1984. Twenty-eight percent of the preterm group reported no health problems compared with 49% of controls. In the preterm group, 16% were in special schools, 1% had severe learning difficulties, 6% had CP, and 2% were blind. Of those mainstreamed into general education classrooms, 7% had severe motor or neurosensory impairment (CP, physical disability, and/or visual impairment). Those in mainstreamed classrooms required academic support in all areas of learning, in cooperativeness, and in team sports. However, they were as likely as controls to report enjoying school, although less likely to plan for college or higher education. Their parents were more likely to report that their child's behavior or health had a serious, negative impact on family functioning, difficulties with emotional well-being, and attention and learning problems (A. Johnson et al., 2003). Others have reported lower school performance, more educational support, and less confidence in their overall abilities and future goals (Hack, Taylor, Klein, & Minich, 2000; Hallin, Hellstrom-Westas, & Stjernqvist, 2010). Adolescents born in 1985–1986 who had no preexisting serious cognitive disability demonstrated poorer full-scale IQ, verbal comprehension, perceptual organization, working memory, processing speed, visual–motor speed, attention, and academic achievement compared with controls. Also, they reported more hearing problems, less athletic participation, and having fewer parents with a university education (Hallin et al., 2010). Minimal neuropsychological dysfunction was reported in a 1984–1986 very preterm cohort without major physical, cognitive, or congenital disabilities. These adolescents performed poorly on backward block tapping. Additionally, shorter digit-span–backward performance was found in those who had intrauterine growth retardation or received neonatal ventilatory assistance. Those who had abnormal neonatal electroencephalograms performed poorly on coding, mental control, and arithmetic tasks; those who had neonatal seizures had poorer verbal IQ, spatial-span–forward abilities, arithmetic skills, coding abilities, and mental control. No differences in working memory or processing speed were reported (Saavalainen et al., 2007).

Several additional reports of survivors from the early era of neonatal care found adaptive functioning in adolescents following preterm-related medical complications and cognitive impairments. Young adults born VLBW in 1971–1974 and 1980–1982, with respective survival rates of 48% and 81%, were compared on perceived quality of life through telephone self-report. It was found that objective quality of life regarding occupational success and social interaction had increased (Dinesen & Greisen, 2001). A prospective questionnaire study of a 1987–1988 preterm cohort and controls at age 20 years found these individuals to have similar perceptions regarding their health, use of tobacco, education, occupation, and lifestyle. However, those with CP, ADHD, or mental retardation had a poorer perception of their physical functioning and health, and those born ELBW or who had bronchopulmonary dysplasia or intraventricular hemorrhage had poorer perceptions about their physical health (Gaddlin, Finnstrom, Sydsjo, & Leijon, 2009).

Thus, earlier birth cohorts consistently show less favorable neuropsychological, behavioral, and adaptive outcomes in adolescence compared with term comparison groups. It remains to be seen how today's newborns will mature into adolescence in the next decade. Newborns today benefit from standards of medical care that lessen the likelihood of severe lifelong disability and, thus, are likely to have an overall lower incidence of severe neurological complications. The reduction in the incidence of visual impairment, blindness, deafness, and CP should provide a basis for a healthier foundation and improved psychological outcome. Additionally, metabolic and nutritional requirements are better integrated into current care protocols, and the strong influences of socioemotional, environmental, and biopsychobehavioral factors on neonatal development are increasingly recognized as influential (Luu, Vohr, et al., 2011).

Adolescent Outcomes of Cohorts Born in the 1990s and 2000s

There are relatively few neuropsychological studies of preterm adolescents born since 1990. However, the studies that do exist are of particular interest because these individuals presumably benefitted from cumulative fetal and neonatal care advances that improved the quality of their care. Neonatal medical complications, brain injury, lower maternal education, and minority status have been strongly associated with lowered intelligence, neuropsychological impairment, and poor behavioral outcomes in adolescence (Luu, Ment, Allan, Schneider, & Vohr, 2011; Luu et al., 2009). Antenatal steroids, higher maternal education, and a two-parent family have been associated with better outcomes (Luu et al., 2009). Additionally, contemporary studies are more likely to include structural or functional imaging, at birth and/or at time of study, that may inform about how brain development proceeds in this at-risk population, as well as brain region-functional outcome relationships. Thus, data obtained from adolescents born in the 1990s and 2000s may ideally elucidate effects of the many advances in care and treatment and provide a more refined appreciation of conditions that either facilitate or impede the development of preterm individuals. Moreover, a different profile of functioning than typified in preterm adolescents born before 1990 is a reasonable expectation.

Longer survival and better outcomes in adolescence and adulthood have already begun to be reported relative to earlier born cohorts (Doyle & Anderson, 2010). A profile of reduced structural abnormalities and less extreme long-term neuropsychological deficit has been predicted. For example, fewer structural abnormalities were found in a cohort of very preterm infants from Sweden followed into adolescence, perhaps attributable to differences in social structure and neonatal care practices, minimally invasive neonatal care, and different social structures in Sweden (Nagy et al., 2009; Nagy & Jonsson, 2009). Severe neurological complications were less prevalent at age 5 years in a 1999–2000 ELBW cohort, and gestational age had a limited association with cognitive and motor function if there was no CP or preterm-associated neurosensory impairment (blindness, deafness) (Leversen et al., 2011).

Higher mean IQ scores are reported with greater frequency in those born since 1990, reaching low-average or average limits across international cohorts. However, even preterm adolescents born in the 1990s had IQ scores below those of controls, and 22%–24% had abnormal basic language skills compared with 2%–4% of controls (Luu et al., 2009). Yet, because IQ measures may not be sufficiently sensitive to the cognitive difficulties of preterm adolescents, academic intervention may be warranted even when IQ is average or better (Narberhaus et al., 2007).

Preterm birth in the 1990s remains an important risk factor of neuropsychological impairment in adolescence, although more recent cohorts often show less severe outcomes than have been reported for those born before 1990. Although all domains may be affected, some are more vulnerable than others. Even without obvious disabilities, greater deficits in verbal fluency, inhibition, cognitive flexibility, planning/organization, working memory, and verbal and visual–spatial memory have been found (Frye, Landry, Swank, & Smith, 2009; Luu, Ment, et al., 2011). However, these functions were mostly unexamined in earlier decades. Moreover, preterm adolescents required more school services in reading, writing, and arithmetic than controls, especially if there was a history of neonatal brain hemorrhage or other neurological complications (Luu et al., 2009). As noted above, Luu and colleagues (2011) examined children born very preterm in 1995, finding that by age 16 years, very preterm adolescents demonstrated a number of cognitive deficits compared with peers, including in overall intelligence and higher-order language skills. However, the adolescents also demonstrated significant catch-up in receptive vocabulary between the ages of 8 years and 16 years compared with term peers. Although this did not result in similar performance between the groups at age 16 years, the importance of interventions to foster preterm individuals' natural ability to "catch up" cognitively during these crucial years was suggested. More optimal outcomes were found in those who had no neurosensory impairment, were from families with higher maternal education level, and who were not an ethnic minority.

An fMRI study of a cohort born between 28 and 35 weeks in 1990–1991 found that adolescents without a history of intraventricular hemorrhage performed well on an experimental test of attention requiring a motor response. However, neonatal complications and pre- and postnatal environmental risk factors were associated with a greater number of errors and slower response times. Those who had fewer birth complications and risk factors had more parietal and temporal lobe activation and better scores. On the attention task, greater activation of the left superior-temporal and left supramarginal gyri was associated with better performance. Medical risk was related to left parietal cortex activation, and environmental risk was related to temporal lobe activation. Early risk appeared to be related to less mature patterns of brain activation including reduced efficiency of processing and responding to stimuli (Carmody et al., 2006).

Thus, although psychological gains have accompanied medical gains, it is increasingly apparent that medical status, birth weight, and gestational age at birth are influential yet insufficient predictors of long-term outcome. Evidence is clear that neonatal intracerebral neurological complications worsen long-term intellectual and neuropsychological outcomes and that more optimal intellectual and neuropsychological functioning results across childhood and adolescent ages in the absence of these adverse events (Baron, Ahronovich, Erickson, Gidley Larson, & Litman, 2009; Luu, Ment, Allan et al., 2011). The significant contributions of environmental, familial, biological, and genetic factors are increasingly being addressed (Luu, Vohr et al., 2011). Recent data showing a slightly improving preterm profile will ideally enable educators to design interventions that better target academic weaknesses more effectively and earlier in their elementary school years. Identification and referral for intervention have resulted in favorable outcomes in preterm adolescents (Luu et al., 2009). Nonetheless, despite seemingly improving outcomes in those born since 1900 due to advantageous effects of current medical protocols, the influence of medical complications remains a concern. However, impairments continue to be documented at adolescence especially now that neuropsychological functioning is being examined more routinely and in finer detail. Overall, it appears appropriate to have an optimistic outlook for today's newborns and tomorrow's adolescents.

FUTURE AIMS AND RESEARCH OPPORTUNITIES

Mixed results about the neuropsychological outcomes of preterm birth have been reported in adolescents and young adults. How well a child born preterm today may be expected to mature into adulthood, and with what profile or extent of neuropsychological dysfunction, continues to be a vibrant area of research. It is crucial to consider that preterm birth is a continuous dynamic process in which each additional gestational week will benefit the immature fetus, although maternal or fetal distress may necessitate early delivery and interrupt the normal in utero gestational course. Of the preterm research conducted to date, the general conclusion is that the results of medical advances are becoming evident in lower rates of severe medical complications, neuromotor compromise, neurodevelopmental delay, higher intelligence scores, and more intact neuropsychological performances. Thus, the most recent birth cohorts are more likely to have mean IQ scores in a low-average to average range, rather than below-average or lower scores, as well as greater overall neuropsychological competence.

Although cohort studies provide indices to set expectations, individual case study remains a valuable means to better understand how a multiplicity of contributing variables may interact to either improve or worsen outcomes as a neonate matures through the preschool and childhood years into adulthood. Instances in which the most at-risk neonate achieves intellectual and neuropsychological competence occur, just as there may be fewer medically at-risk infants who develop unexpectedly profound neuropsychological impairments. A clear evidence-based rationale for understanding which of these preterm infants is most at risk is currently lacking. Although certain medical complications are acknowledged to present greater risk to the preterm neonate, a good outcome may be achieved in the presence of these complications, adding to the controversy about which variables are most meaningful. It is a conundrum that must be solved. Yet, few definitive answers have been found despite many years of preterm studies. The identification of subpopulations that highlight key factors to predict an optimal course and result in minimal deficit is one area of continuing study. For example, the identification of differential outcome between late preterm (34–36 weeks) preschoolers admitted to a neonatal intensive care unit and those not admitted was suggestive that within this particular low-risk preterm group, some forms of medical instability or other related factors may be more relevant regarding prospective neuropsychological outcome (Baron, Erickson, Ahronovich, Baker, & Litman, 2011b). Preterm birth has been a rich source of data with heuristic significance that extends throughout the lifespan. Future studies can be expected to elaborate on the tangible effects of the most recent advances in care and treatment.

REFERENCES

Aarnoudse-Moens, C. S., Weisglas-Kuperus, N., van Goudoever, J. B., & Oosterlaan, J. (2009). Meta-analysis of neurobehavioral outcomes in very preterm and/or very low birth weight children. *Pediatrics, 124,* 717–728.

Ahronovich, M., Baron, I. S., & Litman, F. (2007). Improved outcomes of extremely low birth weight infants. *Pediatrics, 119,* 1044.

Allin, M., Rooney, M., Griffiths, T., Cuddy, M., Wyatt, J., Rifkin, L., & Murray, R. (2006). Neurological abnormalities in young adults born preterm. *Journal of Neurology, Neurosurgery, and Psychiatry, 77,* 495–499. doi: 10.1136/jnnp.2005.075465

Ashton, D. M. (2010). Elective delivery at less than 39 weeks. *Current Opinion in Obstetrics and Gynecology, 22,* 506–510.

Atkinson, J., & Braddick, O. (2007). Visual and visuocognitive development in children born very prematurely. *Progress in Brain Research, 164,* 123–149.

Baron, I. S., Ahronovich, M. D., Erickson, K., Gidley Larson, J. C., & Litman, F. R. (2009). Age-appropriate early school age neurobehavioral outcomes of extremely preterm birth without severe intraventricular hemorrhage: A single center experience. *Early Human Development, 85,* 191–196.

Baron, I. S., Erickson, K., Ahronovich, M., Baker, R., & Litman, F. (2011a). Neuropsychological and behavioral effects of extremely low birth weight at age three. *Developmental Neuropsychology, 36,* 5–21.

Baron, I. S., Erickson, K., Ahronovich, M., Coulehan, K., Baker, R., & Litman, F. (2009). Visuospatial and verbal fluency relative deficits in "complicated" late-preterm preschool children. *Early Human Development, 85,* 751–754.

Baron, I. S., Erickson, K., Ahronovich, M. D., Baker, R., & Litman, F. R. (2011b). Cognitive deficit in preschoolers born late-preterm. *Early Human Development, 87,* 115–119.

Baron, I. S., Litman, F., Ahronovich, M., & Gidley Larson, J. C. (2007). Neuropsychological outcomes of preterm triplets discordant for birthweight: A case report. *The Clinical Neuropsychologist, 21,* 338–362.

Baron, I. S., & Rey-Casserly, C. (2010). Extremely preterm birth outcome: A review of four decades of cognitive research. *Neuropsychology Review, 20,* 430–452.

Baron, I. S., Wills, K., Rey-Casserly, C., Armstrong, K., & Westerveld, M. (2011). Pediatric neuropsychology: Toward subspecialty designation. *The Clinical Neuropsychologist, 25,* 1075–1086.

Bhutta, A. T., Cleves, M. A., Casey, P. H., Cradock, M. M., & Anand, K. J. (2002). Cognitive and behavioral outcomes of school-aged children who were born preterm: A meta-analysis. *Journal of the American Medical Association, 288,* 728–737.

Bode, M. M., D'Eugenio, D. B., Forsyth, N., Coleman, J., Gross, C. R., & Gross, S. J. (2009). Outcome of extreme prematurity: A prospective comparison of 2 regional cohorts born 20 years apart. *Pediatrics, 124*, 866–874.

Caldu, X., Narberhaus, A., Junque, C., Gimenez, M., Vendrell, P., Bargallo, N.,...Botet, F. (2006). Corpus callosum size and neuropsychologic impairment in adolescents who were born preterm. *Journal of Child Neurology, 21*, 406–410.

Carmody, D. P., Bendersky, M., Dunn, S. M., DeMarco, J. K., Hegyi, T., Hiatt, M., & Lewis, M. (2006). Early risk, attention, and brain activation in adolescents born preterm. *Child Development, 77*, 384–394.

Counsell, S. J., Edwards, A. D., Chew, A. T., Anjari, M., Dyet, L. E., Srinivasan, L.,...Cowan, F. M. (2008). Specific relations between neurodevelopmental abilities and white matter microstructure in children born preterm. *Brain, 131*, 3201–3208.

Curtis, C. E. (2006). Prefrontal and parietal contributions to spatial working memory. *Neuroscience, 139*, 173–180.

Deng, W. (2010). Neurobiology of injury to the developing brain. *Nature Reviews Neurology, 6*, 328–336.

Dinesen, S. J., & Greisen, G. (2001). Quality of life in young adults with very low birth weight. *Archives of Disease in Childhood:Fetal and Neonatal Edition, 85*, F165–F169.

Donohue, P. K., Boss, R. D., Shepard, J., Graham, E., & Allen, M. C. (2009). Intervention at the border of viability: Perspective over a decade. *Archives of Pediatrics and Adolescent Medicine, 163*, 902–906.

Doyle, L. W., & Anderson, P. J. (2010). Adult outcome of extremely preterm infants. *Pediatrics, 126*, 342–351. doi: 126/2/342 [pii] 10.1542/peds.2010-0710

Doyle, L. W., & Casalaz, D. (2001). Outcome at 14 years of extremely low birthweight infants: A regional study. *Archives of Disease in Childhood: Fetal and Neonatal Edition, 85*, F159–F164.

Frye, R. E., Landry, S. H., Swank, P. R., & Smith, K. E. (2009). Executive dysfunction in poor readers born prematurely at high risk. *Developmental Neuropsychology, 34*, 254–271.

Gaddlin, P. O., Finnstrom, O., Sydsjo, G., & Leijon, I. (2009). Most very low birth weight subjects do well as adults. *Acta Paediatrica, 98*, 1513–1520.

Gimenez, M., Junque, C., Vendrell, P., Caldu, X., Narberhaus, A., Bargallo, N.,...Mercader, J. M. (2005). Hippocampal functional magnetic resonance imaging during a face-name learning task in adolescents with antecedents of prematurity. *Neuroimage, 25*, 561–569.

Goddeeris, J. H., Saigal, S., Boyle, M. H., Paneth, N., Streiner, D. L., & Stoskopf, B. (2010). Economic outcomes in young adulthood for extremely low birth weight survivors. *Pediatrics, 126*, e1102–e1108.

Grunau, R. E., Whitfield, M. F., & Fay, T. B. (2004). Psychosocial and academic characteristics of extremely low birth weight (< or =800 g) adolescents who are free of major impairment compared with term-born control subjects. *Pediatrics, 114*, e725–e732.

Hack, M., Flannery, D. J., Schluchter, M., Cartar, L., Borawski, E., & Klein, N. (2002). Outcomes in young adulthood for very-low-birth-weight infants. *New England Journal of Medicine, 346*, 149–157.

Hack, M., Taylor, H. G., Klein, N., & Minich, N. (2000). Functional limitations and special health care needs of 10- to 14-year-old children weighing less than 750 grams at birth. *Pediatrics, 106*, 554–559.

Hack, M., Youngstrom, E. A., Cartar, L., Schluchter, M., Taylor, H. G., Flannery, D.,...Borawski, E. (2004). Behavioral outcomes and evidence of psychopathology among very low birth weight infants at age 20 years. *Pediatrics, 114*, 932–940.

Hallin, A. L., Hellstrom-Westas, L., & Stjernqvist, K. (2010). Follow-up of adolescents born extremely preterm: Cognitive function and health at 18 years of age. *Acta Paediatrica, 99*, 1401–1406.

Hille, E. T., Weisglas-Kuperus, N., van Goudoever, J. B., Jacobusse, G. W., Ens-Dokkum, M. H., de Groot, L.,... Verloove-Vanhorick, S. P. (2007). Functional outcomes and participation in young adulthood for very preterm and very low birth weight infants: The Dutch Project on Preterm and Small for Gestational Age Infants at 19 Years of Age. *Pediatrics, 120,* e587–e595.

Indredavik, M. S., Skranes, J. S., Vik, T., Heyerdahl, S., Romundstad, P., Myhr, G. E., & Brubakk, A. M. (2005). Low-birth-weight adolescents: Psychiatric symptoms and cerebral MRI abnormalities. *Pediatric Neurology, 33,* 259–266.

Indredavik, M. S., Vik, T., Evensen, K. A., Skranes, J., Taraldsen, G., & Brubakk, A. M. (2010). Perinatal risk and psychiatric outcome in adolescents born preterm with very low birth weight or term small for gestational age. *Journal of Developmental and Behavioral Pediatrics, 31,* 286–294.

Jaeger, E., Silveira, R. C., & Procianoy, R. S. (2011). Cerebellar growth in very low birth weight infants. *Journal of Perinatology, 31,* 757–759. doi: 10.1038/jp.2011.20

Johnson, A., Bowler, U., Yudkin, P., Hockley, C., Wariyar, U., Gardner, F., & Mutch, L. (2003). Health and school performance of teenagers born before 29 weeks gestation. *Archives of Disease in Childhood: Fetal and Neonatal Edition, 88,* F190–F198.

Johnson, S. B., Blum, R. W., & Giedd, J. N. (2009). Adolescent maturity and the brain: The promise and pitfalls of neuroscience research in adolescent health policy. *Journal of Adolescent Health, 45,* 216–221.

Jonsdottir, G. M., Georgsdottir, I., Haraldsson, A., Hardardottir, H., Thorkelsson, T., & Dagbjartsson, A. (2012). Survival and neurodevelopmental outcome of ELBW children at five years of age. Comparison of two cohorts born ten years apart. *Acta Paediatrica, 101,* 714–718. doi: 10.1111/j.1651-2227.2012.02645.x

Kinney, H. C. (2006). The near-term (late preterm) human brain and risk for periventricular leukomalacia: A review. *Seminars in Perinatology, 30,* 81–88.

Kirby, R. S., & Wingate, M. S. (2010). Late preterm birth and neonatal outcome: Is 37 weeks' gestation a threshold level or a road marker on the highway of perinatal risk? *Birth, 37,* 169–171.

Lawrence, E. J., McGuire, P. K., Allin, M., Walshe, M., Giampietro, V., Murray, R. M.,... Nosarti, C. (2010). The very preterm brain in young adulthood: The neural correlates of verbal paired associate learning. *Journal of Pediatrics, 156,* 889–895.

Lenroot, R. K., & Giedd, J. N. (2010). Sex differences in the adolescent brain. *Brain and Cognition, 72,* 46–55.

Leversen, K. T., Sommerfelt, K., Rønnestad, A., Kaaresen, P. I., Farstad, T., Skranes, J.,... Markestad, T. (2011). Prediction of neurodevelopmental and sensory outcome at 5 years in Norwegian children born extremely preterm. *Pediatrics, 127,* e630–e638.

Limperopoulos, C., Chilingaryan, G., Guizard, N., Robertson, R. L., & Du Plessis, A. J. (2010). Cerebellar injury in the premature infant is associated with impaired growth of specific cerebral regions. *Pediatric Research, 68,* 145–150.

Lohaugen, G. C., Gramstad, A., Evensen, K. A., Martinussen, M., Lindqvist, S., Indredavik, M.,... Skranes, J. (2010). Cognitive profile in young adults born preterm at very low birthweight. *Developmental Medicine and Child Neurology, 52,* 1133–1138.

Lorenz, J. M., Wooliever, D. E., Jetton, J. R., & Paneth, N. (1998). A quantitative review of mortality and developmental disability in extremely premature newborns. *Archives of Pediatric and Adolescent Medicine, 152,* 425–435.

Luu, T. M., Ment, L., Allan, W., Schneider, K., & Vohr, B. R. (2011). Executive and memory function in adolescents born very preterm. *Pediatrics, 127,* e639–e646.

Luu, T. M., Ment, L. R., Schneider, K. C., Katz, K. H., Allan, W. C., & Vohr, B. R. (2009). Lasting effects of preterm birth and neonatal brain hemorrhage at 12 years of age. *Pediatrics, 123,* 1037–1044.

Luu, T. M., Vohr, B. R., Allan, W., Schneider, K. C., & Ment, L. R. (2011). Evidence for catch-up in cognition and receptive vocabulary among adolescents born very preterm. *Pediatrics, 128*, 313–322.

March of Dines. (2011). www.marchofdimes.com/peristats/whatsnewp.aspx

Martin, J. A., Hamilton, B. E., Ventura, S. J., Osterman, M. H. S., Kirmeyer, S., Mathews, T. J., & Wilson, E. (2011). Births: Final data for 2009. *National Vital Statistics Reports, 60*, 1–70.

Martin, J. A., Kirmeyer, S., Osterman, M., & Shepherd, R. A. (2009). Born a bit too early: Recent trends in late preterm births. *NCHS Data Brief, (Nov); 24*, 1–8.

Martin, J. A., Kung, H. C., Mathews, T. J., Hoyert, D. L., Strobino, D. M., Guyer, B., & Sutton, S. R. (2008). Annual summary of vital statistics: 2006. *Pediatrics, 121, 788*–801.

Moster, D., Lie, R. T., & Markestad, T. (2008). Long-term medical and social consequences of preterm birth. *New England Journal of Medicine, 359*, 262–273.

Mulder, H., Pitchford, N. J., Hagger, M. S., & Marlow, N. (2009). Development of executive function and attention in preterm children: A systematic review. *Developmental Neuropsychology, 34*, 393–421.

Mulder, H., Pitchford, N. J., & Marlow, N. (2010). Processing speed and working memory underlie academic attainment in very preterm children. *Archives of Disease in Childhood: Fetal and Neonatal Edition, 95*, F267–F272.

Nagy, Z., Ashburner, J., Andersson, J., Jbabdi, S., Draganski, B., Skare, S.,... Lagercrantz, H. (2009). Structural correlates of preterm birth in the adolescent brain. *Pediatrics, 124*, e964–e972.

Nagy, Z., & Jonsson, B. (2009). Cerebral MRI findings in a cohort of ex-preterm and control adolescents. *Acta Paediatrica, 98*, 996–1001.

Nagy, Z., Lagercrantz, H., & Hutton, C. (2011). Effects of preterm birth on cortical thickness measured in adolescence. *Cerebral Cortex, 21*, 300–306.

Nagy, Z., Westerberg, H., Skare, S., Andersson, J. L., Lilja, A., Flodmark, O.,... Klingberg, T. (2003). Preterm children have disturbances of white matter at 11 years of age as shown by diffusion tensor imaging. *Pediatric Research, 54*, 672–679.

Narberhaus, A., Lawrence, E., Allin, M. P., Walshe, M., McGuire, P., Rifkin, L.,... Nosarti, C. (2009). Neural substrates of visual paired associates in young adults with a history of very preterm birth: Alterations in fronto-parieto-occipital networks and caudate nucleus. *Neuroimage, 47*, 1884–1893.

Narberhaus, A., Pueyo-Benito, R., Segarra-Castells, M. D., Perapoch-Lopez, J., Botet-Mussons, F., & Junque, C. (2007). Long-term cognitive dysfunctions related to prematurity. *Revista de Neurologia, 45*, 224–228.

Narberhaus, A., Segarra, D., Caldu, X., Gimenez, M., Pueyo, R., Botet, F., & Junque, C. (2008). Corpus callosum and prefrontal functions in adolescents with history of very preterm birth. *Neuropsychologia, 46*, 111–116.

Nosarti, C., Al-Asady, M. H., Frangou, S., Stewart, A. L., Rifkin, L., & Murray, R. M. (2002). Adolescents who were born very preterm have decreased brain volumes. *Brain, 125*, 1616–1623.

Parker, J., Mitchell, A., Kalpakidou, A., Walshe, M., Jung, H. Y., Nosarti, C.,... Allin, M. (2008). Cerebellar growth and behavioural & neuropsychological outcome in preterm adolescents. *Brain, 131*, 1344–1351.

Rickards, A. L., Kelly, E. A., Doyle, L. W., & Callanan, C. (2001). Cognition, academic progress, behavior and self-concept at 14 years of very low birth weight children. *Journal of Developmental and Behavioral Pediatrics, 22*, 11–18.

Rushe, T. M., Rifkin, L., Stewart, A. L., Townsend, J. P., Roth, S. C., Wyatt, J. S., & Murray, R. M. (2001). Neuropsychological outcome at adolescence of very preterm birth and its relation to brain structure. *Developmental Medicine and Child Neurology, 43*, 226–233.

Saavalainen, P., Luoma, L., Bowler, D., Maatta, S., Kiviniemi, V., Laukkanen, E., & Herrgard, E. (2007). Spatial span in very prematurely born adolescents. *Developmental Neuropsychology, 32*, 769–785.

Saigal, S., Hoult, L. A., Streiner, D. L., Stoskopf, B. L., & Rosenbaum, P. L. (2000). School difficulties at adolescence in a regional cohort of children who were extremely low birth weight. *Pediatrics, 105*, 325–331.

Saigal, S., Stoskopf, B., Boyle, M., Paneth, N., Pinelli, J., Streiner, D., & Goddeeris, J. (2007). Comparison of current health, functional limitations, and health care use of young adults who were born with extremely low birth weight and normal birth weight. *Pediatrics, 119*, e562–e573.

Saigal, S., Stoskopf, B., Pinelli, J., Streiner, D., Hoult, L., Paneth, N., & Goddeeris, J. (2006). Self-perceived health-related quality of life of former extremely low birth weight infants at young adulthood. *Pediatrics, 118*, 1140–1148.

Saigal, S., Stoskopf, B. L., Streiner, D. L., & Burrows, E. (2001). Physical growth and current health status of infants who were of extremely low birth weight and controls at adolescence. *Pediatrics, 108*, 407–415.

Schothorst, P. F., Swaab-Barneveld, H., & van Engeland, H. (2007). Psychiatric disorders and MND in non-handicapped preterm children. Prevalence and stability from school age into adolescence. *European Child and Adolescent Psychiatry, 16*, 439–448.

Shenkin, S. D., Starr, J. M., & Deary, I. J. (2004). Birth weight and cognitive ability in childhood: A systematic review. *Psychological Bulletin, 130*, 989–1013.

Skranes, J., Vangberg, T. R., Kulseng, S., Indredavik, M. S., Evensen, K. A., Martinussen, M.,...Brubakk, A. M. (2007). Clinical findings and white matter abnormalities seen on diffusion tensor imaging in adolescents with very low birth weight. *Brain, 130*, 654–666.

van de Weijer-Bergsma, E., Wijnroks, L., & Jongmans, M. J. (2008). Attention development in infants and preschool children born preterm: A review. *Infant Behavior and Development, 31*, 333–351.

van Noort-van der Spek, I. L., Franken, M. C., & Weisglas-Kuperus, N. (2012). Language functions in preterm-born children: A systematic review and meta-analysis. *Pediatrics, 129*, 745–754.

Volpe, J. J. (2003). Cerebral white matter injury of the premature infant—more common than you think. *Pediatrics, 112*, 176–180.

Wilson-Costello, D., Friedman, H., Minich, N., Fanaroff, A. A., & Hack, M. (2005). Improved survival rates with increased neurodevelopmental disability for extremely low birth weight infants in the 1990s. *Pediatrics, 115*, 997–1003.

Wilson-Costello, D., Friedman, H., Minich, N., Siner, B., Taylor, G., Schluchter, M., & Hack, M. (2007). Improved neurodevelopmental outcomes for extremely low birth weight infants in 2000–2002. *Pediatrics, 119*, 37–45.

Zayek, M. M., Benjamin, J. T., Maertens, P., Trimm, R. F., Lal, C. V., & Eyal, F. G. (2011a). Cerebellar hemorrhage: A major morbidity in extremely preterm infants. *Journal of Perinatology.* doi: 10.1038/jp.2011.185

Zayek, M. M., Trimm, R. F., Hamm, C. R., Peevy, K. J., Benjamin, J. T., & Eyal, F. G. (2011b). The limit of viability: A single regional unit's experience. *Archives of Pediatric Adolescent Medicine, 165*, 126–133.

13 Sickle Cell Disease

Karen E. Wills

HISTORICAL MEDICAL PERSPECTIVE

The year 2012 was the 100th anniversary of the identification of sickle cells under a microscope, but advances in understanding and treating this devastating disease have been slow to develop. Before 1960, people with sickle cell disease (SCD) were expected to die in early adolescence or young adulthood. When functional, adaptive, or educational problems occurred, they were attributed to chronic pain and school absence, except among patients with obvious cognitive impairment associated with overt stroke. The pervasiveness of neuropsychological compromise, even in milder phenotypes of SCD, was denied or poorly recognized. Deep white matter lacunar strokes, which occur in about one-fourth of people with SCD, were considered functionally benign; however, newer evidence has linked this type of stroke to mild cognitive impairment (Grau-Olivares et al., 2007; Hillery & Panepinto, 2004). Even when neuropathological processes began to be recognized among patients with more severe disease (SS type hemoglobin, or "Hb-SS") in the 1960s, patients with "milder" types of SCD (such as SC-type hemoglobin, or Hb-SC) mistakenly were assumed to be unaffected and were used as a "control group" in research studies. Social and health disparity issues related to race and socioeconomic class were often ignored when discussing SCD outcomes. Finally, SCD often was assumed to be a disease that affected only "black Americans," rather than a genetic variation that affects individuals with a wide variety of skin tones and racial/ethnic heritages. These misunderstandings are gradually being corrected by new knowledge and advances in healthcare. The 1972 National Sickle Cell Disease Control Act, which established funding and organization of collaborative epidemiologic studies, was followed by several waves of clinical trials that led to therapeutic advances for patients with SCD (Bonds, 2005).

The average expected lifespan of North Americans and Europeans with SCD has quadrupled in the past 50 years, thanks to universal newborn screening; improved management of infectious illness, fever, and asthma; and safer blood transfusion procedures and pain medications. Emerging treatments such as hydroxyurea medication to reduce complications and stem cell transplants (a risky but effective cure for abnormal blood cell production) will extend and improve life even further for individuals with SCD. As life expectancy increases, understanding and planning for each phase of living with SCD also must expand.

Neuropsychological and psychological studies on the effects of SCD on everyday functioning and quality of life have become more frequent, and more sophisticated, in recent years. However, at all levels of analysis—from pathophysiology to social policy—many questions remain. Although SCD occurs in every social class, race, and ethnicity, most North American children with SCD are born to African-American or African immigrant families, among whom poverty is disproportionately common compared with European-Americans. Factors related to socioeconomic status (Palermo, Riley, & Mitchell, 2008) as well as racial/ethnic issues and healthcare disparities affect clinical care and research design (Hill, 2003; Tarazi, Grant, Ely, & Barakat, 2007; White & DeBaun, 1998). The first major national survey of patients with SCD was initiated in 1979–1981 when 3619 patients participated in the first Cooperative Study of Sickle Cell Disease (Farber et al., 1985). The study indicated that a higher percentage of adults with SCD were disabled, of low income, or unemployed compared to the general population of black Americans (based on census data) and that more households were headed by single females. Among those adults who were employed, however, the education level was higher than average and they were more likely to have white-collar jobs. These data underscore the diversity of functioning within the SCD adult population in 1980. The Comprehensive Sickle Cell Centers (CSCCs) provided rich information but with high attrition and reliance mainly on survey data.

Much of the current data about neuropsychological consequences of SCD come from the Collaborative Data (C-Data) Project of the CSCC Clinical Trial Consortium, which enrolled 1772 children and adults of African descent from 19 clinics in the United States in 2003–2008 (Dampier et al., 2010). These nationally aggregated data are based on a sample representative of black Americans in the national census. However, the American population of patients with SCD is unevenly distributed across states and cities (Brousseau et al., 2009; Hassell, 2010). This uneven distribution matters because there are significant differences in healthcare and education across states, particularly for minorities and low-income individuals (USDHHS, 2011). Consequently, it is possible that health outcomes for patients with SCD may be affected by state or regional differences. Also, cohort effects, that is, differences related to the era in which patients were born, access to quality healthcare over the individual's lifespan, and the point at which outcomes are measured, clearly influence status and outcomes of people with SCD. Consequently, the current status of older adults may have limited relevance for the prognosis of an infant born today.

CURRENT MEDICAL FACTORS AND TREATMENT AND INTERVENTION UPDATE

SCD is a recessive genetic difference in the gene for globin, part of the hemoglobin (Hb) molecule within red blood cells, which carry oxygen throughout the body (Ashley-Koch, Yang, & Olney, 2000; Wang, 2007). The red blood cells and entire vascular system function less effectively in a person born with SCD, resulting in chronic hemolytic anemia, chronic pain, and episodic vaso-occlusive episodes that cause acute pain and organ damage (described below in more detail).

SCD is endemic to regions where malaria is common because the heterozygous trait (hemoglobin type AS, or, Hb-AS) provides increased resistance to contracting malaria and so confers survival value. SCD occurs with high frequency in Greece, Turkey, and other Mediterranean and Caribbean countries as well as in western Africa. There are an estimated 70,000 Americans with SCD (Wang, 2007). In the United States, due to historical immigration patterns, most people with SCD are of African or Caribbean ancestry (roughly 1 in 350 African American newborns), but a growing number are of Mexican and Central and South American descent.

There are many phenotypes of SCD, about five of which are common in the United States (Ashley-Koch, Yang, & Olney, 2000). Of the many different subtypes of abnormal hemoglobin genotypes, the most commonly occurring in the United States are Hb-SS (65%), Hb-SC (25%), and Hb-S-beta-0-thalassemia (varying, but generally <10%) (Wang, 2007). Outcomes vary by genotype, with Hb-SC generally having less severe complications; however, all are subtypes of SCD and all constitute serious chronic medical conditions. Even among adults with Hb-SA, the sickle cell trait, several studies show an increased risk of exertion-related sudden death, autonomic dysregulation, thromboembolism, and consequent cerebrovascular ischemia and stroke when compared with individuals with normal Hb-AA red blood cell type (Alexy et al., 2010; Austin et al., 2007). This carrier state (Hb-SA) is not associated with increased neuropsychological risk.

The medical effects of SCD that are relevant to neuropsychological outcomes can be summarized by remembering the three B's: blood, breath, and brain. Red blood cells, which are continuously produced from bone marrow, carry oxygen throughout the body, and oxygen is essential to normal function and growth. For people with SCD, newly produced red blood cells appear rounded, malleable, and slippery, similar to cells with normal hemoglobin (Hb-AA). Soon, however, as blood oxygen levels fluctuate, cells with sickle hemoglobin (such as Hb-SS, Hb-SC, or Hb-S-beta-0-thalassemia) form long-chain molecules (polymerize). The process of polymerization changes the cells into rigid, elongated, sticky "sickle" shapes. In a person with untreated Hb-SS, about 90% of red blood cells have "sickled" (on average); in those with Hb-SC, about 50% have sickled (Ashley-Koch, Yang, & Olney, 2000). Compared with normal red blood cells, the sickled cells carry oxygen less efficiently, break down very quickly (hemolysis), and are more likely to damage and adhere to blood vessel walls or form clots (vaso-occlusion).

Normal red blood cells (with Hb-AA) survive about 120 days and are constantly replaced by fresh cells from bone marrow. Sickled cells only survive for 10–12 days. These cells break down faster than they can be replaced, leading to chronic hemolytic anemia. When sickled cells break down, they release free hemoglobin and arginase, both of which inhibit availability of a potent vasodilator, nitric oxide. The consequent vasoconstriction reduces oxygen still further, increasing the sickling process and making blood vessels even more vulnerable to damage and vaso-occlusion by sickled cells. Although there is some dispute about the role and importance of nitric oxide in the pathophysiology of SCD (Bunn et al., 2010), it appears that a complex cascade of hemodynamic factors (not simply vaso-occlusion) contributes to functional disability in SCD (Kato, Gladwin, & Steinberg 2007). Bilirubin, another product of cell breakdown, causes jaundice, making the whites of the eyes appear yellow and further contributing to organ damage if untreated (Wang, 2007).

Sudden, severe vaso-occlusive pain episodes, which occur anywhere in the body but are often localized to hands, feet, back, chest, or abdomen, can be triggered by dehydration, fever, emotional or physical stress, chilling, or sudden changes of body temperature. Crises occur unpredictably, with variable pain intensity and frequency. In addition to chronic and severe acute pain, vasoconstriction and vaso-occlusive events (ischemia and infarcts) cause cumulative organ damage and loss of function. For example, vaso-occlusive events can interfere with bone growth and, if severe, may result in malformed hands and feet in small children (dactylitis, or hand–foot syndrome) or joint necrosis of the hip and lower back in adolescents and adults. Accumulation of sickle cell fragments in the spleen (splenic sequestration) interferes with immune response and often results in splenectomy, which further increases the vulnerability to infectious diseases. About 50% of people with SCD will require gall bladder removal, associated with liver disease. In adults, kidney disease also becomes common. Peripheral neuropathy (particularly loss of sensation in lower limbs) may be increased in adults and may be associated with skin ulcers, particularly over the bony areas of the feet and ankles (Okuyucu et al., 2009). In adults, retinopathy (vascular occlusions of the retina), if severe, can lead to retinal detachment and blindness; vasculopathy also can cause sensorineural hearing loss (Lionnet, 2012).

Universal newborn screening for SCD, now the law in all US states and territories, allows for parent education and early intervention, which reduces later hospitalization costs and saves lives (Kaye et al., 2006). Infants and young children are vaccinated against infectious illness and prescribed prophylactic penicillin from birth through age 5 years, or sometimes longer (since about 2001). Until very recently in the United States and in other parts of the world, infectious illness at age 2–4 years was the most common cause of death for people with SCD.

Red blood cells generated by fetal and infant bone marrow until about 18–24 months postnatal age, termed "fetal hemoglobin," resist sickling (polymerizing). Normally, fetal hemoglobin declines steadily from about age 6 months to about age 2 years. Due to the presence of fetal hemoglobin during the first year, sickle-related pain crises often do not occur until the child is well into the second year of life; often, this postpones enrollment in preventive healthcare. A small percentage of individuals with SCD have persisting fetal hemoglobin throughout life, a genetic feature that seems to protect against the more severe complications of SCD.

Medical management of school-aged children with SCD can be intensive. In comprehensive sickle cell clinics, beginning at around age 5 years, children may be scheduled for annual routine pediatric physical exam, transcranial Doppler (TCD) screening for cerebral blood flow (an indicator of stroke risk) (Mazumdar, Heeney, Sox, & Lieu, 2007), pulmonary function testing to assess lung health (Nelson, Adade, Moquist, McDonough, & Hennessey, 2007), and neuropsychological testing to assess cognitive, emotional, and behavioral development (Wills et al., 2010). At around 10 years, many clinics add an echocardiogram because the vascular anomalies and pulmonary disease in SCD can strain and enlarge the heart.

The kidneys do not concentrate urine as effectively and, as a result, persistent bed-wetting is frequent (42% of 8-year-olds and 9% of young adults). No controlled study of nocturnal enuresis treatment for children with SCD was identified in the literature; however, anecdotally, enuresis in SCD does not seem to respond as well to urine alarm strategies, which work effectively for other children (Field, Austin, An, Yan, & DeBaun, 2008). Pica behavior (chewing and eating nonfood substances such as cloth, foam rubber, or paper) is frequent in children with SCD. The reasons for this behavior are unknown (Issaivanan et al., 2009). In addition, pica increases the risk of lead poisoning.

Pain crises continue to average about one per year through adolescence and adulthood. For adolescents and young adults, priapism (prolonged painful erection) can occur. This is very embarrassing, intensely painful, and rather difficult to treat. Left untreated, priapism can result in permanent erectile dysfunction (Burnett, 2012). Short stature, delayed growth, and delayed onset of puberty (by 2–3 years, on average) are common and may warrant treatment with growth hormone (GH) in early adolescence. Multiple factors including anemia and GH deficiencies contribute to growth delays in SCD (Nunlee-Bland et al, 2004). Studies of GH deficiencies in other populations, including children with thalassemia, revealed consistent problems with memory and attention that were improved by GH replacement therapy (Maruff & Falletti, 2005). GH deficiency and replacement has not been studied in SCD specifically, as yet, but may account for some cases of attention and memory impairment.

Lemanek and colleagues (1999) titled their review of adolescents with SCD, "Too little, too late," emphasizing the often unmet need for a lifespan approach to adolescent transition. There are fewer multidisciplinary "comprehensive clinics" for older adolescents and adults with SCD than for children. Pediatric providers often need to work with adult healthcare providers to increase awareness of specific physical and mental health risks that may emerge in adults with SCD (Kinney & Ware, 1996). Today, the highest risk of serious illness and death occurs in the 19- to 30-year-old age group. This is thought to reflect gaps in continuity of care as adolescents transition their healthcare from pediatric to adult providers and from parent-managed to self-managed planning, a stage when new, unfamiliar, and serious SCD symptoms or risks are emerging (Treadwell et al., 2010). Certain problems that are uncommon in childhood emerge in adolescence and occur with increasing incidence at older ages. These include skin ulcers (especially common around the bony ankles and feet); avascular necrosis (bone breakdown) of the shoulders, hips, or lumbar spine; retinopathy, which at its extreme can lead to retinal detachment and blindness; cardiomegaly and increased risk of heart attacks; liver disease; and kidney disease. Increased frequency and severity of pain episodes are associated with menstruation, pregnancy, and menopause. The childhood complications also increase with age, except for lacunar stroke, which is most common in infants and preschoolers.

With increasing age, there also is an increasing prevalence of Hb-SC type as a proportion of all patients with SCD (because these patients tend to live longer than patients with Hb-SS or Hb-S-beta-0-thalassemia). Hb-SC disease is associated with milder anemia (typical Hgb ~11.5, which is just slightly below normal); however, it carries a very high risk of problems associated with blood viscosity, particularly retinopathy and sensorineural hearing loss, despite much lower risk of problems such as acute chest syndrome (ACS) or stroke (Lionnet et al., 2012).

The second "B" underscores the importance of breath, that is, lung function, in the pathophysiology of SCD. Sleep-disordered breathing (sleep apnea, often signaled by extremely loud, persistent snoring) can lower blood oxygen saturation and increase risk of sickling crises and ACS (Kirkham & Datta, 2006). Although usually not fatal in children, ACS does add to overall mortality risk. The combination of low hemoglobin (blood levels below 7), high lymphocyte count, and one or more episodes of ACS occurring before age 2 years predicts disease severity (pain or death) 10 years later (Miller et al., 2000).

Among adults with SCD, ACS is the leading cause of death and chronic lung disease, including pulmonary hypertension (Boyd, Macklin, Strunk, & DeBaun, 2006; Nelson et al., 2007). Living in poverty is associated with increased asthma risk (Wright & Subramanian, 2007); asthma increases the risk of lung disease such as ACS and pulmonary hypertension (PHT), which, in turn, contributes to cerebrovascular stroke (Henderson, Noetzel, McKinstry, White, Armstrong, & DeBaun, 2003; Hillery & Panepinto, 2004). Thus, economic, environmental, and pulmonary factors all contribute to neuropsychological compromise and mortality risk and provide points of possible medical and behavioral health intervention.

EARLY PSYCHOLOGICAL AND NEUROPSYCHOLOGICAL FINDINGS

Our knowledge of the third "B"—brain dysfunction—has improved since the advent of neuroimaging studies and neuropsychological testing of individuals with SCD. Changes in brain function are associated with anemia and stroke, which are discussed in the following sections.

Effects of Anemia

Hemolytic anemia compromises neuropsychological function among individuals with SCD, absent any neuroimaging evidence of infarcts (Berkelhammer et al., 2007; Kral, Brown, & Hynd, 2001; Wang et al., 2001). Developmental delays among infants and toddlers with SCD and who have lower hemoglobin are more severe (Hogan et al., 2006; Schatz et al., 2008). Neuropsychological deficits occur in children with SCD who have no evidence of cerebrovascular disease on magnetic resonance imaging/magnetic resonance angiogram (MRI/MRA) compared with demographically matched or sibling controls (Hogan et al., 2000; Kral & Brown, 2004; Schatz, Finke, Kellett, & Kramer, 2002; Steen et al., 2005). In a study of 27 children aged 6–16 years, enrolled in a stroke-prevention study, anemia (lower hematocrit) was associated with lower scores on tests of reading, math, sustained attention, and cognitive flexibility. In adolescents (mean age 17.4 ± 4.2) without a history of stroke, the severity of diffuse neuropsychological compromise varied with the severity of anemia and disrupted pulmonary function (Hogan et al., 2006). Scantlebury and associates (2011) identified white matter compromise on diffusion-weighted imaging in brain tissue that appeared normal on MRI. In their small sample of 10 children, differences in white matter microstructure of the cerebellum and right frontal lobe were associated with slower processing speed. Vichinsky and colleagues (2010) reported that one-third of their sample of adults with Hb-SS and low hemoglobin (<10), which excluded those with a history of overt infarcts, had below-average Performance IQ scores (<85 on the Wechsler Adult Intelligence Scale, 3rd. Ed. (WAIS-III), with significantly lower scores for cases than for matched controls. Cases also scored more poorly than controls on indices of executive function, memory, attention, and language, even when MRI showed no abnormalities. In summary, it is clear that chronic hemolytic anemia impairs neuropsychological functioning, and more severe anemia is associated with more severe functional impairment. Therefore, most individuals with SCD are at increased risk of neuropsychological problems. However, as noted above, data from the CSCC national longitudinal study highlight considerable individual variation in functional outcomes among adults who have SCD.

Effects of Silent and Overt Cerebrovascular Infarcts

From 10% to 15% of children with Hb-SS will have an overt stroke by age 15 years, and another 20%–25% will have a silent stroke (DeBaun, Derdeyn, & McKinstry, 2006; Ohene-Frempong et al., 1998; Wang, 2007). A silent stroke (also called covert or subclinical stroke) is defined as lesions detected on MRI without any history of clinical changes in vision, speech, mentation, or movement. Such changes, plus lesions visible on MRI, indicate an overt stroke. In some cases, the silent/overt difference may be more a matter of degree than a difference in neuropathology because minor physical symptoms such as tremor or transient paresis can go unnoticed. However, in other cases, there is a real difference in neuropathology. Many silent strokes are lacunar strokes, that is, a series of tiny round infarcts in the centrum semiovale, which is deep frontal white matter fed by medullary branch arteries (Bogousslavsky & Regli, 1992). Among people with SCD, such lesions may be associated with fluctuations in carotid and basilar artery flow, accompanied by constriction of collateral vessels (Alexy et al., 2010; Ballas, 2010; DeBaun et al., 2006).

Silent strokes occur very early. Wang et al. (2008) reported 13% (3 of 23) of infants aged 10–18 months had experienced silent infarcts, typically located in the deep frontal-subcortical white matter systems; these areas undergo very active growth during infancy. No longitudinal study of infants with silent strokes has been reported. According to longitudinal data on 266 children followed from age 6 years to 19 years in the Cooperative Study of Sickle Cell Disease, few new silent strokes occurred among girls older than 6 years or boys older than 10 years, suggesting that this kind of stroke affects very young children who somehow outgrow the risk for it (Pegelow et al., 2002).

In contrast, the risk of overt hemorrhagic or ischemic stroke increases gradually with age, peaking sharply after age 40 years (Strouse, Lanzkron, & Urrutia, 2011). Anterior infarcts (in the border zone of the anterior and middle cerebral artery distributions) are more common than posterior infarcts at all ages for these types of strokes. However, it is possible for infarcts to occur anywhere. An increased risk of stroke is associated with Hb-SS genotype, hypertension, and lower hemoglobin as well as with increased age. Interestingly, there are no reports of vascular dementia specific to patients with SCD, despite the high incidence of stroke in patients >50 years. Medical advances will allow this population to age beyond 50 years. Therefore, it seems likely that these older individuals will be at higher-than-average risk of cerebrovascular disorders including dementia, in addition to stroke, cardiovascular disease, and kidney and liver diseases.

Most children who have subclinical strokes will never have an overt stroke; yet, their risk of overt stroke is increased compared with children who have normal MRIs. Currently, there is no road map for treating children who have MRI evidence of subclinical stroke, and there is no known way to predict or prevent such strokes from occurring (Miller et al., 2001; Wang, 2007). TCD screening, which measures the rate of blood flow in the carotid and basilar cerebral arteries, is a sensitive predictor of overt stroke, but not of subclinical stroke, in children (Adams, 2007). Abnormal findings on TCD currently trigger initiation of chronic blood transfusion, which reduces the proportion of sickled blood cells and thereby reduces risk of first stroke. Once the child has any infarct history, however, even chronic transfusions do not reduce the risk of another stroke (Wang, 2007). Moreover, the TCD test is sensitive to stroke risk only in children aged 2–16 years, not in adults (Strouse, Lanzkron, & Urrutia, 2011). Stroke prevention in SCD is an area of active ongoing research.

Two recent studies show strong associations between measures of cerebral arterial blood flow and neuropsychological status in SCD, with evidence of hypoperfusion associated with poorer neurocognitive function (Kral & Brown, 2004; Strouse et al., 2006). Kral and colleagues (2006) reported that abnormal TCD predicted more impaired verbal memory in a sample of 27 children without overt stroke, even when age and hematocrit were statistically controlled. Teacher reports of executive function problems on the BRIEF (Behavior Rating Inventory of Executive Function) (Gioia, Isquith, Guy, & Kenworthy, 2000) were associated with the severity of cerebrovascular pathology as indexed by TCD abnormalities among children who were not rated as having behavioral problems in general (Kral and Brown, 2004).

Neuropsychological testing, for example, a computerized test of vigilance and impulsivity (the Test of Variables of Attention [TOVA]) or tests of memorization (California Verbal Learning Test [CVLT]), is sensitive to the presence of subclinical strokes (DeBaun et al., 1998), which are not signaled by TCD abnormalities. Commonly, neuropsychological testing identifies difficulties with verbal fluency, processing speed, initiation, working memory, flexibly shifting attention, and dividing attention or multitasking (Berkelhammer, 2007). In general, the nature and severity of neuropsychological dysfunction in patients with silent or overt stroke are related to the size and location of the infarction (Schatz et al., 1999). For example, Schatz and colleagues (2009) in South Carolina reported semantic, syntactic, and phonological language impairments in 5- to 7-year-olds with SCD that were associated with SCD high-risk subtype and compromised cerebrovascular status. Diminished anterior corpus callosum size was associated with lower scores on measures of attention and executive function, independent of IQ. Greater amount of tissue loss associated with infarct was associated with lower IQ. The lowest IQ scores were seen among those who had both low hematocrit, indicating chronic anemia, and MRI abnormalities (signs of clinical or subclinical stroke or cortical atrophy). In school-age children, the presence of subclinical stroke is associated with specific impairment of executive function and memory on neuropsychological tests as well as mildly diminished general intellectual functioning and academic achievement (Berkelhammer et al., 2007; Bernaudin et al., 2000; Brown et al., 2000; Schatz, Finke, Kellett, & Kramer, 2002).

Researchers at Washington University–St. Louis compared neuropsychological function in children aged 6–18 years with frontal strokes with those with infarcts in other brains areas or no infarcts. Measures of response inhibition and verbal working memory were more severely impaired in those with anterior infarcts, consistent with poor strategic processing of to-be-remembered information (Brandling-Bennet et al., 2003; Christ et al., 2007; Schatz, White, Moinuddin, Armstrong, & DeBaun, 2002). As yet, there is no study of stroke in SCD with samples large enough to permit more fine-grained analysis of individual differences related to age at onset of stroke, age at testing, or length of the interval between the stroke and date of testing.

In one study of silent stroke in adults, individuals with SCD more often had MRI signs of lacunar stroke. However, this finding was not associated with poorer neuropsychological performance (compared with individuals without strokes) in this sample of adults. This is in contrast with most studies of school-age children that suggest adverse impact of lacunar strokes. This lack of findings related to silent stroke may be because Vichinsky's (2010) sample was carefully selected to include only adults of normal intelligence without any overt neurological symptoms or other severe SCD-related medical complications. In populations without SCD, this kind of lesion is seen in cases of carotid artery stenosis, and the overall volume of lacunar lesions is associated with severity of cognitive impairment (Grau-Olivares et al., 2010; Viswanathan et al., 2007).

The impact of neuropsychological problems that are present from early child-hood increases in adolescence and adulthood as environmental demands grow for complex self-directed social problem solving and for increased productivity at faster speeds. Several large studies have reported a decline in IQ scores from childhood to adolescence (Wang et al., 2001; Berkelhammer et al., 2007), but this does not necessarily imply progressive neurologically based deterioration in SCD. It may be that speed and efficiency affect IQ scores, especially Performance IQ, more strongly at older ages. Therefore, lifelong differences in the processing speed of individuals with SCD might have a greater impact on IQ scores of older children and adults than that of young children, producing a decrement in IQ with age. This untested hypothesis might explain why (untimed) Verbal IQ tasks show lesser decrements with age and smaller differences between patients with SCD and matched controls than (timed) Performance IQ tasks.

In summary, on average, children without any MRI abnormalities tend to do better than those who have sustained silent strokes; the latter, in turn, function better than those with a history of overt clinical stroke. There are exceptions to this rule, as case studies in our own clinic have demonstrated. Some bright, high-performing children have had overt or subclinical strokes, whereas some with severe learning problems have not. It is important for clinicians not to overgeneralize predictions based on group averages to individual cases.

SOCIAL, EMOTIONAL, AND CULTURAL CONSIDERATIONS

In addition to the physical complications of blood, brain, and breath, including anemia and cerebrovascular disease, factors that affect functional outcome in SCD include social-emotional adaptation associated with parenting and family functioning, cultural considerations, and individual differences in pain and pain management. These factors are addressed in the following section.

Parents and Families

Many prospective parents do not know they have the recessive gene for the SCD trait (Hb-AS or Hb-AC). This trait is present in 1 of 10 African-Americans but carriers are generally asymptomatic. Efforts to increase awareness are a critical public health issue. A governmental attempt in the 1980s to provide genetic counseling on a population basis was not successful, in part due to inadequate involvement of the sickle cell patient–parent community. That adverse experience has impeded subsequent efforts to develop genetic counseling programs for people at risk, despite studies suggesting that well-designed programs can be accepted and effective (e.g., Atkin, Ahmad, & Anionwu, 1998; Davis, 2011; Wilson et al., 2004).

Pregnancy is intrinsically high risk for women with SCD of any type, and more than one-third of pregnancies terminate without a live infant birth (Dauphin-McKenzie et al., 2006). Pain crises occur in about 50% of pregnant women, and slower fetal growth (intrauterine growth retardation) and premature delivery are common. Availability, access, and funding for specialized prenatal care are critical to outcomes of pregnancy for women with SCD, including maternal survival and child development.

The process of communicating the diagnosis to parents lays a cornerstone for their acceptance and knowledge about SCD. The extent to which parents view the future with hope and a sense of efficacy, that is, the confidence that their actions can make a difference in the course of the child's disease, as well as their inclination and ability to advocate for their child in healthcare, school, and other community settings, clearly affect health outcomes (Atkin, Ahmad, & Anionwu, 1998; Grover, 1989; Hill, 2003). In studies of other populations, these parent/family factors have been shown to affect neuropsychological outcomes as well (Potter et al., 2011). Patient education programs can effectively improve parent knowledge in SCD (Anie & Green, 2002). In turn, parental acceptance, awareness, and advocacy skills may affect child and adolescent development of health-related attitudes and knowledge (Kell et al., 1998; Kelch-Oliver et al., 2007; Thompson et al., 1993; Thompson et al., 2003).

Socioeconomic and Cultural Considerations

Psychosocial risk factors that interfere with typical developmental opportunities also may compromise neuropsychological development. Socioeconomic status was the strongest predictor of neuropsychological function in a recent study of preschool children who had SCD with no history of overt stroke (Tarazi, Grant, Ely, & Barakat, 2007). Disease severity indices were not strongly associated with preschool neuropsychological status. This study underscores that targeting psychosocial risk factors, in conjunction with targeting stroke risk, is critical to supporting development of preschoolers with SCD.

Cultural and linguistic differences between patients and providers are very common in this population and can impede the family's understanding of treatment options as well as the provider's understanding of individual complications. In the United States, immigrant families of patients with SCD speak Spanish, Haitian Creole French, and a variety of African languages. If healthcare providers speak only "medical-ese," communication may break down, even if parents speak English (Hill, 2003; Mahat, Scoloveno, & Donnelly, 2007). Cultural factors play into emotional reactions that may obstruct parents' abilities to accept and learn about their child's SCD (Atkin, Ahmad, & Anionwu, 1998; Hendricks-Ferguson & Nelson, 1999). Grief and fear can be particularly intense if relatives with SCD died young or were severely debilitated, which is a common experience of recent immigrants from rural Africa and grandparents in the United States. Feelings of guilt, self-blame, and blaming the other parent reflect parents' understanding of their own trait or SCD condition. SCD has been viewed as an indication of moral defect, taint, or curse among some families and cultures. The need for vaccinations, medications, and blood transfusions can create a crisis of faith for parents whose religious communities oppose these procedures (even though nearly all religions make compassionate exceptions to preserve health). On the other hand, support from extended family and the community may affect behavioral outcomes that are independent of stressors. For example, in one study of school-age children, parents who reported strong supportive relationships, even if they also reported numerous emotional and financial stressors, had children with better adaptive daily living skills and fewer behavior problems (Wills et al., 2011).

The Impact of Pain and Hospitalization on Social-Emotional Adaptation and Neuropsychological Function. Attachment and autonomy may be disrupted in children with frequent hospitalizations (Hocking & Lochman, 2005; Thompson et al., 2003). The inability to soothe an infant or child in pain is excruciatingly stressful for parents. Pain and illness result in frequent short hospitalizations, disrupting relations among parents and siblings who may or may not have SCD. In theory, alterations in these early social and emotional variables may affect later development of social thinking, behavioral regulation, and executive function (Potter et al., 2011). Employers may have difficulty accommodating a parent's need for time off work when the child's pain crises are frequent but intermittent and unpredictable. Medical bills and time lost from work add economic stress to the impact of the illness.

As the preschooler becomes more active, purposeful, and independent, parents must balance the need for special treatment (maintaining hydration, avoiding temperature extremes, managing pain) against overprotection (restricting play, infantilizing the child, excusing misbehavior "because of" SCD) (Hocking & Lochman, 2005). Early developmental delays sometimes are compounded by lack of early education. Most children can attend Headstart or preschool, but physicians may need to restrict some high-risk children to avoid infectious illness. In such cases, early assessment and referral to in-home early childhood programming can help.

Success in school, sports, and friendships becomes increasingly important for self-esteem and self-reliance during the elementary school years. Children with SCD often raise concerns about pain, short stature, low stamina for sports or recess games, school progress, and parental overprotection. Studies of peer interactions suggest positive adjustment among children with SCD who have not had overt stroke (Noll, Reiter-Purtill, Vannatta, Gerhardt, & Short, 2007). In one study, although peers were aware that children with SCD missed school more often due to illness and were less athletic and had fewer friends, teachers described these children as well behaved, and no group differences in emotional well-being were found (Ievers-Landis et al., 2001). In an interview-based survey, almost all parents of school-aged children with SCD reported problems managing their child's nutrition, helping their child cope with pain, and addressing their child's feelings about having SCD. Issues related to medication adherence and academic and social problems were less frequently reported. In general, however, more than 50% of children aged 5–18 years showed significant academic underachievement (Wills et al., 2010).

For adolescents with SCD, "metacognitive" issues are prominent (e.g., poor planning, difficulty starting and completing multistep tasks), whereas behavioral impulsivity or conduct problems are not typically reported by parents or teachers (Wills et al., 2009). Mood and emotional adjustment are well within normal limits for the average adolescent with SCD (Anie, 2005; Benton, Ifeagu, & Smith-Whitley, 2007; Clay & Telfair, 2007; Kelch-Oliver, Smith, Diaz, & Collins, 2007). Some, however, experience problems with body image and self-esteem associated with short stature, as well as depression and anxiety associated with chronic illness with unpredictable exacerbations (Levenson, 2008). For clinical counseling purposes, it is important to note that youth with SCD face even more severe health consequences than their peers from adolescent behaviors such as smoking tobacco or marijuana (given pulmonary risks), drinking alcohol (given dehydration risk), and having unprotected sex (given increased health risks during pregnancy). Parents' knowledge and perceptions about SCD affect use of emergency and routine healthcare by adolescents (Logan, Radcliffe, & Smith-Whitley, 2002) and presumably affect the adolescents' own development of health literacy and related behavior.

Individual Differences Related to Pain and Pain Management. There is a strong relationship between social–emotional adjustment and pain in children, adolescents, and adults with SCD (Anie, 2005; Levenson, 2008; McClish et al., 2005). Pain in SCD is severe and debilitating at a level comparable to that of patients undergoing hemodialysis (McClish et al., 2005). In general, individual differences in knowledge, attitudes, coping skills, and psychosocial stress may have a greater impact than biomedical factors (including frequency of vaso-occlusive pain events) on the child's long-term psychosocial adjustment (Burlew, Telfair, Colangelo, & Wright, 2000; Casey & Brown, 2003; Kelch-Oliver, Smith, Diaz, & Collins, 2007). Studies differ on the extent to which anxiety and depression influence children's or adolescents' subjective experience of pain (frequency and intensity of reported pain episodes, functional disability associated with pain). On the one hand, some studies suggest that individuals who are depressed or anxious tend to report more pain, whereas optimism and use of active, positive coping strategies reduce reported pain and use of pain medications (Barakat, Schwartz, Simon, & Radcliffe, 2007; Pence, Valrie, Gill, Redding-Lallinger, & Daeschner, 2007). Other studies suggest that pain occurs independent of depression among youth with SCD (Hoff, Palermo, Schluchter, Zebracki, & Drotar, 2006). In reviewing these studies, it appears that the relationship between depressive symptoms and pain complaints is stronger when the psychological and physical symptoms are mild to moderate; the relationship becomes decoupled when pain is more severe, as in SCD pain crises. Thus, in studying this relationship, it seems important to distinguish among different types of SCD pain (e.g., chronic discomfort versus acute crises) (see Stinson & Naser, 2003). Moreover, finding a correlation between emotional distress and physical pain at one point in time does not necessarily imply that one will predict the other longitudinally (see Varni, Burwinkle, & Katz, 2004 for study of these relationships among children with pediatric cancer pain).

The Pain in Sickle Cell Epidemiology study (PiSCES) (Smith et al., 2008) found that 50% of adults with SCD experienced pain on at least 50% of study days. Pain, which was the major contributor to compromised quality of life, was managed mostly at home, not in healthcare settings. Sickle cell pain was not simply a matter of severe intermittent acute crises; rather, chronic pain occurred daily for 1 in 3 patients. Pain is often treated with opioid analgesics, which can improve functioning; however, chronic opioid use can result in tolerance, increased pain sensitivity, and/or physiologic dependence. True addiction is rare but typically overestimated by healthcare providers. Physicians routinely undertreat SCD pain, resulting in pseudoaddiction, that is, patients seeking medication as a result of inadequate pain management (Levenson, 2008). Alcoholism, a problem in 30% of PiSCES participants, may serve as a form of self-medication (Levenson, 2008), as (despite alcohol's dehydrating effect) there were fewer pain reports and no significant risk of increased sickle-cell–related complications among patients reporting alcohol abuse in that self-report survey.

Medical

Hydroxyurea, a medication that inhibits sickling, decreases the frequency of pain episodes and strokes (Brawley et al., 2008; Hagar & Vichinsky, 2008). Puffer and colleagues (2007) reported that 15 children treated with hydroxyurea showed significantly higher scores on tests of verbal comprehension, fluid reasoning, and overall IQ than untreated children. European literature refers to this drug as hydroxycarbamide (Hagar & Vichinsky, 2008). There is a trend toward initiating hydroxyurea therapy early in childhood (as early as 1–2 years of age) rather than waiting for major health crises, such as acute chest syndrome or splenic sequestration, to begin medication management. The protective benefits of hydroxyurea therapy are becoming increasingly apparent, and for most children, adverse effects are minimal or absent; yet, it is not without risk, and its lifelong effects are unknown.

Chronic blood transfusions are another treatment for children with evidence of subclinical stroke who continue to show abnormal cerebral blood flow on TCD screening, particularly when there is evidence of neuropsychological impairment (Mazumdar, Heeney, Sox, & Lieu, 2007). In the most severe cases, the child may be referred for bone marrow or stem cell transplant from a closely matched donor, usually a sibling (Wang, 2007). The stem cell transplant can cure the hemoglobin abnormality, but carries a high risk of morbidity or death at this time.

Psychological and Neuropsychological Therapies

Cognitive rehabilitation to improve executive function in children with SCD has been recommended and piloted by the St. Louis Group (King, DeBaun, & White, 2008; Yerys et al., 2003). However, specific procedures need to be evaluated further, particularly in light of limited effectiveness of similar procedures in children with leukemia (Butler et al., 2008). Children whose self-care and self-advocacy are compromised by excessive pain complaints, executive dysfunction, or derailment of other developmental tasks may benefit from problem-focused interventions by behavioral health providers (Anie, 2005; Anie & Green, 2002).

Educational Interventions

Unfortunately, the one outcome study of educational intervention supported by a hospital team (King et al., 2006) did not show decreased absence or grade retention rates, though it did result in an increased number of students receiving an Individualized Educational Plan (IEP) in the schools. In addition to a school nursing plan, which every child with SCD should have, many will benefit from either a 504 plan or an IEP which is placed under the "Other Health Disabilities" category, to prevent school failure and meet educational needs (King, 2005; see also the Virginia Sickle Cell Awareness Program, 2006). Section 504 of the Civil Rights Act prohibits disability-based discrimination, and a "504 Plan" refers to the contract between a student and a school district, which details "reasonable accommodations" to reduce or prevent educational challenges posed by a student's medical condition. The neuropsychological assessment often will identify educational needs that are not recognized by schools (Herron et al.,

2003; Wills et al., 2010). Clinicians often will need to address parents' negative personal experiences with special education services, as well as their well-founded fears about stigmatization, peer victimization, overidentification of minority children, and low expectations for success. It can be helpful to discuss this using the analogy of a see-saw or teeter-totter that balances risks of neglecting a child's special learning needs (frustration, self-disparagement, academic failure) against the risks of stigmatizing the child, lowering expectations, or fostering overdependency (as parents often put it, "using sickle cell as a crutch"). Because low stamina may contribute to poor physical fitness, adaptive physical education may be important for many children (Moheed, Wali, & El-Sayed, 2007).

American society has no consistent, effective program, nor is there funding, to support adolescent-to-adult transition within the present healthcare system. Educational transition planning systems often are inadequate to meet the needs of youth with chronic health conditions (Barakat, Simon, Schwartz, & Radcliffe, 2008; Wills et al., 2010). From a clinical/rehabilitation perspective, persistent executive dysfunction is a major impediment to successful transition into adult life but may be overlooked or discounted when evaluating adolescents' transition needs. Rules governing Social Security Disability Income (SSDI) are more stringent for adults, disqualifying even some individuals with significant attention, learning, or health needs who qualified for Supplemental Security Income (SSI) as children. In the United States, each state has a client assistance project that can advise families on resources for transition assessment and support services, gratis or at reduced cost (see Resource List at the end of this chapter). Additional state resources can be identified at the disabilities clearinghouse (www.nichcy.org).

Patient Education and Advocacy

Providers can advocate for public policies and provide education and information to help prospective parents obtain genetic counseling; encourage more flexible family leave policies; and educate teachers and school administrators, health insurance payers, and primary care providers about the special educational and health needs of people with SCD. There are books or videos that help explain SCD (see Resource List below).

Community Advocacy and Support Groups

Palermo and colleagues (2008) reported that neighborhood socioeconomic distress affected physical aspects of health-related quality of life among children with SCD, independent of individual family functioning. Like their peers, children with SCD need a safe, supervised, bully-free environment for after-school play. Living in poverty makes this challenging for many. Summer camps specifically for children with SCD help some children gain awareness, coping skills, and peer support. Several studies also have considered spirituality as an important source of hope, optimism, and coping (Cotton et al., 2012). In-person or on-line SCD groups (such as the Sickle Cell Anemia Disease page on Facebook) provide an international forum for networking about common concerns and interests. Providers can guide patients to check the sources and accuracy of health resources online and, at the same time, learn from the concerns and ideas posted in the patient support forums.

CURRENT RESOURCES

Publications:

Platt, A., Eckman, J., & Hsu, L. (2011). *Hope & Destiny: The Patient and Parent's Guide to Sickle Cell Disease and Sickle Cell Trait (3rd Edition)*. Munster, IN: Hilton Publishing.
Internet Links:

1. *National Coordinating and Evaluation Center for Sickle Cell Disease and Newborn Screening Programs* (a coalition of hospitals and the SCDAA), http://www. Sicklecelldisease. Net
2. *Sickle Cell Disease Association of America*, sicklecelldisease. Org
3. *Emory University, Atlanta, Sickle Cell Disease Information*, www. Scinfo. Org
4. *NICHCY*, www. Nichcy. Org (See the "State Resources" sheets for detailed listings of state agencies serving individuals with chronic health conditions or disabilities.)
5. *"Understanding the Child with Sickle Cell Disease, A manual for school personnel"* Virginia Public Health Department, Sickle Cell Awareness Program, 2008. Online at http://www. Vahealth. Org/sicklecell/docs/SchoolHandbook_SickleCellChild_PDF%5B1%5D. Pdf
6. *Transition Manual for Youth and Young Adults with Sickle Cell Disease*, Virginia Public Health Department, 2011. Online at http://www. Vahealth. Org/sicklecell/docs/2011/pdf/Intro_Section1-HealthMaintenance. Pdf

FUTURE AIMS AND RESEARCH OPPORTUNITIES

A dynamic interplay among physical complications, psychosocial stress and support, and neuropsychological function contributes to adaptive outcomes among individuals with SCD. Successful adult outcomes reflect collaboration among multiple providers and settings (parents, extended family, healthcare providers, schools, recreation facilities, community organizations) and across multiple areas of development (physiological, emotional, cognitive, social). In SCD, far more questions remain than there are answers, including:

- Does mandated universal newborn screening save lives and produce higher-functioning (more competent) parents, children, adolescents, and adults with SCD?
- Does training of medical providers to communicate the diagnosis improve parents' adjustment to the SCD diagnosis and ability to advocate for the child?
- When do neurologic and neurodevelopmental problems first emerge in infants or children with SCD? How do they manifest? Can they be treated immediately? Can they be prevented? Do early delays predict lasting neuropsychological impairment? Does early intervention (e.g., earlier initiation of hydroxyurea therapy) allow for "positive plasticity"—healing or catch-up growth from early neurologic compromise?
- Infants and preschoolers with SCD show delays in language skills, but older children and adults tend to show normal verbal abilities. Is this a real developmental difference or an artifact of the different kinds of tests administered? Do early

difficulties with language skill predict later difficulties on tests of fluency, processing speed, working memory, or other aspects of executive function?

- Does educating parents and teachers about what to expect and how to manage SCD across the child's lifespan help to improve the child's age-appropriate adaptive competencies and academic achievement?
- Does establishing hospital–school–community liaisons to develop and provide educational, vocational, and recreational opportunities for youth with SCD improve their access to, and involvement with, age-appropriate activities? And does this involvement help keep them safe, happy, and improve their intellectual and social competence?
- How do pain episodes and hospitalizations during infancy and toddlerhood affect the developing parent–child relationship?
- What strategies work best to minimize the intensity, frequency, and duration of pain in infants, children, adolescents, and adults with SCD? Are there different strategies that work better at different ages or under different individual circumstances?
- Does use of opiate pain medication have any lasting adverse consequences for neuropsychological function in SCD?
- Does cognitive rehabilitation improve concentration, reflection, planning, and other aspects of executive function in children and youth with SCD?
- What indicators (medical, neuropsychological, behavioral, other) best predict successful (versus problematic) transition to adulthood among youth with SCD? Do hospital-based or community-based patient education programs to improve self-awareness, self-acceptance, and self-advocacy promote successful transition to adulthood (as defined by relevant stakeholders) for children and youth with SCD?
- Do medical interventions targeting blood (anemia), lungs (PHT and associated problems with oxygenation), or brain (white matter damage and stroke) yield measureable improvement in children's physical health and neuropsychological status? And does that improvement contribute to successful adult outcomes?
- How do families, youth, and adults with SCD define successful outcomes? And are their definitions congruent with commonly used questionnaires, observation measures, and healthcare providers' assumptions about what constitutes success?
- How can neuropsychologists and other healthcare providers support the community of patients with SCD and their families to advocate for research and clinical care that fosters optimal development and works toward a cure?

REFERENCES

Adams, R. J. (2007). Big strokes in small persons. *Archives of Neurology, 64*, 1567–1574.

Alexy, T., Sangkatumvong, S., Connes, P., Pais, E., Tripette, J., Barthelemy, J. C.,... Coates, T. D. (2010). Sickle cell disease: Selected aspects of pathophysiology. *Clinical Hemorheology and Microcirculation, 44*, 155–166.

Anie, K. A. (2005). Psychological complications in sickle cell disease. *British Journal of Haematology, 129*, 723–729.

Anie, K. A., & Green, J. (2002). Psychological therapies for sickle cell disease and pain. *Cochrane Database Systematic Review, 2*, CD001916.

Ashley-Koch, A., Yang, Q., & Olney, R. S. (2000). Sickle hemoglobin (HbS) allele and sickle cell disease: A HuGE review. *American Journal of Epidemiology, 151*, 839–845.

Atkin, K., Ahmad, W. I. U., & Anionwu, E. N. (1998). Screening and counseling for sickle cell disorders and thalassemia: The experience of parents and health professionals. *Social Science & Medicine, 47*, 1639–1651.

Austin, H., Key, N. S., Benson, J. M., Lally, C., Dowling, N. F., Whitsett, C., & Hooper, W. C. (2007). Sickle cell trait and the risk of venous thromboembolism among blacks. *Blood, 110*, 908–912.

Ballas, S. (2010). Neurocognitive complications of sickle cell anemia in adults. *Journal of the American Medical Association, 303*, 1862–1863.

Benton, T. D., Ifeagwu, J. A., & Smith-Whitley, K. (2007). Anxiety and depression in children and adolescents with sickle cell disease. *Current Psychiatry Reports, 9*, 114–121.

Berkelhammer, L. D., Williamson, A. L., Sanford, S. D., Dirksen, C. L., Sharp, W. G., Margulies, A. S., & Prengler, R. A. (2007). Neurocognitive sequelae of pediatric sickle cell disease: A review of the literature. *Child Neuropsychology, 13*, 120–131.

Bernaudin, F., Verlhac, S., Freard, F., Roudot-Thoraval, F., Benkerrou, M., Thuret, I., … Brugieres, P. J. (2000). Multicenter prospective study of children with sickle cell disease: Radiographic and psychometric correlation. *Child Neurology, 15*, 333–343.

Bogousslavsky, J., & Regli, F. (1992). Centrum ovale infarcts: Subcortical infarction in the superficial territory of the middle cerebral artery. *Neurology, 42*, 1992–1998.

Bonds, D. R. (2005). Three decades of innovation in the management of sickle cell disease: The road to understanding the sickle cell disease clinical phenotype. *Blood Review, 19*, 99–110.

Boyd, J. H., Macklin, E. A., Strunk, R. C., & DeBaun, M. R. (2006). Asthma is associated with acute chest syndrome and pain in children with sickle cell anemia. *Blood, 108*, 2923–2927.

Brandling-Bennett, E. M., White, D. A., Armstrong, M. M., Christ, S. E., & DeBaun, M. (2003). Patterns of verbal long-term and working memory performance reveal deficits in strategic processing in children with frontal infarcts related to sickle cell disease. *Developmental Neuropsychology, 24*, 423–434.

Brawley, O. W., Cornelius, L. J., Edwards, L. R., Gamble, V. N., Green, B. L., Inturrisi, C., … Schori, M. (2008). National Institutes of Health Consensus Development Conference statement: Hydroxyurea treatment for sickle cell disease. *Annals of Internal Medicine, 148*, 932–938.

Brousseau, D. C., Panepinto, J. A., Nimmer, M., & Hoffmann, R. G. (2009). The number of people with sickle-cell disease in the United States: National and state estimates. *American Journal of Hematology, 85*, 77–78.

Bunn, H. F., Nathan, D. G., Dover, G. J., Hebbel, R. P., Platt, O. S., Rosse, W. F., & Ware, R. E. (2010). Pulmonary hypertension and nitric oxide depletion in sickle cell disease. *Blood, 116*, 687–692.

Burlew, A. K., Telfair, J., Colangelo, L., & Wright, E. (2000). Factors that influence adolescent adaptation to sickle cell disease. *Journal of Pediatric Psychology, 25*, 287–299.

Burnett, A. L. (2012). Sexual health outcomes improvement in sickle cell disease: A matter of health policy? *Journal of Sexual Medicine, 9*, 104–113.

Butler, R. W., Copeland, D. R., Fairclough, D. L., Mulhern, R. K., Katz, E. R., Kazak, A. E., … Sahler, O. J. (2008). A multicenter, randomized clinical trial of a cognitive remediation program for childhood survivors of a pediatric malignancy. *Journal of Consulting & Clinical Psychology, 76*, 367–378.

Casey, R. L., & Brown, R. T. (2003). Psychological aspects of hematologic disease. *Child and Adolescent Psychiatric Clinics of North America, 12*, 567–584.

Christ, S. E., Moinuddin, A., McKinstry, R. C., DeBaun, M., & White, D. A. (2007). Inhibitory control in children with frontal infarcts related to sickle cell disease. *Child Neuropsychology, 13*, 132–141.

Dampier, C., Lieff, S., LeBeau, P., Rhee, S., McMurray, M., Rogers, Z.,… Wang, W. for the Comprehensive Sickle Cell Centers (CSCC) Clinical Trial Consortium (CTC). (2010). Health-related quality of life in children with sickle cell disease: A report from the Comprehensive Sickle Cell Centers Clinical Trial Consortium. *Pediatric Blood & Cancer, 55,* 485–494.

Dauphin-McKenzie, N., Gilles, J. M., Jacques, E., & Harrington, T. (2006). Sickle cell anemia in the female patient. *Obstetrical and Gynecological Survey, 61,* 343–352.

DeBaun, M. R., Derdeyn, C. P., & McKistry, R. C. (2006). Etiology of strokes in children with sickle cell anemia. *Mental Retardation and Developmental Disabilities Research Reviews, 12,* 192–199.

DeBaun, M. R., Schatz, J., Siegel, M. J., Koby, M., Craft, S., Resar, L.,… Noetzel, M. (1998). Cognitive screening examinations for silent cerebral infarcts in sickle cell disease. *Neurology, 50,* 1678–1682.

Farber, M. D., Koshy, M., Kinney, T. R., & the Cooperative Study of Sickle Cell Disease. (1985). Cooperative Study of Sickle Cell Disease: Demographic and socioeconomic characteristics of patients and families with sickle cell disease. *Journal of Chronic Disease, 38,* 495–505.

Field, A., An, Y., & DeBaun, M. (2008). Enuresis is a common and persistent problem among children and young adults with sickle cell anemia. *Urology, 72,* 81–84.

Grau-Olivares, M., Bartres-Faz, D., Arboix, A., Soliva, J. C., Rovira, M., Targa, C., & Junque, C. (2007). Mild cognitive impairment after lacunar infarction: Voxel-based morphometry and neuropsychological assessment. *Cerebrovascular Disease, 23,* 353–361.

Grover, R. (1989). Program effects on decreasing morbidity and morality: Newborn screening in New York City. *Pediatrics, 83,* 819–822.

Hagar, W., & Vichinsky, E. (2008). Advances in clinical research in sickle cell disease. *British Journal of Haematology, 141,* 346–356.

Hassell, K. L. (2010). Population estimates of sickle cell disease in the U. S. *American Journal of Preventative Medicine, 38,* S512-S521.

Hendricks-Ferguson, V. L., & Nelson, M. (1999). Update of the health management needs of infants with sickle cell disease. *Journal of Pediatric Health Care, 13,* 217–222.

Henderson, J. N., Noetzel, M. J., McKinstry, R. C., White, D. A., Armstrong, M., & DeBaun, M. R. (2003). Reversible posterior leukoencephalopathy syndrome and silent cerebral infarcts are associated with severe acute chest syndrome in children with sickle cell disease. *Blood, 101,* 415–419.

Herron, S., Bacak, S. J., King, A., & DeBaun, M. R. (2003). Inadequate recognition of education resources required for high-risk students with sickle cell disease. *Archives of Pediatric and Adolescent Medicine, 157,* 104.

Hill, S. (2003). *Managing sickle cell disease in low-income families.* Philadelphia: Temple University Press.

Hocking, M. C., & Lochman, J. E. (2005). Applying the transactional stress and coping model to sickle cell disorder and insulin-dependent diabetes mellitus: Identifying psychosocial variables related to adjustment and intervention. *Clinical Child and Family Psychology Review, 8,* 221–246.

Hogan, A. M., Kirkham, F. J., Prengler, M., Telfer, P., Lane, R., & Vargha-Khadem, F. (2006). An exploratory study of physiological correlates of neurodevelopmental delay in infants with sickle cell anaemia. *British Journal of Haematology, 132,* 99–107.

Hogan, A. M., Pit-ten Cate, I. M., Vargha-Khadem, F., Prengler, M., & Kirkham, F. J. (2006). Physiological correlates of intellectual function in children with sickle cell disease: Hypoxaemia, hyperaemia and brain infarction. *Developmental Science, 9,* 379–387.

Ievers-Landis, C. E., Brown, R. T., Drotar, D., Bunke, V., Lambert, R. G., & Walker, A. A. (2001). Situational analysis of parenting problems for caregivers of children with sickle cell syndromes. *Journal of Developmental and Behavioral Pediatrics, 22*, 169–178.

Issaivanan, M., Ahmed, R., Shekher, M., Esernio-Jenssen, D., & Manwani, D. (2009). Sickle cell disease and plumbism in children. *Pediatric Blood and Cancer, 52*, 653–656.

Kato, G. J., Gladwin, M. T., & Steinberg, M. H. (2007). Deconstructing sickle cell disease: Reappraisal of the role of hemolysis in the development of clinical subphenotypes. *Blood Review, 21*, 37–47.

Kaye, C. I., Committee on Genetics, Accurso, F., La Franchi, S., Lane, P. A., Northrup, H.,… Schaefer, G. B. (2006). Introduction to the newborn screening fact sheets. *Pediatrics, 118*, 1304–1312.

Kelch-Oliver, K., Smith, C. O., Diaz, D., & Collins, M. H. (2007). Individual and family contributions to depressive symptoms in African American children with sickle cell disease. *Journal of Clinical Psychology in Medical Settings, 14*, 376–384.

Kell, R. S., Kliewer, W., Erickson, M. T., & Ohene-Frempong, K. (1998). Psychological adjustment of adolescents with sickle cell disease: Relations with demographic, medical, and family competence variables. *Journal of Pediatric Psychology, 23*, 301–312.

King, A. A. (2005). An education program to increase teacher knowledge about sickle cell disease. *Journal of School Health, 75*, 11–14.

King, A. A., DeBaun, M. R., & White, D. A. (2008). Need for cognitive rehabilitation for children with sickle cell disease and strokes. *Expert Review of Neurotherapeutics, 8*, 291–296.

King, A. A., Herron, S., McKinstry, R., Bacak, S., Armstrong, M., White, D., & DeBaun, M. (2006). A multidisciplinary health care team's efforts to improve educational attainment in children with sickle-cell anemia and cerebral infarcts. *Journal of School Health, 76*, 33–37.

Kinney, T. R., & Ware, R. E. (1996). The adolescent with sickle cell anemia. *Hematology and Oncology Clinics of North America, 10*, 1255–1264.

Kirkham, F. J., & Datta, A. K. (2006). Hypoxic adaptation during development: Relation to pattern of neurological presentation and cognitive disability. *Developmental Science, 9*, 411–427.

Kral, M. C., & Brown, R. T. (2004). Transcranial Doppler ultrasonography and executive dysfunction in children with sickle cell disease. *Journal of Pediatric Psychology, 29*, 185–195.

Kral, M. C., Brown, R. T., & Hynd, G. W. (2001). Neuropsychological aspects of pediatric sickle cell disease. *Neuropsychological Review, 11*, 179–196.

Kral, M. C., Brown, R. T., Connelly, M., Cure, J. K., Besenski, N., Jackson, S. M., & Abboud, M. R. (2006). Radiographic predictors of neurocognitive functioning in pediatric sickle cell disease. *Journal of Child Neurology, 21*, 37–44.

Lemanek, K. L., Steiner, S. M., & Grossman, N. J. (1999). Too little, too late: Primary vs. secondary interventions for adolescents with sickle cell disease. *Adolescent Medicine, 10*, 385–400.

Lionnet, F., Hammoudi, N., Stankovic Stojanovic, K., Avellino, V., Grateau, G., Girot, R., & Haymann, J. P. (2012). Hemoglobin SC disease complications: A clinical study of 179 cases. *Haematologica, 97*, 1136–1141.

Logan, D. E., Radcliffe, J., & Smith-Whitley, K. (2002). Parent factors and adolescent sickle cell disease: Associations with patterns of health service use. *Journal of Pediatric Psychology, 27*, 475–484.

Mahat, G., Scoloveno, M. A., & Donnelly, C. B. (2007). Written educational materials for families of chronically ill children. *Journal of the American Academy of Nurse Practitioners, 19*, 471–476.

Maruff, P., & Falleti, M. (2005). Cognitive function in growth hormone deficiency and growth hormone replacement. *Hormone Research, 64,* 100–108.

Mazumdar, M., Heeney, M. M., Sox, C. M., & Lieu, T. A. (2007). Preventing stroke among children with sickle cell anemia: An analysis of strategies that involve transcranial doppler testing and chronic transfusion. *Pediatrics, 120,* e1107–1116. doi: 10.1542/peds.2006-2002

Miller, S. T., Sleeper, L. A., Pegelow, C. H., Enos, L. E., Wang, W. C., Weiner, S. J.,… Kinney, T. R. (2000). Prediction of adverse outcomes in children with sickle cell disease. *New England Journal of Medicine, 342,* 1612–1613.

Moheed, H., Wali, Y. A., & El-Sayed, M. S. (2007). Physical fitness indices and anthropometrics profiles in schoolchildren with sickle cell trait/disease. *American Journal of Hematology, 82,* 91–97.

Nelson, S. C., Adade, B. B., McDonough, E. A., Moquist, K. L., & Hennessey, J. M. (2007). High prevalence of Pulmonary hypertension in children with sickle cell disease. *Journal of Pediatric Hematology and Oncology, 29,* 334–337.

Noll, R. B., Reiter-Purtill, J., Vannatta, K., Gerhardt, C. A., & Short, A. (2007). Peer relationships and emotional well-being of children with sickle cell disease: A controlled replication. *Child Neuropsychology, 13,* 173–187.

Nunlee-Bland, G., Rana, S. R., Houston-Yu, P. E., & Odonkor, W. (2004). Growth hormone deficiency in patients with sickle cell disease and growth failure. *Journal of Pediatric Endocrinology & Metabolism, 17,* 601–606.

Okuyucu, E. E., Turhanoglu, A., Duman, T., Kaya, H., Melek, I. M., & Yimazer, S. (2009). Peripheral nervous system involvement in patients with sickle cell disease. *European Journal of Neurology, 16,* 814–818.

Ohene-Frempong, K., Weiner, S. J., Sleeper, L. A., Miller, S. T., Embury, S., Moohr, J. W.,… Gill, F. M. (1998). Cerebrovascular accidents in sickle cell disease: Rates and risk factors. *Blood, 91,* 288–294.

Palermo, T. M., Riley, C. A., & Mitchell, B. A. (2008). Daily functioning and quality of life in children with sickle cell disease pain: Relationship with family and neighborhood socioeconomic distress. *Journal of Pain, 9,* 833–840.

Pegelow, C. H., Macklin, E. A., Moser, F. G., Wang, W. C., Bello, J. A., Miller, S. T.,… Kinney, T. R. (2002). Longitudinal changes in brain magnetic resonance imaging findings in children with sickle cell disease. *Blood, 99,* 3014–3018.

Pence, L., Valrie, C. R., Gill, K. M., Redding-Lallinger, R., & Daeschner, C. (2007). Optimism predicting daily pain medication use in adolescents with sickle cell disease. *Journal of Pain Symptom Management, 33,* 302–309.

Potter, J. L., Wade, S. L., Walz, N. C., Cassedy, A., Stevens, M. H., Yeates, K. O., & Taylor, H. G. (2011). Parenting style is related to executive dysfunction after brain injury in children. *Rehabilitation Psychology, 56,* 351–358.

Puffer, E., Schatz, J., & Roberts, C. W. (2007). The association of oral hydroxyurea therapy with improved cognitive functioning in sickle cell disease. *Child Neuropsychology, 13,* 142–154.

Scantlebury, N., Mabbott, D., Janzen, L., Rockel, C., Widjaja, E., Jones, G.,… Odame, I. (2011). White matter integrity and core cognitive function in children diagnosed with sickle cell disease. *Journal of Pediatric Hematology & Oncology, 33,* 163–171.

Schatz, J., Brown, R. T., Pascual, J. M., Hsu, L., & DeBaun, M. (2001). Poor school and cognitive functioning with silent cerebral infarcts and sickle cell disease. *Neurology, 56,* 1109–1111.

Schatz, J., Craft, S., Koby, M., Siegel, M., Resar, L., Lee, R. R.,… DeBaun, M. R. (1999). Neuropsychologic deficits in children with sickle cell disease and cerebral infarction: Role of lesion site and volume. *Child Neuropsychology, 5,* 92–103.

Schatz, J., Finke, R. L., Kellett, J. M., & Kramer, J. H. (2002). Cognitive functioning in children with sickle cell disease: A meta-analysis. *Journal of Pediatric Psychology, 27,* 739–748.

Schatz, J., McClellan, C. B., Puffer, E. S., Johnson, K., & Roberts, C. W. (2008). Neurodevelopmental screening in toddlers and early preschoolers with sickle cell disease. *Journal of Child Neurology, 23,* 44–50.

Schatz, J., Puffer, E. S., Sanchez, C., Stancil, M., & Roberts, C. W. (2009). Language processing deficits in sickle cell disease in young school-age children. *Developmental Neuropsychology, 34,* 122–136.

Schatz, J., White, D. A., Moinuddin, A., Armstrong, M., & DeBaun, M. R. (2002). Lesion burden and cognitive morbidity in children with sickle cell disease. *Journal of Child Neurology, 17,* 891–895.

Steen, R. G., Fineberg-Buchner, C., Hankins, G., Weiss, L., Prifitera, A., & Mulhern, R. K. (2005). Cognitive deficits in children with sickle cell disease. *Journal of Child Neurology, 20,* 102–107.

Stinson, J., & Naser, B. (2003). Pain management in children with sickle cell disease. *Paediatric Drugs, 5,* 229–241.

Strouse, J. J., Cox, C. S., Melhem, E. R., Lu, H., Kraut, M. A., Razumovsky, A.,... Casella, J. F. (2006). Inverse correlation between cerebral blood flow measured by continuous arterial spin-labeling (CASL) MRI and neurocognitive function in children with sickle cell anemia (SCA). *Blood, 108,* 379–381.

Strouse, J. J., Lanzkron, S., & Urrutia, V. (2011). The epidemiology, evaluation, and treatment of stroke in adults with sickle cell disease. *Expert Reviews in Hematology, 4,* 597–606.

Tarazi, R. A., Grant, M. L., Ely, E., & Barakat, L. P. (2007). Neuropsychological functioning in preschool-age children with sickle cell disease: The role of illness-related and psychosocial factors. *Child Neuropsychology, 13,* 155–172.

Thompson, R. J., Fil, K. M., Burbach, D. J., Keith, B. R., & Kinney, T. R. (1993). Roles of child and maternal processes in the psychological adjustment of children with sickle cell disease. *Journal of Consulting and Clinical Psychology, 61,* 468–474.

Thompson, R. J. Jr., Armstrong, F. D., Link, C. L., Pegelow, C. H., Moser, F., & Wang, W. C. (2003). A prospective study of the relationship over time of behavior problems, intellectual functioning, and family functioning in children with sickle cell disease: A report from the Cooperative Study of Sickle Cell Disease. *Journal of Pediatric Psychology, 28,* 59–65.

Treadwell, M., Telfair, J., Gibson, R. W., Johnson, S., & Osunkwo, I. (2011). Transition from pediatric to adult care in sickle cell disease: Establishing evidence-based practice and directions for research. *American Journal of Hematology, 86,* 116–120.

USDHHS (United States Department of Health and Human Services) (2011). *Children with special health care needs in context: A portrait of states and the nation 2007.* Washington, DC: HRSA. Available online at http://www. Eric. Ed.Gov/PDFS/ED530916. Pdf.

Varni, J. W., Burwinkle, T. M., & Katz, E. R. (2004). The PedsQL in pediatric cancer pain: A prospective longitudinal analysis of pain and emotional distress. *Journal of Developmental and Behavioral Pediatrics, 25,* 239–246.

Vichinsky, E. P., Neurmayr, L. D., Gold, J. I., Weiner, M. W., Rule, R. R., Truran, D.,... Armstrong, F. D. (2010). Neuropsychological dysfunction and neuroimaging abnormalities in neurologically intact adults with sickle cell anemia. *Journal of the American Medical Association, 303,* 1823–1831.

Virginia Sickle Cell Awareness Program (2006). *Understanding the child with sickle cell disease: A handbook for school personnel.* Richmond: Virginia Department of Health. Available online at http://www.vdh.virginia.gov/ofhs/childandfamily/childhealth/cshcn/sickleCell/publications.htm.

Viswanathan, A., Gschwendtner, A., Guichard, J. P., Buffon, F., Curmurduc, R., O'Sullivan, M.,... Chabriat, H. (2007). Lacunar lesions are independently associated with disability and cognitive impairment in CADASIL. *Neurology, 69,* 172–179.

Wang, W. C. (2007). Central nervous system complications of sickle cell disease in children: An overview. *Child Neuropsychology, 13,* 103–119.

Wang, W. C., Enos, L., Gallagher, D., Thompson, R., Guarini, L., Vichinsky, E.,... Armstrong, F. D., for the Cooperative Study of Sickle Cell Disease. (2001). Neuropsychologic performance in school-aged children with sickle cell disease: A report from the Cooperative Study of Sickle Cell Disease. *Journal of Pediatrics, 139,* 391–397.

Wang, W. C., Pavlakis, S. G., Helton, K. J., McKinstry, R. C., Casella, J. F., Adams, R. J., & Rees, R. C. for the BABY HUG Investigators. (2008). MRI abnormalities of the brain in one-year-old children with sickle cell anemia. *Pediatric Blood and Cancer, 51,* 643–646.

White, D. A., & DeBaun, M. (1998). Cognitive and behavioral function in children with sickle cell disease: A review and discussion of methodological issues. *Journal of Pediatric Hematology/Oncology, 20,* 458–462.

Wills, K., Nwaneri, O., Nelson, S., & the SCD-PLANE team. (February 19, 2009). *Early Findings from SCD-PLANE (Sickle Cell Disease Program for Learning and Neuropsychological Evaluation, Children's Hospitals and Clinics of Minnesota).* Presented at the Third Annual Sickle Cell Disease Scientific Meeting, Fort Lauderdale, FL.

Wills, K. E., Nelson, S. C., Hennessy, J., Nwaneri, M. O., Miskowiec, J., McDonough, E., & Moquist, K. (2010). Transition planning for youth with sickle cell disease: Embedding neuropsychological assessment into comprehensive care. *Pediatrics, 126,* S151–S159.

Wilson, B. J., Forrest, K., van Teijlingen, E. R., McKee, L., Haites, N., Matthews, E., & Simpson, S. (2004). Family communication about genetic risk: The little that is known. *Community Genetics, 7,* 15–24.

Wright, R. J., & Subramanian, S. V. (2007). Advancing a multilevel framework for epidemiologic research on asthma disparities. *Chest, 132,* 757S–769S.

Yerys, B. E., White, D. A., Salorio, C. F., McKinstry, R., Moinuddin, A., & DeBaun, M. (2003). Memory strategy training in children with cerebral infarcts related to sickle cell disease. *Journal of Pediatric Hematology/Oncology, 25,* 495–498.

14 Spina Bifida/ Hydrocephalus

T. Andrew Zabel, Lisa Jacobson, and
E. Mark Mahone

HISTORICAL MEDICAL PERSPECTIVE

Spina bifida refers to an incomplete closure of the the spinal canal, and frequently requires surgical correction of a protrusion of the meninges (i.e., meningocele) and the spinal cord itself (i.e., myelomeningocele) outside of the spinal column. It is the only neural tube defect compatible with life. Spina bifida is frequently accompanied by significant neurologic complications including hydrocephalus, Chiari malformations, callosal dysgenesis, and posterior white matter disruption, as well as substantial medical complications such as neurogenic bowel and bladder (Charney, 1992; Northrup & Volcik, 2000). The prognosis associated with spina bifida has changed markedly over the past 50 years, particularly with respect to mortality, cognitive functioning, and quality of life. During the 1950s, the vast majority of infants born with myelomeningocele died within the first year of life (Laurence, 1974). Improvements in care and medical technologies in the 1960s resulted in a reduction in mortality rate, with infant and/or early childhood mortality rates reported to be between 30% and 40% (Smith & Smith, 1973; Oakeshott, Hunt, Poulton, & Reid, 2010). This increased survival rate was due in great part to critical breakthroughs in the care of individuals with spina bifida occurring during this period. The first of these involved the treatment of hydrocephalus, which changed dramatically with the collaborative innovation of a high-school–educated mechanic, John Holter, and a neurosurgeon, Eugene Spitz. In the late 1950s, their pioneering valve design (combined with the simultaneous invention of silicone) resulted in the development of an implantable one-way shunt to treat hydrocephalus (Aschoff, Kremer, Hashemi, & Kunze, 1999; Boockvar, Loudon, & Sutton, 2001). Because approximately 80% of individuals with spina bifida have hydrocephalus (McLone, 1989), the development of an effective shunting method was a major contribution to further increased survival rates in spina bifida in the 1970s, particularly with respect to a reduction of death during infancy (Davis et al., 2005).

Reductions in mortality rates shifted attention to functional outcomes, with retrospective case series from the 1960s and early 1970s reportedly showing associations between poor prognostic indicators (e.g., gross paralysis of the legs, thoracolumbar lesions, grossly enlarged head, other birth injuries or congenital abnormalities) and severe levels of impairment, defined as "extensive, crippling, multisystem handicaps" and/or intellectual disability (Lorber, 1971; Lorber, 1972). Based upon these data and other prognostic indicators, neurosurgeons frequently faced the controversial decision of treatment versus selective nontreatment of infants born with spina bifida, involving the withholding of surgical intervention and other types of treatment in cases identified with an "unfavorable prognosis" (Lorber & Salfield, 1981). This disputed practice declined in the United States in the 1980s due to improving medical technologies combined with rising ethical and legal challenges presented to selective treatment practices. Controversy peaked (Freeman, 1984; McLone, 1986) following the scientific publication of the "Oklahoma Experiment" (Gross, Cox, Tatyrek, Pollay, & Barnes, 1983) in which 22 infants with myelomeningocele died after the decision was made to provide only "supportive care." Although now largely prohibited by legislation in the United States and elsewhere, the practice of selective infant euthanasia remains legal in the Netherlands, with 22 cases reported in the late 1990s and early 2000s. Each case involved a child with a severe form of spina bifida and was justified under the Groningen Protocol, that is, the presence of "hopeless and unbearable suffering" (Verhagen & Sauer, 2005).

Mortality rates continued to decline from the late 1970s through the late 1990s with respect to congenital hydrocephalus (66% mortality decline) and spina bifida with hydrocephalus (30% mortality decline) (Chi, Fullerton, & Gupta, 2005). Several additional breakthroughs in treatment of co-occurring conditions are thought to have greatly increased survivability. First, the introduction of clean intermittent catheterization practices by Lapides and colleagues (1976) in the 1970s provided an effective way to manage the complications of a neurogenic bladder as well as reduce the life-threatening risk of urinary tract infections and related renal complications. Second, the introduction of widespread use of a vaccine to combat *Haemophilus influenzae* type B (Hib), the leading cause of meningitis in the United States in the 1980s, spurred a >99% decline in Hib disease (Centers for Disease Control and Prevention, 2008). This vaccine proved to be of protective benefit to children, in general, but particularly to children with shunted hydrocephalus who were at elevated risk for meningitis due to frequent surgical interventions. Third, the ongoing development and refinement of neuroimaging technologies were instrumental in rapid identification of ventricular, brainstem, and spinal cord complications. The advent of magnetic resonance imaging in the mid-1980s (Vogl, Ring-Mrozik, Baierl, Vogl, & Zimmermann, 1987) represented a particularly important step forward. Emerging technologies and practices may further improve both survival and prognosis. One recent development is the prenatal surgical correction of myelomeningocele. Although initial results indicated improved motor outcome and a reduction in the need for shunting in these patients (Adzick et al., 2011), the procedure increases risk of preterm birth and is controversial.

Coupled with the increased survivability of spina bifida as a condition, the rate of births with neural tube defects (including spina bifida) has declined significantly since the late 1990s (Williams, Rasmussen, Flores, Kirby, & Edmonds, 2005). This reduction has been linked to the US Food and Drug Administration's requirement that folic acid be added to all cereal grain products beginning in 1998 (Centers for Disease Control and Prevention, 2004). Data from the National Birth Defects Prevention Network from 2003 to 2004 indicate an overall prevalence of 3.39 cases of spina bifida per 10,000 live births in the "mandatory fortification" era (Boulet et al., 2008). Comparison of "pre-fortification" and "mandatory fortification" incidence estimates of spina bifida suggests declines for Hispanics (6.49–4.18 per 10,000 live births), non-Hispanic whites (5.13–3.37 per 10,000), and non-Hispanic blacks (3.57–2.90 per 10,000) (Tennant, Pearce, Bythell, & Rankin, 2010). In addition to nutritional fortification, improvements in prenatal testing and detection and subsequent elective pregnancy termination have also contributed to the decline in incidence of spina bifida.

Estimates based on longitudinal research beginning in the late 1990s suggest that 75% of individuals born with spina bifida (myelomeningocele) can now be expected to survive into early adulthood (Bowman, McLone, Grant, Tomita, & Ito, 2001). Although encouraging, this still represents a much higher mortality rate than the national average (Strauss, 2010). Survival rate disparities have been noted in youth with spina bifida at age 1 year based upon the presence (56.2%) or absence (87.8%) of hydrocephalus, and these discrepancies continued to be noted at the 20-year follow-up (survival rates of 50% and 86.7%, respectively) (Tennant et al., 2010). Between the ages of 5 years and 40 years, Oakeshott and colleagues (2010) found the highest mortality rates in individuals with spina bifida having high lesion levels; the most common causes of death were epilepsy, pulmonary embolus, acute hydrocephalus, and acute renal sepsis.

In short, the incidence of spina bifida has declined over time and the life expectancy of individuals with this condition has increased considerably. Although transition issues such as education (Welbourn, 1975), independent living (Castree & Walker, 1981), and employment (Tew, Laurence, & Jenkins, 1990) received early attention in the research literature, recently there has been a more concentrated effort to understand and address the complex condition-related impact of spina bifida upon adolescent and young adult development. Notably, governmental resources were formally allocated to these transition issues in 2003 via the establishment of the National Spina Bifida Program at the National Center for Birth Defects and Developmental Disabilities at the Centers for Disease Control and Prevention (Thibadeau, Alriksson-Schmidt, & Zabel, 2010).

EARLY PSYCHOLOGICAL AND NEUROPSYCHOLOGICAL FINDINGS

With increased rates of survival, the focus shifted from mortality to morbidity, with a growing emphasis on the cognitive development of children with spina bifida. Early research on cognitive functions associated with spina bifida focused mostly on gross assessment of function such as IQ. Over the past 20 years, however, it has become clear that the cognitive profiles of these individuals are complex, dynamic, and at times unstable (Mahone & Slomine, 2008). Published research has begun to emphasize the broader range of neuropsychological functioning in these children.

Early research found the intellectual functioning of many youth with spina bifida to fall largely within normal limits (Mawdsley, Rickham, & Roberts, 1967; Laurence & Tew, 1971), and recent evidence continues to confirm this finding (Fletcher et al., 2005). Early studies of brain–behavior relationships in those diagnosed as having spina bifida during the 1970s mostly focused on characteristics of spina bifida that might explain intellectual variability between individuals. For instance, linkages were proposed and demonstrated between intelligence and the presence/ absence of hydrocephalus in youth with spina bifida (Smith & Smith, 1973; Tew, 1977), and shunted hydrocephalus has remained a robust variable in more current spina bifida research examining cognitive and intellectual functioning (e.g., Iddon, Morgan, Loveday, Sahankian, & Pickard, 2004). Associations between high spinal lesion level and low IQ were also identified in the early 1970s (Hunt, Lewin, Gleave, & Gairdner, 1973), and higher level lesions in spina bifida continue to be linked with poorer neurocognitive outcomes (Fletcher et al., 2005). Other early brain–behavior hypotheses were less fruitful, including the proposed relation between IQ and the thickness of the cerebral mantle in those patients with hydrocephalus (Ivan, Stratford, Gerrard, & Weder, 1968; Young, Nulsen, Weiss, & Thomas, 1973). In general, ventricular volume and thickness of cerebral mantle have not proven to be as strongly correlated with intelligence in spina bifida patients as originally proposed (Hommet et al., 2002; Warf et al., 2009), although more sophisticated imaging methods have recently revealed brain–behavior relationships involving reduced cortical volume in some regions and increased cortical thickness in others (Juranek et al., 2008).

A somewhat more refined neuropsychological approach that emerged in the late 1970s identified specific deficits in perceptual–motor functioning (Soare & Raimondi, 1977). This was followed shortly thereafter by additional inquiry into variation within the intellectual profile of youth with spina bifida and/or hydrocephalus, that is, Verbal IQ (VIQ) being stronger than Performance IQ (PIQ) (Dennis et al., 1981; Hurley, Laatsch, & Dorman, 1983; Fletcher, Francis, Thompson, Davidson, & Miner, 1992). The profile associated with shunted hydrocephalus (e.g., VIQ>PIQ, poor visual perceptual skills) was soon subsumed under the broader construct of nonverbal learning disability (NLD) (Fletcher, Brookshire, Bohan, Brandt, & Davidson, 1995), and to a great extent spina bifida was also included in the NLD conceptual model. In some individuals with spina bifida, the nonverbal learning disability model has been found to be a good "fit" (Yeates, Loss, Colvin, & Enrile, 2003; Ris et al., 2007; Yeates et al., 2007). However, the appropriateness of the NLD model for spina bifida continues to be debated due to variability in the pattern of cognitive deficits and assets frequently seen in individuals with spina bifida as well as their significant phenotypic heterogeneity.

At least a portion of the debate over the appropriateness of the NLD model for spina bifida comes from the evidence of language-based deficits observed with some frequency in this condition. As spina bifida became an increasingly survivable condition beginning in the 1970s, verbal deficits and/or difficulties were described, including the now infamous "cocktail party syndrome" (Tew & Laurence, 1979), which is characterized by a pattern of reduced meaningful language content despite prolific speech production. Over time, research continued to highlight language-based deficits in those with spina bifida, including in verbal narrative (Dennis, Jacennik, & Barnes,

1994), verb generation accuracy (Dennis et al., 2008), and verbal learning (Cull & Wyke, 1984; Scott et al., 1998).

In response to the mixed pattern of functional assets and deficits in both verbal and nonverbal content seen in spina bifida, Dennis and colleagues proposed a specific "phenotype of spina bifida" (Dennis, Landry, Barnes, & Fletcher, 2006; Dennis & Barnes, 2010). Both the NLD and spina bifida phenotype models link cognitive deficits in spina bifida to the commonly occurring symptom triad of hydrocephalus, posterior white matter disruption, and abnormalities of the corpus callosum. However, the spina bifida phenotype model also links general and domain-specific cognitive deficits to brain dysmorphology specific to individuals with spina bifida, that is, abnormal midbrain and cerebellar structures associated with the Chiari II malformation (Dennis & Barnes, 2010). The contributing role of the Chiari II malformation may be unique to the neuropsychological presentation of spina bifida (Vinck, Maassen, Mullaart, & Rotteveel, 2006) and not related to other conditions typically subsumed under the umbrella of NLD. As such, the debate between proponents of generalized (NLD) and specific (spina bifida phenotype) models to explain the learning needs and functional deficits of individuals with spina bifida is ongoing.

Another recent development in spina bifida research has been an increased focus on executive function. Executive dysfunction in individuals with spina bifida and shunted hydrocephalus was originally noted by Fletcher and colleagues (1995) and has subsequently been demonstrated via parent report methods by Mahone and colleagues (Mahone, Zabel, Levey, Verda, & Kinsman, 2002; Tarazi, Zabel, & Mahone, 2008; Zabel et al., 2011) as well as by Brown et al. (2008). Research utilizing parent report methodology has frequently identified deficits in "cognitive" aspects of executive functioning (e.g., initiation, working memory, planning and organization), while behavioral and affective regulation is less frequently identified as an area of concern (Mahone et al., 2002). Performance-based measures (Rose & Holmbeck, 2007) of executive functioning have also revealed deficits in youth with spina bifida, with executive findings linked to social difficulties characteristic of this medical population.

RECENT PSYCHOLOGICAL AND NEUROPSYCHOLOGICAL FINDINGS

Increased survivability of spina bifida and obstructive hydrocephalus has permitted a conceptual shift in thinking within neuropsychology, with these now largely considered lifespan conditions rather than exclusively pediatric conditions. The majority of research on spina bifida, however, has been conducted in children and adolescents, with only a recent focus on neuropsychological functioning of adults with spina bifida. The learning disorders associated with childhood spina bifida have lifespan implications. As this research literature has accrued, developmental trends and trajectories have been identified, allowing for early identification of neuropsychological issues as well as increasing understanding of distal outcomes of these early deficits. Longitudinal research suggests that youth with spina bifida acquire the majority of general functional autonomy skills between 2 and 5 years later than typically developing youth (Davis, Shurtleff, Walker, Seidel, & Duguay, 2006). To date, the trajectories of "lifespan" neuropsychological delays and deficits have been best demonstrated in reading, math, and attention/executive functioning; these are presented below as well as in Table 14.1.

Table 14.1 Quick reference sheet for educators of individuals with spina bifida

	Summary	Preschool/Early Elementary School	Later Elementary School	Middle School/High School	College/Young Adulthood
Reading	While sight word reading and decoding can be a problem, they are often much better developed than reading comprehension skills. Isolated reading disability (achievement <25%ile) in children with SB is rare (~3%), while patterns of combined reading/math disabilities are common (26%)	Letter knowledge, sight word reading, and pseudoword decoding are often areas of relative strength in SB. These strengths in basic reading often mask the emergence of reading comprehension difficulties at later ages.	Sight word reading and decoding remain relative strengths for children with SB during elementary school, but difficulties in reading comprehension often become increasingly apparent with grade. Reading comprehension skills are typically strongest at the sentence level, but can be quickly overwhelmed by the integrative demands of reading paragraphs and longer texts.	Word reading strengths typically persist in later grades. Reading comprehension difficulties, however, remain common when youth with SB are required to construct meaning, integrate information, and draw inferences from paragraphs and longer texts.	Reading comprehension often remains less developed than word reading accuracy in many adults with SB. Problems with inferential comprehension may persist. Functional reading skills are often adequate for daily adult life. Stronger reading and math skills are associated with a broader range of life experiences in adulthood for individuals with SB.
Math	Math disability is a common area of lifetime difficulty in SB. Estimates suggest that 29% of children with SB have an isolated math learning disability (achievement <25%ile), and an additional 26% have math and reading disabilities. Math disability can be identified at an early age.	One-to-one counting correspondence, rote counting, and matching-based-on-quantity are common areas of early math difficulty. Preschool screening of these number sense skills is a useful way to identify children with SB at risk for math disability who may require intervention.	Math fact retrieval is often intact in youth with SB, but may be performed more slowly or performed using less-mature counting strategies (e.g., finger counting, "counting up"). Math procedures (e.g., "borrowing from zero" during subtraction) can be areas of difficulty, and may result from periodic attentional "slips" and/or from an overt lack of procedural math knowledge.	Math becomes increasingly complex in higher grades, and topics such as geometry and estimation place increased demands upon common areas of cognitive weakness in SB, e.g., working memory, executive functions, mental manipulation of visual / spatial information.	Difficulties in computation accuracy, speed, math problem solving, and functional numeracy can persist, and can interfere with "real world" functional skills such as price comparisons, value of coins, banking and budgeting, and time concepts. To a greater extent than functional literacy, functional math skills are related to self-reported levels of social and personal autonomy in SB.

Executive Functions				
ADHD in youth with SB falls at around 33%, with inattentive type most frequently noted. Many youth with SB struggle with task initiation, planning, and organization.	Children with SB often respond well to the routine of early classroom structures, including "built-in" prompts and step-by-step directions.	The transition into third and fourth grades (e.g., "reading to learn" instead of "learning to read") places additional organizational demands upon children with SB, and this change in expectations often "unmasks" underlying difficulties in executive functions.	Transition into middle school puts added organizational demands upon youth with SB, and often includes extra tasks (e.g., catheterization) they must "remember" to remember" to complete.	Executive functioning difficulties appear to persist into young adulthood in many individuals with SB, and should be actively accounted for in the process of transition into college or work settings.
Processing				
Strength is often seen in the ability to form associations (e.g., _associative processing_) such as forming associations between words and their definitions. Weaknesses often occur in the ability to integrate information (e.g., _assembled processing_).	Strengths in _forming associations_ often support the development of good functional language skills, categorical knowledge, and age-appropriate word reading abilities in children with SB.	In early adolescence, youth with SB often find it increasingly difficult to comprehend complex oral and written language. This is most evident when oral or written communication requires the active construction of meaning and the _integration_ of multiple sources of information, e.g., word definitions, social context, etc.	Difficulty _integrating_ information can disrupt social competence, particularly if the adolescent with SB has trouble using past and current social experiences to assess how well he or she is being received by others.	While young adults with SB often report high quality of life, many also report social participation restrictions, unemployment, and difficulty moving into more independent living arrangements. For these reasons, school-based efforts to address processing concerns and learning difficulties prior to young adulthood are essential.

Source: Zabel, T.A., & Raches, D. (2010). Used with permission of the Spina Bifida Association

Reading

Considerable research has focused on reading skills in individuals with spina bifida. Isolated reading disability (achievement <25th percentile) in children with spina bifida is rare (~3%), while patterns of combined reading/math disabilities are far more common (26%) (Fletcher et al., 2005). Basic reading skills and reading "mechanics" such as letter knowledge, sight word reading, phonological decoding, and reading fluency are often areas of relative strength in students with shunted hydrocephalus and spina bifida (Barnes & Dennis, 1992; Barnes, Faulkner, & Dennis, 2001). Interestingly, there is emerging evidence for possible structural and functional brain reorganization in this condition to preserve language and word decoding abilities. For example, reductions in inferior parietal and posterior temporal volumes and increases in left middle frontal areas as well as increased left posterior temporal and inferior parietal gyral complexity have been identified (Simos et al., 2011). Because the acquisition of early basic reading skills often follows typical educational trajectories in children with spina bifida, reading concerns are frequently not evident or identified in early elementary school grades.

These strengths in basic reading, however, often mask the emergence of substantial reading comprehension difficulties at later ages, and many such difficulties frequently go un- or underrecognized across the educational process. Sight word reading and decoding may remain relative strengths during elementary school, but difficulties in reading comprehension often become increasingly apparent as children advance through school (Barnes & Dennis, 1992; Barnes, Dennis, & Hetherington, 2004). Further complicating identification of problems in this area, reading comprehension skills are typically strongest at the sentence level but markedly weaker for reading paragraphs and longer texts (Barnes & Dennis, 1996; Barnes & Dennis, 1998; Barnes et al., 2004). During middle and high school, reading comprehension difficulties become particularly evident when youth with spina bifida are required to construct meaning, integrate information, and draw inferences from paragraphs and longer texts (Barnes et al., 2004). Although the reading skills of adults with spina bifida have received less attention, the same pattern persists into adulthood: reading comprehension often remains less well developed than word reading accuracy (Barnes et al., 2004). Encouragingly, functional reading skills in individuals with spina bifida are often adequate for daily adult life, and reading comprehension skills can approach age-appropriate levels by adulthood (Barnes et al., 2004). Development of these skills is critical because stronger reading and math skills have been associated with a broader range of life experiences in adulthood for individuals with spina bifida (English, Barnes, Taylor, & Landry, 2009).

Math

Math disability is a common area of lifetime difficulty in spina bifida and appears to have a pervasive and persistent pattern of disruption to academic progress of many individuals with spina bifida (Ayr, Yeates, & Enrile, 2005), even among those who are good readers (Barnes et al., 2002). Estimates suggest that 29% of children with spina bifida have an isolated math learning disability (achievement <25th percentile) and an additional 26% have math and reading disabilities (Fletcher et al., 2005), resulting in the staggering estimate of math learning difficulties in more than half of all individuals with spina bifida. Development of math abilities is postulated to depend upon intact visual–perceptual and visuospatial skills (Raghubar, Barnes, & Hecht, 2010), visual–spatial working memory (e.g., Bull, Espy, & Wiebe, 2008), fine motor dexterity and coordination (Alibali & DiRusso, 1999; Penner-Wilger et al., 2007), and language-based skills such as vocabulary knowledge, verbal working memory, and phonological skills (Raghubar, Barnes, & Hecht, 2010). These skills depend in large part upon a combination of intact posterior parietal, posterior temporal, and prefrontal areas, as well as cerebellar structures, with clear involvement of the white matter connections that link these areas into an efficient problem-solving network. Notably, many of these regions have been implicated in spina bifida, with cerebellar and posterior white matter disruptions quite common. Not surprisingly, many of the skills believed to be critical for development of foundational math competence are areas of particular weakness in spina bifida.

One of the more important research achievements in this area has been the development of methods of early identification of math disability, particularly early indicators that can be screened prior to or near the beginning of formal education. These early indicators include weaknesses in early number sense, one-to-one counting correspondence, rote counting, and matching-based-on-quantity. Preschool screening of these skills has been shown to be a useful way to identify children with spina bifida at the highest risk for math disability and who may require intervention to prevent later failure (Barnes, Smith-Chant, & Landry, 2005). During elementary school, although math fact retrieval is often intact in youth with spina bifida, it may be performed more slowly or performed using less mature counting strategies (e.g., finger counting, "counting up") (Barnes et al., 2006). Procedural math skills (e.g., subtraction with regrouping) frequently continue to be areas of difficulty, resulting from periodic attentional "slips" and/or from an overt lack of procedural math knowledge (Barnes et al., 2006). Although basic word reading is thought to become less effortful over time as skills become increasingly automatic, Barnes and colleagues (2009) have proposed that math actually becomes increasingly complex over time, with increasing demands placed upon executive processes in higher-level curricula. Thus, as topics such as geometry and estimation place greater demands upon common areas of cognitive weakness in spina bifida, for example, working memory, executive functions, and mental manipulation of visual–spatial information (Dennis & Barnes, 2002; English, Barnes, Taylor, & Landry, 2009), students with spina bifida may fall further and further behind in these math content areas.

Growing evidence suggests that early math is the skill area most predictive of later academic success (e.g., Duncan et al., 2007), putting children with spina bifida who have math difficulties at substantial risk for poor academic outcomes. During the adult years, specific difficulties in computation accuracy, speed, math problem-solving, and functional numeracy may persist and interfere with "real-world" functional skills such as price comparisons, value of coins, banking and budgeting, and time estimation (English, Barnes, Taylor, & Landry, 2009). To a greater extent than functional literacy, functional math skills in adults with spina bifida have been shown to be related to self-reported levels of social and personal autonomy as well as adaptive competence (English, Barnes, Taylor, & Landry, 2009; Hetherington, Dennis, Barnes, Drake, & Gentili, 2006). Although both reading and math can be areas of difficulty in spina bifida, the majority of evidence suggests that math disabilities are more pervasive in this clinical population and have a more profound negative impact upon functioning both during childhood and at older ages. Thus, although assessment of learning disabilities is typically considered to fall within the purview of pediatric specialists, these areas of difficulty have far-reaching effects on young adults with spina bifida and should be of concern to providers across the lifespan.

Attention and Executive Functions

Attention difficulties, particularly those implicating posterior attentional systems (Brewer, Fletcher, Hiscock, & Davidson, 2001), and executive dysfunction (Brown et al., 2008) have been well documented in children and adolescents with spina bifida (Fletcher et al., 1996) and appear to be linked to a wide range of behavioral, academic, and social difficulties (Loss, Yeates, & Enrile, 1998). Further, the incidence of attention-deficit/hyperactivity disorder (ADHD) in those with spina bifida is approximately 30% (Fletcher et al., 2005), with the primarily inattentive type most frequent. Moreover, the parents of many youth with spina bifida report significant concerns with specific areas of executive functioning consistent with those seen in youth with ADHD, including task initiation, planning, and organization (Mahone et al., 2002; Brown et al., 2008; Tarazi et al., 2008). This combination of attentional and executive deficits put youth with spina bifida at particular risk of negative outcomes, including social difficulties (Rose & Holmbeck, 2007) because executive skills, particularly inhibitory control and working memory, have been shown to be critical to young children's intellectual development (Hongwanishkul, Happeney, Lee, & Zelazo, 2005) and both early and later academic success (Barkley, Grodzinsky, & Du Paul, 1992; Blair & Razza, 2007; Jacobson, Williford, & Pianta, 2011).

The traditional school setting demands an increasingly complex array of executive skills from children, including attentional regulation (i.e., attending to instruction and ignoring distractions), inhibition of impulsive responding, verbal working memory (i.e., multitasking or remembering multi-step instructions), and task approach skills (i.e., determining how to initiate a task or to break more complex tasks into manageable pieces). The structure of the classroom in the primary grades is often explicitly designed to support children's developing ability to transition smoothly between activities and events: teachers provide clear advance warning of upcoming transitions, give specific reminders of expected behavior, and anticipate areas of difficulty and plan accordingly. Often, these behavioral strategies are accompanied by concrete language, single-step directions, wait time between tasks, and assistance as needed. All these supports serve to reduce concurrent executive functioning demands and increase students' readiness and availability for learning (Jacobson & Mahone, 2012). Children with spina bifida often respond well to the routine of early classroom structure, including automatization of basic skills over time via frequent repetition and practice, "built-in" prompts, and step-by-step directions. By third and fourth grade, however, instruction shifts from a "learning to learn" or "learning to read" model to a model requiring application and integration of prior knowledge ("reading to learn"). By fourth grade, assignments routinely require multiple steps, narrative responses, integration of oral language and writing, and inferential ("beyond the text") thinking (Holmes, 1987). Similarly, fourth grade textbooks typically rely on expository rather than narrative language, with no explicit template to aid comprehension and recall. These more complex tasks and assignments place an increased demand on children's developing executive functioning skills (Jacobson & Mahone, 2012). These changes place additional executive demands upon children with spina bifida, often "unmasking" underlying difficulties in executive functions and creating a diagnostic question of decline in functioning versus inability to meet age-typical increases in environmental expectations.

As youth with spina bifida transition into middle school, already at risk by virtue of academic and executive difficulties, expectations increase sharply for independent management of materials, assignments, work completion, and belongings (Akos, Queen, & Lineberry, 2005; Rudolph, Lambert, Clark, & Kurlakowsky, 2001). These changes also include increases in the number of teachers, decreases in perceived teacher support, increases in class size, changes in peer networks, and increased expectations for individual responsibility, along with increased exposure to the potential for delinquent behavior (Akos, Queen, & Lineberry, 2005; Rudolph, Lambert, Clark, & Kurlakowsky, 2001), which place even greater executive demands upon youth with spina bifida. Additionally, those with spina bifida often have the additional executive burden of managing their self-care appropriately via extra tasks (e.g., catheterization) that they must "remember to remember" to complete. Executive functioning difficulties appear to persist into young adulthood in many individuals with spina bifida (Tarazi et al., 2008; Zabel et al., 2011) and should be actively accounted for in the process of transition into college or work settings.

Investigations are ongoing with regard to the neurologic correlates of attentional and executive dysregulation common with spina bifida. Recent evidence suggests that although there appears to be substantial heterogeneity in the nature and severity of structural abnormalities in youth with spina bifida, myelination defects and deterioration of axonal structure are evident, with particular impact upon long-range white matter connections including the arcuate fasciculus and uncinate fasciculus (Hasan et al., 2008). Furthermore, the findings of cerebellar, callosal, and posterior white matter disruptions in spina bifida suggest that there are differences in intra- and inter-hemispheric regulation and communication. Because intact cognitive control of information and behavioral reactions requires efficient communication among multiple brain regions, evidence suggests both structural and functional differences in brain connectivity put individuals with spina bifida at greater risk for executive dysfunction.

Medical Self-Management

Although most children with spina bifida now survive into young adulthood (Wong & Paulozzi, 2001), they remain at high risk for a number of co-occurring conditions, including hydrocephalus, tethered cord, neurogenic bladder and bowel, lower extremity paralysis, and seizures (Charney, 1992; Northrup & Volcik, 2000). These conditions create a unique, spina bifida disease-specific constellation of challenges that add additional self-care burden to the functioning of these individuals. For example, prevention of bladder voiding complications often requires clean intermittent catheterization at regular intervals to maintain bladder and kidney function. Furthermore, lower extremity sensory loss frequently necessitates regular self-inspection for pressure ulcers as well as proactive implementation of prophylactic exercises (e.g., wheelchair push-ups).

The atypical self-care competencies associated with spina bifida combined with the features of executive dysfunction create a unique medical self-management dilemma. Specifically, individuals with spina bifida are faced with increased adaptive skill requirements, while presenting with impairments in the executive abilities thought to be necessary for consistent self-care implementation in general.

For example, difficulties with "remembering to remember" to initiate skills such as clean intermittent self-catheterization are commonly reported by parents. These self-care "lapses" may be more likely to occur when naturally occurring cues are not available (e.g., on the weekend when the youth with spina bifida has difficulty remembering to complete catheterization in the afternoon, even though he or she routinely does so upon returning home from school). Parents may help compensate for lack of naturally occurring cues for completing spina bifida–related self-care competencies via verbal prompts or reminders. However, this may leave the youth ill equipped to assume self-care responsibilities upon moving out of a supportive family home. Further complicating the clinical picture, demands for executive function skills typically increase with older age, as greater levels of independent problem solving and behavioral self-regulation are expected as the adolescent approaches adulthood (Tarazi et al., 2008). Thus, finding ways to use novel technologies to provide continued cues and "executive assistance" for young adults with spina bifida may help them to better manage their medical self-care needs independently, improving adaptive outcomes generally.

CURRENT RESOURCES

Due to higher survival rates and lifespans extending into adulthood, increased attention has been given to the development of self-management and independence skills and the transition into older adolescence and young adulthood (e.g., Buran, Brei, Sawin, Stevens & Neufeld, 2006; Mukherjee, 2007). At present, transition is a major source of concern for the spina bifida community in general because approximately two-thirds of young adults with spina bifida are unemployed, compared with approximately one-fourth of typical young adults between the ages of 18 and 29 years (Blomquist, 2006; Johnson, Dudgeon, Kuehn, Walker, 2007). Furthermore, the majority of adults with spina bifida live with their parents or in other supportive settings (Boudos & Mukherjee, 2008; Johnson et al., 2007). Level of adaptive competence and need for assistance with medical self-care (especially mobility and continence) are key variables of interest (Cate, Kennedy, & Stevenson, 2002) because they have been linked with health-related quality of life and employment status in youth and young adults with spina bifida (Bier, Prince, Tremont, & Msall, 2005; Tew, Laurence, & Jenkins, 1990). For example, early development of locomotion (with or without use of aids) is associated with increased competence in visuospatial skills, compared to those dependent on wheelchairs (Rendeli et al., 2002). As they grow older, individuals with spina bifida who do not achieve an adequate level of adaptive competence are at risk for continued problems as they move into young adulthood, including underemployment, limited independence, limited access to social opportunities, poor self-esteem, and reliance upon federal and state support programs (Boudos & Mukherjee, 2008; Hunt & Oakeshott, 2003; Young et al., 2006). Even those individuals with spina bifida who are able to perform activities of daily living independently often do not engage in the full range of adolescent activities necessary to facilitate the skill development required for the successful transition to adulthood (Buran, Sawin, Brei, & Fastenau, 2004).

Developmental studies suggest that early indications of delays in acquisition of autonomy skills may underlie eventual patterns of underemployment and increased dependence in adulthood, including delays in the development of independent toileting/catheterization (Davis et al., 2006; Schoenmakers, Gulmans, Gooskens, & Helders, 2004). The variables that underlie these delays are likely multifactorial, including physical characteristics of the individual, level of individual knowledge and skill, and cognitive abilities, as well as family supports and knowledge. Executive functioning, especially those skills that support planning, initiating, and problem-solving, have recently been shown to mediate the impact of neurological severity on functional independence (Heffelfinger et al., 2008). Although surgical advances may reduce complications associated with continence procedures and other aspects of self-management, cognitive and executive difficulties will likely continue to affect the initiation and implementation of any atypical self-care tasks that do not present with naturally occurring cues (e.g., sensation of a full bladder). Therefore, a developmental approach remains important in considering normative acquisition of self-care competence across methods of self-management to assist the families of adolescents and young adults with spina bifida to determine needs for intervention and support during the transition into adulthood.

Areas of Need, Future Aims, and Research Opportunities

The growing body of literature describing the incidence and high base rate of learning disabilities in this clinical population justifies increased and possibly universal screening of individuals with spina bifida for specific learning problems, especially those involving math. As noted, estimates suggest that up to half of individuals with spina bifida may have isolated or combined problems in reading and math. Because specific learning disabilities have been associated with less favorable distal outcomes in young adulthood, it must be a priority that learning problems be identified as early as possible in development. Advances in screening methodologies have greatly improved the capability of neuropsychologists and school psychologists to detect early indicators of these learning disabilities in the early elementary grades, and use of these methods is strongly endorsed to facilitate early intervention and/or accommodation. Moreover, targeted screening of math and reading disabilities across the lifespan in individuals with spina bifida (especially around periods of transition) is strongly suggested because specific learning disabilities can manifest in an increasingly disruptive manner with age and changes in age-related educational expectations (e.g., those changes associated with the transition into fourth grade, middle school, high school, and adulthood).

Given the high incidence of learning disabilities in this population, it is unrealistic to presume that all youth with spina bifida can be initially screened for learning problems or executive dysfunction by a neuropsychologist. Moreover, many state and/or private insurance policies do not provide a neuropsychological assessment benefit for individuals with spina bifida. As such, advocacy and lobbying efforts must continue to increase the access of individuals with spina bifida to neuropsychologists familiar with their condition. Moreover, there is also a need for assessment professionals in general to develop a stronger understanding of the "neuropsychology of spina bifida," an improved ability to screen for spina bifida–related cognitive disorders, and an increased appreciation for when referral for additional neuropsychological assessment is necessary. Advocacy groups such as the Spina Bifida Association have made neuropsychological information available to the lay public, including the information presented in Table 14.1, which is reproduced here with their permission.

Additionally, Table 14.2 has been included in this chapter as an example of a means by which parents, physicians, and other invested parties can bring the commonly occurring learning and executive problems of spina bifida to the attention of

Table 14.2 Spina bifida academic riskassessment

Child's Name: _____

	Neurological
• Chiari II Malformation • Shunted Hydrocephalus • Upper spinal lesion level • None of the above	Youth with spina bifida who have any or all of the neurologic features to the left are at risk for intellectual, memory, and academic difficulties.

Check any that apply

	Preschool/Kindergarten
• Math Concerns	During the preschool years, early learning difficulties can be identified before academic performance and/or confidence suffers. Studies show that preschoolers/kindergarteners with spina bifida often have math problems, particularly with early number sense (e.g., counting procedures, quantity comparisons, etc.). It is recommended that school based assessment investigate early number sense using the Test of Early Math Abilities—Third Edition (TEMA-3).
• Reading Concerns	Youth with spina bifida rarely have *isolated* problems in word reading or decoding, but frequently have co-occurring math *and* reading disorders. If math concerns are suspected, early reading skills should be screened as well via a measure of phonological awareness and rapid naming.

Check any that apply

	Elementary School
• Math Concerns	Studies show that elementary school-age youth with spina bifida are at significant risk for math problems, particularly in terms of their math fluency (i.e., math speed) and their ability to learn and/or consistently use math procedures (e.g., renaming, regrouping, division). It is recommended that school based assessment investigate these and others areas of mathematics functioning.
• Reading Concerns	Elementary school-age youth with spina bifida are at significant risk for reading comprehension difficulties, and it is recommended that school-based assessment include a thorough investigation of reading comprehension skills.

Check applicable	Middle/High School
• Math Concerns	Studies show that middle/high school youth with spina bifida are at significant risk for math problems, particularly in terms of math applications such as estimating, problem solving, and geometry. Testing in these and other areas of math functioning is recommended.
• Reading Concerns	Middle/high school-age youth with spina bifida are at significant risk for reading comprehension difficulties, and it is recommended that school-based assessment include a thorough investigation of reading comprehension skills.
	Attention
• Concerns	Recent estimates of the prevalence of ADHD in youth with spina bifida fall around 33%, and this possibility should be carefully considered in school-based assessment.
• No Concerns	
	Executive Functions
• Concerns	Executive functions such as initiation, working memory, organization, and planning are often areas of vulnerability in many youth with spina bifida, and it is recommended that these types of skills be assessed in school-based evaluation.
• No Concerns	
	Depression/Anxiety
• Concerns	Adolescents with spina bifida have fewer positive contexts at school, which may place them at risk for higher levels of depressive symptoms. Screening of mood is recommended.
• No Concerns	

Source: Zabel, T. A. & Day, L., 2011.

community-based assessment providers, such as school psychologists, and facilitate screening efforts. Increased public understanding of the learning and executive problems associated with spina bifida will help bring attention to the need for early identification and intervention/accommodations.

There is a significant need for the development and funding of evidence-based intervention and treatment procedures for those issues most disruptive to the adaptive functioning and life satisfaction of individuals with spina bifida. From an educational perspective, research is needed to further determine whether the reading and math problems experienced by individuals with spina bifida can be addressed with commonly utilized math and reading intervention programs or whether intervention programs specific to spina bifida are necessary. From a self-management perspective, it will be essential to develop intervention and accommodation techniques to help youth and young adults with spina bifida continue to assume greater responsibility for their specialized self-care, despite persisting symptoms of executive dysfunction. Because more "cognitive" aspects of executive functioning are thought to underlie much of the difficulty experienced in assuming full responsibility for specialized self-care tasks (e.g., inconsistent initiation of self-catheterization), it is reasonable to think that rehabilitation technologies focused upon initiation deficits in general may be of considerable use to individuals with spina bifida (Studer, 2007). Rehabilitation technologies may further facilitate the development of self-management skills using technological advances to provide in vivo cueing to accommodate for initiation and prospective memory deficits. Commercially available products, such as smart phones, tablet computing devices, and associated applications, may serve a useful cueing role and could potentially reduce the executive burden associated with spina bifida–related self-management tasks. Moreover, specialized and integrated telemedicine programs such as the Telerehabilitation Enhanced Wellness Program for Spina Bifida, being developed by Andrea Fairman and Brad DiCianno at the University of Pittsburgh, may have an intervention role for the management of this condition as well.

The lack of neuropsychological research involving individuals with spina bifida in their thirties and forties is a major research gap. Unfortunately, spina bifida represents a developmental condition typically characterized as a "childhood disorder," and neuropsychologists specializing in adult and geriatric practice are often unfamiliar with the medical and clinical needs of this population. Although well served by the efforts of pediatric-focused neuropsychology labs, individuals with spina bifida have yet to benefit from a research concentration focused upon aging processes, particularly now that life expectancy has extended well beyond the typical focus of pediatric neuropsychologists. Unfortunately, the neuropsychological deficits frequently noted in individuals with spina bifida hold a high potential for disruption of adult functioning as well as a potential contribution to dementia processes and premature aging. Conceptualizing spina bifida as a "lifespan" condition is an important starting point to focusing the attention and specialized research and assessment practices of both pediatric and adult/geriatric neuropsychologists upon this condition.

Finally, although there have been multiple iterations in the development and refinement of shunt technologies, there has been only minimal improvement made in terms of the failure rate of shunts over time. At the time this chapter was written, a large proportion of shunts continue to fail within several years of being surgically implanted, and it is not uncommon for individuals with different etiologies of hydrocephalus to undergo multiple brain surgeries in their lifetimes (Berry et al., 2008; Cochrane &

Kestle, 2002; Stein & Guo, 2007). Not surprisingly, frequency of shunt revision after age 2 years has been associated with poorer long-term outcome (Hunt, Oakenshott, & Kerry, 1999), although the reason for needing revision may be more pertinent than the number of revisions. This finding represents both a personal and public health burden, and improvements in technology developed nearly 50 years ago are sorely needed.

REFERENCES

Adzick, N. S., Thom, E. A., Spong, C. Y., Brock, J. W., Burrows, P. K., Johnson, M. P., ... Farmer, D. L. (2011). A randomized trial of prenatal versus postnatal repair of myelomeningocele. *New England Journal of Medicine, 364,* 993–1004.

Akos, P., Queen, J. A., & Lineberry, C. (2005). *Promoting a successful transition to middle school.* Larchmont, New York: Eye on Education.

Alibali, M. W., & DiRusso, A. A. (1999). The function of gesture in learning to count: More than keeping track. *Cognitive Development, 14,* 37–56.

Aschoff, A., Kremer, P., Hashemi, B., & Kunze, S. (1999). The scientific history of hydrocephalus and its treatment. *Neurosurgical Review, 22,* 67–93.

Ayr, L. K., Yeates, K. O., & Enrile, B. G. (2005). Arithmetic skills and their cognitive correlates in children with acquired and congenital brain disorder. *Journal of the International Neuropsychological Society, 11,* 249–262.

Barkley, R. A., Grodzinsky, G. M., & Du Paul, G. (1992). Frontal lobe functions in attention deficit disorder with and without hyperactivity: A review and research report. *Journal of Abnormal Child Psychology, 20,* 163–188.

Barnes, M., & Dennis, M. (1992). Reading in children and adolescents after early onset hydrocephalus and in normally developing age peers: Phonological analysis, word recognition, word comprehension, and passage comprehension skill. *Journal of Pediatric Psychology, 17,* 445–465.

Barnes, M. A., & Dennis, M. (1996). Reading comprehension deficits arise from diverse sources: Evidence from readers with and without developmental brain pathology. In C. Cornoldi & J. V. Oakhill (Eds.), *Reading comprehension difficulties: Processes and interventions* (pp. 251–278). Hillsdale, NJ: Erlbaum.

Barnes, M. A., & Dennis, M. (1998). Discourse after early-onset hydrocephalus: Core deficits in children of average intelligence. *Brain & Language, 61,* 309–334.

Barnes, M., Dennis, M., & Hetherington, R. (2004). Reading and writing skills in young adults with spina bifida and hydrocephalus. *Journal of the International Neurological Society, 10,* 655–663.

Barnes, M. A., Faulkner, H. J., & Dennis, M. (2001). Poor reading comprehension despite fast word decoding in children with hydrocephalus. *Brain and Language, 76,* 35–44.

Barnes, M., Pengelly, S., Dennis, M., Wilkinson, M., Rogers, T., & Faulkner, H. (2002). Mathematic skills in good readers with hydrocephalus. *Journal of the International Neuropsychological Society, 8,* 72–82.

Barnes, M. A., Smith-Chant, B., & Landry, S. H. (2005). Number processing in neurodevelopmental disorders: Spina bifida myelomeningocele. In J. D. Cambell (Ed.), *Handbook of mathematical development* (pp. 299–313). New York: Psychology Press.

Barnes, M. A., Wilkinson, M., Khemani, E., Boudesquie, A., Dennis, M., & Fletcher, J. M. (2006). Arithmetic processing in children with spina bifida: Calculation accuracy, strategy use, and face retrieval fluency. *Journal of Learning Disabilities, 39,* 174–187.

Berry, J. G., Hall, M. A., Sharma, V., Goumnerova, L., Slonim, A. D., & Shah, S. S. (2008). A multi-institutional, 5-year analysis of initial and multiple ventricular shunt revisions in children. *Neurosurgery, 62,* 445–453.

Bier, J. B., Prince, A., Tremont, M., & Msall, M. (2005). Medical, functional, and social determinants of health-related quality of life in individuals with myelomeningocele. *Developmental Medicine & Child Neurology, 47,* 609–612.

Blair, C., & Razza, R. P. (2007). Relating effortful control, executive function, and false-belief understanding to emerging math and literacy ability in kindergarten. *Child Development, 78,* 647–663.

Blomquist, K. B. (2006). Health, education, work, and independence of young adults with disabilities. *Orthopedic Nursing, 25,* 168–187.

Boockvar, J. A., Loudon, W., & Sutton, L. N. (2001). Development of the Spitz-Holter value in Philadelphia. *Journal of Neurosurgery, 95,* 145–147.

Boudos, R. M., & Mukherjee, S. (2008). Barriers to community participation: Teens and young adults with spina bifida. *Journal of Pediatric Rehabilitation Medicine: An Interdisciplinary Approach, 1,* 303–310.

Brewer, V. R., Fletcher, J. M., Hiscock, M., & Davidson, K. C. (2001). Attention processes in children with shunted hydrocephalus versus attention deficit-hyperactivity disorder. *Neuropsychology, 15,* 185–198.

Brown, T. M., Ris, M. D., Beebe, D., Ammerman, R. T., Oppenheimer, S. G., Yeates, K. O., & Enrile, B. G. (2008). Factors of biological risk and reserve associated with executive behaviors in children and adolescents with spina bifida myelomeningocele. *Child Neuropsychology, 14,* 118–134.

Boulet, S. L., Yang, Q., Mai, C., Kirby, R. S., Collins, J. S., Robbins, J. M., Meyer, R., Canfield, M. A., & Mulinare, J. (2008). Trends in the postfortification prevalence of spina bifida and anecephaly in the United States. *Birth Defects Research. Part A, Clinical and Molecular Teratology, 82,* 527–532.

Bowman, R. M., McLone, D. G., Grant, J. A., Tomita, T., & Ito, J. A. (2001). Spina bifida outcome: A 25-year prospective. *Pediatric Neurosurgery, 34,* 114–120.

Bull, R., Espy, K. A., & Wiebe, S. A. (2008). Short-term memory, working memory, and executive functioning in preschoolers: Longitudinal predictors of mathematical achievement at 7 years. *Developmental Neuropsychology, 33,* 205–228.

Buran, C. F., Brei, T. J., Sawin, K. J., Stevens, S., & Neufeld, J. (2006). Further development of the adolescent self-management and independence scales: AMIS II. *Cerebrospinal Fluid Research, 3,* S37.

Buran, C., Sawin, K., Brei, T., & Fastenau, P. S. (2004). Adolescents with elomeningocele: Activities, beliefs, expectations, and perceptions. *Developmental Medicine & Child Neurology, 46,* 244–252.

Castree, B. J., & Walker, J. H. (1981). The young adult with spina bifida [special issue]. *British Medical Journal (Clinical Research Edition), 283,* 1040–1042.

Centers for Disease Control and Prevention (2004). Spina bifida and anencephaly before and after folic acid mandate—United States, 1995–1996 and 1999–2000. *Morbidity and Mortality Weekly Report, 53,* 362–365.

Centers for Disease Control and Prevention. (2008). *Haemophilus influenzae* serotype b (Hib) disease. Retrieved June 24, 2011, from http://www.cdc.gov/ncidod/dbmd/diseaseinfo/haeminfluserob_t.htm.

Charney, E. (1992). Neural tube defects: Spina bifida and myelomeningocele. In M. Batshaw & Y. Perret (Eds.), *Children with disabilities: A medical primer,* third edition (pp. 471–488). Baltimore: Brookes Publishing Co.

Chi, J. H., Fullerton, H. J., & Gupta, N. (2005). Time trends and demographics of deaths from congenital hydrocephalus in children in the United States: National Center for Health Statistics data, 1979 to 1998. *Journal of Neurosurgery, 103,* 113–118.

Cochrane, D. D., & Kestle, J. (2002). Ventricular shunting for hydrocephalus in children: Patients, procedures, surgeons and institutions in English Canada, 1989–2001. *European Journal of Pediatric Surgery, 12*, 6–11.

Cull, C., & Wyke, M. A. (1984). Memory function of children with spina bifida and shunted hydrocephalus. *Developmental Medicine and Child Neurology, 26*, 177–183.

Davis, B. E., Daley, C. M., Shurtleff, D. B., Duguay, S., Seidel, K., Loeser, J. D., & Ellenborgen, R. (2005). Long-term survival of individuals with myelomeningocele. *Pediatric Neurosurgery, 41*, 186–191.

Davis, B. E., Shurtleff, D. B., Walker, W. O., Seidel, K. D., & Duguay, S. (2006). Acquisition of autonomy skills in adolescents with myelomeningocele. *Developmental Medicine & Child Neurology, 48*, 253–258.

Dennis, M., & Barnes, M. (2002). Math and numeracy in young adults with spina bifida and hydrocephalus. *Developmental Neuropsychology, 21*, 141–155.

Dennis, M., Fitz, C. R., Netley, C. T., Sugar, J., Harwood-Nash, D. C., Hendrick, E. B.,...Humphreys, R. P. (1981). The intelligence of hydrocephalic children. *Archives of Neurology, 38*, 607–615.

Dennis, M., Jacennik, B., & Barnes, M. A. (1994). The content of narrative discourse in children and adolescents after early-onset hydrocephalus and in normally developing age peers. *Brain and Language, 46*, 129–165.

Dennis, M., Jewell, D., Hetherington, R., Burton, C., Brandt, M. E., Blaser, S. E., & Fletcher, J. M. (2008). Verb generation in children with spina bifida. *Journal of International Neuropsychology Society, 14*, 181–191.

Dennis, M., Landry, S. H., Barnes, M., & Fletcher, J. M. (2006). A model of neurocognitive function in spina bifida over the life span. *Journal of the International Neuropsychological Society, 12*, 285–296.

Duncan, G. J., Dowsett, C. J., Claessens, A., Magnuson, K., Huston, A. C., Klebanov, P.,...Duckworth, K. (2007). School readiness and later achievement. *Developmental Psychology, 43*, 1428–1446.

English, L. H., Barnes, M. A., Taylor, H. B., & Landry, S. H. (2009). Mathematical development in spina bifida. *Developmental Disabilities Research Reviews, 15*, 28–34.

Fletcher, J. M., Brookshire, B. L., Bohan, T. P., Brandt, M. E., & Davidson, K. C. (1995). Early hydrocephalus. In B. P. Rourke (Ed.), *Nonverbal learning disabilities: Neurodevelopmental manifestations* (pp. 206–233). New York: Guilford.

Fletcher, J. M., Brookshire, B. L., Landry, S. H., Bohan, T. P., Davidson, K. C., Francis, D. J.,...Morris, R. D. (1996). Attentional skills and executive functions in children with early hydrocephalus. *Developmental Neuropsychology, 12*, 53–76.

Fletcher, J. M., Copeland, K., Fredercick, J. A., Blaser, S. E., Kramer, L. A., Northrup, H....Dennis, M. (2005). Spinal lesion level in spina bifida: A source of neural and cognitive heterogeneity. *Journal of Neurosurgery, 102*, 268–279.

Freeman, J. M. (1984). Early management and decision making for the treatment of myelomeningocele: A critique. *Pediatrics, 73*, 564–566.

Gross, R. H., Cox, A., Tatyrek, R., Pollay, M., & Barnes, W. A. (1983). Early management and decision making for the treatment of myelomeningocele. *Pediatrics, 72*, 450–458.

Hasan, K. M., Eluvathingal, T. J., Kramer, L. A., Ewing-Cobbs, L., Dennis, M., & Fletcher, J. M. (2008). White matter microstructural abnormalities in children with spina bifida myelomeningocele and hydrocephalus: A diffusion tensor tractography study of the association pathways. *Journal of Magnetic Resonance Imaging, 27*, 700–709.

Heffelfinger, A. K., Koop, J. I., Fastenau, P. S., Brei, T. J., Conant, L., Katzenstein, J.,...Sawin, K. J. (2008). The relationship of neuropsychological functioning to adaptation outcome in adolescents with spina bifida. *Journal of the International Neuropsychological Society, 14,* 793–804.

Hetherington, R., Dennis, M., Barnes, M., Drake, J., & Gentili, F. (2006). Functional outcome in young adults with spina bifida and hydrocephalus. *Childs Nervous System, 22,* 117–124.

Holmes, J. M. (1987). Natural histories in learning disabilities: Neuropsychological difference/environmental demand. In S. J. Ceci (Ed.), *Handbook of cognitive, social and neuropsychological aspects of learning disabilities* (pp. 303–320). Hillsdale, NJ: Lawrence Erlbaum Associates.

Hommet, C., Cottier, J. P., Billard, C., Perrier, D., Gillet, P., De Toffol, B.,…Autret, A. (2002). MRI morphometric study and correlation with cognitive functions in young adults shunted for congenital hydrocephalus related to spina bifida. *European Neurology, 47,* 169–174.

Hongwanishkul, D., Happaney, K. R., Lee, W. S. C., & Zelazo, P. D. (2005). Assessment of hot and cool executive function in young children: Age-related changes and individual differences. *Developmental Neuropsychology, 28,* 617–644.

Hunt, G., Lewin, W., Gleave, J., & Gairdner, D. (1973). Predictive factors in open myelomeningocele with special reference to sensory level. *British Medical Journal, 4,* 197–201.

Hunt, G. M., & Oakeshott, P. (2003). Outcome in people with open spina bifida at age 35: Prospective community based cohort study. *British Medical Journal, 326,* 1365–1366.

Hunt, G. M., Oakeshott, P., & Kerry, S. (1999). Link between the CSF shunt and achievement in adults with spina bifida. *Journal of Neurology, Neurosurgery, and Psychiatry, 67,* 591–595.

Iddon, J. L., Morgan, D. J. R., Loveday, C., Sahakian, B. J., & Pickard, J. D. (2004). Neuropsychological profile of young adults with spina bifida with or without hydrocephalus. *Journal of Neurology, Neurosurgery, and Psychiatry, 75,* 1112–1118.

Ivan, L. P., Stratford, J. G., Gerrard, J. W., & Weder, C. H. (1968). Surgical treatment of infantile hydrocephalus: Ten years' experience in the use of ventriculoatrial shunts with the Holter value. *Canadian Medical Association Journal, 98,* 337–343.

Jacobson, L. A., & Mahone, E. M. (2012). Educational implications of executive dysfunction. In S. J. Hunter & E. P. Sparrow (Eds.), *Executive function and dysfunction: Identification, assessment and treatment* (pp. 232–246). New York: Cambridge University Press.

Jacobson, L. A., Williford, A., & Pianta. R. C. (2011). The role of executive function in children's competent adjustment to middle school. *Child Neuropsychology, 17,* 255–280.

Johnson, K. L., Dudgeon, B., Kuehn, C., Walker, W. (2007). Assistive technology use among adolescents and young adults with spina bifida. *American Journal of Public Health, 97,* 330–336.

Juranek, J., Fletcher, J. M., Hasan, K. M., Breier, J. I., Cirino, P. T., Pazo-Alvarez, P.,…Papanicolaou, A. C. (2008). Neocortical reorganization in spina bifida. *Neuroimage, 40,* 1516–1522.

Lapides, J., Diokno, A. C., Gould, F. R., & Lowe, B. S. (1976). Further observations on self-catheterization. *The Journal of Urology, 116,* 169–171.

Laurence, K. M. (1974). Occasional Survey: Effect of early surgery for spina bifida cystica on survival and quality of life. *Lancet, 303,* 301–304.

Laurence, K. M., & Tew, B. J. (1971). Natural history of spina bifida cystica and cranium bifidum cysticum: Major central nervous system malformations in South Wales, part iv. *Archives of Disease in Childhood, 46,* 127–138.

Lorber, J. (1971). Results of treatment of myelomeningocele: An analysis of 524 unselected cases, with special reference to possible selection for treatment. *Developmental Medicine & Child Neurology, 13,* 279–303.

Lorber, J. (1972). Spina bifida cystica: Results of treatment of 270 consecutive cases with criteria for selection for the future. *Archives of Disease of in Childhood, 47,* 854–873.

Lorber, J., & Salfield, S. A. (1981). Results of selective treatment of spina bifida cystica. *Archives of Disease in Childhood, 56,* 822–830.

Loss, N., Yeates, K. O., & Enrile, B. G. (1998). Attention in children with myelomeningocele. *Child Neuropsychology, 4,* 7–20.

Mahone, E. M., Zabel, T. A., Levey, E., Verda, M., & Kinsman, S. (2002). Parent and self-report ratings of executive function in adolescents with myelomeningocele and hydrocephalus. *Child Neuropsychology, 8,* 258–270.

Mawdsley, T., Rickham, P. P., & Roberts, J. R. (1967). Long-term results of early operation of open myelomeningoceles and encephaloceles. *British Medical Journal, 3541,* 663–666.

McLone, D. G. (1986). Treatment of myelomeningocele: Arguments against selection. *Clinical Neurosurgery, 33,* 359–370.

McLone, D. G. (1989). The cause of Chiari II malformation: A unified theory. *Pediatric Neuroscience, 15,* 1–12.

Mukherjee, S. (2007). Transition to adulthood in spina bifida: Changing roles and expectations. *The Scientific World Journal, 7,* 1890–1895.

Northrup, H., & Volcik, K. A. (2000). Spina bifida and other neural tube defects. *Current Problems in Pediatrics, 30,* 313–332.

Oakeshott, P., Hunt, G. M., Poulton, A., & Reid, F. (2010). Expectation of life and unexpected death in open spina bifida: A 40-year complete, non-selective, longitudinal cohort study. *Developmental Medicine & Child Neurology, 52,* 749–753.

Penner-Wilger, M., Fast, L., LeFevre, J., Smith-Chant, B. L., Skwarchuk, S., Kamawar, D., & Bisanz, J. (2007). The foundations of numeracy: Subitizing, finger gnosia, and fine-motor ability. In D. S. McNamara & J. G. Trafton (Eds.), *Proceedings of the 29th Annual Cognitive Science Society* (pp. 1385–1390). Austin, TX: Cognitive Science Society.

Pit-ten Cate, I. M., Kennedy, C., & Stevenson, J. (2002). Disability and quality of life in spina bifida and hydrocephalus. *Developmental Medicine & Child Neurology, 44,* 317–322.

Raghubar, K. P., Barnes, M. A., & Hecht, S. A. (2010). Working memory and mathematics: A review of developmental, individual difference, and cognitive approaches. *Learning and Individual Differences, 20,* 110–122.

Rendeli, C., Salvaggio, E., Sciascia-Cannizzaro, G., Bianchi, E., Caldarelli, M., & Guzzetta, F. (2002). Does locomotion improve the cognitive profile of children with meningomyelocele? *Child's Nervous System, 18,* 231–234.

Rose, B. M., & Holmbeck, G. N. (2007). Attention and executive functions in adolescents with spina bifida. *Journal of Pediatric Psychology, 32,* 983–994.

Rudolph, K. D., Lambert, S. F., Clark, A. G., & Kurlakowsky, K. D. (2001). Negotiating the transition to middle school: The role of self-regulatory processes. *Child Development, 72,* 929–946.

Schoenmakers, M. A. G. C., Gulmans, V. A. M., Gooskens, R. H. J. M., & Helders, P. J. M. (2004). Spina bifida at the sacral level: More than minor gait disturbances. *Clinical Rehabilitation, 18,* 178–185.

Scott, M. A., Fletcher, J. M., Brookshire, B. L., Davidson, K. C., Landry, S. H., Bohan, T. C.,...Francis, D. J. (1998). Memory functions in children with early hydrocephalus. *Neuropsychology, 12,* 578–589.

Simos, P. G., Papanicolaou, A., Castillo, E. M., Juranek, J., Cirino, P. T., Rezaie, R., & Fletcher, J. M. (2011). Brain mechanisms for reading and language processing in spina bifida meningomyelocele: A combined magnetic source- and structural magnetic resonance imaging study. *Neuropsychology, 25,* 590–601.

Smith, G. K., & Smith, E. D. (1973). Selection for treatment in spina bifida cystica. *British Medical Journals, 4,* 189–197.

Soare, P. L., & Raimondi, A. J. (1977). Intellectual and perceptual-motor characteristics of treated myelomeningocele children. *American Journal of Diseases of Children, 131*, 199–204.

Strauss, D. (2010). Evidence-based life expectancy. *Developmental Medicine & Child Neurology, 52*, 695.

Stein, S. C., & Guo, W. (2007). A mathematical model of survival in a newly inserted ventricular shunt. *Journal of Neurosurgery, 107*, 448–454.

Studer, M. (2007). Rehabilitation of executive function: To err is human, to be aware—divine. *Journal of Neural Transplantation and Plasticity, 31*, 128–134.

Ris, M. D., Ammerman, R. T., Waller, N., Walz, N., Oppenheimer, S., Brown, T. M.,…Yeates, K. O. (2007). Taxonicity of nonverbal learning disabilities in spina bifida. *Journal of International Neuropsychological Society, 13*, 50–58.

Rose, B. M., & Holmbeck, G. N. (2007). Attention and executive functions in adolescents with spina bifida. *Journal of Pediatric Psychology, 32*, 983–994.

Tarazi, R. A., Zabel, T. A., & Mahone, E. M. (2008). Age-related changes in executive function among children with spina bifida/hydrocephalus based on parent behavior ratings. *The Clinical Neuropsychologist, 22*, 585–602.

Tennant, P. W. G., Pearce, M. S., Bythell, M., & Rankin, J. (2010). 20-year survival of children born with congenital anomalies: A population-based study. *Lancet, 375*, 649–656.

Tew, B., Laurence, K. M., & Jenkins, V. (1990). Factors affecting employability among young adults with spina bifida and hydrocephalus [Special issue]. *Zeitschrift fur Kinderchirurgie, 45*, 34–36.

Thibadeau, J. K., Alriksson-Schmidt, A. I., & Zabel, T. A. (2010). The national spina bifida program transition initiative: The people, the plan, and the process. *Pediatric Clinics of North America, 57*, 903–910.

Verhagen, E., & Sauer, P. J. J. (2005). The Groningen protocol—euthanasia in severely ill newborns. *New England Journal of Medicine, 352*, 959–962.

Vinck, A., Maassen, B., Mullaart, R., & Rotteveel, J. (2006). Arnold-Chiari-II malformation and cognitive functioning in spina bifida. *Journal of Neurology, Neurosurgery, and Psychiatry, 77*, 1083–1086.

Vogl, D., Ring-Mrozik, E., Baierl, P., Vogl, T., & Zimmermann, K. (1987). Magnetic resonance imaging in children suffering from spina bifida. *Zeitschrift fur Kinderchirurgie, 42*, 60–64.

Warf, B., Ondoma, S., Kulkarni, A., Donnelly, R., Ampeire, M., Akona, J.,…Nsubuga, B. K. (2009). Neurocognitive outcome and ventricular volume in children with myelomeningocele treated for hydrocephalus in Uganda. *Journal of Neurosurgery: Pediatrics, 4*, 564–570.

Welbourn, H. (1975). Spina bifida children attending ordinary schools. *British Medical Journals, 1*, 142–145.

Williams, L. J., Rasmussen, S. A., Flores, A., Kirby, R. S., & Edmonds, L. D. (2005). Decline in the prevalence of spina bifida and anencephaly by race/ethnicity: 1995–2002. *Pediatrics, 116*, 580–586.

Wong, L. C., & Paulozzi, L. J. (2001). Survival of infants with spina bifida: A population study, 1979–1994. *Paediatric Perinatal Epidemiology, 15*, 374–378.

Yeates, K. O., Loss, N., Colvin, A. N, & Enrile, B. G. (2003). Do children with myelomeningocele and hydrocephalus display nonverbal learning disabilities? An empirical approach to classification. *Journal of the International Neuropsychology Society, 9*, 653–662.

Young, H. F., Nulsen, F. E., Weiss, M. H., & Thomas, P. (1973). The relationship of intelligence and cerebral mantle in treated infantile hydrocephalus (IQ potential in hydrocephalic children). *Pediatrics, 52*, 38–44.

Young, N. L., McCormick, A., Mills, W., Barden, W., Boydell, K.,...& Law, M. (2006). The transition study: A look at youth and adults with cerebral palsy, spina bifida, and acquired brain injury. *Physical and Occupational Therapy in Pediatrics, 26,* 25–45.

Zabel, T. A., Jacobson, L. A., Zachik, C., Levey, E., Kinsman, S., & Mahone, E. M. (2011). Parent- and self-ratings of executive functions in adolescents and young adults with Spina Bifida. *The Clinical Neuropsychologist, 25,* 926–941.

Zabel, T. A., & Raches, D. (2011). Quick Reference Sheet for Educators of Individuals with Spina Bifida. [Brochure]. Retrieved July 15, 2011, from http://www.spinabifidaassociation.org/atf/cf/%7BEED435C8-F1A0–4A16-B4D8-A713BBCD9CE4%7D/Spina BifidaA_Overview_FactSheet.pdf.

Zabel, T. A., & Day, L., (2011). Spina bifida academic risk assessment. Unpublished questionnaire.

15 Traumatic Brain Injury

Michael W. Kirkwood, Robin L. Peterson, and Keith Owen Yeates

Traumatic brain injury (TBI) is a leading cause of morbidity and mortality in youth worldwide. In the United States, among children aged 0–14 years, TBI accounts for approximately 2200 annual deaths, 35,000 hospitalizations, and 474,000 emergency department visits (Faul, Xu, Wald, & Coronado, 2010). The incidence of TBI varies by severity, with mild TBI comprising 80%–90% of all treated pediatric cases (Cassidy et al., 2004). Most children who sustain mild TBI recover well and relatively quickly, although exceptions exist, especially when injuries fall on the more severe end of the mild TBI spectrum; comprehensive reviews of the mild TBI literature are available elsewhere (Kirkwood & Yeates, 2012). This chapter focuses on pediatric moderate to severe TBI, which is associated with broad-based consequences that can persist for years, including into adulthood. The chapter provides a brief snapshot of TBI from a historical perspective, then reviews recent scientific literature relevant to understanding and managing the consequences of pediatric TBI over both the short and long term.

HISTORICAL MEDICAL PERSPECTIVE

Historically, much of the scientific literature on TBI has focused on adults; attention has shifted to pediatric TBI much more recently. The historical emphasis on adult patients undoubtedly arose, at least in part, because the main advances in TBI treatment have occurred in the context of major wars (Bell, Neal, Lettieri, & Armonda, 2008). Until early in the 20th century, severe TBI was usually fatal (Langfit, 1978). Under the leadership of Dr. Harvey Cushing during World War I, battlefield neurosurgery reduced mortality rates of patients with severe penetrating TBI to 35% (Gurdjian, 1973). The increased numbers of injured survivors led to the development of rehabilitation centers in both the United States and Europe. The best of these centers emphasized some of the principles that continue to characterize rehabilitation today, including integrated service models and vocational training geared toward community reentry.

Attention to civilian TBI burgeoned in the last decades of the 20th century, in part, because of the increase in injuries resulting from high-speed motor vehicle collisions (Cifu, Cohen, Lew, Jaffee, & Sigford, 2010). This time period also marked the establishment of modern rehabilitation medicine, including the founding of permanent, independent rehabilitation hospitals and the development of TBI rehabilitation as a subspecialty. Beginning in the late 1970s, data informing evidence-based medical management of severe TBI were accrued through the Traumatic Coma Data Bank, a longitudinal prospective study funded through the National Institute of Neurological Disorders and Stroke (Marshall et al., 1983). Since then, a number of guidelines for the management of adult TBI have been published. Those of the Brain Trauma Foundation (BTF) are the most widely accepted internationally and were updated most recently in 2007 (Bell et al., 2008). Treatment of TBI in children has historically relied heavily on information derived from adult patients or on physicians' clinical experience. The BTF guidelines served as the template for the only existing evidence-based guidelines devoted exclusively to the management of severe pediatric TBI, which were published by Adelson and colleagues in 2003 and are discussed in more detail below.

CURRENT MEDICAL MANAGEMENT

The pathological effects of TBI are typically classified as either primary or secondary. Primary injury occurs at the time of trauma as a direct result of the impact or acceleration–deceleration forces applied to the head. Common primary effects include skull fractures, contusion, and focal bleeding. Though therapeutic options to address primary injury could emerge in the future (e.g., stem cell technologies), prevention efforts are the only current means by which these injuries can be fundamentally addressed. The general focus of medical management for TBI is on avoiding or treating secondary effects, which can be particularly deleterious after more severe TBI. Secondary effects include additional insults (e.g., brain swelling and edema, hypoxia, hypotension, hydrocephalus, seizures) that follow primary injury and serve to compound the initial effects. The primary injury also leads to a secondary pathophysiological cascade that can include impaired blood flow, increased intracranial pressure (ICP), excitotoxity, energy failure, inflammation, and cell death.

The 2003 management guidelines provided practitioners with a comprehensive set of empirically based recommendations to guide treatment of severe pediatric TBI, including a suggested first tier clinical pathway or acute medical management algorithm. However, the document also served to highlight the low level of evidentiary support for nearly all specific interventions in this population. In keeping with customary practice of evidence-based medicine, the authors classified interventions as "standards" (accepted principles based on strong data), "guidelines" (moderate clinical certainties derived from moderately strong data), or "options" (treatments with limited empirical support and hence of unclear clinical significance). Only three recommendations approached a high level of support: avoid propofol as a continuous infusion, avoid hyperventilation chronically for the management of ICP, and avoid prophylactic use of antiepileptic medication for the treatment of late posttraumatic seizures (Adelson, 2010). Thus, nearly all widely accepted therapies for the treatment of pediatric TBI were supported only at a guideline or option level. Some of the specific recommendations from the guidelines are summarized below, as are several areas in which new evidence has accumulated since 2003.

One set of recommendations focuses on preventing hypoxia and hypotension and correcting these quickly if they arise through administration of supplemental oxygen and fluid resuscitation. Endotracheal intubation to secure the airway is recommended in patients with severe TBI. Early sedation is also suggested to help avoid fluctuations in ICP and blood pressure. Evidence supports transferring children to pediatric trauma centers whenever possible because survival rates are better than when children are treated in adult trauma centers.

The management of ICP following severe TBI illustrates the complexities of evidence-based medicine. Children with severe TBI are at high risk for developing elevated ICP, and sustained elevations in ICP are prognostic of poor outcome. Close monitoring of ICP and aggressive treatment of intracranial hypertension (ICH) have become standard practice in both pediatric and adult trauma centers and are widely believed to have contributed to improved outcomes. However, no randomized clinical trial (RCT) has investigated the efficacy of ICP monitoring, and such a study would now pose serious ethical challenges. Most of the recommendations related to management of ICP and cerebral perfusion pressure (CPP) in the 2003 guidelines are at the "option" level, though the space dedicated to these topics (13 of 19 chapters) highlights their perceived importance in treatment.

ICP monitoring is recommended for infants, children, and adolescents with severe TBI, with the goal of maintaining ICP <20 mmHg. Although the ideal threshold to institute treatment of ICH likely varies by age, insufficient data are available currently to understand what these levels actually are. Researchers have made progress in identifying age-related changes in optimal CPP since 2003, and targets of 50 mmHg (2–6 years), 60 mmHg (7–10 years) and 65 mmHg (11–16 years) have recently been proposed (Bell & Kochanek, 2008). First-line treatments for ICH include raising the head of the bed to 30 degrees, sedation, cerebrospinal fluid drainage, hyperosmolar therapy, and mild to moderate hyperventilation. Aggressive hyperventilation should be avoided if possible because of the risk of ischemia. Refractory ICP is treated with higher risk procedures including barbiturate coma, hypothermia, aggressive hyperventilation, and craniectomy.

Many of these second-tier therapies for refractory ICP have been the focus of increased research attention since publication of the guidelines (Emeriaud, Pettersen, & Ozanne, 2011). In general, recent data support their efficacy in at least some contexts, though evidence remains limited (Bell & Kochanek, 2008). Particular interest has been given to the possible neuroprotective effects of hypothermia following severe TBI because of its established efficacy following other kinds of neurologic insult. However, results of an initial RCT suggested that the risks may actually outweigh the benefits following pediatric TBI, although the disappointing results were thought initially to relate perhaps to the specific cooling and rewarming protocols used (Koch & Kernie, 2011).

EARLY PSYCHOLOGICAL AND NEUROPSYCHOLOGICAL FINDINGS

Intense interest in the psychological sequelae of acquired brain damage dates to the 19th century, as illustrated by one of the most famous TBI patients of all time, Phineas Gage. Margaret Kennard studied the effects of brain lesions within a developmental context through her research on young monkeys in the 1930s. The Kennard principle, which holds that earlier age at injury predicts better functional outcome, has been offered as a summary for her work, although this view represents a gross oversimplification (Dennis, 2010). Rather than supporting a simplistic age–outcome relationship, Kennard demonstrated complex interactions among age at injury, lesion location, and total lesion burden. The Kennard principle was in some sense created in the 1970s amid a wave of interest in brain development and plasticity. In fact, a large body of research on pediatric TBI and other types of diffuse brain injury demonstrates that younger age is a robust risk factor for poorer outcome (Taylor & Alden, 1997). Nonetheless, two late 20th century studies found that many practicing neuropsychologists continued to believe young children would recover from TBI better than older children or adults (Hart & Faust, 1988; Webb, Rose, Johnson, & Attree, 1996).

Specific attention to the neuropsychological effects of pediatric TBI is fairly recent, beginning with the seminal Isle of Wight studies published by Sir Michael Rutter and colleagues in the early 1980s. This work demonstrated that following moderate to severe TBI, children displayed deficits in both intellectual and emotional–behavioral functioning (Chadwick, Rutter, Brown, Shaffer, & Traub, 1981; Brown, Chadwick, Shaffer, Rutter, & Traub, 1981). Early findings suggested that nonverbal IQ was more vulnerable to the effects of TBI than verbal IQ, with particular problems seen in speeded visual–motor and visual–spatial tasks (Chadwick, Rutter, Shaffer, & Shrout, 1981).

RECENT PSYCHOLOGICAL AND NEUROPSYCHOLOGICAL FINDINGS

Since these early studies, numerous international research groups have further elucidated the neurobehavioral consequences of pediatric TBI, which can be classified into several broad-based domains including cognitive, psychosocial, functional, educational, and familial. Compared to outcome work in the initial post-injury years, fewer studies have followed children into adulthood, though an increasing amount of data are available in this regard, as summarized below.

Cognitive Outcomes. Childhood TBI results in a multitude of well-documented cognitive effects, which are strongly related to injury severity. Partial cognitive recovery is often seen within the first months to years postinjury, although longitudinal work demonstrates persistent cognitive deficits thereafter, especially following more severe injury (Anderson, Catroppa, Haritou, Morse, & Rosenfeld, 2005; Babikian & Asarnow, 2009). In general, cognitive effects become more prominent as effortful processing increases. Thus, overlearned knowledge and automatized skills can be relatively unaffected by TBI in older children, whereas tasks more dependent upon attention, speeded processing, executive functioning, and new learning reveal more problems.

On measures of IQ, severe injuries and injuries occurring in infancy or the preschool years are associated with a broad-based diminution in scores and/or less rapid growth over time (Babikian & Asarnow, 2009; Ewing-Cobbs et al., 2006). For less severe injury and as children become older, IQ effects become more heterogeneous but are greatest on speeded tasks, at least postacutely. For instance, research with both the third and fourth editions of the Wechsler Intelligence Scale for Children has documented that the processing speed factor has the best criterion validity after TBI (Donders & Janke, 2008; Tremont, Mittenberg, & Miller, 1999).

In terms of more specific cognitive skills, TBI has been found to result in persistent problems with discourse, pragmatics, and other higher-level communication skills. In contrast, vocabulary, syntax, and other basic linguistic skills can be relatively spared, especially after the early stages of recovery and in children injured later in development (Ewing-Cobbs & Barnes, 2002). TBI can also undermine a range of nonverbal capacities, including spatial orientation and perceptual–motor functioning (Lehnung et al., 2001; Yeates et al., 2002), although visual perceptual skills overall are likely to be less affected by injury than many other domains (Babikian & Asarnow, 2009). Negative effects on a wide variety of learning and memory tasks have been documented as well (Allen et al., 2010; Ward, Shum, McKinlay, Baker, & Wallace, 2007).

Attentional processes are also frequently compromised, especially divided and sustained attention (Ginstfeldt & Emanuelson, 2010). Postinjury deficits on tasks that tap executive functioning include problems with working memory (Mandalis, Kinsella, Ong, & Anderson, 2007), monitoring (Ornstein et al., 2009), self-regulation and inhibition (Anderson, Catroppa, Morse, Haritou, & Rosenfeld, 2005a; Ganesalingam, Sanson, Anderson, & Yeates, 2006), planning (Levin, Song, Ewing-Cobbs, & Roberson, 2001), and concept formation and verbal fluency (Anderson et al., 2005a). These performance-based executive functioning difficulties correspond to executive problems observed in everyday settings (Mangeot, Armstrong, Colvin, Yeates, & Taylor, 2002).

Psychosocial Outcomes. Pediatric TBI also increases the risk for a variety of psychosocial and functional problems, which are not necessarily linked to its cognitive consequences. Compared with the cognitive effects, psychosocial outcomes are more multifactorially determined, depending in part on injury severity but also heavily on noninjury-related factors such as family stress, coping, and socioeconomic status. Moreover, in contrast with many cognitive difficulties that show recovery in the initial months after injury, psychosocial difficulties are more likely to show a stable or even worsening pattern over time (Taylor et al., 2002). In general, social outcomes have received relatively little attention after pediatric TBI, though the conceptual groundwork for future work exists (Yeates et al., 2007). Extant studies have documented poorer social problem solving and less social competence in children with TBI compared with noninjured peers (Yeates et al., 2004). Numerous studies have also documented that moderate to severe TBI increases the risk for a wide range of behavioral problems. For example, in a prospective controlled study, Schwartz et al. (2003) found that 36% of the severe TBI group displayed significant behavioral problems at 4 years postinjury, compared with 22% of the moderate TBI group, and 10% of the orthopedic control children.

Pediatric TBI is also associated with a variety of psychiatric symptoms and disorders. Generally speaking, novel disorders occur more commonly after severe TBI and much less frequently after moderate injuries when aspects of the disorder are not present premorbidly. Personality change is a frequent psychiatric consequence of more severe TBI. Changes involving lability, aggression, and disinhibition are most common, whereas apathy and paranoia occur less frequently (Max et al., 2000). "Secondary" attention-deficit/hyperactivity disorder (S-ADHD) has been found to develop in approximately 15%–20% of children with TBI who did not display premorbid ADHD (Levin et al., 2007; Yeates et al., 2005). TBI also increases the risk for other disruptive behavioral disorders such as oppositional defiant disorder (Max et al., 1998). Depressive and anxiety symptoms and disorders are also observed more frequently in children with TBI than in controls (Luis & Mittenberg, 2002; Max et al., 2011). In contrast, manic and psychotic symptoms are documented much less frequently after childhood injury.

Functional Outcomes. Moderate or severe TBI is also associated with persistent deficits in adaptive behavior (e.g., poorer communication and daily living skills) and functional limitations (Anderson, Catroppa, Haritou, et al., 2005; Fay et al., 2009; Taylor et al., 2002). In addition, declines in children's health-related quality of life are often apparent (Rivara et al., 2011).

Following milder TBI, a variety of somatic, cognitive, and behavioral complaints are often reported; these are commonly referred to as "post-concussive symptoms." After severe TBI, the onset or exacerbation of similar symptomatology is seen, typically with more persistence than after milder injury. Yeates et al. (2001) found that in comparison to children with orthopedic injury or moderate TBI, children with severe TBI reported more frequent cognitive/somatic symptoms (e.g., headache, fatigue, attention and memory problems) and emotional/behavioral symptoms (e.g., moodiness, impulsivity, aggressiveness) through 12 months postinjury.

Educational Outcomes. Children injured during infancy or the preschool years are at risk for difficulties in the acquisition of a broad range of academic skills (Ewing-Cobbs et al., 2006). In contrast, TBI in later childhood or adolescence can be associated with age-appropriate basic academic achievement (Ewing-Cobbs, Barnes, et al., 2004). Despite adequate performance on many standardized academic tests, however, children injured at any age often display poor everyday classroom functioning. Across development, pediatric TBI significantly increases the risk for failing grades, need for special education services, and parental and teacher concerns about academic competence (Ewing-Cobbs et al., 2004; Ewing-Cobbs et al., 2006). Although the entire range of factors contributing to these classroom difficulties remains to be elucidated, post-injury compromise of neuropsychological capacities (e.g., attention, self-regulation, speeded responding, memory) that are necessary for effective everyday school performance can be expected to play a major role, as can the student's emotional and behavioral adjustment (Yeates & Taylor, 2006).

Familial. Research examining the effects of moderate to severe pediatric TBI on families has been accumulating quickly in recent years. TBI increases the risk for psychological symptoms in parents and siblings and contributes significantly to marital conflict and family distress, burden, and negativity (Sambuco, Brookes, & Lah, 2008; Wade et al., 2002). Family-related problems can persist for years post-injury and may become especially apparent during periods of developmental transition (Wade et al., 2005). Families with increased stress and fewer resources appear to be most likely to develop post-injury problems (Stancin, Wade, Walz, Yeates, & Taylor, 2010).

Long-term Outcomes of Injury in Childhood

Advances in medical care and increased life expectancy have led to greater attention in recent years on long-term outcomes after TBI. Unfortunately, few high-quality studies have focused on adult outcomes of pediatric TBI. Most available research has used cross-sectional designs, examining former pediatric patients evaluated at a single follow-up point in adulthood. Available data do suggest that individuals who sustain TBI in childhood are at much higher risk for struggling in adulthood, even if some individuals make a positive adjustment to adult life (Todis, Glang, Bullis, Ettel, & Hood, 2011). Beauchamp and colleagues (2010) provided a recent summary of much of this work. As these authors highlight, many of the difficulties apparent in the initial months to years post-injury persist into adulthood, especially after severe injury, although lasting gross neurobehavioral impairment is rare. Cognitively, persistent deficits are most common in the dynamic areas frequently affected in the pediatric years, including attention, processing speed, and memory (Beauchamp et al., 2010). The psychosocial costs of childhood TBI are often quite visible in the adult years and have been found to include social maladjustment, mood disturbance, family problems, and high rates of involvement with the criminal justice system (Hoofien, Gilboa, Vakil, & Donovick, 2001; Klonoff, Clark, & Klonoff, 1993; Newman et al., 2011). Educationally, students with TBI are enrolled in postsecondary opportunities at significantly lower rates than their peers in the general population and need life-skills training much more frequently than many others with disabilities (Wagner, Newman, Cameto, Garza, & Levine, 2005). Childhood TBI is also associated with relatively high rates of unemployment and greater need for sheltered employment opportunities and other vocational services (Koskiniemi, Kyykkä, Nybo, & Jarho, 1995; Nybo, Sainio, & Müller, 2004; Wagner et al., 2005).

Influences on Outcome

The specific consequences of pediatric TBI for a given individual are difficult to predict, even relatively soon after injury, with substantial variance unaccounted for in outcome studies. The variables that have been found to influence outcome up to 5 years after pediatric TBI can be classified into three broad categories: injury related, contextual, and developmental. The few studies examining outcome variance into adulthood tend to emphasize injury-related predictors more exclusively.

Injury-related. The relationship between injury severity and outcome has been investigated in many studies, resulting in the identification of a clear dose–response relationship. Uncomplicated mild TBI (i.e., mild TBI without intracranial pathology on imaging) has typically been found to produce transient neuropsychological effects. Although subjectively reported postconcussive complaints may linger in a minority of children, deficits on cognitive/psychoeducational tests are generally not apparent, particularly after the initial days or weeks post injury (Carroll et al., 2004). As the severity of TBI increases, however, so do the risks for a host of neurobehavioral problems, with severe injuries responsible for the greatest morbidity (Babikian & Asarnow, 2009).

The Glasgow Coma Scale (GCS), or a modified version for infants and toddlers, has probably been investigated more than any other severity measure in pediatric studies, with lower scores associated with worse early and long-term outcomes. In contrast to static measurements such as a one-time GCS score, however, markers that are presumed to index neurobiological recovery, such as duration of coma, length of impaired consciousness, or duration of PTA, may serve as even better predictors of neurobehavioral outcome (Yeates, 2010).

Data from neuroimaging studies indicate that the greater the lesion burden, the greater the morbidity. Studies have also documented an anterior–posterior gradient in the focal lesions associated with pediatric TBI, with larger and more numerous lesions found in the frontal and anterior temporal regions (Wilde et al., 2005). This frontotemporal susceptibility to injury relates to how these regions are positioned in the skull and has long been assumed to be the basis of the core neurobehavioral problems seen after TBI. In pediatric populations, multiple studies have found expected brain–behavior associations supporting this assumption. Levin and Hanten (2005) reviewed much of this literature as it pertains to executive functioning, highlighting relationships between frontal lobe pathology and neuropsychological deficits in children that match well with predictions based on adult-based models of brain–behavior relationships.

Several studies have also made it clear, however, that classic brain-behavior relationships cannot be assumed after childhood TBI. For example, in a population of school-aged children with TBI, Slomine and colleagues (2002) found that frontal lesion volume failed to predict performance on any measure of executive function. Power and colleagues (2007) failed to find a relationship between frontal lesion severity and performance on measures of attentional control. Salorio and colleagues (2005) found that performance on a list-learning memory measure was more strongly related to lesions outside the frontotemporal regions than lesions within those regions. Taken together, these studies support the position that pediatric brain–behavior relationships differ from those of adults, likely reflecting the differences in maturation of cortical regions at different stages of development.

Contextual. The need to consider variables beyond injury severity in predicting postinjury outcomes is now well appreciated, including the importance of a number of contextual factors. In general, such variables have been found to have a greater effect on psychosocial and academic outcomes than physical and cognitive outcomes. Socioeconomic status, family resources, and both pre-injury and postinjury family functioning have all been shown to be important moderators of long-term outcome (Anderson, Catroppa, Haritou et al., 2005; Taylor et al., 2002; Todis et al., 2011).

Brain injuries in children are not randomly distributed in the general population: different patterns of pre-injury functioning are associated with increased risk for injury. Inattentive or impulsive children engage in more risky behavior that increases their likelihood of injuries, including head injuries. The rate of pre-injury ADHD in children who go on to suffer TBI is likely at least twice as high as that seen in the general population. Rates of premorbid cognitive and academic difficulties and familial stressors may also be higher in children who sustain TBI (Goldstrohm & Arffa, 2005). For the clinician, this means that behaviors attributed to the injury must be scrutinized carefully to determine precisely what is new, changed, or unexpected in the child's post-injury functioning.

The mechanisms by which the broader environment exerts its effect on TBI outcome have not yet been clarified. Families from disadvantaged environments could lack the resources or availability to enhance the child's recovery or to optimally manage post-injury neurobehavioral problems; family adversity could also differentially affect neurologically compromised children because these children may be more dependent on the environment because of their limitations (Taylor et al., 2002). In any case, the relationships between child and environment are likely to prove bidirectional in at least some situations. Taylor and colleagues (Taylor et al., 2001) found that higher family distress at 6 months post-injury predicted worse child behavior at 12 months and also that increased child behavior problems at 6 months predicted poorer family outcomes at 12 months.

Developmental. A number of developmental variables have been shown to influence outcomes as well. At a general level, developmental skills and functional status of the child prior to the injury can strongly impact post-injury adaptive and behavioral functioning (Catroppa, Anderson, Morse, Haritou, & Rosenfeld, 2008; Schwartz et al., 2003; Yeates et al., 2005). Post-injury psychiatric problems are also predicted by a number of pre-injury child variables, including intellectual status, adaptive skills, and psychiatric condition (Anderson et al., 2005; Max et al., 2006).

Several time-specific developmental variables have also been studied as moderators. Age at injury, time since injury, and age at testing have all received scientific attention, although age at injury has clearly been investigated the most thoroughly. As discussed above, historically, earlier age at injury was thought to produce better outcomes because of the young brain's "plasticity." Better outcomes can indeed be seen in immature nonhuman animals under certain well-defined conditions (Kolb & Gibb, 2007) and in humans after early focal or discrete injuries such as perinatal stroke (Bates et al., 2001). Nonetheless, more recent investigations have demonstrated that the immature child brain is more vulnerable, not more accommodating, to diffuse, evolving injuries such as TBI (Anderson et al., 2005b; Ewing-Cobbs et al., 2006). Skills that have not yet developed or are currently in development at the time of injury may be particularly susceptible to injury effects and may show an altered course of post-injury development (Catroppa et al., 2007; Ewing-Cobbs, Prasad, Landry, Kramer, & DeLeon, 2004). Few studies have examined whether earlier injury results in worse long-term outcomes than later injury, though initial work suggests that earlier injury is associated with lower postsecondary education attainment, lack of independent living, and increased need for legal guardianship (Donders & Warschausky, 2007; Todis et al., 2011). Explanations to account for the general vulnerability in younger versus older children include potential restrictions on functional recovery imposed by the injured child's narrower repertoire of skills, the damaging impact of diffuse injury on systems responsible for later skill acquisition and maintenance (e.g., self-regulation, learning, and memory), and the potentially limiting effects of prolonged hospitalization and treatment on learning.

INTERVENTION AND TREATMENT GAINS

Assessment

With increasingly sophisticated acute medical care and technology, neuropsychologists are rarely asked to assist in making an initial diagnosis of TBI, except perhaps in certain cases of milder TBI, when the medical or neuroimaging evidence for injury may be less clear. Of course, neuropsychological assessment has value above and beyond simply diagnosing TBI. Neuropsychological assessment can be used to delineate the neurobehavioral consequences of injury, disentangle injury effects from other factors that may be contributing to or moderating post-injury functioning, assist with post-injury diagnostic decision making, and develop rehabilitation and educational management plans appropriate to the individual's needs and circumstances. Given the persistence of some neurobehavioral problems after pediatric TBI, evaluation and management often needs to continue into adulthood in order to allow progress to be tracked and interventions to be tailored to the many changing demands that occur across development.

Empirical investigation of the value of neuropsychological assessment after pediatric TBI is still in its infancy, and thus few interventions or recommendations are as yet evidence based. However, the general "neurological" validity of psychometric testing has been demonstrated throughout the extensive outcome literature, that is, numerous tests and certain rating scales have been shown to discriminate youth with moderate to severe TBI from other children. This discriminatory power clearly provides support for the utility of neuropsychological testing in characterizing the impact of TBI. The ability of tests to predict or change specific functional outcomes—the "ecological" validity of the tests—has received far less study.

In addition to a thorough history and systematic observation, well-standardized, performance-based psychological and psychoeducational tests are indispensable to understanding the postinjury neuropsychological profile. The worth of testing is unlikely to derive exclusively from a specific test or test battery, which will change as psychometric technology evolves. Rather, the primary value of testing stems from the fact that TBI is known to impact a variety of neurobehavioral domains, and psychometric testing is the most well-validated methodology to evaluate neurobehavioral performance relative to age expectations.

After pediatric TBI, no particular battery of tests has been shown to be more or less sensitive or valid. However, the TBI outcome literature does indicate that clinicians should avoid an over-reliance on tests of automatized information or functioning (e.g., many academic tests) and ensure sufficient coverage of more dynamic processes such as speeded processing, learning and memory, and attention/executive control. Given the differences in outcome expected at different ages, clinicians should consider targeting different skills depending on the age at injury. For example, in terms of language skills, clinicians may want to conduct a more thorough evaluation of basic linguistic skills (e.g., phonological awareness and lexical skills) when evaluating a child injured in infancy or the preschool years, while focusing on higher-level communication skills for older children. Numerous resources are available to assist in the development of a comprehensive test battery. Baron (2004) and Strauss, Sherman, and Spreen (2006) may be especially worthwhile because they include coverage of both the general and TBI-related psychometric properties of many commonly used tests.

Management

Empirical work that can be expected to have most application to neuropsychological management following pediatric TBI can be grouped into several areas: rehabilitation, pharmacological, psychosocial, and educational/vocational.

Rehabilitation. In adult populations, considerable evidence supports the efficacy of rehabilitation in addressing cognitive deficits after TBI (Cicerone et al., 2011). In children, only a few class I or class II rehabilitation studies exist. A review by Laatsch and colleagues (2007) resulted in the following practice guidelines: service providers should consider providing attention remediation to assist recovery after acquired brain injury and comprehensive pediatric rehabilitation programs should consider involving the family members as active treatment providers in the rehabilitation treatment team. These guidelines were based largely on the TBI work of van't Hooft and colleagues (2005, 2007) in Sweden and Braga and colleagues (2005) in Brazil, as well as Butler and colleagues (2008) work focused on pediatric cancer. The literature on pediatric rehabilitation has continued to evolve in recent years, with at least some support at this point for interventions focused on memory, unilateral neglect, speech/language, and executive functioning (Slomine & Locascio, 2009; Wade et al., 2010), even if the strength of this support pales in comparison to that available for adult populations.

Pharmacological intervention. In the last decade, attention has been given to developing evidence-based guidelines for the use of psychopharmacological agents in managing the neurobehavioral consequences of TBI in adults (Warden et al., 2006). Treatment with psychotropic medication after pediatric TBI is not well studied, despite common use in practice. Psychostimulants are the most researched agent, likely because of the frequency of attention/regulatory problems after TBI and the success of stimulants in treating developmentally based ADHD. However, even with stimulants, results of TBI-focused studies have been mixed. Existing studies suggest that treatment effects on behavior (hyperactivity, impulsivity) may be greater than on cognition and that effects overall may be less apparent than those seen in developmental ADHD populations (Jin & Schachar, 2004).

Psychosocial intervention. Few randomized, controlled studies have investigated psychosocial interventions after pediatric TBI, though management concepts can be garnered from the psychology literature generally and a number of TBI-specific models and case studies. The limited pediatric TBI-specific research does suggest that interventions derived from traditional applied behavioral analysis methodologies, as well as those grounded in the provision of proactive, antecedent-focused support, may be most effective in reducing behavioral problems after TBI (Ylvisaker et al., 2007). Assisting parents in becoming better advocates for their children who have sustained TBI has also been investigated in an RCT by Glang and colleagues (2007). Although training parents in a CD-based program improved TBI knowledge and attitudes, parents who received the training did not differ in their intention to actually use the skills or their feelings of self-efficacy.

The randomized controlled studies of Wade and colleagues, which are aimed at improving family functioning, deserve particular mention, given their quality and the contribution of familial-related variables to psychosocial outcomes after pediatric TBI. Wade and colleagues developed a family problem-solving program to provide information to families about TBI, as well as training in problem-solving skills, family communication, and antecedent behavior management. The intervention was provided originally in face-to-face sessions that included parents, children with TBI, and siblings over a 6-month period. This intervention resulted in improvements in childhood internalizing symptoms, depression/anxiety, and withdrawal. The intervention was then adapted to be provided in an online format, which was found in a small nonrandomized study to reduce childhood behavioral problems and improve parent–child conflict (Wade, Wolfe, Brown, & Pestian, 2005). These researchers also reported on an RCT involving 40 families assigned to receive the online intervention or general Internet resource support (Wade, Carey, & Wolfe, 2006). The intervention group displayed reduced parental levels of global distress, depressive symptoms, and anxiety. These findings were consistent with a small study by Singer and colleagues (1994), which also found that a skills-based stress management group was more effective in reducing parental anxiety and depression than simply providing information during a parent-based support group meeting. Wade and colleagues (2011) also investigated the value of a teen-only version of the Web-based problem-solving intervention in a recent RCT. The intervention group reported significantly less parent–teen conflict and fewer internalizing symptoms than the comparison group.

The work by Wade and colleagues serves to illustrate a broader trend in medicine that utilizes telecommunication technologies to meet health needs, particularly for those who have difficulty accessing care through traditional routes. Given the lack of specialized care for TBI available in many communities, telecommunication or Web-based service delivery options are apt to be invaluable for linking both professionals and families with state-of-the-art information and care by reducing barriers such as cost, geographical distance, and stigma associated with seeking treatment. In this regard, multiple Web-based resources focused on TBI are now available, although the value of most of these resources has yet to be established empirically. An example of a well-conceptualized resource aimed at clinicians is PsycBITE (www.psycbite.com), which catalogues studies of cognitive, behavioral, and other treatments for psychological problems occurring as a consequence of acquired brain injury. Studies are rated for their methodological quality to assist clinicians in making decisions about intervention options. An example of a reputable Web-based resource geared toward parents and educators is LEARNet (www.projectlearnet.org), which provides a problem-solving system and numerous informational and advocacy resources geared toward improving understanding and outcomes after pediatric brain injury.

Educational/Vocational Support. In the United States, the average length of a hospital stay after pediatric TBI has been decreasing in recent years, and the availability of comprehensive outpatient rehabilitation programs has declined. Thus, much rehabilitation and support after pediatric TBI is now expected to occur within the educational system. Unfortunately, quality research examining specific educational interventions after TBI is strikingly absent, perhaps in part because of the significant variability in the needs and settings of each student. Given the lack of direct empirical support at this time, empirically backed school intervention following TBI must rely largely on indirect studies conducted with populations who may display similar manifest problems (e.g., ADHD). Ylvisaker and colleagues (2001) and Glang and colleagues (2008) have summarized much of this research in pediatric populations. Very little research on TBI has focused on supporting individuals in navigating the transition from school to work or from family-centered pediatric systems to more traditional self-directed adult-based services. Nonetheless, many older teens will clearly require structured assistance in identifying appropriate vocational goals, as well as support from vocational counselors and employers in meeting these goals. In adulthood, self-awareness skills appear particularly important in determining vocational success and have been successfully targeted in several studies (e.g., Goverover, Johnston, Toglia, & Deluca, 2007).

FUTURE AIMS AND RESEARCH OPPORTUNITIES

Clinical neuropsychologists currently have sufficient data to anticipate and evaluate the common consequences of pediatric TBI, examine plausible factors affecting individual outcomes, and assist in developing scientifically informed management plans. Despite this solid research foundation, considerable work remains.

Neuropsychological outcome studies have recently moved away from the historical emphasis on cognition to consider the broader impact of TBI. Nonetheless, ongoing investigation will be necessary to better capture the socioemotional effects of injury as well as the everyday functional consequences for children, families, and the educational and healthcare systems. Further delineation of the mechanisms by which neural, contextual, and developmental variables serve as risk and protective factors will also be necessary and should be especially valuable in identifying those in need of intervention. Initial data suggest that brain–behavior relationships will differ at least to some extent after TBI in childhood as compared to adulthood. Increasingly sophisticated models will be needed to clarify these relationships, with an eye toward developmentally minded evaluation and treatment prioritization.

Given the limited amount of sound long-term longitudinal research available, studies that follow children prospectively into adulthood should continue to be a high priority. Even if such work is costly and methodologically demanding, it will be necessary to more fully appreciate the evolving consequences of pediatric TBI and how patient and family needs change over different developmental periods. Finally, one of the most glaring areas of need continues to be TBI-specific intervention; relatively few efficacy studies exist, let alone RCTs that could be used to drive evidence-based practice. Clearly, much more study will be required to understand which treatments are most effective after pediatric TBI and which aspects of the treatment benefit whom under what circumstances and at what time points post-injury. A particularly important question for neuropsychologists will be how neuropsychological data can help to identify effective intervention by, for example, classifying individuals and/or families into groups using evaluation results and then demonstrating group by treatment interactions. A theory-based, developmentally driven approach that addresses psychological and socioenvironmental factors will likely be most productive in this effort.

REFERENCES

Adelson, P. D. (2010). Clinical trials for pediatric TBI. In V. Anderson & K. O. Yeates (Eds.), *Pediatric traumatic brain injury: New frontiers in clinical and translational research* (pp. 54–67). Cambridge: Cambridge University Press.

Adelson, P. D., Bratton, S. L., Carney, N. A., Chesnut, R. M., du Coudray, H. E., Goldstein, B.,...Wright, D. W. (2003). Guidelines for the acute medical management of severe traumatic brain injury in infants, children, and adolescents. Chapter 1: Introduction. *Pediatric Critical Care Medicine, 3*, S2–S4.

Allen, D. N., Leany, B. D., Thaler, N. S., Cross, C., Sutton, G. P., & Mayfield, J. (2010). Memory and attention profiles in pediatric traumatic brain injury. *Archives of Clinical Neuropsychology, 25*, 618–633.

Anderson, V. A., Catroppa, C., Haritou, F., Morse, S., & Rosenfeld, J. V. (2005). Identifying factors contributing to child and family outcome 30 months after traumatic brain injury in children. *Journal of Neurology, Neurosurgery, and Psychiatry, 76*, 401–408.

Anderson, V., Catroppa, C., Morse, S., Haritou, F., & Rosenfeld, J. (2005a). Attentional and processing skills following traumatic brain injury in early childhood. *Brain Injury, 19*, 699–710.

Anderson, V., Catroppa, C., Morse, S., Haritou, F., & Rosenfeld, J. (2005b). Functional plasticity or vulnerability after early brain injury? *Pediatrics, 116*, 1374–1382.

Babikian, T., & Asarnow, R. (2009). Neurocognitive outcomes and recovery after pediatric TBI: Meta-analytic review of the literature. *Neuropsychology, 23*, 283–296.

Baron, I. S. (2004). *Neuropsychological evaluation of the child.* Oxford: Oxford University Press.

Bates, E., Reilly, J., Wulfeck, B., Dronkers, N., Opie, M., Fenson, J.,...Herbst, K. (2001). Differential effects of unilateral lesions on language production in children and adults. *Brain & Language, 79*, 223–265.

Bell, M. J., & Kochanek, P. M. (2008). Traumatic brain injury in children: Recent advances in management. *Indian Journal of Pediatrics, 75*, 1159–1165.

Bell, R. S., Neal, C. J., Lettieri, C. J., & Armonda, R. A. (2008). Severe traumatic brain injury: Evolution and current surgical management. *Medscape Emergency Medicine.* Retrieved November 1, 2011, from http://www.medscape.org/viewarticle/575753

Beauchamp, M., Dooley, J., & Anderson, V. (2010). Adult outcomes of pediatric traumatic brain injury. In J. Donders & S. J. Hunter (Eds.), *Principles and practice of lifespan developmental neuropsychology* (pp. 315–328). Cambridge: Cambridge University Press.

Braga, L. W., Da Paz, A. C., & Ylvisaker, M. (2005). Direct clinician-delivered versus indirect family-supported rehabilitation of children with traumatic brain injury: A randomized controlled trial. *Brain Injury, 19*, 819–831.

Brown, G., Chadwick, O., Shaffer, D., Rutter, M., & Traub, M. (1981). A prospective study of children with head injuries: III. Psychiatric sequelae. *Psychological Medicine, 11*, 63–78.

Butler, R. W., Copeland, D. R., Fairclough, D. L., Mulhern, R. K., Katz, E. R., Kazak, A. E.,...Sahler, O. J. (2008). A multicenter, randomized clinical trial of a cognitive remediation program for childhood survivors of a pediatric malignancy. *Journal of Consulting and Clinical Psychology, 76*, 367–378.

Carroll, L. J., Cassidy, J. D., Peloso, P. M., Borg, J., von Holst, H., & Holm, L.,...Pepin, M. (2004). Prognosis for mild traumatic brain injury: Results of the WHO collaborating centre task force on mild traumatic brain injury. *Journal of Rehabilitation Medicine, 43 Suppl*, 84–105.

Cassidy, J. D., Carroll, L. J., Peloso, P. M., Borg, J., von Holst, H., Holm, L.,...Coronado, V. G. (2004). Incidence, risk factors and prevention of mild traumatic brain injury: Results of the WHO Collaborating Centre Task Force on Mild Traumatic Brain Injury. *Journal of Rehabilitation Medicine, 43 Suppl*, 28–60.

Catroppa, C., Anderson, V. A., Morse, S. A., Haritou, F., & Rosenfeld, J. V. (2008). Outcome and predictors of functional recovery 5 years following pediatric traumatic brain injury (TBI). *Journal of Pediatric Psychology, 33*, 707–718.

Chadwick, O., Rutter, M., Brown, G., Shaffer, D., & Traub, M. U. (1981). A prospective study of children with head injuries: II. Cognitive sequelae. *Psychological Medicine, 11*, 49–61.

Chadwick, O., Rutter, M., Shaffer, D., & Shrout, P. E. (1981). A prospective study of children with head injuries: IV. Specific cognitive deficits. *Journal of Clinical Neuropsychology, 3*, 101–120.

Cicerone, K. D., Langenbahn, D. M., Braden, C., Malec, J. F., Kalmar, K., Fraas, M.,...Ashman, T. (2011). Evidence-based cognitive rehabilitation: Updated review of the literature from 2003 through 2008. *Archives of Physical Medicine & Rehabilitation, 92*, 519–530.

Cifu, D. X., Cohen, S. I., Lew, H. L., Jaffee, M., & Sigford, B. (2010). The history and evolution of traumatic brain injury rehabilitation in military service members and veterans. *American Journal of Physical Medicine and Rehabilitation, 89*, 688–694.

Dennis, M. (2010). Margaret Kennard (1899–1975): Not a "principle" of brain plasticity but a founding mother of developmental neuropsychology. *Cortex, 46*, 1043–1059.

Donders, J., & Janke, K. (2008). Criterion validity of the Wechsler Intelligence Scale for Children-Fourth Edition after pediatric traumatic brain injury. *Journal of International Neuropsychological Society, 14*, 651–655.

Donders, J., & Warschausky S. (2007). Neurobehavioral outcomes after early versus late childhood traumatic brain injury. *Journal of Head Trauma Rehabilitation, 22*, 296–302.

Emeriaud, G., Pettersen, G., & Ozanne, B. (2011). Pediatric traumatic brain injury: An update. *Current Opinion in Anaesthesiology, 24*, 307–313.

Ewing-Cobbs, L., & Barnes, M. (2002). Linguistic outcomes following traumatic brain injury in children. *Seminars in Pediatric Neurology, 9*, 209–217.

Ewing-Cobbs, L., Barnes, M., Fletcher, J. M., Levin, H. S., Swank, P. R., & Song, J. (2004). Modeling of longitudinal academic achievement scores after pediatric traumatic brain injury. *Developmental Neuropsychology, 25*, 107–133.

Ewing-Cobbs, L., Prasad, M. R., Kramer, L., Cox, C. S., Jr., Baumgartner, J., Fletcher, S.,...Swank, P. (2006). Late intellectual and academic outcomes following traumatic brain injury sustained during early childhood. *Journal of Neurosurgery, 105,* 287–296.

Ewing-Cobbs, L., Prasad, M. R., Landry, S. H., Kramer, L., & DeLeon, R. (2004). Executive functions following traumatic brain injury in young children: A preliminary analysis. *Developmental Neuropsychology, 26,* 487–512.

Faul, M., Xu, L., Wald, M. M., & Coronado, V. (2010). *Traumatic brain injury in the United States: Emergency department visits, hospitalizations and deaths, 2002–2006.* Atlanta, GA: Centers for Disease Control and Prevention, National Center for Injury Prevention and Control.

Fay, T. B., Yeates, K. O., Wade, S. L., Drotar, D., Stancin, T., & Taylor, H. G. (2009). Predicting longitudinal patterns of functional deficits in children with traumatic brain injury. *Neuropsychology, 23,* 271–282.

Ganesalingam, K., Sanson, A., Anderson, V., & Yeates, K. O. (2006). Self-regulation and social and behavioral functioning following childhood traumatic brain injury. *Journal of International Neuropsychological Society, 12,* 609–621.

Ginstfeldt, T., & Emanuelson, I. (2010). An overview of attention deficits after paediatric traumatic brain injury. *Brain Injury, 24,* 1123–1134.

Glang, A., McLaughlin, K., & Schroeder, S. (2007). Using interactive multimedia to teach parent advocacy skills: An exploratory study. *Journal of Head Trauma Rehabilitation, 22,* 198–205.

Glang, A., Ylvisaker, M., Stein, M., Ehlhardt, L., Todis, B., & Tyler, J. (2008). Validated instructional practices: Application to students with traumatic brain injury. *Journal of Head Trauma Rehabilitation, 23,* 243–251.

Goldstrohm, S. L., & Arffa, S. (2005). Preschool children with mild to moderate traumatic brain injury: An exploration of immediate and post-acute morbidity. *Archives of Clinical Neuropsychology, 20,* 675–695.

Goverover, Y., Johnston, M. V., Toglia, J., & Deluca, J. (2007). Treatment to improve self-awareness in persons with acquired brain injury. *Brain Injury, 21,* 913–923.

Gurdjian, E. S. (1973). Prevention and mitigation of head injury from antiquity to the present. *Journal of Trauma, 13,* 931–945.

Hart, K., & Faust, D. (1988). Prediction of the effects of mild head injury: A message about the Kennard Principle. *Journal of Clinical Psychology, 44,* 780–782.

Hoofien, D., Gilboa, A., Vakil, E., & Donovick, P. J. (2001). Traumatic brain injury (TBI) 10–20 years later: A comprehensive outcome study of psychiatric symptomatology, cognitive abilities and psychosocial functioning. *Brain Injury, 15,* 189–209.

Jin, C., & Schachar, R. (2004). Methylphenidate treatment of attention-deficit/hyperactivity disorder secondary to traumatic brain injury: A critical appraisal of treatment studies. *CNS Spectrums, 9,* 217–226.

Lehnung, M., Leplow, B., Herzog, A., Benz, B., Ritz, A., & Stolze, H.,...Ferstl, R. (2001). Children's spatial behavior is differentially affected after traumatic brain injury. *Child Neuropsychololgy, 7,* 59–71.

Kirkwood, M. W., & Yeates, K. O. (2012). *Mild traumatic brain injury in children and adolescents: From basic science to clinical management.* New York: Guilford Press.

Klonoff, H., Clark, C., & Klonoff, P. S. (1993). Long-term outcome of head injuries: A 23 year follow up study of children with head injuries. *Journal of Neurology Neurosurgery Psychiatry, 56,* 410–415.

Koch, J. D., & Kernie, S. G. (2011). Protecting the future: Neuroprotective strategies in the pediatric intensive care unit. *Current Opinion in Pediatrics, 23,* 275–280.

Kolb, B., & Gibb, R. (2007). Brain plasticity and recovery from early cortical injury. *Developmental Psychobiology, 49,* 107–118.

Koskiniemi, M., Kyykkä, T., Nybo, T., & Jarho, L. (1995). Long-term outcome after severe brain injury in preschoolers is worse than expected. *Archivos of Pediatric Adolescent Medicine, 149,* 249–254.

Laatsch, L., Harrington, D., Hotz, G., Marcantuono, J., Mozzoni, M. P., Walsh, V., & Pike, K. (2007). An evidence-based review of cognitive and behavioral rehabilitation treatment studies in children with acquired brain injury. *Journal of Head Trauma Rehabilitation, 22,* 248–256.

Langfit, T. W. (1978). Measuring the outcomes from head injuries. *Journal of Neurosurgery, 48,* 673–678.

Levin, H. S., & Hanten, G. (2005). Executive functions after traumatic brain injury in children. *Pediatric Neurology, 33,* 79–93.

Levin, H., Hanten, G., Max, J., Li, X., Swank, P., Ewing-Cobbs, L., & Dennis, M. (2007). Symptoms of attention-deficit/hyperactivity disorder following traumatic brain injury in children. *Journal of Developmental and Behavioral Pediatrics, 28,* 108–118.

Levin, H. S., Song, J., Ewing-Cobbs, L., & Roberson, G. (2001). Maze performance following traumatic brain injury in children. *Neuropsychology, 15,* 557–567.

Luis, C. A., & Mittenberg, W. (2002). Mood and anxiety disorders following pediatric traumatic brain injury: A prospective study. *Journal of Clinical Experimental Neuropsychology, 24,* 270–279.

Marshall, L. F., Becker, D. P., Bowers, S. A., Cayard, C., Eisenberg, H., Gross, C. R.,... Warren, J. (1983). The National Traumatic Coma Data Bank. Part 1: Design, purpose, goals, and results. *Journal of Neurosurgery, 59,* 276–284.

Mandalis, A., Kinsella, G., Ong, B., & Anderson, V. (2007). Working memory and new learning following pediatric traumatic brain injury. *Developmental Neuropsychology, 32,* 683–701.

Mangeot, S., Armstrong, K., Colvin, A. N., Yeates, K. O., & Taylor, H. G. (2002). Long-term executive function deficits in children with traumatic brain injuries: Assessment using the Behavior Rating Inventory of Executive Function (BRIEF). *Child Neuropsychology, 8,* 271–284.

Max, J. E., Castillo, C. S., Bokura, H., Robin, D. A., Lindgren, S. D., Smith, W. L. Jr.,... Mattheis, P. J. (1998). Oppositional defiant disorder symptomatology after traumatic brain injury: A prospective study. *Journal of Nervous and Mental Disease, 186,* 325–332.

Max, J. E., Keatley, E., Wilde, E. A., Bigler, E. D., Levin, H. S., Schachar, R. J.,... Yang, T. T. (2011). Anxiety disorders in children and adolescents in the first six months after traumatic brain injury. *Journal of Neuropsychiatry and Clinical Neurosciences, 23,* 29–39.

Max, J. E., Koele, S. L., Castillo, C. C., Lindgren, S. D., Arndt, S., Bokura, H.,... Bokura, Y. (2000). Personality change disorder in children and adolescents following traumatic brain injury. *Journal of the International Neuropsychological Society, 6,* 279–289.

Max, J. E., Levin, H. S., Schachar, R. J., Landis, J., Saunders, A. E., Ewing-Cobbs, L.,... Dennis, M. (2006). Predictors of personality change due to traumatic brain injury in children and adolescents six to twenty-four months after injury. *Journal of Neuropsychiatry and Clinical Neurosciences, 18,* 21–32.

Newman, L., Wagner, M., Knokey, A. M., Marder, C., Nagle, K., Shaver, D.,... Schwarting, M. (2011). *The post-high school outcomes of young adults with disabilities up to 8 years after high school.* A Report from the National Longitudinal Transition Study-2 (NLTS2) (NCSER 2011-3005). Menlo Park, CA: SRI International.

Nybo, T., Sainio, M., & Müller, K. (2004). Stability of vocational outcome in adulthood after moderate to severe preschool brain injury. *Journal of the International Neuropsychological Society, 10,* 719–723.

Ornstein, T. J., Levin, H. S., Chen, S., Hanten, G., Ewing-Cobbs, L., Dennis, M.,...Schachar, R. (2009). Performance monitoring in children following traumatic brain injury. *Journal of Child Psychology & Psychiatry, 50*, 506–513.

Power, T., Catroppa, C., Coleman, L., Ditchfield, M., & Anderson, V. (2007). Do lesion site and severity predict deficits in attentional control after preschool traumatic brain injury (TBI)? *Brain Injury, 21*, 279–292.

Rivara, F. P., Koepsell, T. D., Wang, J., Temkin, N., Dorsch, A., Vavilala, M. S.,...Jaffe, K. M. (2011). Disability 3, 12, and 24 months after traumatic brain injury among children and adolescents. *Pediatrics, 128*, e1129–e1138.

Salorio, C. F., Slomine, B. S., Grados, M. A., Vasa, R. A., Christensen, J. R., & Gerring, J. P. (2005). Neuroanatomic correlates of CVLT-C performance following pediatric traumatic brain injury. *Journal of the International Neuropsychological Society, 11*, 686–696.

Sambuco, M., Brookes, N., & Lah, S. (2008). Pediatric traumatic brain injury: A review of siblings' outcome. *Brain Injury, 22*, 7–17.

Schwartz, L., Taylor, H. G., Drotar, D., Yeates, K. O., Wade, S. L., & Stancin, T. (2003). Long-term behavior problems following pediatric traumatic brain injury: Prevalence, predictors, and correlates. *Journal of Pediatric Psychology, 28*, 251–263.

Singer, G. H. S., Glang, A., Nixon, C., Cooley, E., Kerns, K. A., Williams, D.,...Powers, L. (1994). A comparison of two psychosocial interventions for parents of children with acquired brain injury: An exploratory study. *Journal of Head Trauma Rehabilitation, 9*, 38–49.

Slomine, B., & Locascio, G. (2009). Cognitive rehabilitation for children with acquired brain injury. *Developmental Disabilities Research Reviews, 15*, 133–143.

Slomine, B. S., Gerring, J. P., Grados, M. A., Vasa, R., Brady, K. D., Christensen, J. R., & Denckla, M., B. (2002). Performance on measures of executive function following pediatric traumatic brain injury. *Brain Injury, 16*, 759–772.

Stancin, T., Wade, S. L., Walz, N. C., Yeates, K. O., & Taylor, H. G. (2010). Family adaptation 18 months after traumatic brain injury in early childhood. *Journal of Developmental and Behavioral Pediatrics, 31*, 317–325.

Strauss, E., Sherman, E. M. S., & Spreen, O. (2006). *A compendium of neuropsychological tests: Administration, norms, and commentary* (3rd ed.). Oxford: Oxford University Press.

Taylor, H. G., & Alden, J. (1997). Age-related differences in outcomes following childhood brain insults: An introduction and overview. *Journal of the International Neuropsychological Society 3*, 555–567.

Taylor, H. G., Yeates, K. O., Wade, S. L., Drotar, D., Stancin, T., & Burant, C. (2001). Bidirectional child-family influences on outcomes of traumatic brain injury in children. *Journal of the International Neuropsychological Society, 7*, 755–767.

Taylor, H. G., Yeates, K. O., Wade, S. L., Drotar, D., Stancin, T., & Minich, N. (2002). A prospective study of short- and long-term outcomes after traumatic brain injury in children: Behavior and achievement. *Neuropsychology, 16*, 15–27.

Todis, B., Glang, A., Bullis, M., Ettel, D., & Hood, D. (2011). Longitudinal investigation of the post-high school transition experiences of adolescents with traumatic brain injury. *Journal of Head Trauma Rehabilitation, 26*, 138–149.

Tremont, G., Mittenberg, W., & Miller, L. J. (1999). Acute intellectual effects of pediatric head trauma. *Child Neuropsychology, 5*, 104–114.

van't Hooft, I., Andersson, K., Bergman, B., Sejersen, T., Von Wendt, L., & Bartfai, A. (2005). Beneficial effect from a cognitive training programme on children with acquired brain injuries demonstrated in a controlled study. *Brain Injury, 19*, 511–518.

van 't Hooft, I., Andersson, K., Bergman, B., Sejersen, T., von Wendt, L., & Bartfai, A. (2007). Sustained favorable effects of cognitive training in children with acquired brain injuries. *NeuroRehabilitation, 22*, 109–116.

Wade, S. L., Carey, J., & Wolfe, C. R. (2006). An online family intervention to reduce parental distress following pediatric brain injury. *Journal of Consulting and Clinical Psychology, 74*, 445–454.

Wade, S. L., Taylor, H. G., Drotar, D., Stancin, T., Yeates, K. O., & Minich, N. M. (2002). A prospective study of long-term caregiver and family adaptation following brain injury in children. *Journal of Head Trauma Rehabilitation, 17*, 96–111.

Wade, S. L., Taylor, H. G., Yeates, K. O., Drotar, D., Stancin, T., Minich, N. M., & Schluchter, M. (2005). Long-term parental and family adaptation following pediatric brain injury. *Journal of Pediatric Psychology, 31*, 1072–1083.

Wade, S. L., Walz, N. C., Carey, J., McMullen, K. M., Cass, J., Mark, E., & Yeates, K. O. (2011). Effect on behavior problems of teen online problem-solving for adolescent traumatic brain injury. *Pediatrics, 128*, e94/–e953.

Wade, S. L., Walz, N. C., Carey, J., Williams, K. M., Cass, J., Herren, L.,... Yeates, K. O. (2010). A randomized trial of teen online problem solving for improving executive function deficits following pediatric traumatic brain injury. *Journal of Head Trauma Rehabilitation, 25*, 409–415.

Wade, S. L., Wolfe, C., Brown, T. M., & Pestian, J. P. (2005). Putting the pieces together: Preliminary efficacy of a web based family intervention for children with traumatic brain injury. *Journal of Pediatric Psychology, 30*, 437–442.

Wagner, M., Newman, L., Cameto, R., Garza, N., & Levine, P. (2005). *After high school: A first look at the postschool experiences of youth with disabilities*. A Report from the National Longitudinal Transition Study-2 (NLTS2). Menlo Park, CA: SRI International.

Ward, H., Shum, D., McKinlay, L., Baker, S., & Wallace, G. (2007). Prospective memory and pediatric traumatic brain injury: Effects of cognitive demand. *Child Neuropsychology, 13*, 219–239.

Warden, D. L., Gordon, B., McAllister, T. W., Silver, J. M., Barth, J. T., Bruns, J.,... Zitnay, G. (2006). Guidelines for the pharmacologic treatment of neurobehavioral sequelae of traumatic brain injury. *Journal of Neurotrauma, 23*, 1468–1501.

Webb, C., Rose, F. D., Johnson, D. A., & Attree, E. A. (1996). Age and recovery from brain injury: Clinical opinions and experimental evidence. *Brain Injury, 10*, 303–310.

Wilde, E. A., Hunter, J. V., Newsome, M. R., Scheibel, R. S., Bigler, E. D., Johnson, J. L.,... Levin, H. S. (2005). Frontal and temporal morphometric findings on MRI in children after moderate to severe traumatic brain injury. *Journal of Neurotrauma, 22*, 333–344.

Yeates, K. O. (2010). Traumatic brain injury. In K. O. Yeates, M. D. Ris, H. G. Taylor, & B. F. Pennington (Eds.), *Pediatric neuropsychology: Research, theory, and practice* (2nd ed.) (pp. 112–146). New York: The Guilford Press.

Yeates, K. O., Armstrong, K., Janusz, J., Taylor, H. G., Wade, S., Stancin, T., & Drotar, D. (2005). Long-term attention problems in children with traumatic brain injury. *Journal of the American Academy of Child and Adolescent Psychiatry, 44*, 574–584.

Yeates, K. O., Bigler, E. D., Dennis, M., Gerhardt, C. A., Rubin, K. H., Stancin, T.,... Vannatta, K. (2007). Social outcomes in childhood brain disorder: A heuristic integration of social neuroscience and developmental psychology. *Psychological Bulletin, 133*, 535–556.

Yeates, K. O., Swift, E., Taylor, H. G., Wade, S. L., Drotar, D., Stancin, T., & Minich, N. (2004). Short- and long-term social outcomes following pediatric traumatic brain injury. *Journal of the International Neuropsychological Society, 10*, 412–426.

Yeates, K. O., & Taylor, H. G. (2006). Behavior problems in school and their educational correlates among children with traumatic brain injury. *Exceptionality, 14*, 141–154.

Yeates, K., Taylor, H., Barry, C., Drotar, D., Wade, S., & Stancin, T. (2001). Neurobehavioral symptoms in childhood closed head injuries: Changes in prevalence and correlates during the first year postinjury. *Journal of Pediatric Psychology, 26*, 79–91.

Yeates, K. O., Taylor, H. G., Wade, S. L., Drotar, D., Stancin, T., & Minich, N. (2002). A prospective study of short- and long-term neuropsychological outcomes after traumatic brain injury in children. *Neuropsychology, 16*, 514–523.

Ylvisaker, M., Todis, B., Glang, A., Urbanczyk, B., Franklin, C., DePompei, R.,...Tyler, J. S. (2001). Educating students with TBI: Themes and recommendations. *Journal of Head Trauma Rehabilitation, 16*, 76–93.

Ylvisaker, M., Turkstra, L., Coehlo, C., Yorkston, K., Kennedy, M., Sohlberg, M. M., & Jack, A. (2007). Behavioural interventions for children and adults with behaviour disorders after TBI: A systematic review of the evidence. *Brain Injury, 21*, 769–805.

SECTION II
IMPACT ON EDUCATIONAL SYSTEMS

16 The Changing Face of Public Education

Meeting the Needs of Medically Challenged Children

Ellen Goldberger, Irene Meier, and Mary Ann Panarelli

Diego is of age to transition to kindergarten this fall. He presents as a friendly, interactive, and curious little boy with a high energy level. Diego is the product of a 23 gestational week pregnancy. At birth he weighed 1 pound and 1 ounce. He remained in the neonatal intensive care unit for 5 months. His medical status was extremely compromised. Diego has undergone heart surgery, laser surgery to repair a severe retinopathy of prematurity, bilateral cataract surgery, has been diagnosed with chronic lung disease, required respiratory support, and received multiple total blood transfusions. Diego continues to have an unsteady gait and requires ankle-foot orthotics to safely navigate his environment.

Throughout his three years in preschool, teachers have adapted all materials for Diego so that he is able to access the curriculum. Diego's compromised visual skills and poor attention have been challenging. Teachers have consistently used verbal cues and gestural prompts to help Diego learn to scan his visual environment methodically. Vision, physical, occupational, and speech therapists have all been provided to improve his skills, and his teachers have formulated strategies to allow him to engage in the academic environment.

Diego has been receiving language-rich special education services in a small group setting for three years. He has made impressive gains. Diego is at a turning point in his academic development and he will move into elementary school this fall. Visual complications due to his prematurity and his cognitive profile will present challenges as he enters elementary school and begins to integrate into larger classes. Teachers and therapists will need to develop new strategies with a strong evidence base to sustain Diego's positive academic trajectory as the demands of school become increasingly complex and as the pace of instruction increases and the curriculum becomes more prescribed by the need to prepare for mandatory state assessments.

In 1975, a federal law was passed requiring local educational agencies to provide a free, appropriate public education to all children, regardless of physical, mental, or emotional disability. This law, reauthorized and amended most recently as the Individuals with Disabilities Education Act (IDEA) in 2004, requires all states to provide early intervention, special education, and related services for infants, toddlers, and school-aged children. In 2010 the number of children aged 3–21 years receiving special education services exceeded 6.6 million, at an annual cost of approximately $50 billion above the base cost of general education (New America Foundation, 2011). The number of students receiving special education services increased 37% during the 25-year period from 1980–2005, while the total student population increased only 20% during the same period of time. Currently, approximately 14% of the educational population receives some form of special education support, which is an increase from the 10% of the population that received services in 1980 (National Center for Educational Statistics, 2011).

A number of factors contributed to both the increasing number of students receiving special education services and the per pupil cost of providing these services during the past 25 years. Schools began actively working with parents, physicians, and others in the community to identify students in need of special education support as early as possible. Identification criteria changed as more was learned about how disabilities present at different developmental stages. In addition, since the passage of the No Child Left Behind Act in 2000, the annual assessment of students on high-stakes testing has led to the identification of more students who are struggling to meet grade-level expectations. These changes resulted in earlier identification and longer periods of eligibility for special education services.

During the same time period, case law regarding the implementation of IDEA (*Cedar Rapids Community School District v. Garret F, 1999*) resulted in school divisions being responsible for nursing support and provision of a range of medical procedures to enable students to receive education in the least restrictive environment possible. Evolving interpretations of special education law based on court decisions, as well as advances in medical technology to create smaller and more portable medical devices, resulted in the inclusion of increasing numbers of children with significant medical, physical, and severe cognitive disabilities in the typical school setting versus placement in the private centers of the past. Required services during school hours expanded to include tube feeding, colostomy care, suctioning, ventilator management, catheterization, tracheostomy care, and the administration of oxygen, inhalants, and insulin (Heller, Frederick, Dykes, & Cohen, 2002). In this chapter we examine the processes used to determine whether a child is eligible for special education services in the school setting. We also explore the educational practices that have evolved specifically for children affected by low birth weight, respiratory disorders, childhood cancers, neurological disorders, autism, and chronic health conditions.

In a study completed by the Progressive Policy Institute (Berman, Davis, Koufman-Frederick, & Urion, 2001), researchers found that the number of children enrolled in special education preschool programs was increasing at a rate that exceeded the increase previously reported in school-aged special education and that the children in this population had more severe disabilities than those seen earlier. Reviewing one study completed in Massachusetts, they reported that the number of children served in special education preschool had increased 105% and that the number of children in this program with moderate to severe disabilities had increased 86% during the 10-year period from 1990 to 2000. The study also found that in 1980, approximately 2% of school-aged children had a medical condition that affected daily classroom functioning; by 2001 this number had increased to 7.5%. Changes in medical technology and outcomes during the same period provide a context for the increase seen in the need for special education services. Survival rates for children born weighing <3.3 pounds increased from 52% in 1980 to 73% in 1990 and to more than 90% today. Of these surviving children, approximately 10% develop severe spastic motor deficits and seizure disorders, and 50% experience significant cognitive difficulties, ranging from severe retardation to various learning disabilities. The authors note that prematurity and its consequences are not evenly distributed across the country, with children born in multigenerational poverty experiencing the greatest percentage of poor outcomes. This results in a disproportionate incidence of disabilities in poor urban and rural communities.

Studies conducted using national data from the United States and Canada demonstrated outcomes that are consistent with the Massachusetts findings. While the need for more costly services may vary by geographical location, all studies reported significant increases in the number of children surviving premature birth and a correlated increase in the number of students requiring special education services. In a study examining the relationship between birth conditions and special education eligibility in kindergarten, Roth et al. (2004) found that 50% of children born weighing <2500 grams required special education by kindergarten, as did 60% of children weighing <1500 grams. Special education services and staff ratios also vary by need, resulting in varying costs related to services provided. The cost of educating premature children is closely related to birth weight and associated medical complications, with children born weighing <2500 grams costing 22% more than average to educate in kindergarten, those weighing <2000 grams costing 49% more than average, and those weighing <1500 grams with 71% higher educational costs. Congenital abnormalities, separate from birth weight, resulted in 29% higher costs, with complications during delivery resulting in approximately 5% higher costs. As with the Massachusetts study, maternal poverty and low maternal education exacerbated the poor outcomes for low birth weight children, resulting in the need for additional special education services. Short and colleagues (2003) studied children at age 8 years who had experienced bronchopulmonary dysplasia (BPD) in addition to low birth weight and found that BPD and duration of the use of oxygen following birth predicted the need for special education services at an increased level, even among children of very low birth weight. More than 50% of the BPD children required special education services by age 8 years. Even when neurologically compromised children were removed from the analysis, 40% of the children with a history of BPD were receiving services. Similarly, Resnick and colleagues (1998) reported that within a population of Florida neonatal intensive care graduates, physical disabilities were positively correlated with birth weight; sensory impairments in vision and hearing were associated with very low (750–999 grams) and extremely low (500–749 grams) birth weight only; severe to moderate intellectual disabilities were associated with medical complications across all birth weight categories; and mild intellectual disabilities and learning disabilities were associated with medical conditions, ventilation, maternal education below high school graduate, and family income of less than $12,000 per year.

Medical treatment and ongoing pharmaceutical management have also broadened the number of children who are able to attend school and increased the range of conditions addressed at school each day. Although the number of full-term babies asphyxiated during delivery has remained fairly constant at 2 per 1000 births, the survival rate during the newborn period after asphyxia has increased from approximately 65% to close to 100% today (Berman, Davis, Koufman-Frederick, & Urion, 2001). Similarly, the percent of students with epilepsy who were able to attend school without significant interruptions has increased from 60% to 95% during the last 30 years. Although only 1% of school-aged children experience epilepsy, 85% of these children require special education services to maintain academic functioning, with all of the children requiring specialized training for staff in management of antiseizure medications and emergency seizure response.

Improved treatment outcomes and survival rates for children with childhood cancers have also increased dramatically in the past 25 years. Data from the Surveillance, Epidemiology, and End Results Program (1999) show that 5-year survival rates for all childhood cancers improved from 56% in 1974 to 75% by 1995, with an update indicating that by 2004 the survival rate was 80%. The same study found 81% of patients with acute lymphoblastic leukemia and 93% of patients with Hodgkin's disease or Wilms tumors survive. In a comparative study of young cancer survivors and their siblings, 23% of the survivors required special education services compared with 8% of their siblings. The highest rates of need for special education were among those diagnosed before age 6 years, especially survivors of central nervous system tumors and Hodgkin's disease (Mitby et al., 2003). Use of intrathecal methotrexate and cranial radiation therapy administered separately or in combination significantly increased use of special education services. Survivors of leukemia, central nervous system tumors, non-Hodgkin's lymphoma, and neuroblastoma were less likely to finish high school when compared with siblings. However, when these children received special education support, they were as likely to graduate as any of their siblings who had also needed special education services.

The number of children with chronic medical conditions attending public schools has also increased significantly in the past 25 years. Taras and Brennan (2008) report that 12.8% of school-aged children meet the definition for a special healthcare need. They report peak childhood prevalence in many Western nations for insulin-dependent diabetes, severe food and insect allergies, and asthma, especially among black, Hispanic, and poor children. Their study indicated that 26% of children in early-childhood special education programs were taking medications, and 16% were using some sort of medical equipment such as nebulizer machines and breathing monitors.

In addition, several disorders that may previously have been viewed as rooted in social–emotional development are now understood to have their genesis in neurological or biological differences. These include autism spectrum disorders and emotional disabilities such as depression, bipolar disorder, and anxiety disorder. As with other medical conditions, the incidence of these disorders has increased in the school population. A conservative estimate by Rutter (2005), based on a meta-analytic review of multiple epidemiological and clinical studies, suggests an increase in autism spectrum disorders from 1 in 10,000 to 30–60 in 10,000 during the past 40 years. Although Rutter attributes the increase both to better diagnostic evaluations and expansion of the definition of autism, he also indicates that the incidence of more severe forms of autism with concomitant social limitations, nonverbal or severe limitations in communication, and aggressive or self-injurious behaviors has also increased significantly. In 2010, the Centers for Disease Control and Prevention estimated the incidence of autism spectrum disorders to be 1 in 110, suggesting the incidence continues to climb and creating ongoing challenges for today's educators.

ACCOMMODATIONS TO GENERAL EDUCATION INSTRUCTION

Students with learning, physical, or medical needs secondary to a resolved or chronic health condition may receive accommodations under Section 504 of the Federal Rehabilitation Act of 1973, as amended in the Americans with Disabilities Amendment Act of 2008. This act expanded the definition of disability and guarantees that an individual with a disability cannot be denied participation in or excluded from the benefits of any program receiving federal assistance. Under the provisions of this act, a knowledgeable committee, including the student's parents or guardian, review medical documentation of a disability or history of suspected disability and current student performance to determine if accommodations are needed to ensure student access to all school activities. Evaluations may be completed to assess the extent of the educational impact of the condition, if necessary, or to determine if special educational services may also be required. If the committee determines accommodations are needed, these are written into a 504 plan and reviewed annually. Accommodations may include specialized transportation, adjustments in the school day, additional access to computers or other assistive technology, or specification that the student requires a specialized health plan. The health plan may be developed separately, in collaboration with the student's physicians, the public health nurse, and others who may be providing specialized health-related interventions. Often students who have experienced typical development but who also have chronic health conditions receive accommodations through Section 504.

Attendance is often an issue for these students due to frequent doctor or hospital visits or disease and treatment limitations such as immune system suppression. Sexson and Madan-Swain (1995) highlighted other factors that may affect peer interactions for students with chronic medical conditions, including changes in physical appearance due to illness or treatment; medication-related mood changes; and increased need to use the bathroom due to use of steroids, diuretics, and gastrointestinal problems such as those found with Crohn's disease. The recent increase in the incidence of disability related to Lyme disease and syndrome disorders related to auto-immune diseases, as well as less invasive cancer treatments, have challenged schools to provide flexible homebound services that allow students to attend school when they are feeling well and to receive services at home on a part-day or intermittent basis. Schools are beginning to encourage use of the Internet to help students stay in touch with instruction and peers during periods of absence. HopeCam is a nonprofit organization that provides laptops, Web cameras, and high speed Internet connections at no cost to children with cancer so they can stay connected.

Although the cost of providing homebound services and accommodations for students with chronic illnesses has not been calculated at a national level, parent advocacy for the needs of these children is increasing. Guidelines for parents, doctors, and other advocates created by a task force of national medical and nonprofit organizations, and published by the National Institutes of Health (2003), stresses the need for confidentiality and the appropriate sharing of information, acceptance and elimination of stigma, and thorough training and protocols for school personnel. In addition to asthma, diabetes, epilepsy, and allergies, this report addresses the unique needs of students with contagious conditions such as HIV/AIDS and methicillin-resistant staphylococcus aureus infections.

EVALUATION AND ELIGIBILITY FOR SPECIAL EDUCATION SERVICES

In addition to accommodations in general education provided under Section 504, some students require specialized instructional materials and strategies and additional accommodations that cannot reasonably be provided by a general education teacher. These students may be eligible for special education services under IDEA. The decision to evaluate to determine if the student is in need of services is made by a committee that includes the parents, classroom teacher, a special education teacher, and a school administrator. This team first reviews data collected over time by the classroom teacher, documenting the student's rate of progress in reading, mathematics, and written language, as well as response to any accommodations or interventions that have been tried prior to consideration for special education. If evaluation appears to be necessary, a multidisciplinary team that includes a school psychologist, social worker, educational specialist, and speech, language, vision, hearing, physical, or occupational therapists, as appropriate, complete evaluations and share data to determine patterns of performance and areas of strength and difficulty. The evaluations are intended to both identify deficits and strengths in processing and to determine the impact of this pattern of cognitive skills on the child's ability to access and make progress in the general curriculum.

Evaluations include observation of the child in the classroom setting and a review of any medical, developmental, and academic records that were collected prior to the decision to test for an educational disability. Specific evaluation tools vary with suspected area of disability but commonly include tests of intelligence and cognitive processing; tests of academic achievement in reading, mathematics, and written language, including speed, accuracy, and developmentally appropriate comprehension; problem solving; and oral and written communication skills. A complete sociocultural case history, including review of medical records and extensive input on parent perceptions of the student's challenges and desired educational interventions, is completed by interview with the parent or guardian. Additional medical evaluations to identify possible sensorineural or neurological conditions are completed as needed. If the parent has previously obtained neuropsychological or other evaluations, the findings of these evaluations are also considered; if current, these findings may replace an assessment typically completed by the school.

Evaluation of Cognitive Processes

Evaluations are completed to determine intellectual ability and identify the underlying cognitive processes that are deficient and creating barriers to learning and success in the educational setting. The goal of assessment in public schools is to delineate the presence or absence of skills needed for successful functioning in the classroom and provide information that will guide specific teaching strategies. These assessments are not intended to describe all cognitive processes involved in day-to-day functioning.

Evaluations completed in the school setting typically include an overall assessment of cognitive abilities followed by specific measures to explore areas of deficit (Baron, 2004). This approach, initially described by Wilson (1986), is labeled "the branching hypothesis testing model." It has been used successfully with both preschool and school-aged populations. The underlying presumption of this model is that children have multifaceted cognitive abilities and these abilities should be probed in isolation using tests that examine each multivariate skill set that is used to complete diverse academic tasks.

Overall tests of cognitive functioning such as the Wechsler tests (Wechsler, 2003) and the Differential Ability Scales–Second Edition (Elliott, 2007) as well as others are typically used for the initial portion of the evaluation. Tests targeting speech and language, visual–motor, visual–perceptual, visual–spatial, fine–motor, and gross–motor functioning are then utilized depending on the outcome of the subtests from the initial measure. Targeted evaluation tools such as the NEuro PSYchological Assessment-II (Korkman, Kirk, & Kemp, 2007) make the branching hypothesis model more accessible within the school setting where testing time is significantly constrained. This assessment tool partially has its theoretical underpinnings in Luria's theory (1973) of brain organization and of cognitive development. It is comprised of subtests that tap the underlying functional domains of attention and executive functioning, language, memory and learning, sensorimotor skills, social perception, and visuospatial processing. The authors indicate that the whole test does not need to be administered; selected subtests can be used to probe a suspected area of disability. This flexibility of test administration lends itself to Wilson's assessment model. Further, in addition to testing completed by the psychologist, information collected by team other members help derive a more precise profile of the student.

In addition to the assessment of discrete processes described above, the evaluation of executive function and the subset of attention and self-regulation are essential components of the school-based evaluation. Within this portion of the assessment, metacognitive processes are examined because they are essential for the successful acquisition of academics. Specifically, this domain concerns the brain's overarching ability to integrate individual cognitive functions, coordinate incoming information, and apply working memory abilities to analyze and respond to information from the brain's discrete regions (Zelazo, Carlson, & Keesak, 2008). Not surprisingly, executive functions are especially vulnerable in children with severely challenged neonatal and medical histories.

Development of executive function skills throughout childhood is critical for academic success, especially the area of self-regulation (Blair et al., 2005; Carlson, 2005). In the academic setting, students are expected to plan and execute assignments, often together with other students and in response to instruction from many teachers with different deadlines. Thus, understanding challenges that the student faces in this domain is especially important and will aid the development of strategies that can be used to access and organize information in a timely manner.

As noted above, with the introduction of Public Law 94–142 in 1975, age-appropriate and early intervention to allow access to the entire curriculum has become a major focus, along with the need for precise assessment of possible disabling conditions that result in appropriate interventions for preschoolers. Both Wilson's hypothesis branching model and Heffelfinger's clinical research (Mrakotsky & Heffelfinger, 2006) and work with preschoolers at the Medical College of Wisconsin provided tools and underlying developmental analyses that aid in the comprehension of strengths and deficits presented by the youngest children.

It is also essential that the student's physician or other healthcare provider and the school team communicate and collaborate on behalf of the student. Through this partnership, a more informed understanding of the student's school behavior, medical history, and medical concerns will be possible. In additon, each professional will gain a more comprehensive picture of the child's cognitive abilities across environments. Information from the physician regarding anticipated fluctuations in performance, stamina, and attention secondary to illness or treatment helps teachers appropriately plan the pace and type of instruction needed. This, in turn, allows the team to determine where along the spectrum of disability the child functions, as well as the intervention approaches that may be most effective.

Once evaluations are completed, the parents meet with the evaluation team members, the classroom teacher, and the school administrator to determine if the student meets established criteria for 1 of 14 possible disability areas. Both evidence of the disability and the impact of the disability on the student's ability to access and benefit from instruction are considered. Children with complex medical histories may be found eligible for services under a range of categories. Some may be eligible as students with intellectual or physical disabilities or with sensory impairments. Others may need services to address more subtle learning disabilities that do not affect intellect but may impair reading, writing, mathematics, memory, or executive functioning skills. Still others may receive special education services under the Other Health Impaired category to address neurological side effects such as attentional disorders, fluctuations in mood, changes in fine- or gross-motor coordination, or need for medical intervention within the school setting. Often students in this latter category learn at expected rates but need targeted instruction, practice, and support in order to increase independence, work completion, endurance, or attention.

SPECIAL EDUCATION SERVICES

To assist the IEP team in determining the types of services and the class placement that would best support Diego in the kindergarten setting, a developmental evaluation was completed to describe the precise nature of Diego's strengths and deficits. After the assessment data were gathered, the team convened to discuss the results. The findings indicated that with accommodations in place to give Diego clear structure and extra cues for the examination of visual materials, he demonstrated language conceptual skills within the low-average to average range. Functioning in the spatial analytic domain fell in the very low range. Educational testing indicated that Diego was learning age-appropriate pre-academic skills in the classroom because he performed within the average range on measures of general knowledge and applied problem solving. Results from graphomotor tasks revealed performance in the low range. The conclusion was that Diego presented as a student with relatively intact conceptual language skills but severely compromised spatial analytic functioning. Executive functioning was negatively impacted as well; Diego demonstrated considerable challenges in his ability to self-regulate and focus his attention. Organizational (sequencing) abilities were also delayed. Despite evidence of average cognitive functioning, Diego's learning profile suggested that he would require carefully designed instruction to continue to progress as the number of students in his class and the pace of instruction increased with entry into kindergarten.

Following eligibility determination, the IEP team develops an educational plan. This document includes goals in all areas of need and defines how progress will be measured. These goals take into consideration grade-level expectations and the child's current level of functioning in each domain and establish expected progress during the coming year. For some, the annual goal may be to develop foundational skills that underlie the more complex grade-level skills. For others, the aim may be to close the gap between current and expected levels of performance. The IEP identifies accommodations and services that should allow the child to progress. Depending on the severity of the child's disability, special education services to meet these goals may be provided in the regular classroom or in smaller group settings.

INSTRUCTIONAL MODELS FOR STUDENTS WITH SEVERE COGNITIVE DISABILITIES

Prior to the passage of Public Law 94–142, students with severe disabilities were often institutionalized or kept at home and cared for by relatives. In the mid-twentieth century schools created special classes where teachers focused instruction on each child's apparent mental age level, as determined by developmental assessment (Spooner & Browder, 2006). In the mid 1970s, Brown and colleagues (1976) rejected the developmental model in favor of a more functional curriculum. They argued that the developmental model for a student whose maximum developmental age might be 2 years or less limited instruction for the student and did not maximize opportunities to develop independent living skills. Typical instruction in the developmental model might, for example, have engaged the student using toys appropriate for a 2-year-old even if the student was in high school. Using a functional model, the teacher would have targeted a skill, such as doing laundry, and taught the student to sort whites from dark-colored clothing.

From the 1970s through the turn of the century, the acquisition of functional skills was considered to be the primary outcome of educational programming for students with moderate to severe disabilities (Snell & Brown, 2006). The rationale was that functional skills would enable students to live with maximum independence and was based on the belief that academic skills were of little use for a child who would likely need supervision and support into adulthood. Westling and Fox (2004) recommended teaching functional skills on a daily basis and noted that functional objectives should be incorporated into a student's IEP. Brown and colleagues (1976) referred to four domains in the functional curriculum: community, domestic, vocational, and recreational. Classroom time addressed each domain in order to increase independent daily living skills.

Effective functional skill instruction focused on increasing independence by teaching practical skills in natural settings. Instructional strategies included practice to ensure that skills could be applied, maintained, and generalized across multiple settings. A critical component of effective functional skill instruction was the collection of data about student performance, which guided decisions about when the student had mastered a target skill and was ready to learn more complex skills (Westling & Fox, 2004). Areas of need that have an impact on the student's life were incorporated into the curriculum (Gee, 2004). Advocates also began to request that students with a range of disabilities have the opportunity to interact with their typically developing peers so they could practice their newly acquired functional skills in a natural setting.

Beginning in the late 1990s and into the current decade, a shift occurred in the instruction of students with disabilities. While acknowledging that functional skills were critically important, parents and educators began advocating for functional activities that also provided a context for learning academic skills as well (Spooner & Browder, 2006). In addition to promoting the inclusion of students with disabilities in general education settings to enhance social skills, educators and parents began to focus on improving academic skills in these settings as well.

ACADEMIC FOCUS

The legal mandates of the No Child Left Behind (NCLB) Act (2001) and IDEA (2004) together changed the focus of instruction for students with disabilities across the nation. These two statutes included mandates for the provision of evidenced-based instruction for students with disabilities and required that all students, including those with disabilities, participate in statewide accountability measures (Wakeman, Browder, Meier, & McColl, 2007). With the reauthorization of IDEA (2004), it was no longer sufficient for students to have access to the general curriculum. The legislation mandated they should also "make progress" in the general curriculum. This applied to all students, from those with the most profound cognitive disabilities to those with more subtle but significant learning difficulties.

Instructional practices evolved in response to greater understanding of the potential of students with disabilities and to changes in the law. In order for students with disabilities to progress in the general curriculum, strategies with a foundation in research were developed. These strategies were proven effective with many students, including those with severe cognitive impairments, but must be implemented with fidelity, and progress must be continually assessed to ensure mastery and determine the appropriate pace of instruction.

Past instruction focused on mastery of discrete basic reading and writing skills and often limited student exposure to higher-level concepts in diverse academic domains. In the area of literacy, Koppenhaver and Yoder (1993) reported that students with severe disabilities did not have sufficient opportunities to participate in literacy activities in school. This was further demonstrated in a literature review by Browder, Wakeman, et al. (2006) who identified 128 studies in literacy between 1975 and 2003. This review indicated that the majority of studies focused on sight word vocabulary and fluency. Less than one-fourth of the studies assessed comprehension, phonemic awareness, or phonics. These results suggested that reading instruction for students with disabilities did not include instruction in all critical components of reading.

According to Browder, Ahlgrim-Delzell, et al. (2006), mathematics instruction for students with moderate to severe disabilities focused on instruction of the functional skill of money management. In 2005, Browder and colleagues conducted a comprehensive review of 55 mathematics studies since 1975 that involved students with moderate to severe disabilities and found that 27, almost half, involved a form of money management skills. Although mathematics focuses on five content areas of "number and operations, algebra, geometry, measurement, data analysis and interpretation" (Browder, Ahlgrim-Delzell et al., 2006, p.192), most studies involving students with significant cognitive disabilities focused on purchasing skills. Similar limitations in curriculum were seen in science and social studies (Spooner, DiBiase, & Courtade-Little, 2006), with most instruction focusing on weather and basic earth sciences, famous Americans, and basic civic responsibilities.

Since 2000, when all students with disabilities had to take state assessments of reading and mathematics, instruction has shifted to include a broader exposure to grade-level concepts, even for the most disabled students. McGrew and Evans (2004) report that in a 4-year span, rates of students with disabilities meeting grade-level benchmarks increased from 26% to 50% in reading and from 36% to 58% in math, suggesting that when higher standards are set, and appropriate interventions and materials used to teach these students, many will succeed at higher levels than previously demonstrated. In addition, passing the state exams also opens up a route to enrollment in high school course work that will lead to a standard diploma or GED.

ASSISTIVE TECHNOLOGY

Students with significant disabilities often require the use of assistive technology in order to access the general curriculum and derive benefit from special education services. Assistive technology devices and services are delineated in the statute separately. An assistive technology device can be defined as "any item, piece of equipment, or product system, whether acquired commercially off the shelf, modified, or customized, that is used to increase, maintain, or improve functional capabilities of children with disabilities" [20 U.S.C. § 1401, 25–26]. Examples of assistive technology devices include communication boards, voice output augmentative communication, word processing devices, and iPads and other mobile devices. The use of the latter devices has enabled some students with disabilities to better access the general curriculum.

One use of assistive technology for students with severe disabilities is to provide a means of communication for students who cannot speak. Cosbey and Johnston (2006) showed the benefits of assistive technology for students aged 3–6 years who had severe and multiple disabilities. The children were taught to use a voice output communication aid (VOCA) to request access to peers or preferred items during play; there was an increase in all participants' correct use of the VOCA when unprompted. The participants obtained access to toys in all opportunities and obtained access to social intervention with peers in 96% of the opportunities. These results indicated target skill acquisition for all participants even though they had severe developmental disabilities that affected communication and motor skills.

The Assistive Technology Act of 2004 provides for increased access to technology for individuals with disabilities and requires that school districts use assistive technology resources to improve transition services. It also ensures that students with disabilities have support as they apply for loans for devices. In addition, under IDEA, a central repository of digital versions of all textbooks published in the United States was created. The law requires that publishers provide a digital copy of all textbooks to the national center. These can then be converted into Braille, or other electronic format to allow students with a range of disabilities to access instructional materials. IDEA

2004 also requires that school divisions consider the concept of Universal Design for Learning (UDL), which integrates multiple ways to access materials for all students so that special accommodations are not required for learners with challenges. With the correct instructional support, including UDLs, students with disabilities can successfully access and make progress in the general curriculum.

BEST PRACTICES IN INSTRUCTION FOR STUDENTS WITH DISABILITIES

Systematic Instruction

Students with disabilities, even those with significant cognitive and sensory disabilities, have been able to acquire new skills and behaviors through by using systematic instruction. Systematic instruction is "teaching focused on specific, measurable responses...that are established through the use of defined methods of prompting and feedback based on the principles and research of applied behavior analysis" (Browder & Lim, 2001, p. 95). Systematic instruction can be used to increase attention span. Through prompting and reinforcing approximations of desired behaviors, severely disabled students can begin to master self-help and communication skills. Systematic instruction also includes the use of task analysis to identify the specific skills required to execute a given behavior or task. Teachers conduct task analysis to break down desired behaviors into a sequence or chain of tasks that can be taught individually and then completed in a sequence. Utilizing fundamental behavioral strategies, teachers gradually move from constant reinforcement of desired behaviors to intermittent delays prior to reinforcing. They then gradually fade prompts until the behavior is self-sustaining, generalized across environments, and reinforced by naturally occurring consequences. Utilizing these techniques, students with significant cognitive disabilities as well as students with autism are taught reading, mathematics, communication, and social skills.

Literacy Instruction

More than 50% of students with speech and language disorders develop a reading disability (Hamilton & Glascoe, 2006), and a majority of students identified as disabled have difficulty learning to read. Although students with cognitive disabilities may struggle with all aspects of reading, from letter and sound recognition to comprehension and writing skills, students with processing deficits may have difficulty mastering one skill, such as decoding unfamiliar vocabulary, but may have no difficulty with higher-order skills such as comprehension. Others may decode easily and read fluently but struggle to remember or comprehend inferences in what they read. These deficit areas can be overcome through the use of instruction that is direct, systematic, and explicit (Archer & Hughes, 2011). Rosenshine (1987) described explicit instruction as "a systematic method of teaching with emphasis on proceeding in small steps, checking for student understanding, and achieving active and successful participation by all students" (p.34). Based on several US Department of Education reports (Gersten et al., 2009; Kamil et al., 2008), the evidence level for explicit instruction such as modeling, guided practice, corrective feedback, and review was found to be strong. According to Archer and Hughes (2011), "explicit methodology...is absolutely essential for struggling or disadvantaged learners" (p. 17).

According to Archer and Hughes (2011) the teacher effectiveness literature has described the following six principles of effective instruction: (1) optimizing engaged time on task, (2) promoting high success levels, (3) increasing content coverage, (4) increasing time in instructional groups, (5) scaffolding instruction, and (6) addressing the different forms of knowledge. In addition to the use of explicit instruction, the use of effective instructional practices, as outlined above, is essential for teaching students with disabilities and struggling learners.

Inclusive Practices

Another best practice is to include students with disabilities with their nondisabled peers. IDEA requires that the IEP team consider the least restrictive environment possible when determining where the student will receive special education services. As noted earlier, the commitment to ensuring that all students have the maximum possible opportunity to interact with their peers has resulted in students with a range of medical needs being served in general education school settings. Teachers and assistants are trained to perform a number of personal or medically related tasks from administering Diastat for seizures to suctioning a tracheostomy tube.

In inclusive education, students with disabilities attend the district school they would attend if they were not disabled, appropriate supports are available in both special and general education settings, and all students are welcome in the general education program (Giangreco, 2006). Students with disabilities are educated with age-appropriate peers and shared educational experiences take place in general education classes and integrated community settings. Over the course of the day, it is important to ensure that students with more severe disabilities have varied educational experiences that are designed to meet individual needs for a balance of academic, functional, and social–personal domains of learning. Ryndak (1996) outlined instructional strategies such as cooperative learning strategies, small group instruction, and peer partnering, including peer tutoring and study buddies, as effective strategies to facilitate inclusion of students with significant cognitive disabilities.

The benefits of inclusion for students with significant disabilities have been established. Alper and Ryndak (1992) found that students with significant cognitive disabilities who are included had more opportunities for social interaction, appropriate behavior models, improved communication and social skills, and friendships. Teachers develop higher expectations as students access more age-appropriate curricular content. Finally, students increase their chances for participation in life-long integrated activities.

The utilization of peer supports has been a viable alternative strategy to support students with significant cognitive disabilities in the general education classroom (Cushing & Kennedy, 1997). Carter et al. (2005) investigated the impact of altering the number of participating peers on social and academic outcomes of students with significant cognitive disabilities. The participants were three middle school students with significant cognitive disabilities and six general education students. Peers were taught strategies including how to adapt materials, provide instruction on IEP goals, implement behavior plans, give feedback to the student, and promote communication between the students with disabilities and their peers in the classroom. Results indicated that students with disabilities increased their social interaction when two peers were provided versus one peer, but this did not affect their interactions with other students in the class. Peer supports encouraged the students to engage in activities that were aligned with the general curriculum. Neither configuration of peer supports had a negative effect on the general education student's curricular access. Therefore, it was not detrimental for the general education students to serve as peer supports for student with disabilities. These studies illustrate a body of research that supports inclusive practices for students with significant cognitive disabilities (Giangreco, 2006).

Strong Family and School Collaboration

Another best practice found to be effective for students with disabilities is to build a strong relationship between home and school. Chen and Miles (2004, p. 31) wrote that, "teachers not only must have instructional skills for teaching children but also must have the competency to work effectively with families." The 1997 amendments to IDEA increased the parent's responsibility to be an active partner in making decisions with the schools and agencies. Under this amendment, parents have the right to informed consent as it relates to assessment, goals, objectives, and services and also to participate in all decisions that relate to eligibility and placement.

Although today's schools are generally child focused, there is a need to be more family focused and to utilize a family-centered approach when working with students with significant cognitive disabilities (Childre, 2004). Family and educator collaborative practices are more likely to be positive when using a family-centered approach. According to Powell, Batsche, Ferro, Fox, and Dunlap (1997), major principles for establishing a family-centered approach include the following: building trust, establishing open communication, enabling and empowering family and student, and using a collaborative problem-solving approach.

Conflicts may arise between parents and educators when educational priorities are discussed (Browder & Lim, 2001). In a study by Hamre-Nietupski, Nietupski, and Strathe (1992), parents of students with moderate to severe and profound disabilities were asked to rate the value they placed on functional life skills, social relationship/ friendship skills, and functional academics. Parents of students with moderate disabilities ranked functional life skills at the highest level, followed by functional academics and social relationship/friendship skills. Parents of students with severe and profound disabilities ranked social relationship/friendship skills at the highest level, followed by functional life skills and functional academics. In another study, Lim, Tan, and Quah (2000) surveyed Singaporean parents of students with mild, moderate, and severe disabilities. Parents of students with moderate and severe disabilities ranked self-help functional life skills highest, followed by community-based life skills, social relationship, and functional academics. Because differences exist among parents of varying cultures in terms of educational priorities, educators must be aware of both parental preferences and cultural influences when collaborating with families to achieve optimum outcomes for students.

Collaborative Learning and Teaching Teams

Another highly effective practice is collaborative teaming among school personnel. For students with disabilities to experience school success, a certain degree of collaborative teaming among professionals is required (Ryndak, 1996). This teaming is necessary in order to meet the student's needs in many environments, including school, home, and the community. The team shares roles and responsibilities and treats the student as a "whole" rather than just focusing on the student's needs in their particular discipline. Collaborative teams plan services in locations that would be considered "natural." For example, collaborative services are delivered in a location where the target skill may naturally occur (e.g., the cafeteria) rather than working on skills in isolation. A benefit of collaborative teaming is that the students have an increased number of practice trials during the instructional day that may result in a faster acquisition and generalization of skills. A second benefit is that collaborative teams provide information to parents relative to instructional strategies and application to real-life situations. Third, members of the collaborative team consider solutions and provide technical and moral support to each other and to the classroom teacher, family, and student (Ferguson, Meyer, Jeanchild, Juniper, & Zingo, 1992). The use of collaborative teaming, including cross-disciplinary instruction and flexible scheduling, has been supported by expert opinion as a best practice for this population of students (Ryndak, 1996; Snell & Brown, 2006; Westling & Fox, 2004).

Positive Behavior Supports

Positive behavior support (PBS) has been cited as an evidence-based practice that is used to manage challenging behaviors in students with disabilities, including those with significant cognitive disabilities (Snell & Brown, 2006). Positive behavior support strategies have also been proven effective for students with autism (Horner et al., 2002) and those with developmental disabilities (Carr et al., 1999). It applies positive strategies to decrease inappropriate behaviors and increase appropriate behaviors (Horner et al., 2006). Snell (2005) reported that although PBS has experienced success, there is a research-to-practice gap for students with significant cognitive disabilities. Carr et al. (1999) conducted a review of 107 studies involving PBS. Two hundred and twenty-two participants, with the largest percentage having mental retardation, were identified in study years 1985–1996. The investigation focused on the following variables: demographics, assessment, interventions, and outcomes. Results indicated that the field has been growing over the years primarily in the areas of assessment and interventions focused on remediating environmental deficiencies. PBS strategies can be utilized for people with serious behavioral problems and are effective in reducing behavioral problems in 50%–66% of cases. Success rates almost double when the intervention is predicated upon functional assessment.

SELF-DETERMINATION

The importance of self-determination for students with disabilities has been substantiated in the literature, although students with significant cognitive disabilities have not always had the opportunity to learn these skills (Algozzine, Browder, Karvonen, Test, & Wood, 2001; Martin, Van Dycke, Christensen, Greene, Gardner, et al., 2006; Wehmeyer & Schwartz, 1998; Wood, Fowler, Uphold, & Test, 2005). Self-determination has been defined as "a combination of skills, knowledge, and beliefs that enable a person to engage in goal-directed, self-regulated, autonomous behavior" (Field, Martin, Miller, Ward, & Wehmeyer, 1998, p. 2). These skills include choice making, decision making, goal setting and attainment, problem solving, self-awareness, self-regulation, and participation in the IEP process (Agran, Blanchard, Wehmeyer, & Hughes, 2001; Allen,

Smith, Test, Flowers, & Wood, 2001; Van Reusen & Bos, 1990). Wehmeyer (2005) has proposed that the definition of self-determination for students with significant cognitive disabilities be that "self-determined behavior refers to volitional acts that enable one to act as the primary causal agent in one's life and to maintain or improve one's quality of life" (p. 117).

Self-determination practices evolved as a result of the normalization and deinstitutionalization efforts of the 1970s. Self-determination relates to teaching individuals with disabilities to make choices, as well as teaching individuals without disabilities to respect those choices (Algozzine et al., 2001). Regardless of the severity of disability, all individuals should be active participants in exercising choice over the decisions affecting their lives (Brown, Belz, Corsi, &Wenig, 1993). According to Wehmeyer and Schwartz (1998), people who are self-determined have better quality of life. Research has demonstrated that students of varying ages and disabilities can be taught self-determination and self-advocacy skills (Algozzine et al., 2001; Wood et al., 2005).

Wood et al. (2005) reviewed 20 single-subject designs and one qualitative study focusing on interventions in self-determination for students with significant cognitive disabilities. Results of both Algozzine et al. (2001) and Wood et al. (2005) indicate that research on self-determination for students with significant disabilities is limited; in both reviews, the most common self-determination component was choice making.

The school team had the opportunity to consult with Diego's physicians. The ophthalmologist explained that Diego experiences significantly decreased visual acuity and also appears to have cortical involvement, which may help explain his compromised spatial analytic skills. Executive functioning was discussed with Diego's pediatrician. She believed, based on data from the school and home environments, that a trial of medication for ADHD might be useful. In fact, it resulted in improved self-regulation and focus on academics. The school-based physical therapist and the orthopedist discussed issues surrounding Diego's safety within the school environment due to his unsteady gait and poor motor planning. As a result, more precise accommodations were put in place at school. The school team has also been crafting interventions based on the results of all assessments. Based on collaborative team discussions, a literacy program has been selected, and instructional strategies and accommodations tailored for Diego are in place for the upcoming school year.

CONCLUSION

The initiation of the 1976 federal law that mandated local educational agencies to provide a free, appropriate public education to all children, regardless of physical, mental, or emotional disabilities has altered public school systems. This law, further refined, has been reauthorized as part of the IDEA, most recently in 2004. It delineates the responsibilities for all states to provide early intervention, special education, and related services for infants, toddlers, and school-aged children. This mandate has vast implications for the public education system not only because of the increase in the number of services that must be provided by these institutions but also because of the significant increase in the number of children with special needs requiring individualized instruction.

Federal law mandates that all children have equal access to participation in the least restrictive educational environment. This directive has caused school systems to adapt their programs to meet the needs of diverse populations. School teams must use the expanded definition of disabilities that now includes both Section 504 plans executed in the general education environment and special education plans delivered in both the general and special education environments when determining how to give all students equal access to the educational curriculum.

In 2010, the number of students receiving special education services in the United States exceeded 6.6 million. With more sophisticated medical technology, the number of children surviving premature births has increased dramatically. The correlation between the increased number of students requiring special education services and these survival rates is apparent; 50% of children born weighing <2500 grams require special education. Medical treatments have also made it possible for more physically compromised students to attend school. Moreover, improved treatment outcomes and survival rates from childhood cancers contribute to the growing number of children in this group. In addition, the incidence of autism spectrum disorders as well as other biologically based emotional disorders has grown larger.

Understanding the educational needs and necessary accommodations for these students in the public school is multifaceted and requires detailed targeted assessments by school teams. These evaluations may include an overall examination of cognitive processes within the linguistic–conceptual, spatial–conceptual, and executive–function domains; social and emotional assessments; speech and language evaluations; academic testing; physical and occupational assessments as well as sociocultural interviews to document the child's developmental history. In addition, consultation with the student's physicians and other outside providers is, at times, imperative. In this way a thorough understanding of the child's medical status and performance in other settings can be incorporated into the school team's understanding of the student's strengths and weaknesses as well as his or her ability to sustain academic functioning throughout the school day.

When the team has reaches an understanding of the child's overall developmental status, including the student's strengths and challenges, they are then able to develop an IEP plan that will address the goals the child is expected to reach within all academic and behavioral domains, within a year's time. The IEP is data driven and can be revised at any point if goals are determined to have been reached or are too difficult for the student to attain.

With this document as a guide, teachers are required to facilitate their students' educational progress. Due to the complexity of the students' cognitive, social, emotional, and physical challenges, diverse data-driven teaching strategies are put in place and constantly adapted to meet the students' changing needs. Much research in pedagogy has influenced teaching strategies with systematic direct instruction focused on targeted skills at the core of strategies used to teach students with disabilities. All students are exposed to academic skills, and their understanding of presented concepts is evaluated through formative assessments at least weekly, as well as by summative assessments at the end of the year.

Due to the changing nature of federal mandates, the increase in the number of challenged students entering the public education system, and the diverse teaching strategies necessary to accommodate their needs, flexibility and individualization are key components of modern education. Professionals who work with students with disabilities must be trained and willing to perform a range of personal help and medically related procedures. Collaboration is essential, and everyone must be willing to make mid-course corrections as dictated by the data indicating the effectiveness of a given strategy or to accommodate changing medical needs. Despite the demands inherent in the field, few would deny that every step was worth the effort it took when watching a student who has overcome many obstacles graduate with his peers.

REFERENCES

Agran, M., Blanchard, C., Wehmeyer, M., & Hughes, C. (2001). Teaching students to self-regulate their behavior: The differential effects of student vs. teacher-delivered reinforcement. *Research in Developmental Disabilities, 22*, 319–332.

Algozzine, B., Browder, D., Karvonen, M., Test, D. W., & Wood, W. M. (2001). Effects of interventions to promote self-determination for individuals with disabilities. *Review of Educational Research, 71*, 219–277.

Allen, S. K., Smith, A. C., Test, D. W., Flowers, C., & Wood, W. M. (2001). The effects of self-directed IEP on student participation in IEP meetings. *Career Development for Exceptional Individuals, 24*, 107–120.

Alper, S., & Ryndak, D. (1992). Educating students with severe handicaps in regular classroom settings. *The Elementary School Journal, 92*, 373–387.

Archer, A. L., & Hughes, C. A. (2011). Explicit instruction: Effective and efficient teaching. In K. R. Harris & S. Graham (Eds.), *What works for special needs learners* (pp. 1–22). New York: Guilford Press.

Baron, I. S. (2004). *Neuropsychological Evaluation of the Child.* New York: Oxford University Press.

Berman, S., Davis, P., Koufman-Frederick, A., & Urion, D. (2001). The rising cost of special education in Massachusetts: Causes and effects. In C. E. Finn, A. J. Rotherham, & C. R. Hokanson (Eds.), *Rethinking special education for a new century* (pp. 183–211). The Thomas B. Fordham Foundation and Public Policy Institute. Retrieved December 1, 2011, from http://www.edexcellencemedia.net/publications/2001/200105_rethinking-specialed/special_ed_final.pdf

Blair, C., Zelazo, P. D., & Greenberg, M. T. (2005). Measurement of executive function in early childhood. *Developmental Neuropsychology, 28*, 561–571.

Browder, D. M., & Lim, L. (2001). Family-centered planning: A multicultural perspective. In D. M. Browder (Ed.), *Curriculum and assessment for students with moderate and severe disabilities* (pp. 116–147). New York: The Guilford Press.

Browder, D. M., Ahlgrim-Delzell, L., Pugalee, D., & Jimenez, B. (2006). Enhancing numeracy. In D. M. Browder & F. Spooner (Eds.), *Teaching language arts, math, and science to students with significant cognitive disabilities.* (pp. 171–196). Baltimore, MD: Paul H. Brookes.

Browder, D. M., Wakeman, S. Y., Spooner, F., Ahlgrim-Delzell, L., & Algozzine, B. (2006). Research on reading for students with significant cognitive disabilities. *Exceptional Children, 72*, 392–408.

Brown, L., Belz, P., Corsi, L., & Wenig, B. (1993). Choice diversity for people with severe disabilities. *Education and Training in Mental Retardation, 28*, 318–326.

Brown, L., Nietupski, J., & Hamre-Nieutupski, S. (1976). The criterion of ultimate functioning and public school services for severely handicapped students. In M. A. Thomas (Ed.), *Hey, don't forget about me: Education's investment in the severely, profoundly, and multiply handicapped* (pp. 2–15). Reston, VA: Council for Exceptional Children.

Carter, E. W., Cushing, L. S., Clark, N. M., & Kennedy, C. H. (2005). Effects of peer support interventions on students' access to the general curriculum and social interactions. *Research and Practice for Persons with Severe Disabilities, 30*, 15–25.

Carr, E. G., Horner, R. H., Turnbull, A. P., Marquis, J. G., McLaughlin, D. M., McAtee, M. L.,...Braddock, D. (1999). *Positive behavior support for people with developmental disabilities: A research synthesis.* Washington, DC: American Association on Mental Retardation.

Cedar Rapids Community School District v. Garret F., 526 U.S. 66, 1999.

Center for Disease Control Autism and Developmental Disabilities Monitoring Network. http://www.cdc.gov/ncbddd/autism/addm.html

Chen, D., & Miles, D. (2004). Working with families. In: F. P. Orelove, D. Sobsey, & R. K. Silberman (Eds.), *Educating children with multiple disabilities: A collaborative approach* (pp. 31–65). Baltimore, MD: Paul H. Brookes Publishing Co, Inc.

Childre, A. L. (2004). Families. In C. H. Kennedy & E. M. Horn (Eds.), *Including students with severe disabilities* (pp. 78–99). Boston: Pearson.

Cosbey, J. E., & Johnston, S. (2006). Using a single-switch voice output communication aid to increase social access for children with severe disabilities in inclusive classrooms. *Research and Practice for Persons with Severe Disabilities, 31,* 144–156.

Cushing, L. S., & Kennedy, C. H. (1997). Academic effects of providing peer support in general education classrooms on students without disabilities. *Journal of Applied Behavior Analysis, 30,* 139–151.

Elliott, C. D. (2007). *Differential Ability Scales-Second Edition,* San Antonio, TX: Harcourt Assessment.

Ellis, E. S., & Worthington, L. A. (1994). *Research synthesis on effective teaching principles and the design of quality tools for educators* (Technical Report No. 5). Eugene: University of Oregon, National Center to Improve the Tools of Educators.

Ferguson, D., Meyer, G., Jeanchild, J., Juniper, L., & Zingo, J. (1992). Figuring out what to do with the grown-ups. How teachers make inclusion "work" for students with disabilities. *Journal of the Association for Persons with Severe Handicaps, 17,* 218–228.

Field, S., Martin, J., Miller, R., Ward, M., & Wehmeyer, M. (1998). *A practical guide for teaching self-determination.* Reston, VA: Council for Exceptional Children.

Gee, K. (2004). Developing curriculum and instruction. In: F. P. Orelove, D. Sobsey, & R. K. Silberman (Eds.), *Educating children with multiple disabilities: A collaborative approach* (pp. 67–114). Baltimore, MD: Paul H. Brookes.

Gersten, R., Beckmann, S., Clarke, B., Foegen, A., Marsh, L., Star, J. R., et al. (2009). *Assisting students struggling with mathematics: Response to intervention (RtI) for elementary and middle schools* (NCEE No. 2009-4060). Washington, DC: National Center for Education Evaluation and Regional Assistance, Institute of Education Sciences, U. S. Department of Education.

Giangreco, M. (2006). Foundational concepts and practices for educating students with severe disabilities. In M. E. Snell & F. Brown (Eds.), *Instruction of students with severe disabilities* (6th ed) (pp. 1–27). Upper Saddle River, NJ: Pearson.

Hale, J. B. (2004). *School neuropsychology: A practitioner's handbook* (2nd ed.). New York: Guilford Press.

Hamre-Nietupski, S., Nietupski, J., & Strathe, M. (1992). Functional life skills, academic skills, and friendship/social relationship development: What do parents of moderate/severe /profound disabilities value? *Journal of the Association for Persons with Severe Handicaps, 17,* 53–58.

Heller, K. W., Frederick, L. D., Best, S., Dykes, M. K., & Cohen, E. T. (2002). Specialized health care procedures in the schools: Training and services. *Exceptional Children, 66,* 173–186.

Horner, R. H., Carr, E. G., Strain, P. S., Todd, A. W., & Reed, H. K. (2002). Problem behavior interventions for young children with autism: A research synthesis. *Journal of Autism and Developmental Disorders, 32,* 423–446.

Individuals with Disabilities Education Improvement Act (2004). 20 U. S.C. § 1400 et seq.

Lim, L., Tan, A. G., & Quah, M. L. (2000). Singaporean parents' curriculum priorities for their children with disabilities. *International Journal of Development, Disability, and Education, 47,* 77–87.

Kamil, M. L., Borman, G. D., Dole, J., Dral, C. C., Salinger, T., & Torgesen, J. (2008). *Improving adolescent literacy: Effective classroom and intervention practices: A practice guide* (NCEE No. 2008-4027). Washington, DC: National Center for Education Evaluation and Regional Assistance, Institute of Education Sciences, U.S. Department of Education.

Korkman, M., Kirk, U., & Kemp, S. (2007). *NEPSY-II*. San Antonio: The Pyschological Corporation.

Koppenhaver, D., & Yoder, D. (1993). Classroom instruction for children with severe speech and physical impairment (SSPI): What is and what might be. *Topics in Language Disorders, 13,* 1–15.

Luria, A. R. (1973). *The working brain: An introduction to neuropsychology*. New York. Basic Books Inc.

Mrakotsky, C. M., & Heffelfinger, A. K. (2006). Neuropsychological assessment of preschoolers. In J. L. Luby (Ed.), *Handbook of preschool mental health: Development, disorders and treatment* (pp. 1–27). New York: Guilford Press.

Martin, J. E., Van Dycke, J. L., Christensen, W. R., Greene, B. A., Gardner, J. E., & Lovett, D. L. (2006). Increasing student participation in their transition IEP meetings: Establishing the self-directed IEP as an evidence-based practice. *Exceptional Children, 72,* 299–316.

McGrew, K. S., & Evans, J. (2004). *Expectations for students with cognitive disabilities: Is the cup half empty or half full? Can the cup flow over?* (Synthesis Report 55). Minneapolis, MN: University of Minnesota, National Center on Educational Outcomes. Retrieved 11/22/11: http://education.umn.edu/NCEO/OnlinePubs/Synthesis55.html

Mitby, P. A., Robison, L. L., Whitton, J. A., Zevon, M. A., Gibbs, I. C., Tersak, J. M. ... Mertens, A. C. (2003). Utilization of special education services and educational attainment among long-term survivors of childhood cancer: A report from the Childhood Cancer Survivor Study. *Cancer, 97,* 1115–1126.

Nations Center for Educational Statistics. Retrieved June, 2011, from http://nces.ed.gov/programs/digest/d08//tables/d08_052.asp

National Institutes of Health (2003). *Health, mental health, and safety guidelines for schools.* Retrieved 11/12/11: http://www.nationalguidelines.org/chapter_full.cfm?chap=0

New America Foundation (2011). *Individuals with Disabilities Act: Cost impact on local school districts,* Retrieved 11/12/11: http://febp.newamerica.net/background-analysis/individuals-disabilities-education-act-cost-impact-local-school-districts#footnoteref1_7jls1z5)

No Child Left Behind Act of 2001, Pub. L. No. 107–110, 115, Stat. 1425 (2002).

Powell, D. S., Batsche, C. J., Ferro, J., Fox, L., & Dunlap, G. (1997). A strength-based approach in support of multi-risk families: Principles and issues. *Topics in Early Childhood Special Education, 17,* 1–26.

Resnick, M. B., Gomatam, S. V., Carter, R. L., Ariet, M., Roth, J., Kilgore, K. L., ... Eitzman, D. V. (1998). Educational disabilities of neonatal intensive care graduates. *Pediatrics, 102,* 303–314.

Rosenshine, B. (1987). Explicit teaching and teacher training. *Journal of Teacher Education, 38,* 34–36.

Roth, J., Figlio, D. N., Chen, Y., Carter, R. L., Ariet, M., Resnick, M. B., & Morse, S. B. (2004). Maternal and infant factors associated with excess kindergarten costs. *Pediatrics, 114,* 720–728.

Rutter M. (2005). Incidence of autism spectrum disorders: Changes over time and their meaning. *Acta Paediatrica, 94,* 2–15.

Ryndak, D. (1996). *Curriculum content for students with moderate and severe disabilities in inclusive settings*. Boston: Allyn & Bacon.

Sexson, S., & Madan-Swain, A. (1995). The chronically ill child in the school. *School Psychology Quarterly, 10*, 359–368.

Short, E. J., Klein, N. K., Lewis, B., Fulton, S., Eisengart, S., Kercesmar, C.,... Singer, L. T. (2003). Cognitive and academic consequences of broncho-pulmonary dysplasia and very low birth weight: 8 year old outcomes. *Pediatrics, 112*, 359–366.

Snell, M. E. (2005). Fifteen years later: Has positive programming become the expected technology for addressing problem behavior? A commentary on Horner et al. (1990). *Research and Practice for Persons with Severe Disabilities, 30*, 11–14.

Snell, M. E., & Brown, F. (Eds.). (2006). *Instruction of students with severe disabilities* (6th ed.). Upper Saddle River, NJ: Pearson Merrill/Prentice Hall.

Spooner, F., & Browder, D. M. (2006). Why teach the general curriculum. In D. M. Browder & F. Spooner (Eds.), *Teaching language arts, math, and science to students with significant cognitive disabilities* (pp. 1–37). Baltimore, MD: Paul H. Brookes.

Spooner, F., DiBiase, W., & Courtade-Little, G. (2006). Science standards and functional skills: Finding the links. In D. M. Browder & F. Spooner (Eds.), *Teaching language arts, math, and science to students with significant cognitive disabilities* (pp. 229–244). Baltimore, MD: Paul H. Brookes.

Surveillance, Epidemiology, and End Results (SEER) Program (1995) *Cancer Incidence and Survival Among Children and Adolescents: United States SEER Program 1975–1995*, at http://seer.cancer.gov/publications/childhood/

Taras, H., & Brennan, J. J., (2008) Students with chronic diseases: The nature of school physician support. *Journal of School Health, 78*, 389–396.

The Improving Access to Technology Act of 2004. 29 U. S. C. § 2202 (2).

Van Reusen, A. K., & Bos, C. S. (1990). IPLAN: Helping students communicate in planning conferences. *Teaching Exceptional Children, 22*, 30–32.

Wakeman, S. Y., Browder, D. M., Meier, I., & McColl, A. (2007). The implication of No Child Left Behind on students with developmental disabilities. *Mental Retardation and Developmental Disabilities Research Review, 13*, 143–150.

Wechsler, D. (2003). *Wechsler Intelligence Scale for Children–Fourth Edition*. San Antonio, TX: Harcourt Assessment, Inc.

Wehmeyer, M. L. (2005). Self-determination and individuals with severe disabilities: Re-examining meanings and misperceptions. *Research and Practice for Persons with Severe Disabilities, 30*, 113–120.

Wehmeyer, M. L., & Schwartz, M. (1998). The self-determination focus of transition goals for students with mental retardation. *Career Development for Exceptional Individuals, 21*, 75–86.

Westling, D., & Fox, L. (2004). *Teaching students with severe disabilities* (3rd ed.). Upper Saddle River, NJ: Pearson/Merrill Prentice-Hall.

Wilson, B. C. (1986). An approach to the neuropsychological assessment of the preschool child with developmental deficits. In S. B. Fiskov & T. J. Boll (Eds.), *Handbook of clinical neuropsychology* (Vol. 2, pp. 121–171), New York; Wiley.

Wood, W. M., Fowler, C. H., Uphold, N. M., & Test, D. W. (2005). A review of self-determination interventions with individuals with severe disabilities. *Research and Practice for Persons with Severe Disabilities, 30*, 121–146.

Zelazo, P. D., Carlson, S. M., & Kesek, A. (2008). The development of executive function in childhood. In C. Nelson & M. Luciana (Eds.), *Handbook of developmental cognitive neuroscience* (2nd ed., pp. 553–571). Cambridge, MA: The MIT Press.

17 Transition to Higher Education for Youth with Disabilities

Lorraine E. Wolf and Sarah Kroesser

INTRODUCTION

Advances in medical and critical care over the past two decades have resulted in enhanced survival (and concomitant quality of life) for many children with low-incidence and severe conditions (Plioplys, 2003). Children with very low birth weight, severe head trauma, neuromuscular and neurological disorders, childhood cancers, and heart disease, to name only a few, who may not have survived childhood previously are now considering college as a viable option. Elementary and secondary school districts have begun to understand how to model services, for example, for children in wheelchairs or those using augmented communication devices. Gains in special education services coupled with enhanced survivability have resulted in a nationwide increase in the number of college students with the types of conditions (Fairweather & Shaver, 1990) that are the focus of this volume. Like public school districts, colleges have become more sophisticated in determining what services are required for these youths. However, families and clinicians also need to understand the transition process in order to plan optimally.

The transition from comprehensive, often clinic-based, wraparound medical services for children to more fragmented options available to adults can be difficult for families dealing with a severe or chronic medical condition. They do not always understand that the transition from high school to higher education will be similar. Along with a high school diploma comes a sea change in the ways individuals with disabilities access their civil rights. College students are considered adults. As such, they must actively seek the services they require. Students are likely to have received school-based interventions for the administration of medication, provision of medical equipment, access to door-to-door transportation, personal aides, curricular modification, and extensive accommodations. These services change in both degree and kind when the student moves to higher education. In this chapter we discuss the areas that need to be considered by clinicians caring for college-bound students with severe and low-incidence disabilities in order to help them anticipate and adapt to their new environment.

Families, along with the educational and clinical team, need to be prepared to ask detailed questions when transitioning a student with medical compromise to college. For example, what levels of service are provided in terms of tutoring and assistance with learning self-advocacy skills? How is the Office of Disability Services staffed? What experience does the office have with a particular condition or with the student's functional needs? What are the admissions procedures, and is the process accommodated? What documentation is required when the student requests accommodations? Are there policies on waivers and substitutions of academic requirements? What assistive and adaptive technology is available, and who is responsible for procuring equipment and training the student? What are the housing and transportation options? Are there any special programs or fees? And perhaps most importantly—how will the student succeed, and who will be available to help him or her?

Gauging Readiness

Along with pride, excitement, and expectations, clinicians, parents, and students typically raise many concerns when approaching college transition. As a society we assume that all children can and should go to college, and certainly that is the case for students with disabilities as well. However, the entire family (including the student) needs to understand that the process—from the decision to go to college to the search and application process—and certainly the transition will be much more challenging for a student with a disability compared with his or her peers without disabilities. Therefore, the first steps must include a realistic appraisal of the student's readiness for higher education. The student, family, and outside providers must assess readiness before the actual college transition (Thierfeld Brown, Wolf, King, & Bork, 2012). Questions at the outset focus on the following student skills, needs, or attributes:

Is the student…

- Cognitively ready for higher education?
- Medically able to live independently?
- Prepared to disclose disability and seek assistance when needed?
- Able to manage medical needs and activities of daily living (ADLs)?
- Able to self-advocate with minimal assistance?

Students for whom the answer to any of the above questions is "no" may not be ready for college. Some families decide that college immediately after high school is not in the best interest of their child and opt to take advantage of the 18–21 transition or bridge programs available in many states. Other families decide their child can take some general academic classes at a local community college and live at home for the first year of school. In this way, the student continues to utilize familiar medical supports while he or she explores community resources and solidifies independent living skills. Other families decide that an online environment or a supported living facility is a better option. Whatever the decision, clinicians are most helpful during this process by offering guidance, suggesting additional functional assessments, and providing a realistic picture of whether an individual student is up to the challenge of higher education.

Many fairly straightforward (but often overlooked) factors must be examined when considering a college. For example, is the student going to stay close to home or live away from home? Is the campus urban or rural, cold or warm, flat or hilly? Is there a good residence life situation for the student (such as dietary options or cooking facilities)? Is the academic curriculum too demanding or too inflexible to meet the student's needs? Families often do not realize that they can and should ask such questions well in advance of applying to a specific college.

There is a host of other more individual issues that families and clinicians need to consider when researching colleges for a student with a disability. For example, a student who is a survivor of a severe traumatic brain injury often has resulting deficits in executive functioning and concept formation (Slomine et al., 2002), which preclude the advanced degree of reasoning expected in a college-level course (Wolf, Thierfeld Brown, & Bork, 2009). That student might be better served in a community college or self-paced online environment. A student who depends on a ventilator and a power wheelchair has more complex medical needs and might not be able to independently care for him- or herself. For that student, a residential college might be too difficult without the assistance of a full-time personal care attendant (PCA) for whom arrangements will need to be made (see discussion later in this chapter). Students with mobility impairments, chronic fatigue as a result of compromised respiratory or cardiac capacities, or sensitive immune systems are likely to be challenged by a cold, snowy, or hilly campus where transportation options are limited. There are as many different considerations as there are students, and the decisions should not be undertaken lightly.

Families also need to research the specific disability services that each school offers. There is no standardization in terms of policies and procedures for determining eligibility, processing service requests, or notifying faculty. In addition, different colleges offer different levels of service to students with disabilities. Some are more familiar with students living with certain disabilities, while others are known for a particularly supportive faculty or student body. The details of the search and application process are not discussed in this chapter. However, the interested reader can reference Thierfeld Brown and colleagues (2012) for a detailed discussion of the application and selection process (the volume is geared toward autism spectrum disorder but is applicable to students with other disabilities as well).

Once a school has been selected, the actual transition process begins. This process should start as early as middle school to allow more time for the student to assume more responsibility for managing his or her needs and accommodations in school (to the extent that is possible). However, it is still better to begin in the last months of high school than to wait until the student has left home to matriculate at college. For example, a student who requires a PCA should begin to appreciate some of the scheduling and personnel management issues that they will be taking on independently in college (this is discussed in more detail below). Accommodations that were seamlessly handled behind the scenes in high school would be something the student learns to arrange for him- or herself. In this way, students begin to learn basic self-advocacy skills that will become more crucial in college. As discussed above, students who are not up to this task may not be prepared for certain college environments and will need to consider other options such as a commuter school or an online curriculum while they develop independent living skills.

In order to better understand the transition to college, it is helpful for clinicians to recall where families have been and the hurdles they have previously faced in the educational arena. Also see Chapter 16 for a more detailed discussion of special education and the kindergarten to secondary school experience.

The Primary and Secondary Experience

It is difficult to come to grips with a situation that by its nature is wrought with heartache, confusion, and complexity. Adjusting to a child with a chronic medical condition, whether it is an illness, injury, or developmental disability, is difficult for everyone involved. Families have grieved the loss of a future once held dear and now must adapt to a new reality. Medical or financial decisions are likely to have taken precedence over school issues for some of this period. Hospital and point-of-service–based assistance has been available in the acute stages of an accident or during the evaluation and diagnostic stages, and this involves some educational planning. However, families quickly become familiar with the available educational services in order to advocate for what their child needs. Parents have learned to be the expert on their child's condition, the boss and CEO of their medical and educational needs, and their child's chief advocate. Many families have battled for their child's needs and are shocked to learn that higher education works differently. Clinical teams play a valuable role in preparing families for what will come next.

Special Education

Throughout elementary and secondary school (up to age 21 years or high school graduation in most states, though this varies for certain conditions), the educational rights of children with disabilities are governed under federal special education law. Although these are federal laws, individual states and even individual school districts vary considerably in how they interpret and apply the statutes. The Individuals with Disabilities Education Act (www.idea.gov; also see www.wrightslaw.com) and its recent reauthorization (Individuals with Disabilities Educational Improvement Act [IDEIA] www.in.gov/ipas/2411.htm) mandate free and appropriate public education for children with disabilities. By law, the educational setting and process must be made accessible to these students. The details of the special education system are beyond the scope of this chapter, and the reader is referred to Chapter 14 for more information. However, it is important to discuss aspects of the law that will change radically when a student graduates from high school.

Under IDEIA, public schools are mandated to identify, evaluate, accommodate, and remediate students with disabilities. A student with medical needs may be eligible for additional support services such as skilled nurses, transportation, and aides; the need is determined based on the student's condition and its impact on access to an education. Some students receive tutoring, instruction, or adaptive equipment that is home based, while others are transported (at the school district's expense) to needed adjunct clinical services such as occupational therapy, speech therapy, or rehabilitation services. Schools work with government entitlement programs (such as Medicaid or Medicare) to offset some of the expenses the district incurs. However, two features are inherent in the statute and in the process, and these change after high school graduation. The first is that the school assumes responsibility for providing these services. The second is that the parents are highly involved in the decision-making and oversight processes to ensure the services are actually delivered.

The Higher Education Experience

During the transition from high school to college, the student and his or her parents begin to change roles. Parents who have previously been their child's educational and medical advocate need to step back. After high school graduation (or age 21 years, whichever comes first), a student's rights and responsibilities change. By law, most of the process of securing accommodations and services in higher education must be initiated and carried out by the adult student. Students are no longer entitled to an education; they are only protected from discrimination and provided equal access. An adult student must be able to formally disclose that he or she has a disability in order to receive accommodations. In addition, accommodations are no longer automatically based on a diagnosis of disability.

Perhaps most surprising to families and clinicians is the degree of confidentiality to which colleges must adhere. Often, parents do not have access to their child's information, regardless of whether they are paying for college, nor can they call the school office(s) in place of their students. Confidentiality is stricter in this new milieu, and the student has complete control over the flow of information. Student privacy and confidentiality are guaranteed under the Family Educational Rights and Privacy Act (FERPA) (see www2.ed.gov/policy/gen/guid/fpco/ferpa). This statute protects the disclosure of personal student information, including educational records such as grades, and disciplinary actions. Realistically, this also means that different campus offices are prohibited from sharing information about a student with a disability without the student's written consent. It is typically the case that student needs are acted on only to the extent that the student has put the process into place.

The legal protection for adults with disabilities in higher education falls under the umbrella of federal disability laws. These statutes prohibit discrimination in employment, education, and facilities by public entities (including colleges and universities) solely on the basis of disability (see below) and thus protect individuals with disabilities from discrimination. College students with disabilities are no longer entitled to an education, but rather are protected from discrimination based on their disability in the educational setting. This right is governed by a pair of related civil rights statutes. Because the laws are closely related and interpreted together, most colleges refer to them as "ADA/504" (Macurdy & Geetter, 2008).

Access to educational programs and provision of accommodations on college campuses in the United States are mandated under Section 504 of the Rehabilitation Act of 1973 (see www.hhs.gov/ocr/504.pdf; also see wrightslaw.com). This civil rights statute prohibits discrimination on the basis of disability in programs and activities that receive federal financial assistance. There is no funding (government or otherwise) to the student or the school under 504. Specifically, Section 504 states that:

No otherwise qualified individual with a disability in the United States, as defined in section 7(20), shall, solely by reason of her or his disability, be excluded from the participation in, be denied the benefits of, or be subjected to discrimination under any program or activity receiving Federal financial assistance or under any program or activity conducted by any Executive agency or by the United States Postal Service. (Sec 504, a)

In practical terms, this means that schools must make accommodations for students with disabilities in order to render the educational process accessible. Accommodations include ramps and accessible seating for a student using a wheelchair, extra time on exams for a student with slow processing speed, permission to have a note taker or to audio record exams for a student with an attention impairment, digital audio textbooks for a student with a visual impairment, or a sign language interpreter for a classroom lecture for a student with a hearing impairment. In some instances, "accommodation" means altering policies or procedures, for example, allowing a student in a full-time program to register at a reduced course load or to extend the statute of limitations on completing a degree program. Accommodations are always individually tailored to the student's needs. This is discussed in more detail below.

The Americans with Disabilities Act (ADA, 1990) (www.ada.gov) and its recent amendment (Americans with Disabilities Amendment Acts) (ADAAA, 2008, effective 2009) guarantee that places of public accommodation (e.g., government buildings, medical facilities, movie theaters, sports arenas, college campuses) are accessible for individuals with disabilities. This not only means that buildings must be physically accessible with ramps, elevators, and adaptive restrooms, but also that programs must be accommodated so that a person with a disability enjoys the benefits of the activity (www.ada.gov). Achieving physical access to college campuses is challenging, particularly where there is older architecture (buildings constructed pre-ADA may be exempt from modification to render them accessible) (www.ada.gov). Program access can be even more difficult. ADA and ADAAA outline the areas of functional impairment (defined as "major life activity" such as breathing, walking, seeing) that are affected by a disability. The original ADA was fairly restricted; however, the recent amendments broadened these categories to include such areas as bodily functions, ability to care for oneself, and ability to pay attention, just to name a few (see www.eeoc.gov/laws/regulations/adaaa-summary.cfm).

The Accommodation Process

Students making the transition to college need to become their own advocate and learn to speak the language of disability services. They must know the policies and procedures that govern disability access on their campus and must seek out and utilize the resources of the Disability Services Office if they intend to use accommodations. Disability Services is the official office charged with making decisions, setting policy, and overseeing access for students with disabilities. Transitioning students must learn to work with this office closely because they will be responsible for requesting the accommodations they need.

Below are the steps customary in the accommodation process:

1. Student formally discloses to the designated office or individual that he or she has a disability. This office is usually called the Office of Disability Services, Disabled

Student Support, or something similar. All colleges are required to have either an office or an individual designated to be in charge of accommodations and access.

2. Student provides medical documentation as requested by the school. Medical documentation will vary depending on the type of disability; however, clinicians should be prepared to provide a current and comprehensive statement of diagnosis and objective evidence of functional impairment in the educational environment. This will be the justification for the accommodations the student will request. Even a student with a longstanding or permanent condition may be required to document their current functional status and needs. Some specific documentation issues are discussed below.

3. Student requests accommodations and/or services. By law and by policy, the student directly engages in the self-disclosure step. Clinicians and families can (and often do) send medical documentation; however, each student must approach and engage the official agent on campus in what is referred to as an "interactive process." As the name implies, this is (usually) a face-to-face meeting between the student and the disability provider at which the student discloses his or her disability and discusses related needs. Inherent in the process is a joint discussion of the reasonable and appropriate accommodations the student wishes to request.

4. Designated office/individual (the Office of Disability Services is usually that agent) reviews the student's eligibility according to established procedures within that office. There are no common metrics for this eligibility review; however, the documentation must establish that the student has a significant limitation in a major life activity (as defined in the law; see www.ada.gov) and that the impairment is relevant to the current academic environment and to the accommodation the student is requesting. For example, a student with a seizure disorder whose documentation only addresses limitations relative to driving may not be found eligible to receive academic accommodations such as extra time for exams unless those needs are specifically addressed and justified.

5. Designated office/individual familiar with course, program, and degree requirements in their school determines reasonable accommodations relative to the school, program, or course. Accommodations must be relevant to the disability but do not need to be made to the extent that they compromise essential features of a course or program (this is discussed below).

6. Designated office/individual facilitates the implementation of accommodations. This means that after the office clears accommodations, the student is assisted in communicating his or her needs to their faculty. A letter, memo, or email is used for this communication. In most cases, the student assumes the responsibility for requesting the accommodation and making specific arrangements directly with the faculty. The Office of Disability Services is involved to a greater or lesser degree. Students using adaptive or assistive technology, for example, need the office to assist with digitizing exams to be read by a text-to-voice program. This is discussed in more detail below.

College Responsibilities and Rights

Under the laws discussed above, the school clearly has the responsibility to provide access to their facilities, services, and programs for students with disabilities. All schools are required to provide reasonable accommodations (defined as academic adjustments and/or auxiliary aids and services) to make a program accessible. Schools are also required to maintain student confidentiality, as discussed above, and to establish and enforce written policies and procedures, including grievance procedures should a student feel that he or she has been the victim of discrimination based on his or her disability.

However, along with that mandate come rights, such as the right to determine academic requirements and to maintain academic integrity. The college maintains the right to determine fundamental requirements of courses and programs and the right to maintain and enforce conduct codes. Courts have historically given great weight to decisions made by colleges in regard to academic requirements and policies (Macurdy & Geetter, 2008).

The law does not require accommodations to be made that would compromise fundamental requirements or essential features of a course (www.ada.gov) (see Macurdy & Geetter, 2008). This means that if a program requires math or English, accommodations that excuse a student from meeting this requirement (e.g., waivers) are not necessary and possibly not allowed. For example, a student with a dense language disorder subsequent to resection of a brain tumor would be required to fulfill a foreign language requirement despite difficulties using their primary language. Students with disabilities that affect one or more basic academic skills or functions are advised to look carefully at all required courses that would be impacted. Clinicians should not assume that requests for waivers or prolonged absences from classes will necessarily be granted, no matter how compelling the student's situation.

Student Responsibilities and Rights

In order to maintain enrollment (e.g., active student status), all students, including those with disabilities, are expected to assume the full responsibility of complying with school regulations. For example, students are required to self-disclose if they need services related to their disability or disorder. They must follow policies for documenting the disability. It is the student's responsibility to request accommodations and to monitor the effectiveness of those adjustments. They must follow all policies and procedures set forth by the college and continue to meet required academic and behavioral standards.

All college students, including those with disabilities, must learn to impose structure on their free time, organize their academic and personal lives, and advocate for themselves in times of need. Accordingly, students are held responsible for their independent living needs. In other words, students are expected to behave like adults regardless of their individual medical situations.

Students need to determine how they will do their laundry, use the toilet and shower, and negotiate the dining facilities. Students with medical needs often require outside assistance with some aspects of these needs, but ultimately it is the student's responsibility to figure out how that will be accomplished. Unlike the high school environment, a college is not going to hire or pay for an aide and will not be responsible for maintaining personal medical or electronic equipment that the student requires. However, the school is responsible for facilitating the student's use of an aide (e.g., allowing access to classrooms and residence halls or providing a parking pass). For example, if a student has a class in a building with limited elevator access, it is the college's responsibility to move the class to an accessible space. It is, however, up to the student to notify the designated office of his or her specific access need and any problems he or she encounters. The school would, for example, need to reconfigure a lab station for a student. If the same student also has manual dexterity impairments, the school would arrange for a lab aide to manage manual tasks that the student cannot do independently. However, in creating access for a student with a physical or motor impairment, the school will not alter or lower the expectation for a fundamental component of a course as an accommodation.

Student rights always intersect with their responsibilities. Students have the right to have access to school programs, facilities and activities, reasonable and appropriate accommodations, privacy and confidentiality, and grievance and due process. Failure to comply with responsibilities, however, can compromise the student's rights.

Special Considerations

Residence life and housing. Most students live in some type of residence hall during their freshman year of college. Many colleges make this a requirement because it is a valuable social and cocurricular part of the college experience. Some colleges allow students with disabilities to opt out of this requirement; however, many students enjoy living in a dormitory. If a student with special needs plans to live on campus, the student and his or her family must examine residence life and housing options and seek assistance from the campus residence and disability offices. For example, a student with mobility impairments would require either elevator access or a ground-floor room. However, although colleges must offer different types of accessibility options, not every room in every residence hall must be accessible. Newer buildings are usually up to code in terms of access; however, some campuses have only small, pre-ADA residence halls. In some instances, the residence a student wants is not accessible and cannot be made so. Because these arrangements take time, special housing needs are best arranged early.

The bathrooms in residence halls must be accessible and meet individual needs such as appropriately placed grab bars, roll-in showers, or large doors. Bath seats and shower chairs are often considered personal medical devices to be provided by the student. A student with a bowel regimen may need a private bathroom. By the same token, beds must be accessible for students with disabilities (many residences use bunk beds). If a student needs a hospital bed, however, the student must negotiate who will provide it; the school usually considers this a personal medical device. Transfer equipment to baths or showers may or may not be provided by the school.

Roommates are part of the experience of living in a residence hall. However, students and families must understand that it is not appropriate, for example, to expect a roommate to perform personal duties such as assisting with ADLs or serving as an emergency back-up in the event a PCA does not show up. Roommates are not recruited to be social coaches for a student with an autism spectrum disorder, nor are they expected to push a wheelchair or carry food in the dining hall on a routine basis. Many peers will voluntarily assume some of these responsibilities; however, part of the transition is understanding that a student who cannot assume responsibility for his or her own self-care will either need professional assistance (e.g., a PCA) or a different college environment.

Personal medical equipment. Students are directly responsible for bringing and maintaining their own medical equipment. For example, if a student in a residence hall requires an oxygen compressor, it is his or her responsibility to arrange for and pay for such. Colleges have strict regulations on electric and electronic devices in residence halls, and families must check that the device meets fire and safety codes. For example, refrigerators for storing medications may need to be of a specific size and brand. Air conditioners or humidifiers may not be allowed at all. If large medical equipment will occupy space in the room, negotiations must include the size of the space and whether a roommate is feasible. Items such as lifts and transfer equipment may or may not be provided by the school, and the negotiations for such equipment cannot be accomplished at the last minute.

Dietary and food services. Most students who elect to live on campus must also enroll in a meal plan. There are several things that need to be taken into consideration with regard to food plans and similar services. Students with special dietary needs may opt out of food plans as an accommodation; however, that student will need to explore whether safe cooking options are available. Many residence halls have communal kitchens; however, a student with allergies may not be able to share the facility. For example, although a student who has severe food allergies or autoimmune disorders, such as celiac disease, will need to cook his or her own meals, he or she likely will not be able to safely share a kitchen because of the risk of cross-contamination. This needs to be considered and negotiated with the housing office prior to move-in. However, clinicians can assist students in developing the awareness and skills necessary to choose and shop for food. Finally, on-campus dining and nutrition services are increasingly sophisticated in their ability to respond to students with life-threatening food allergies, inflammatory bowel disease, and similar conditions, and their expertise should be sought.

Personal care attendants. As mentioned previously, many issues need to be resolved if a student requires a PCA to attend school. This includes recruiting, funding, and supervising the PCA or making arrangements for the individual to get around campus. For example, if the student is a male and the PCA is a female, which bathroom will be used? Will a single-use bathroom be needed? How will the PCA eat? Will the PCA require use of a kitchen or will he or she be allowed to pay for a meal plan? Will a parking pass be issued, and will this provide handicap access? How will the PCA be integrated on campus? Students need to understand that they are responsible for deciding how the PCA will be integrated into academic life. For example, PCAs are usually not permitted to act as academic aides, test readers, scribes for exams, or note takers. However, PCAs often assist with page turning or getting in and out of a classroom. It is up to the student to set some of the guidelines for his or her relationship with their PCA. This will be more important in terms of integrating the PCA into residential and cocurricular life. For example, will the PCA feed the student in public? Will he or she accompany the student to social events or on dates?

Families and students must work with the housing and public safety office to make arrangements for a PCA to live on campus. A larger room might be needed to accommodate medical equipment as well as space for the PCA. Certain buildings do not have large rooms or accessible single-use bathrooms. Colleges will not cover the costs for a PCA to live or eat on campus. Families should understand that housing a PCA is likely to impact overall college costs. Also, students must understand that they are responsible for ensuring that their PCAs comply with residence hall policies, such as rules related to guests, alcohol and drug use, and conduct.

Assistive and adaptive technology. For many students, assistive and adaptive technology is an important tool for college success. Examples include adaptive hardware such as joysticks, foot switches, headgear, and enlarged keyboards. Dictation (voice-to-text) and read-back (text-to-voice) software, and webbing and concept mapping software are useful for students with a variety of physical and cognitive disabilities. For example, many students with disabilities benefit from digital audio textbooks. Students who need technology to access academic materials must consider these needs well in advance of the start of classes. Some schools provide both hardware and software options for students needing these accommodations. Students must be clear on what is considered a personal device provided by the student (e.g., a computer with necessary modifications) and what is an accommodation provided by the school (e.g., permission to use this device on a test).

The Office of Disability Services provides certain equipment as an accommodation; however, it is up to the student to request and document the need. Training for students to use assistive and adaptive products needed to access the academic program is provided by schools under Section 508 of the Rehabilitation Act (Section 508, n.d.). Advanced or specialized training, however, may be beyond this mandate.

For some students, these technologies are funded through vocational rehabilitation services, their prior school districts or are offered free of charge by the college. For other students, the technologies must be purchased out-of-pocket. At some schools, training in the use of these products is provided on-site or through the office that handles disability services. In any case, the Office of Disability Services provides clearance for these special technologies to be used in class or exam situations. If something breaks or is malfunctioning, students must know where to go for maintenance and repair. Similarly, if a student is experiencing an unanticipated problem, he or she should know where to turn for help.

A new initiative for many schools is to provide access to Web sites, videos, and other media that are part of the academic curriculum. This often involves digital access, read-back software for Web sites, text enlargement, captioning, and describing films. The interface between adaptive technology and computer systems on campus is vital for students with many disabilities to achieve access.

Behavior and conduct. Often students with disabilities either have difficulty moderating their behavior or lack the awareness of how their conduct affects the people and environment around them. Certain conditions such as traumatic brain injuries and autistic spectrum disorders may result in problems with behavior regulation and impulse control. It is important to note that behavioral problems (e.g., outbursts, aggression) are never tolerated in a higher education setting, even if the behavior is directly tied to a disabling condition. This is a stark contrast to K–12 educational settings, where the policy of manifestation determination protects a student with a disability from discipline for such behaviors. Manifestation determination (Huefner, 2000) goes into effect when any public school student with a documented disability is charged with misconduct in order to determine whether the student's disability played a part in an inability to control his or her behavior. If this is the case, the student might be excused from sanctions for that behavior. However, in a college environment, a student who violates a conduct or academic code will be subject to judicial sanction, even if the behavior was directly related to his or her disability. For example, a student with an autism spectrum disorder who stalks a peer could be brought up on whatever charges a college associates with that behavior and suffer the same consequences as a student without a disability (see Wolf, Thierfeld Brown, & Bork, 2009).

Medical issues. Students with complicated medical conditions face financial and insurance issues as they become adults. Most colleges require students to be covered by the school's medical insurance. However, these insurance policies are often not sufficiently comprehensive for a student with medical needs. If the school insurance does not cover a student's specific needs, he or she will need to consider alternative health insurance plans and provide the school with proof of insurance. Students are also responsible for locating, following up with, and arranging transportation to necessary medical specialists. For example, if a college has a student health center, that center must ensure that all students are seen for routine medical issues. However, the student health service is not responsible for providing specialty care (although they may refer to an outside provider for such). Students needing specialized medical care (such as infusion treatments or injectable medications) must make their own arrangements for accessing that care.

Students must know how to obtain, store, and administer their own medications. It is often helpful for students to use mail order pharmacy services (if allowable), which lower the costs of medications. Perhaps more important in the life of a student, medications delivered to a mailbox or dorm room relieve the need to go to the pharmacy each month. Students need to start school with a system that works for them, whether it is pillboxes or scheduled alerts on a cellular device, to ensure that they manage their medications safely and responsibly.

Students with medical or mobility needs must have an emergency plan that is feasible in their current living situation. This could entail wearing a medical alarm bracelet, having other forms of identification visible on their person, or making their resident assistant aware of their condition. Finally, students with medical needs must consider what activities are and are not accessible to them. For example, it would be appropriate to request that a van transporting a student with a heart condition to a required field-trip have a defibrillator on board. It is not reasonable to request a nurse to accompany the student on the trip.

Emergency preparedness and safety planning. Emergency preparedness, including evacuation planning, is the student's responsibility. The means by which this is accomplished differs from school to school. Emergency preparedness is especially crucial for students in wheelchairs or those with mobility and sensory disabilities. Alarms must be accessible, safety routes must be clearly marked, and students must be oriented to the safety procedures each school has established. Students, however, are also responsible for maintaining emergency numbers, carrying appropriate medical alerts (if necessary), and demonstrating an understanding of what to do in an emergency.

Documentation. As discussed above, some students with chronic or longstanding disorders are required to provide current and comprehensive documentation of their disability. This will, of necessity, vary according to the specific clinical condition. Neuropsychological evaluation is the documentation of choice in neurodevelopmental, neurocognitive, and neurobehavioral disorders, including autism spectrum disorders, psychiatric disorders, neurological disorders, survivors of childhood cancers that include radiation to the head, and learning and attention disorders. All college-bound students who have experienced learning or educational difficulties are likely to benefit from a careful educational evaluation as well. Children for whom neurobehavioral or psychiatric symptomatology have been present should pursue a psychiatric or behavioral neurology assessment. Functional assessments of individual capabilities are very useful in determining the most effective choice among available accommodations. For example, a functional motor assessment highlights assistive technology needs for a student with cerebral palsy.

SPECIFIC CLINICAL CONDITIONS

It is beyond the scope of this chapter to discuss each condition covered in this volume. Rather, we present a few to highlight postsecondary issues that illustrate the level of analysis that the accommodation process entails.

Traumatic Brain Injury

Colleges are handling an increasing number of students with long-term effects of significant head trauma. Students with traumatic brain injury (TBI) commonly experience residual difficulties in the areas of executive functioning and self-regulation due to involvement of the frontal lobe and associated subcortical structures (Stuss, 2011; also see this volume chapter 15). Deficits typically depend on the age at which the injury occurred as well as the area of the brain impacted by the lesion(s). Longstanding cognitive problems that will impact higher education include slow processing speed, working memory deficits, confusion, disorientation, alterations in judgment, changes in attention, and changes in decision-making ability (Gordon, Haddad, Brown, Hibbard, & Sliwinski, 2000). Behavioral deficits associated with TBI include impatience, anger, frustration, confrontational behaviors, impulsivity, increased avoidance, and withdrawal (Stuss, 2011; Dennis, Guger, Roncadin, Barnes, & Shachar, 2001). Psychiatric conditions that are comorbid with TBI include posttraumatic stress disorder, depression, and anxiety (Bryant & Harvey, 1999). Students with TBI often have difficulties with emotional control, transitions, and adapting to novelty due to the changes in behavioral regulation that often occur following a TBI (Dennis et al., 2001). Such difficulties therefore inform where (and if) a student goes to college and their ability to comply with behavioral codes.

Students with TBI are likely to be eligible for accommodations in college, including academic accommodations to mitigate the impact of the condition, as well as housing or facilities access. Extended time for exams, breaks during exams without time penalty, reduced credit loads, extensions on statues of limitations to obtain degrees, assistive or adaptive technology, memory aids, and scribes or note takers are all possible accommodations. Colleges also provide referrals to psychiatric rehabilitation facilities, psychological services, tutoring services, and career counseling services.

Mobility Impairment

Students with mobility impairments (MIs) face academic as well as physical barriers in higher education. Access for these students is shared between the student and the school. For example, a student who uses a wheelchair must bring his or her own chair and must make arrangements for repair and maintenance. It is the school's responsibility to provide ramps, elevators, wheelchair-accessible desks, and tables as well as other means of physical access to classrooms and buildings.

A number of different conditions impact mobility, including chronic or acute health impairments such as arthritis, orthopedic conditions, cancer with or without amputation, and surgery. Other students have neuromuscular conditions such as cerebral palsy and muscular dystrophy. Some students with MIs use wheelchairs, while others use assistive devices such as crutches, motorized scooters, walkers, and canes. These students require an evacuation and safety plan to be conducted by the appropriate school official, as well as an assessment of access needs in terms of locations of residence halls, classrooms, and other important academic buildings.

Many students with MIs have reduced energy, either as a concomitant of their disorder or secondary to the effort it takes to get around campus. These students are likely to require accommodations such as extended time for exams, breaks during exams, and exams to be spaced apart. Others have limited writing ability due to limited use of their arms or hands and will require computer assistance, scribes, or both in order to complete in-class and out-of-class work. Some students require full- or part-time aides or PCAs, assistive and adaptive technology, and transportation assistance.

Both on- and off-campus transportation must be considered; transportation to classes often involves walking or a shuttle service. Public transportation may also be involved. A student with a physical disability must consider whether these options are accessible and, if not, if there are other alternatives. In many cases, shuttle services are provided on large campuses; however, students must be able to get to a bus stop.

Autism Spectrum Disorders

The percentage of people diagnosed with autism spectrum disorders (ASDs) has dramatically increased in the last 20 years (see Chapter 2). Consequently, the number of college students with ASD has also increased (Wolf, Thierfeld Brown, & Bork, 2009). These students have challenges in many aspects of college life, including social interaction, residential life, and executive functioning. The interested reader is referred to Wolf and colleagues (2008) and Thierfeld Brown et al. (2012) for detailed discussions of college services for students with ASDs.

Social skills training is often helpful for those diagnosed with ASD. In college, the typical student is able to rely on his or her social skills to adapt to college life and integrate into the community. For students with ASD, this is a challenge and often leads to social isolation and, in some cases, depression and anxiety. Social skills training during the adolescent years can help to mitigate these challenges and enable greater success in the college environment. In terms of residential life, students diagnosed with ASD sometimes find it difficult to live with a roommate. Some students find it helpful to disclose their disability to their roommate as an opener to negotiating difficult situations such as bed time, the amount of social activity to take place in the room, guidelines around sharing personal items, and rules about overnight guests.

Some colleges offer special programs designed for students on the autistic spectrum (see Thierfeld Brown et al., 2012). These programs often include mentors, organized social activities and support groups, and executive functioning coaching. It is worthwhile to look into these special programs when deciding on a postsecondary placement. Because they often cost more than the general tuition, finances play a part in choosing a school with these special programs. Finally, the choice of college for a student with an ASD is critical, and clinicians can assist families in gauging what sort of academic setting would be most appropriate and provide the desired level of support (see Thierfeld Brown et al., 2012).

Other Disorders

Seizure disorders. Depending on the nature and severity of the seizure disorder, students may struggle in different aspects of higher education. Students who have had surgeries to alleviate seizure frequency and subsequent brain disease (Hermann & Seidenberg, 2007) are likely to have a variety of focal or diffuse residual symptoms that necessitate assistive or adaptive technology or academic accommodations. Memory or language disorders secondary to seizures will necessitate accommodations such as fact sheets to mitigate the effects of seizure on short- and long-term memory. Other students have relatively few symptoms but take medication that must be managed carefully. Postseizure fatigue as well as the side effects of many antiepileptic medications necessitate accommodations such as breaks or rescheduling of exams. Students with residual seizures as a concomitant of another condition such as TBI need to be accommodated accordingly. Finally, all students who are prone to active seizures must be aware of the school policy for emergency transport should they have a seizure on campus and should carry appropriate identification.

Childhood cancer survivors. Children who underwent extensive chemotherapy or radiation therapy for childhood cancers present with a host of academic difficulties that persist into college age (Mitby et al., 2003; see Chapter 3). Nonverbal learning disorders and difficulties with executive function have been reported in children with leukemia who were treated with intrathecal chemotherapy agents and cranial radiation (Mitby et al., 2003; see Chapter 1). These conditions need to be documented by neuropsychological assessment in order to secure appropriate accommodations. Other children who have had cancers of the brain or eyes require accommodations for focal deficits or low vision (Al-Mefty, Kersh, Routh, & Smith, 1990).

Prematurity and very low birth weight. Educational outcome in terms of high school completion and postsecondary enrollment is often reduced in survivors of very low birth weight (Hack et al., 2002). Lower IQ and executive deficits have been reported in adolescents who were born premature (Anderson, Doyle, & Victorian Infant Collaborative Study Group, 2004; also see Chapter 12). The most commonly reported long-term effect is learning disorder, ranging from mild to severe (Anderson, Doyle, & Victorian Infant Collaborative Study Group, 2004). Youth with mild to moderate learning disorder and/or executive dysfunction do attend college (Wolf & Kaplan, 2008). As with any student with a learning disorder, accommodations would focus on the cognitive difficulties. Other students have visual, motor, or neuromuscular difficulties and are accommodated accordingly. Again, clinical intervention should include careful neuropsychological and functional assessment of residual impairments geared toward supporting accommodations, technology needs, housing, and similar issues.

Cerebral palsy. Cerebral palsy affects motor, sensory, and cognitive functioning in young adults (Krigger, 2006; Murphy, Molnar, & Lankasky, 1995; see Chapter 4). Some students with motor or sensory manifestations require housing accommodations or assistive and adaptive technology, as discussed above. Others require PCAs to assist with daily care (e.g., care of breathing or feeding tubes or equipment, assistance with dressing and bathing), scribes, computers or note takers to assist with writing, or digital text or live readers to assist with course readings or exams. Milder cognitive impairments in executive function, for example (Straub & Obizut, 2009), are sometimes not recognized or appropriately accommodated due to the more striking manifestation of other functional difficulties. In these cases, neuropsychological documentation clarifies whether a student also requires additional academic assistance. Students who have difficulty communicating require communication aids, devices, or interpreters. Some students experience pain and fatigue (Murphy, Molnar, and Lankasky, 1995) and require reduced course load, breaks, or modified schedules in order to attend college.

FUTURE AIMS AND RESEARCH OPPORTUNITIES

In this chapter, we have discussed the transition of students with disabilities from high school to college, including where they have come from, where they are going, and the specific legal responsibilities of the student as well as the individual college. We have discussed individual issues such as housing, medical equipment and emergency planning as well as some specific conditions that warrant additional attention. We have provided information for clinicians about the nature and level of services a student with a severe medical disability can expect and provided some guidance about documenting such conditions. We hope that this will assist clinical teams in preparing capable young people to launch into the next steps of their educational lives.

The process of adjusting to college can be challenging for a student with a disability. In a sense, a student with a disability must become a mature adult much faster than the average college student. He or she has learned to cope with challenges in a way that other students have not, and usually comes to college with a set of adaptive skills that will be critical for him or her to adapt to the new environment. The parent and the clinical team who make sure the student is so armed have done that young person a great service.

In order to be successful, students with disabilities must both understand and accept their conditions. In order to request and use accommodations, for example, students need to be able to discuss their medical condition and provide insights as well as specific details about how the condition impacts them. They must be aware of their strengths and weaknesses and must have accepted themselves for (and sometimes in spite of) them. It is asking a lot of an adolescent, but college students need to be able to advocate for themselves as well as care for their individual personal and medical needs. Successful students know how to locate and use resources on campus, and how to access training in additional skills and strategies that they need. Finally, students must know their rights and responsibilities as college students with disabilities (see Thierfeld Brown, Wolf, King, Bork, 2012). This is a huge developmental leap for a young person who must be supported by their family as well as their entire clinical team. Only in this way will they obtain the independent life skills they will carry into college and beyond that into the world of work.

The needs of young adults with severe disabilities who attend college have been under-researched. Available data do show us that students with disabilities are less likely to go to college and significantly less likely to complete four-year degree programs (Horn, Berktold, & Bobbit, 1999; Wagner, Newman, Cameto, Garza, & Levine, 2005) compared with peers without disabilities. Very little outcome data or information regarding specific predictive factors exist on individuals who will be successful; most studies are comprised of anecdotal experience or analysis of the results of the practices at one site (Collins, Hedrick, & Stumbo, 2007; Tincani, 2004) and in some instances merely present college completion rates for students with disabilities (Harvey, 2002).

The lack of predictive data broken down by student variables or disability type clearly limits the development of best practices to support the developmental, educational, and personal needs of these students. Many schools are struggling to meet basic housing and access issues that an increasing (and complex) cohort of students brings to college and have not expended resources to investigate student and college characteristics that predict success.

A promising model to meet the needs of larger numbers of students with disabilities within a mainstream framework is that of Universal Instructional Design (UID; www. washington.edu/doit/CUDE) (Pliner, Johnson, 2004). UID is based on instructional design that embeds certain modifications in the curriculum available to all students. For example, student competency can be assessed in several modalities such as combining different formats (e.g., multiple choice, short answer, essay, matching) into a single examination. In addition, the combination of exams with papers, presentations, or portfolios enables students with disabilities to excel in certain areas. Presentations of course content and material in multiple formats, such as traditional lecture accompanied by visual supplements such as Power Points or videos, live or online modeling, or demonstration, provide access to the information through alternate learning routes for students with impairments. Embedding captions into lecture materials and presenting readings in digital audio format accommodate students with different disabilities as well as different types of learners. Successful UID allows students with disabilities to utilize less in terms of formal accommodation because many of their access needs can be accomplished in the integrated setting. Moreover, UID benefits all students as they have the opportunity to use their strengths to learn and demonstrate mastery. However, encouraging faculty to explore and utilize UID is a time-consuming and costly effort that must be supported by school administrators. Data on the effectiveness of UID are just beginning to become available (Higbee, Goff, 2008).

Another under-researched area is the design of programs that support the transition of youth with disabilities from college into employment (USGAO, 2003; Transition to Adulthood, 2009). School-to-work programs are well funded; however, many concentrate on high school students and not on college graduates (Williamson, Robertson, & Casey, 2010). Consequently, approximately 34%–45% of college graduates with disabilities remain unemployed (New England ADA Center, n.d.).

Clearly we have advanced in our knowledge of how to care for and educate children with severe and low incidence disabilities. The next steps must include preparing the work world to meet the needs of employees with disabilities.

REFERENCES

Al-Mefty, O., Kersh, J., Routh, A., & Smith, R. (1990). The long-term side effects of radiation therapy for benign brain tumors in adults. *Journal of Neurosurgery, 73*, 502–512.

Americans with Disabilities Act of 1990. §42 U.S.C.A. 12101-213. www.ada.gov.

Americans with Disabilities Amendments Act of 2008. www.ada.gov; www.eeoc.gov/laws/regulations/adaaa-summary.cfm.

Anderson, P., Doyle, L., & Victorian Infant Collaborative Study Group. (2004). Executive functioning in school-aged children who were born very preterm or with extremely low birth weight in the 1990s. *Pediatrics, 114*, 50–57.

Bryant, R. A., & Harvey, A. G. (1999). Post-concussive symptoms and posttraumatic stress disorder after mild traumatic brain injury. *Journal of Nervous & Mental Disease, 187,* 302–305.

Center for Universal Design in Education. (n.d.). Retrieved December 1, 2011, from http://www.washington.edu/doit/CUDE/

Dennis, M., Guger, S., Roncadin, S., Barnes, M., & Shachar, R. (2001). Attentional-inhibitory control and social–behavioral regulation after childhood closed head injury: Do biological, developmental, and recovery variables predict outcome? *Journal of the International Neuropsychological Society, 7,* 683–692.

Family Educational Rights and Privacy Act. 20 U.S.C. § 1232g; 34 CFR Part 99. www2.ed.gov/policy/gen/guid/fpco/ferpa.

Fairweather, J., & Shaver, D. (1990). A troubled future? Participation in postsecondary education by youths with disabilities. *Journal of Higher Education, 61,* 332–348.

Gordon, W., Haddad, L., Brown, M., Hibbard, M., & Sliwinski, M. (2000). The sensitivity and specificity of self-reported symptoms in individuals with traumatic brain injury. *Brain Injury, 14,* 21–33.

Hack, M., Flannery, D. J., Schluchter, M., Cartar, L., Borawski, E., & Klein, N. (2002). Outcomes in young adulthood for very-low birth-weight infants. *New England Journal of Medicine, 346,* 149–57

Hermann, B., & Seidenberg, M. (2007). Epilepsy and cognition. *Epilepsy Current, 7,* 1–6.

Higbee, J., & Goff, E. (Eds.). (2008). Pedagogy and student services for institutional transformation: Implementing universal design in higher education. Minnesota: University of Minnesota. http://cehd.umn.edu/passit/docs/PASS-IT-BOOK.pdf

Huefner, D. S. (2000). *Getting comfortable with special education law: A framework for working with children with disabilities* (2nd ed.). Norwood, MA: Christopher-Gordon Publishers, Inc.

Individuals with Disabilities Education Act of 2004. Public Law No. 108-446, 20 U.S.C. §1400 et seq. (2004).

Krigger, K. W. (2006). Cerebral palsy: An overview. *American Family Physician, 73,* 91–100

Macurdy, A., & Geetter, E. (2008). Legal issues for adults with learning disabilities in higher education. In L. Wolf, H. Schreiber, & J. Wasserstein (Eds.). *Adult learning disorders: Contemporary issues* (pp. 415–432). New York: Psychology Press.

Mitby, P. A., Robison, L. L., Whitton, J. A., Zevon, M. A., Gibbs, I. C., TeraK, J. M.,…Mertens, A. C. (2003). Utilization of special education services and educational attainment among long-term survivors of childhood cancer: A report from the Childhood Cancer Survivor Study. *Cancer, 97,* 1115–1126.

Murphy, K.P., Molnar, G. E., & Lankasky, K. (1995). Medical and functional status of adults with cerebral palsy. *Developmental Medicine and Child Neurology, 37,* 1075–1084.

New England ADA Center. (n.d.). Project Director's Report. Retrieved December 1, 2011, from http://www.adaptenv.org/neada/site/2007_winter_pd_report

Pliner, S., & Johnson, J. (2004). Historical, theoretical, and foundational principles of universal design in higher education. *Equity of Excellence in Education, 37,* 105–113.

Plioplys, A. (2003). Survival rates of children with severe neurological disabilities: A review. *Seminars in Pediatric Neurology, 10,* 120–129.

Rehabilitation Act of 1973, Section 504. 29 U.S.C. §7-1-96 (i) (2001). http://www2.ed.gov/about/offices/list/ocr/504faq.html.

Rehabilitation Act, Section 508. 29 U.S.C. 794d, as amended by the Workforce Investment Act of 1998 (P.L. 105–220). www.section508.gov/index.cfm?fuseAction=1998Amend.

Slomine, B., Gerring, J., Grados, M., Vasa, R., Brady, K., Christensen, J., & Denckla, M. B. (2002). Performance on measures of "executive function" following pediatric traumatic brain injury. *Brain Injury, 16,* 759–772.

Straub, K., & Obrzut, J. E. (2009). Effects of cerebral palsy on neuropsychological function. *Journal of Developmental and Physical Disability, 21,* 153–167.

Stuss, D. (2011). Traumatic brain injury: Relation to executive dysfunction and the frontal lobes. *Current Opinions in Neurology, 24,* 584–589.

Thierfeld Brown, J., Wolf, L. E., King, L., & Bork, R. (2012). *The parents' guide to college for students on the autism spectrum.* Shawnee Mission, KS: Autism Asperger Publishing Co.

Transition to Adulthood. (2009). http://nichcy.org/schoolage/transitionadult.

University of Washington DOIT. www.washington.edu/doit/CUDE

Wolf, L. E., Thierfeld Brown, J., & Bork, R. (2009). *Students with asperger syndrome: A guide for college personnel.* Shawnee Mission, KS: Autism Asperger Publishing Co.

Wolf, L. E., & Kaplan, E. (2008). Executive functioning and self-regulation in young adults: Implications for neurodevelopmental learning disorders. In: L. E. Wolf, H. Schreiber, & J. Wasserstein (Eds.). *Adult learning disorders: Contemporary issues* (pp. 219–246). New York: Psychology Press.

SECTION III
METHODOLOGICAL AND LIFESPAN DEVELOPMENTAL CONSIDERATIONS

18 Insignificant Statistical Significance and Other Common Methodological Oversights

Brandi A. Weiss

My first consulting job as a methodologist was for a client conducting a study in the veterinary medical sciences. The client's manuscript had been determined to need "major revisions" and was rejected by a journal for improper use of statistics and a lack of statistically significant findings. The authors had conducted a longitudinal study to investigate the effects of a vaccine in water buffalo. Data were collected from 30 water buffalo, each randomly assigned to one of five treatment groups (six water buffalo per group). Measures were taken from the water buffalo at eight time points over a 27-week period. Data were missing at multiple time points (at times, zero to three water buffalo had complete data within a group), measurements were taken at inconsistent times in each group, and baseline measurements were not taken for many of the variables. During our first meeting the client told me, "I need to say something is statistically significant." I drew him a graph.

Statistical inference has come a long way since the early days of Ronald A. Fisher, Jerry Neyman, and Egon Pearson. Trends are moving away from tests of "statistical significance" and toward the reporting of effect sizes and "practical significance." Although the ideas in this chapter have previously been presented in the social sciences literature, researchers still continue to misuse statistical significance tests and report results based on methodological flaws. This chapter is divided into three sections. The first section focuses on the limitations of statistical significance testing and the benefits of effect sizes. The second section contains information on frequently overlooked methodological pitfalls. The chapter concludes with a list of methodological recommendations for

STATISTICAL SIGNIFICANCE VERSUS PRACTICAL SIGNIFICANCE

Statistical Significance

Over the years many people have criticized the use and interpretation of statistical significance testing (e.g., Carver, 1993; Cohen, 1990; Cohen, 1994; Kirk, 1996; Mills, 2003; Shaver, 1993; Thompson, 1999). Some limitations are incorrect interpretations of what the p value actually represents, claims that statistical significance tests are just tests of whether or not you have a large sample, the argument that the null hypothesis is always false, and the dichotomous significant/nonsignificant decision.

First, the p value obtained from statistical significance tests is often incorrectly interpreted to represent the probability that the null hypothesis is true. For analyses comparing groups this can be thought of as the probability that the means of the two groups do not differ. This may be what researchers want to know, but it is incorrect. The p value represents the probability that one would have seen these data, given that the null hypothesis is true. Falk and Greenbaum (1995) refer to this as "the illusion of probabilistic proof by contradiction" and in their article discuss this common misconception in depth.

Second, with a large enough sample size, any hypothesis test may be statistically significant. To examine this criticism, recall that test statistics are a function of two values: the amount of sampling error (denominator) and the magnitude of the effect (numerator). These two numbers, however, are more informative when interpreted separately rather than in combination. First, consider sampling error. Sampling error is an estimate of how much the sample differs from the population. As the variability of scores increases and sample size decreases, the amount of sampling error increases. Thus, with a small sample, a large effect must be present in order to find statistically significant results. Similarly, with a large enough sample, statistically significant results may be found even when a very small effect exists in the population. For this reason, statistical significance tests are often criticized because they are essentially just tests of whether or not you have a large sample (Cohen, 1994; Thompson, 1999).

Third, some researchers have argued that the null hypothesis is always false (e.g., Cohen, 1994; Kirk, 1996; Tukey, 1991). Tukey (1991), for example, stated, "the effects of A and B are always different—in some decimal place—for any A and B. Thus asking 'Are the effects different?' is foolish" (p. 100). This statement implies that rather than asking if the effects are different, researchers should be asking, "What is the magnitude of the difference?

Finally, when conducting statistical significance tests researchers draw conclusions about whether or not their results were "statistically significant." By doing so, a dichotomous decision is made (i.e., results were either statistically significant or they were not). If a researcher concludes that his or her findings were not "statistically significant," then nothing has been learned about the data. In cases of statistically nonsignificant findings, all you can say is that the direction of the mean difference is uncertain (Tukey, 1991; Cohen, 1994). On the other hand, concluding that the test is statistically significant does not necessarily mean that the findings were practically meaningful. That is, statistical significance testing does not inform researchers about the magnitude of effects.

For example, in 2011 Cable News Network (CNN) Health published an article quoting, "The length of a mother's employment is associated with an increase in her child's body mass index [BMI], according to a study in the journal *Child Development*." This finding suggests that as the amount of time a mother works increases, the BMI of her children also increases. Of course, this finding may anger the 71% of US mothers reported in the article as working. Although multiple methodological criticisms can be made about the study, one stands out more than others. The article continues to report, "We found quite a small, but (statistically) significant increase in the body mass index of children." This statement suggests that although BMI and maternal employment were statistically significantly related, the magnitude of the relation was quite small and perhaps not practically meaningful. Perhaps the small effect was statistically significant due to the large sample of 990 children examined in the study. For these reasons, researchers should always consider effect sizes and power when interpreting results from statistical significance tests (discussed in more detail in the next section).

Effect Sizes

Effect sizes are values that quantify the magnitude of the effect within the collected sample. They inform researchers about whether the observed results are meaningful or not. Sometimes this is referred to as "practical significance." Usually the effect of interest is the amount that the independent variable(s) relates to the dependent variable. However, effect sizes can be any number that is of interest to researchers, for example, mean values, mean changes, proportions, percents, and standardized difference values. They can be on a standardized metric or a raw score metric. Two of the most frequently reported types of effect sizes are standardized mean differences and measures of association.

When making comparisons between two groups, effect sizes quantifying the mean difference are most appropriate. The two most common standardized effect sizes of this type are Cohen's d and Hedges' g. These are standardized using the metric of the dependent variable and can be interpreted as the number of standard deviations difference between the two groups. For example, a d value of .50 indicates that the means of the two groups differed by half of a standard deviation. Larger values indicate larger mean differences between the groups. Cohen (1988) suggested benchmarks for his d statistic in social science research in which 0.2 could be interpreted as a small effect, 0.5 represents a medium effect, and 0.8 or larger represents a large effect size. Caution should be used when interpreting these benchmarks. Researchers should note that these cut-values are rules-of-thumb and thus should not be considered absolute. The metric of the dependent variable should also be taken into consideration along with research findings from previous studies in the same construct area.

For two-group comparisons it is also useful to report effect sizes in the form of raw group differences. For example, a useful effect size could be obtained by taking the difference of the two group means. Consider average birth head circumference in which group A reports a value of 23 centimeters and group B reports a value of 35 centimeters. In this case the unstandardized effect size is 12 centimeters. The sixth edition of the *APA Publication Manual* (2009) encourages researchers to report effect sizes for two-group comparisons in both standardized mean difference format and in raw group differences whenever possible and meaningful (APA Publication Manual, 2009; Cumming & Fidler, 2010). The standardized form of effect sizes is necessary in order to make comparisons across studies and to enable others to conduct meta-analyses. Formulas for calculating effect sizes are available in many textbooks, including Grissom and Kim (2004).

When making comparisons between three or more groups or when conducting studies in which the independent variable(s) is(are) measured on a continuous scale, measures of association are the most appropriate type of effect size. Frequently reported measures of association include (but are not limited to) the following: r^2, R^2, eta squared, omega squared, partial-eta squared, and partial-omega squared. For regression analyses, r^2 and R^2 are typically reported, while for analysis of variance (ANOVA)-based analyses some form of eta squared or omega squared is typically reported. Although the calculation for each measure is slightly different, the interpretation is the same. They represent the proportion of variance in the dependent variable that the effect of interest explains. Because they are proportions, possible values range from zero to 1, with larger values being indicative of a stronger relation between the effect of interest and the dependent variable.

Benchmarks for measures of association have been recommended by Cohen (1988) in which .01 is considered to be small, .09 is a medium-sized effect, and .25 is a large effect size. However, these are only rough guidelines, and researchers should interpret the size of the effect along with the variable(s) of interest and previous research. The size of an effect depends on many features in a study including the number of independent variables. A larger effect size may be needed to be meaningful in studies with a large number of independent variables. For example, if trying to predict freshman college grade point average (GPA) solely from high-school GPA, an R^2 effect size of .05 may be practically important (i.e., high-school GPA explains 5% of the variance in freshman college GPA). However, if predictors also include SAT-quantitative, SAT-verbal, recommendation letters, and the number of extracurricular activities a student engages in, then an R^2 effect size of .05 may be considered to be small.

Statistical Significance and Effect Sizes

The *APA Publication Manual* (1994) was the first edition to mention effect sizes and "encourage" researchers to report effect sizes along with tests of statistical significance. In 1994 *Educational and Psychological Measurement* was the first social sciences journal that required authors to report effect sizes (Capraro & Capraro, 2002). The fifth edition of the *APA Publication Manual* (2001) more strongly stated that it is, "almost always necessary to include some index of effect size."

With all the limitations of statistical significance testing and the increasing encouragement for researchers to report effect sizes, why not just get rid of statistical significance testing? Recommendations about the use of statistical significance tests have ranged from those who encourage researchers to report both tests of statistical significance as well as effect sizes (*APA Publication Manual*, 2009; Hyde, 2001) to researchers who suggest statistical significance tests should never be reported (Carver, 1993). The answer to this question has to do with the types of conclusions that can be drawn from each of these. Effect sizes are descriptive statistics, meaning that they only describe the sample. On the other hand, statistical significance tests are inferential statistics, meaning they allow us to make inferences back to the population. If the purpose of a researcher's study includes both of these, then the researcher should report results from both statistical significance tests, as well as effect sizes.

One way to use effect sizes to make inferences about a population may be to report adjusted effect sizes. Because effect sizes are computed based on a sample, they are fit to the idiosyncrasies of the data. This means they are positively biased and the effect in the population is smaller than what is observed in the sample. This concept is known as shrinkage because the effect "shrinks" in the population. When conducting descriptive studies meant solely to describe the given sample, effect sizes reported in an unadjusted format make sense. However, adjusted forms of effect sizes may make more sense for interpretation when inferences are to be made back to the population or when results will be used for prediction purposes.

Power and Power Analyses

Power is the probability that one will correctly reject a false null hypothesis. It can be thought of as the power to detect statistically significant results if an effect truly exists in the population. Because power is a probability, possible values range from zero to 1 in which higher values are indicative of a test having greater power to detect effects.

Power cannot be directly set by a researcher the way that alpha (the probability of making a type I error) can be. Instead, power is indirectly influenced by the alpha level, the sample size, and the effect size in the population. To increase the power of a statistical test, a researcher can increase the value of alpha or increase the sample size. Statistical tests also have more power to detect large effect sizes in the population. Because these four features are all mathematically related, one can choose values for three and the fourth is mathematically determined. As such, the following two types of power analysis are used by researchers: sample size determination and post-hoc power analysis.

Sample size determination occurs when a researcher conducts a power analysis in order to determine what sample size he or she needs to collect in order to have adequate power for a particular type of hypothesis test. Post-hoc power analysis is conducted when a researcher already knows the sample size that he or she will be able to obtain and thus wants to know the power of the statistical test given a particular sample size. Of note, power analysis should be conducted prior to collecting data and/ or conducting analyses. For more information about how to conduct power analyses, refer to Cohen (1988).

Researchers typically want the power of a test to range from .70 to .90. If resources are limited (e.g., time and money), then lower values of power may be acceptable. If, however, researchers are concerned about making type II errors (e.g., concluding that a medicine results in improvement of patient symptoms when in truth it has no effect or a negative effect), then larger values of power may be desirable.

Of note, each statistical test to be conducted has different power associated with it. Researchers should conduct a power analysis for all types of planned analyses. For example, if a researcher has several hypotheses and plans on conducting an independent t-test and a two-way ANOVA, each statistical test has an associated power value. In this case, the researcher should conduct two types of power analysis (note that the two-way ANOVA will have power for the two main effects and the interaction effect).

Each power analysis may result in a different necessary sample size in order to have the desired value of power. For example, the researcher in the scenario just presented will have obtained four necessary sample sizes (t-test, two ANOVA main effects, and one ANOVA interaction). The researcher conducts power analyses to determine what sample size is necessary for each of these two types of tests and finds that to have power of .80, samples of 40, 50, 60, and 120 are needed, respectively. Which sample size should be chosen? In this case, the researcher needs to consider the purpose of the study in conjunction with the power analysis results. Researchers should note that there is no harm in exceeding the desired value of power (other than one may have too much power, causing all of the statistical tests to be statistically significant).

Considering Statistical Significance, Effect Sizes, and Power

When interpreting results from studies, researchers need to take into consideration statistical significance, effect sizes, and the power of the statistical tests. Studies that have small samples (e.g., the water buffalo study) may result in nonsignificant test statistics due to low power but could have large effect sizes that are practically meaningful. If the researcher fails to consider effect sizes and power, the effects may go undetected. On the other hand, studies with extremely large samples may have too much power and thus all statistical tests would be concluded as statistically significant, even if the accompanying effect size was small and not practically meaningful.

OTHER COMMON METHODOLOGICAL OVERSIGHTS

Dichotomization and Categorization

One commonly encountered pitfall in measurement is the act of dichotomizing or categorizing continuously measured variables. Categorization occurs when a researcher takes a continuous variable and classifies it into different categories. For example, a teacher administers a math test with scores on a 100-point scale. For purposes of discussing students as "high," "average," and "low" ability, the teacher divides the scores so that those with 90+ are put in the "high" group, 70–89 are put in the "average" group, and 069 are put in the "low" ability group. Dichotomization is a specialized case of categorization in which the construct of interest is classified into only two groups. Because much of the methodology literature in this area focuses on dichotomization, that will be the focus of this section. However, the same drawbacks exist when categorizing continuous variables into more than two groups.

Numerous studies have provided evidence that researchers should not dichotomize continuous variables (Allison, Gorman, & Primavera, 1993; Cohen, 1983; MacCallum, Zhang, Preacher, & Rucker, 2002; Maxwell & Delaney, 1993; Streiner, 2002). The primary drawback with dichotomization is the substantial loss of information. This process essentially throws away information by treating individuals on the same side of the cut-point as identical (MacCallum et al., 2002; Maxwell & Delaney, 1993; Streiner, 2002). As a result, dichotomization leads to a loss in measurement precision because it introduces systematic measurement error into the data (Cohen, 1983; MacCallum et al., 2002; Maxwell & Delaney, 1993). The loss of information can be observed in several ways, for example, decreased variabilities, incorrect estimation of effect sizes, and reduction in power and effective sample sizes.

First, discarding information about individual differences can lead to a reduction in variability (MacCallum et al., 2002). Second, numerous studies have demonstrated how dichotomization underestimates statistical significance tests and effect sizes (Cohen, 1983; MacCallum et al., 2002; Streiner, 2002). Cohen (1983) claimed that the practice of dichotomization results in a loss of between one-fifth and two-thirds of the variance accounted for by the original continuous variables. More recently, however, it was found that dichotomization could actually lead to spuriously high correlations and effect sizes (MacCallum et al., 2002; Maxwell & Delaney, 1993). In particular, simulation studies have shown that dichotomization sometimes leads to an artificial increase in the correlation coefficient, particularly when the sample size is small and the original correlation between the two variables is small (MacCallum et al., 2002). This is particularly problematic for researchers in the social sciences because small correlations and small samples are frequently encountered. This overestimation of relationships can be conceptualized as an increase in type I errors.

Finally, the actual reduction of effect size caused by dichotomization can be effectively interpreted as a reduction of statistical power (Cohen, 1983; MacCallum et al., 2002). This loss of power can be illustrated in the relationships among the four conditions that affect statistical inferences described earlier, that is, a designated alpha level, sample size, the population effect size, and the power of the statistical test (Cohen, 1983; Cohen, 1988; Cohen, 1990; Cohen, 1992a; Cohen, 1992b). All four conditions are a function of one another such that any can be determined by knowing the values of the other three. Therefore, a reduced effect size results in a loss of statistical power, which can further be conceptualized as an effective loss in sample size. In sum, dichotomization can be equivalent to discarding between one-third and two-thirds of a sample size (Cohen, 1983).

There are some circumstances in which dichotomization may be appropriate, however. MacCallum et al. (2002) stated that it is, "rarely defensible and often will yield misleading results" (p. 19). However, they provide two scenarios in which researchers may desire to dichotomize their variables. First, when data are highly skewed and bimodal, it may suggest the presence of two distinct groups. The example provided by MacCallum et al. (2002) is of smokers and nonsmokers. When asking individuals about the quantity of cigarettes they smoke per day, a large number of individuals would most likely select zero. In this instance, the data would be positively skewed, and consequently the presence of two distinct groups is clear (i.e., two modes). Researchers should keep in mind, however, that if categorizing these data, all information regarding the variability among smokers would be lost (MacCallum et al., 2002).

Second, when taxometric analyses (e.g., latent class analyses and latent profile analyses) show a clear point that differentiates between two groups, it may be an indication that dichotomization is acceptable. Allison and colleagues (1993) state that if a statistical test (e.g., latent class analyses and latent profile analyses) shows that a significant bimodal distribution and strong theoretical rationale support the distribution, then dichotomization may be appropriate.

Additionally, there may be circumstances in which it is unethical or implausible to ask participants to report exact values of variables on a continuous measurement scale. For example, some people do not want to report their exact age but they may feel comfortable checking a box that contains age ranges. Another example is income. It is unreasonable to expect participants to report exact income values, and thus asking them to identify which income range they fall in may be more feasible. In these cases, it is important for researchers to keep equal distance between the categories. For example, when asking participants to report their age, options such as 0–9, 10–19, 20–29, and 30–39 would be better than 0–19, 19–25, and 26–40.

Latent Variable Analyses

Traditional measured-variable analyses, such as t-tests, ANOVA, and multiple regression, are based on the assumption that variables are measured perfectly without error. For variables such as years of education, age, height, and weight, this is true because they can be measured directly and thus do not contain measurement error. In contrast, most social science researchers hypothesize relations between latent variables. Latent variables are variables that must be measured indirectly and consequently contain measurement error. For example, consider the psychological construct depression, which cannot be measured directly. Beck's depression inventory (BDI) is commonly used to indirectly measure the severity of depression in adults. This instrument contains a series of questions relating to symptoms of depression in which participants respond on a Likert-type scale. The latent variable (depression) is what causes scores on the measured variables (the BDI questions). Scores on a survey measure may vary as a function of social desirability bias, respondent bias, or differences in interpretation of the questions. All of these are examples that contribute to measurement error. Other examples of latent variables include extroversion, fluency, happiness, health, knowledge, motivation, intelligence, and quality of life.

When the traditional measured-variable analyses are conducted using variables that contain measurement error, standard error estimates will be biased and result in weak statistical significance tests. Conceptually this can be thought of as a loss of power for statistical significance tests. Additionally, when independent variables contain measurement error, the parameter estimates of how the independent variable and dependent variable are related will be biased. In in the case where there is more than one independent variable, the bias could be negative or positive.

When relations are hypothesized between latent variables, latent variable analyses such as structural equation modeling (SEM) are more appropriate than the traditional measured-variable analyses. Examples of other latent variable analyses include latent class analysis, mixture modeling, and Bayesian statistics. Latent variable analyses incorporate measurement error into the statistical model. Modeling error allows the analyses to estimate the amount of measurement error that exists in the measured variables. Effects between latent variables can then be estimated free from error.

In comparison with measured-variable analyses, SEM requires a much larger sample size. The question, "how large of a sample size is needed," is difficult to answer. Some researchers roughly recommend using a ratio of cases to the number of parameters you wish to estimate, but these ratios range from 5:1 (Bentler & Chou, 1987) to 20:1 recommendations (Tanaka, 1987). Gerbing and Anderson (1984) found that at least 150 cases were necessary for a model to converge to a proper solution, while Hu and Bentler (1998, 1999) found that a sample size of 250 or more was needed in order to estimate whether or not a theoretical model fit the observed data. An even larger sample size may be needed to obtain accurate and stable parameter estimates. As such, SEM is often considered to be a large-sample data analysis.

Small Sample Sizes

Similar to the client with the 30 water buffalo, I frequently hear researchers say they plan to collect a sample of 30 participants. My response is always, "Why 30? You need to justify your choice in sample size." The myth that one need only obtain a sample size of 30 most likely comes from the central limit theorem discussed in introductory statistics courses. The central limit theorem states that as sample size increases, the sampling distribution of the mean becomes more normally distributed. Generally, the magic number 30 is recommended as being "large enough" for scores to approximate a normal distribution. Two important points should be considered in regards to this. First, this means that in order to approximate a normal distribution, you need a sample of 30 or more for each arithmetic mean you plan to estimate (i.e., you need at least 30 cases per group, not 30 total). Second, approximating a normal distribution and having enough power to detect a true effect are not equivalent. Thus, just because you have a sample size of 30 does not necessarily mean you have adequate power to detect true effects.

There are many situations in which it is not feasible to collect large sample sizes, for example, the client with the 30 water buffalo (6 water buffalo per treatment group). This does not mean the researcher should abandon his or her small studies. Instead there are several ways researchers can examine their hypotheses using small samples.

First, the majority of statistical significance tests taught in introductory statistics courses are considered to be parametric tests (e.g., t-tests, ANOVA, and multiple regression). Parametric tests require researchers to meet a series of assumptions, at least one of which is that the data must approximate a known distribution. There are, however, a series of distribution-free nonparametric tests that, generally speaking, require fewer assumptions than their parametric counterparts. When researchers cannot approximate a known distribution due to small samples, then nonparametric tests may be an attractive alternative. Nonparametric tests often use rank-order data and medians instead of equal-interval data and means, which are used in most parametric tests. Most introductory statistics and ANOVA textbooks discuss some types of nonparametric tests.

Second, researchers should not diminish the capability of descriptive statistics, especially effect sizes. When the sample size is small, researchers can still use descriptive statistics such as the mean, median, and range. Because effect sizes are a type of descriptive statistic, they should be examined whenever possible. Graphs also provide an effective way of describing data collected for studies. Except in the case of nonparametric tests, statistical significance testing should most likely be avoided when sample sizes are small. Do you really want to make inferences back to the population based on a sample size of six water buffalo?

Nine Recommendations for Applied Researchers

The previous two sections in this chapter focused on how effect sizes and power should be considered in conjunction with results from statistical significance tests and other common methodological oversights that researchers frequently don't consider. This section summarizes the ideas already presented into a list of recommendations that researchers should consider when conducting studies and when reading other researcher's studies.

1. When reporting the results from statistical significance tests, use the term "statistically significant" rather than just "significant" (Carver, 1993; Cumming & Fidler, 2010). This will communicate to readers what your statement means. For explaining effect sizes, terms such as "practically significant," "practically important," "clinically important," or "educationally important" are appropriate terms to use (Cumming & Fidler, 2010).

2. For every statistical significance test there is an effect size. Always report effect sizes along with the results from statistical significance tests. Even post-hoc tests and planned comparison follow-up tests have effect sizes associated with them (usually Cohen's d).

3. Report effect sizes in the metric of the original measurement scale of the dependent variable and in standardized form (*APA Publication Manual*, 2009; Cumming & Fidler, 2010; Durlak, 2009). Effect sizes in the original metric are helpful for interpretation purposes, and standardized effect sizes are helpful because they enable researchers to compare them across studies and conduct meta-analyses. For example, a researcher wants to compare the intelligence (IQ) of two groups. The researcher finds a Cohen's d value of .33. This .33 value indicates that there is one-third of a standard deviation difference in the mean IQ of the two groups. Although the standardized Cohen's d is useful for comparing this effect across studies, it is also helpful to state that this is equivalent to a 5-point difference in IQ (the standard deviation of IQ scales is 15, and one-third of 15 is 5).

4. Conduct power analyses before conducting a study. A sample size resulting in power between .7 and .9 for your planned statistical significance tests is ideal. Knowing how much power a test has helps researchers know how much weight they should give statistical significance tests when interpreting results. You want enough power to detect effects if they exist, but not too much power so that all tests appear to be statistically significant. If you have data from many people already collected, you do not necessarily want to discard cases. You still want the sample to be representative of the demographics in the population. The more people you have from the population, the better you can generalize your inferences back to the population (i.e., you will have less shrinkage). In these cases, put less weight in the results from statistical significance tests and more weight in effect sizes when interpreting the results from your study.

5. Consider the relationships between statistical significance, effect sizes, power, and sample sizes when interpreting results of studies. For example, a nonstatistically significant finding based on a small sample (and thus low power) accompanied by a practically significant effect size should not be disregarded as unimportant. Similarly, a statistically significant test based on a large sample (and thus very high power) accompanied by a practically unimportant effect size should not be regarded as important.

6. Do not categorize or dichotomize continuous variables. Whenever possible, variables should be measured in their natural form and left in that form when conducting analyses. There are some situations in which it is acceptable to categorize continuous variables, such as when data are highly skewed and bimodal, when taxometric analyses reveal two distinct groups, or when it is unethical or not feasible to ask participants to respond with exact values.

7. If the underlying variables of interest are latent and you have an adequately large sample size, consider using latent variable methods.

8. If you have a small sample size, consider using nonparametric tests. When samples are small, focus the interpretation of your results on effect sizes rather than the results from statistical significance tests. Don't underestimate the power of descriptive statistics and graphs.

9. Before conducting a study, researchers should consider obtaining a copy of Hancock and Mueller's (2010) reference book. This book contains detailed information about the type of information that researchers should be reporting in their studies. There is a separate chapter on each type of data analysis currently used in social sciences. Each chapter contains a table of desiderata along with detailed explanations of key elements that should be included in any study using the method discussed within the chapter.

REFERENCES

Allison, D. B., Gorman, B. S., & Primavera, L. H. (1993). Some of the most common questions asked of statistical consultants: Our favorite responses and recommended readings. *Genetic, Social, and General Psychology Monographs, 119*, 155–185.

American Psychological Association. (1994). *Publication Manual of the American Psychological Association* (4th ed.). Washington, DC: American Psychological Association.

American Psychological Association. (2001). *Publication Manual of the American Psychological Association* (5th ed.). Washington, DC: American Psychological Association.

American Psychological Association. (2009). *Publication Manual of the American Psychological Association* (6th ed.). Washington, DC: American Psychological Association.

Bentler, P. M., & Chou, C. P. (1987). Practical issues in structural modeling. *Sociological Methods & Research, 16*, 78–117.

Cable News Network. (2011). *Study: Kids' weight increases when mom works more*. Retrieved March 1, 2011, from http://www.cnn.com/2011/HEALTH/02/04/children.bmi.moms/index.html?hpt=C2

Capraro, R. M., & Capraro, M. M. (2002). Treatments of effect sizes and statistical significance tests in textbooks. *Educational and Psychological Measurement, 62*, 771–782.

Carver, R. P. (1993). The case against statistical significance testing, revisited. *Journal of Experimental Education, 61*, 287–292.

Cohen, J. (1983). The cost of dichotomization. *Applied Psychological Measurement, 7*, 249–253.

Cohen, J. (1988). *Statistical power analysis for the behavioral sciences* (2nd ed.). Hillsdale, NJ: Erlbaum.

Cohen, J. (1990). Things I have learned (so far). *American Psychologist, 45*, 1304–1312.

Cohen, J. (1992a). A power primer. *Psychological Bulletin, 112*, 155–159.

Cohen, J. (1992b). Statistical power analysis. *Current Directions in Psychological Sciences, 1*, 98–101.

Cohen, J. (1994). The earth is round (p <.05). *American Psychologist, 49*, 997–1003.

Cumming, G., & Fidler, F. (2010). Effect sizes and confidence intervals. In G. R. Hancock, & R. O. Mueller (Eds.), *The reviewer's guide to quantitative methods in the social sciences* (pp. 79–91). New York: Routledge.

Durlak, J. A. (2009). How to select, calculate, and interpret effect sizes. *Journal of Pediatric Psychology, 34*, 917–928.

Falk, R., & Greenbaum, C. W. (1995). Significance tests die hard: The amazing persistence of a probabilistic misconception. *Theory & Psychology, 5*, 75–98.

Gerbing, D. W., & Anderson, J. C. (1984). On the meaning of within-factor correlated measurement errors. *Journal of Consumer Research, 11*, 572–580.

Grissom, R. J., & Kim, J. J. (2004). *Effect sizes for research: A broad practical approach.* Mahwah, NJ: Erlbaum.

Hancock, G. R., & Mueller, R. O. (Eds.) (2010). *The reviewer's guide to quantitative methods in the social sciences.* New York: Routledge.

Hu, L., & Bentler, P. M. (1998). Fit indices in covariance structure modeling: Sensitivity to underparameterized model misspecification. *Psychological Methods, 3*, 424–453.

Hu., L., & Bentler, P. M. (1999). Cutoff criteria for fit indexes in covariance structure analysis: Conventional criteria versus new alternatives. *Structural Equation Modeling: A Multidisciplinary Journal, 6*, 1–55.

Hyde, J. S., (2001). Reporting effect sizes: The roles of editors, textbook authors, and publication manuals. *Educational and Psychological Measurement, 61*, 225–228.

Kirk, R. E., (1996). Practical significance: A concept whose time has come. *Educational and Psychological Measurement, 56*, 746–759.

MacCallum, R. C., Zhang, S., Preacher, K. J., & Rucker, D. D. (2002). On the practice of dichotomization of quantitative variables. *Psychological Methods, 7*, 19–40.

Maxwell, S. E., & Delaney, H. D. (1993). Bivariate median-splits and spurious statistical significance. *Psychological Bulletin, 113*, 181–190.

Mills, S. R. (2003). Statistical practices: The seven deadly sins. *Child Neuropsychology, 9*, 221–233.

Shaver, J. P. (1993). What statistical significance testing is, and what it is not. *Journal of Experimental Education, 61*, 293–316.

Streiner, D. L. (2002). Breaking up is hard to do: The heartbreak of dichotomizing continuous data. *Research Methods in Psychiatry, 47*, 262–266.

Tanaka, J. S. (1987). "How big is big enough?": Sample size and goodness of fit in structural equation models with latent variables. *Child Development, 58*, 134–146.

Thompson, B. (1999). If statistical significance tests are broken/misused, what practices should supplement or replace them? *Theory and Psychology, 9*, 165–181.

Tukey, J. W. (1991). The philosophy of multiple comparisons. *Statistical Science, 6*, 100–116.

19 Bridging the Gap

Transitioning from Developmental Healthcare to Adult Healthcare

Jane Holmes Bernstein and
Celiane Rey-Casserly

Advances in healthcare (surgical, medical, pharmacologic, psychosocial) have changed the mortality and morbidity landscape for a wide variety of medical conditions and, in turn, have increased the number of individuals now living with chronic illness throughout childhood and into adult life. Not only are we seeing an increase in the number of survivors of previously lethal or cognitively devastating illnesses, but there has also been a substantial increase in the number of children with chronic health conditions reaching adulthood. As chronically ill children live into adulthood, unanticipated new health and adaptive function issues emerge. "Rapid increases in childhood chronic conditions will lead to large numbers of younger adults with chronic illness and disabilities, dependent on public programs and expenditures, and experiencing lower quality of life, poorer social interactions and less community participation" (Perrin, Bloom, & Gortmaker, 2007, p. 2758). The number of children receiving Supplementary Security Income exceeded 1 million in 2005, more than tripling over the prior 20 years (Perrin et al., 2007).

Study of these individuals and their developmental progress—capacities, limitations, and medical and psychosocial needs—combined with rapid advances in the biological and neurological sciences relating to the processes that underlie neural structure and function has led to paradigm shifts in how we view both acute and chronic illness in the developing child. A major shift in thinking about the impact of childhood conditions is the understanding that in a developing organism, any insult (disease, acquired injury, adverse experience) can be expected to affect the integrity of the central nervous system, irrespective of the actual site (brain or body) of insult. This results from the complex interaction between the nature and the timing of disease/injury (and treatment) with developmental processes (experience, plasticity, learning) over the extended course of childhood and adolescence. The basic principle is that any perturbation of expectable developmental processes becomes part of the developmental course thereafter and is manifest in changed trajectories for both brain and behavioral development. Changes in the neural infrastructure can be expected to result in limited and/or atypical functional capacities that undermine the achievement of the expected goals of childhood and adolescence, those of autonomy, self-efficacy, and social competence.

Changed trajectories can be seen not only as an outcome of brain injury or systemic medical illness but also as a result of early trauma and adverse social experiences that may play a significant role in the provocation of later-onset adult disease (Barker, 2001; Bauer & Boyce, 2004). The American Academy of Pediatrics recently issued a policy statement on the impact of adversity and toxic stress on the development and health of children (Committee on Psychosocial Aspects of Child and Family Health et al., 2012), highlighting the expanding knowledge base documenting the effects of toxic stress on brain development. Quoting Frederick Douglas, "It is easier to build strong children than to repair broken men" (p. e224), the statement exhorts the pediatrics community to incorporate advances in science and advocacy efforts in order to reduce adversity and risk in young children and to promote their well-being and that of society.

We frame the discussion in this chapter in the context of a developmental integrative approach to conceptualizing the ongoing lifespan effects of childhood conditions. We highlight the role of the neuropsychologist as a member of the developmental care team, the challenges in the transition to adulthood, and the neuropsychologist's contribution in the adult healthcare setting. We use the label "parents" or "family members" to refer to the full range of potential caretakers of a child, recognizing that siblings, grandparents, and legal guardians may be included.

BRAIN–BEHAVIOR DEVELOPMENT

Broadly speaking, there are two primary sources of neuropathology: neurodevelopmental disorders (NDD) and acquired disorders (AcqD). The NDD comprise genetic syndromes such as Down, Turner, Prader-Willi, fragile-X, Williams, neurofibromatosis-1 (NF-1), and sickle cell disease; complex genetic syndromes such as autism, specific language impairment, dyslexia, and attention deficit/hyperactivity disorder; and structural abnormalities such as congenital hydrocephalus, a/dysgenesis of the corpus callosum, Dandy-Walker, Arnold-Chiari, Sturge-Weber conditions, congenital cardiac malformations, myelodysplasias, and cerebral palsies. The AcqD include traumatic conditions such as missile injury, motor vehicle accidents, falls, and physical injury; neurological conditions such as brain tumors, brain infections, cerebrovascular accidents, and anoxia; and medical conditions such as leukemias, infectious disease, prematurity, liver disease, kidney disease, endocrine disease, and gastrointestinal conditions. A given medical condition may not have a direct impact on the brain; it can nonetheless have major indirect effects on brain–behavior development secondary to (unavoidable) treatment agents/modalities (radiation, chemotherapy, steroids, other toxic agents), disrupted metabolic or endocrine status, and/or increased vulnerability to specific neuropathologic outcomes such as neonatal hypoxic/ischemic encephalopathy or silent stroke in sickle cell disease.

The change in neurobehavioral trajectories that is characteristic of both NDD and AcqD is not, as noted above, limited to known perturbations of the biological substrate for behavior. Importantly, it also may occur when developmental processes are directly undermined. Adverse life events can significantly limit the "expectable experience" (nurturing, language, exploration) of the infant and young child at critical developmental epochs (Shonkoff, 2010). In so doing, there is potential compromise of critical brain–experience transactions that are needed to sculpt both brain and behavior, thus setting the stage for subsequent derailment of behavioral outcomes (Fox, Levitt, & Nelson, 2010). Psychiatric disorders can also take a child "out of the (learning) loop" for shorter or longer periods of time, compromising developing neural substrates for behavior and constraining knowledge acquisition, social skills development, and regulatory capacities.

The NDD–AcqD distinction is critical for understanding how neural systems are constructed and shaped throughout development. As a general principle, in NDD there is no period of typical development; the brain is sculpted according to nonstandard principles. This may limit both the acquisition of brain capacity and the ability to engage effectively with the expectable experiences that are necessary for learning. Thus, for example, the structural developmental changes in the brain of the child with spina bifida have specific consequences for the child's interaction with the environment (Dennis & Barnes, 2010; Juranek et al., 2008). This condition is associated with motor limitations affecting the lower extremities. This limits the independent locomotion needed for exploration. The lack of exploratory capacity in turn limits the experience available for specific types of learning because the neural networks subserving the learning are changed. The subsequent profile of neuropsychological assets and deficits that the child acquires is thus shaped not only by biological variables but also by experiential factors.

In AcqD, in contrast, there is a period of typical brain development. This may be relatively short in developmental terms, as in the case of injury in infancy, or relatively lengthy, as for a teenager. Age at time of injury or disease onset is an important variable. Traditionally, age has been viewed as a "placeholder," or marker. In a developmental context, however, it must be conceptualized more dynamically. Chronological age is not simply an index of time passing; it must be understood as an indication of "amount-of-time-in-the-world-having-experiences." Constant brain–world interactions shape emerging behavioral capacities with different experiences during different periods building on each other. Age is then construed as a marker for the developmental processes and specific vulnerabilities in play at a particular time in development (Dennis, 2011). Thus, brain tumors in children with NF-1 form and grow not only due to genetic errors but because of the molecular changes in nonneoplastic cells, which create a permissive environment at particular stages in development (Crouse, Dahiya, & Gutmann, 2011). Hypoxic-ischemic injury in the premature infant has different pathophysiology and consequences than in the term infant (Ferriero, 2004). The timing of injury/disease onset interacts with developmental brain processes and the trajectories of expectable experiences in critical developmental epochs. Derailment of early experience that undermines the foundations of behavior can be expected to change behavioral outcomes thereafter as the individual seeks to learn from experience not only with "nonstandard" neural systems but from experiences that are themselves potentially constrained by the limitations of the changed neural system. The type of derailment that occurs is related to the developmental status of the organism at the time of injury.

Even a very solid early foundation of neurobehavioral development may not be sufficient to counter the impact of later severe injury. Traumatic brain injury in adolescence, for example, can be devastating—not only by damaging the brain directly but by also undermining critical developmental processes that sculpt neural systems at this age. The expectable experiences of adolescence/young adulthood support the fine-tuning of social cognition, executive processes, and regulatory capacities that are the hallmark of adolescent development. Any disruption of opportunities for expected learning in this period has significant potential for undermining successful independent functioning in adulthood (Blakemore, 2008).

Critical to the understanding of brain construction over time is the balance between specialization and plasticity. Specialization provides stability, and plasticity provides the flexibility needed to respond to novel environments/challenges (Dennis, 2011). In general, earlier acquired skills are dependent on evolutionarily conserved systems that are critical for survival. They are typically stable and have limited, if any, capacity for plastic change. More recently acquired systems, evolutionarily speaking, have greater capacity for flexible response to changing environmental conditions. The extent to which such flexibility is available for recovery varies significantly. Plasticity of the developing brain may provoke specific vulnerabilities given the increased susceptibility to excitatory neurotransmitters (Johnston, 2009).

Where the acquired disorders are concerned, understanding the variables associated with the behavioral outcomes of alternative development pathways is made more complex by the need to integrate the co-occurring trajectories of maturation and recovery. This is most salient when the insult that alters subsequent brain–environment transactions also damages brain directly and involves a period of physical recovery. The course of immediate recovery from the new insult involves regaining biological function to the extent possible, but this may be limited and further constrain new learning by a now altered brain in its ongoing interactions with the environment. Indeed, in the presence of alternative or changed developmental trajectories for both brain and behavior, there are significant sources of constraint on behavioral outcomes. These can be directly related to changes and/or adjustments in the neural substrate in terms of re-organization or re-engagement of disrupted circuits. Equally, they can result from behavioral accommodations that solve one set of adaptive problems by alternate—compensatory—means, but may limit effective solutions for other adaptive problems. In analyzing behavioral outcomes to evaluate the potential response to different interventions, the neuropsychologist will focus on the interaction between the child's learning trajectory and the time of injury: Has all learning from the beginning of life been done atypically? Were some skills developed or developing prior to the insult and subsequently available for recovery and development thereafter? Are compensatory strategies available? Have they been mastered/used? To what extent might the learning capacity of the overall system be constrained or potentiated by derailed structures, limited resources, or available opportunities for successful adaptation?

Another important distinction to be made when working with individuals with chronic conditions is that between adaptive capacities that enable more or less effective daily functioning and higher-order thinking skills that are required for more abstract knowledge acquisition, conceptual reasoning, problem solving, insight, and judgment. Independence in both of these domains of behavioral function is important, and neither predicts the other. Nor does the ability to demonstrate a (relatively) successful functionally adaptive skill in a specific domain necessarily entail success in apparently related domains; in all situations, transfer of skills and generalization need to be demonstrated. In the context of altered developmental trajectories, the ability to function effectively may be dependent on the recruitment and activation of alternative neural pathways and circuitry that may be less efficient, demand more resources, or simply be inadequate to support other related capacities (Park & Reuter-Lorenz, 2009).

GROWING UP WITH A CHRONIC CONDITION

For the purpose of this discussion, "chronic condition" encompasses both conditions that date from birth and conditions that have been acquired in childhood/adolescence. The notion of "chronicity" is not limited to the persistence of a given disease or condition over time; it is extended to include the ongoing impact of a given condition as disease, treatment, and experience interact with fundamental developmental processes over childhood and adolescence. The chronicity of the condition is entailed by the fact that any perturbation at any point in the ongoing development of a dynamically changing system (such as supports brain–behavior development) will then become part of the developmental course itself—and will shape the way in which the organism interacts with its environment and thus influence the subsequent organization of the system. Thus, when the primary disease can be considered cured, as in, for example, many childhood leukemias, the impact of the disease and of its treatment at a critical developmental epoch will persist in the form of altered developmental trajectories and changed organization of neural circuitry and behavioral architecture (Iuvone et al., 2002; Lesnik, Ciesielski, Hart, Benzel, & Sanders, 1998). This is true for neurobehavioral development, but may also affect the subsequent maturation of biological structures as the child matures, changing outcomes and setting up different risk profiles with respect to future cardiac or endocrine status. The potential for "late effects" of early-occurring disease has been well articulated for childhood leukemias and brain tumors (Rey-Casserly & Meadows, 2008). The concept is equally applicable to any condition that interacts with developmental processes; specific effects will not be seen until the child is required to meet later developmental challenges and has difficulty doing so in optimal fashion.

For the clinical team taking on the care of an individual in early adulthood who has a chronic condition that first presented in childhood/adolescence, there are three variables that play a major role in the developmental outcome and thus in the individual's behavioral adjustment to the adult healthcare setting. These are the variables associated with the insult (condition/disease/injury/adverse events, timing, severity); the variables associated with the treatment (agents, procedures, side effects, hospitalization); and the variables associated with the experience of insult and treatment—and ongoing developmental challenges (coping skills, resilience/cognitive reserve, physical/social/psychological resources). An important component of the latter is the psychological impact of the child's potentially limited capacities for meeting expectable challenges. In addition, the successful progress of the individual will depend not only on the resource capacities of the family, the community, and relevant societal structures, but will also be influenced by attitudes and beliefs associated with human development in general and issues of disability in particular (Pledger, 2003).

Two major aspects of the child and family's experience with a chronic condition impact the transition from the childhood healthcare setting to the adult healthcare system. One is the nature of developmental healthcare itself and what this entails; the second is the impact, both neuropsychological and psychological, of a disorder on the child's development across the childhood and adolescent period.

Developmental healthcare

Systems that provide adult healthcare have largely been shaped by a medical model that conceptualizes "almost all ailments as the consequence of episodic, endogenous factors" (Hochstein, Halfon, & Inkelas, 1998). As such, the medical team assumes a certain degree of "normal" functioning on the part of the patient and focuses on the condition or disease, an approach considered "condition- (or disease-) centered." Likewise, the pediatric practitioner monitors a child's acquisition of developmental milestones through "wellness visits" but (all other things being equal) assumes a generally adequate level of normal development and functioning against which to evaluate symptoms of disease as necessary.

The chronic conditions of childhood have a different starting point. With advances in medical care, individuals with these conditions are "survivors" of diseases that were previously incompatible with life and/or led to high levels of morbidity. Management of these conditions in survivors requires a wide range of medical and psychosocial care strategies to promote health and well-being. In addition, a core feature of these various conditions is that they undermine normal trajectories of development. The major focus of the developmental healthcare team is "normalizing lives" while providing needed medical services. This has led to a different conceptualization of developmental healthcare: "The state of the art is the provision of care by interdisciplinary teams that balance the needs for healthcare services for the child with other needs of the social family unit and that work with families as full partners in providing care. These teams are designed to maximize quality of life, to provide long-term continuity, and to integrate and balance biomedical and psychosocial issues" (Stein, 1998, pp. 732–733). Developmental care is thus child-and-family centered, rather than condition/disease centered. Providing healthcare in this framework means that parents and the clinical care team are following the developmental course of a child, rather than the natural history of a condition. The family together with all care team members have an investment in the individual child, and all monitor how the child matures and achieves developmental milestones over time. The parental investment is that their child becomes as successful an adult as possible. The care team also has an investment in the success of their clinical contribution to the child's progress and well-being. These strong relationships are repeatedly reinforced as development proceeds.

The developmental care experience is founded on the following:

- A clinical team: comprised of medical, technological, psychological, and social service specialists and with child–family relationships with care providers that can be extensive;
- Repeated close contacts: the child and family and the team create enduring relationships;
- Experience of life-threatening situations: relationships will be forged in intense circumstances;
- Frequent decision making under often critical conditions: already emotionally stretched parents can be rapidly overwhelmed with information and must rely on the care team for guidance;
- Repeated and/or extended periods of treatment/hospitalization: these can change the child's developmental experience, limiting opportunities for exploration, learning, and mastery of both neuropsychological and psychosocial skills;

- Multiple organ impact: many chronic conditions, neurodevelopmental and acquired, affect multiple organs systems, increasing both the number of individuals in the complex web of relationships between the child and family and the care team and the number of contacts needed to address and follow all aspects of the condition; and
- Treatment planning: needed treatment modalities have the potential for serious side effects; parents must make more decisions.

A family cannot realistically undertake the complexity of the child's care. The need for medical, psychological, and social support creates dependency in the child and family unit that binds the team even closer together. The history of shared challenges, reinforced over time, creates in both child and family an often intense psychological commitment to an institution/care team, a commitment that is reciprocated. The members of clinical care teams may also have major issues around the transition of "their patients" from their care and may, unwittingly or otherwise, reinforce any reluctance on the part of the individual or the family to move on. A significant element in this regard is the challenge of locating adult providers who are willing to care for young adults with chronic health conditions; this is a significant barrier in transition planning (McManus et al., 2011). The transition from child care to adult care must involve individualized, developmentally centered care that requires active coordination and communication (Cooley & Sagerman, 2011). Best practices in this regard remain to be developed for adolescents and young adults with complex medical needs (Watson, Parr, Joyce, May, & Le Couteur, 2011).

The psychosocial dynamic

A primary goal when working with children with chronic conditions and their families is to "normalize life" to the fullest extent possible. The impact of a disorder on development across the childhood and adolescent period should be evaluated in all domains of life. The psychological perspective is crucial. Members of the psychosocial team (e.g., psychologist, neuropsychologist, social worker) are major contributors to achievement of this goal. Psychologically, the fundamental developmental dynamic of dependence-to-separation-to-autonomy is central and encompasses both the experiences of nurturing adults and the development of self-control and self-efficacy in the child.

Typically, as children proceed toward independent adulthood, the primary responsibilities in the developmental "dance" between child and caretaker(s) shift from the parent to the child. Initially, parents are totally responsible for an infant. As children grow, they become more independent in mastering the developmentally referenced tasks of childhood and adolescence. Parents support this increasing independence by moving from being nurturing and protective developmental partners who provide security and limit to ones who gradually stand back to let the increasingly competent youngster learn for him/herself, only providing limits and support as needed. Promoting this movement from being looked after to looking after self is central to the parenting role. It is this child–parent "dance" that promotes child independence that is the most vulnerable to disruption by a chronic condition. When confronted with disease and/or treatments, parents may find it intensely difficult to "parent" the child who "has been through so much" and/or who has compromised functioning. They may avoid imposing limits, fail to encourage the child to "do for him- or herself," talk for the child rather than wait for the child to answer questions, or be worried that the child will "fail" or that other children will be cruel. Their biggest challenge is leaving the protective role in the "young child-nurturing adult" equation so that the adolescent/young adult has the opportunity to begin to take on adult responsibilities. This is made much more difficult when parents have had to be more protective and nurturing due to their child's medical disorder and its treatments.

Not surprisingly, an intensely protective stance by parents reinforces the lack of control for self that is associated with medical treatment. The outcome may be a young person who has not learned to regulate his/her behavior or emotions, has limited problem-solving skills, and has been unable to take responsibility for self, resorting to a passive role and/or learned helplessness stance in the face of any challenge.

From the perspective of the child or adolescent, expectable opportunities for participating in the moment-to-moment experiences that are important to ongoing developmental mastery are often curtailed. This may be a direct effect of the disease/treatment undermining relevant brain systems. It may also result from an inability to participate because of limitations in relevant skills (physical, neuropsychological, social, psychological) or it may be a consequence of intense parental concerns and fears, as noted above. Children may also feel, and/or be treated as, "different" and withdraw from participation or not be invited to participate by others, thus further limiting opportunity. They are at risk for being continually overwhelmed by experiences that are not congruent with their cognitive and/or emotional processing capacities and may repeatedly resort to ineffective and/or maladaptive coping strategies. Their exposure to major adversity at a young age has the potential to undermine the development of a sense of mastery and efficacy and contribute to social isolation, limiting opportunity for sustaining peer relationships.

What does the neuropsychologist contribute?

Comprehensive education and support that address the impact of changed neuropsychological status on functional outcomes (e.g., adaptive, vocational, academic, social, emotional) with the goal of promoting an individual's ability to meet ongoing developmental expectations are central to the neuropsychologist's contribution to the transition process. This will be based on the following:

- Detailed analysis of individual goals as the basis for supporting ongoing developmental progress;
- Detailed description of the nature and source of neuropsychological capacities and weaknesses;
- Understanding of the role of neuropsychological variables in the individual's capacities for independence, insight, managing emotions, ability or inability to meet age-expected social expectations with both peers and adults, and the contribution of these to ongoing risk for psychological distress; and
- Appreciation of psychological variables, the impact of the psychological experience of the medical condition and treatment, lack of expectable developmental experiences that promote ongoing learning secondary to curtailed opportunities to learn as compared to peers, and sense of "difference" as compared to peers.

An understanding of the contributions, and interactions, of neuropsychological and psychological variables to the individual's ability to manage specific situations is central to the formulation of strategies to meet everyday expectations for age-congruent functioning (social, cognitive, emotional, and behavioral). There is a need to promote optimal educational experience and effective psychological functioning. The immediate goals of intervention planning are those of optimal social adjustment and schooling. The requirements include access to learning opportunities (social, behavioral, adaptive/vocational, academic), educational placement decisions, targeted instructional programming, and psychotherapeutic support. Addressing systems issues such as family functioning, social–environmental context, and access to resources is also an important component of developmental healthcare.

What does this mean for the adult care team?

As a young person transitions to an adult healthcare setting, new primary care and specialty care teams will encounter an unfamiliar set of decisions regarding patient medical management. No less challenging, the team must negotiate with an individual who may not be able to communicate symptoms effectively, may expect to be told what to do, and may not be compliant with instructions. It is also likely that the team will have to negotiate a relationship with a parent or caretaker who has historically been the primary player in making healthcare decisions for the individual. In this context, patient-centered adult care needs to adopt many of the characteristics of family-centered care in order to promote optimal transition (Duke & Scal, 2011; Kuhlthau et al., 2011). Furthermore, optimal transition planning requires a dynamic and integrative approach that does not merely focus on the skills and disease knowledge of the adolescent/young adult but also incorporates an understanding of social–ecological, familial, and developmental factors. Schwartz et al. (2011) describe such a model that addresses social/cultural factors, access to resources, individual issues related to medical disorder, neuropsychological functioning, development, and psychosocial adjustment. The individual's knowledge base as related to health and disease in general as well as an understanding of one's own condition, available skills/self-efficacy, belief/expectations, and personal goals must also be incorporated into the care framework, as must the nature and impact of relationships with family and providers.

THE TRANSITION CHALLENGE

Individuals with chronic conditions require healthcare throughout adulthood and must navigate adult healthcare systems. To do so effectively requires a relatively high degree of autonomy and independence. To the extent that such individuals may lack necessary skills to achieve these critical goals secondary to the developmental impact of their condition, they are likely to be seriously challenged in meeting the expectations of the adult system.

Access to care. A primary challenge is access to healthcare. In the United States, this challenge extends to access to the insurance that underwrites care and types of benefits. Typically, families have not been faced with the full impact of the costs of care during childhood and may not anticipate the limitations in the adult setting. The young person with a chronic condition transitioning to adult care may not have the educational capacities to move to a tertiary education setting that would allow for extended insurance coverage until age 25 years. His or her functioning may, however, not be impaired enough to qualify for social benefits. The adult care provider can expect to be recruited to provide assistance in obtaining access to needed services.

Legal responsibility for healthcare. Responsibility for healthcare must also be addressed. In modern North American society, maximum autonomy as an adult is a civil right that is governed by law. The challenges of transition can be framed in terms of the following three broad independent-function outcomes of chronic disease in childhood: the need for legal guarantees for the individual, full responsibility for self, and conservatorship or guardianship.

Beyond age 18 years, the law presumes that the responsibility for self with respect to societal obligations belongs to the individual. If the individual cannot fulfill this responsibility, specific safeguards are required to protect the individual's civil rights. Evaluation is required for guardianship (full decision-making capacity by others) or conservatorship (e.g., limited decision-making capacity by others for financial affairs, healthcare). The adult care team cannot treat a patient who lacks the capacity to make medically relevant decisions on their own behalf without such legal safeguards in place. The fact that autonomy holds such a central place in civil rights, however, means that the requirements for guardianship or conservatorship are stringent. Not all individuals who are limited in managing their own affairs will fulfill the requirements; they will be considered as competent to manage their affairs and treated accordingly. This will require additional education and support from the adult care team through participation in ongoing healthcare with respect to decisions, regimens, procedures, and follow-up. Parents and family members may also need help and support in recognizing that they are no longer "in charge" and, indeed, cannot even be present without the patient's consent and/or formal legal conservatorship/guardianship.

The shift in responsibility for healthcare and the safeguards that protect the individual's rights and permit delivery of needed healthcare occurs at age 18 years. The necessary decisions, procedures, and documentation cannot, however, wait until the individual's eighteenth birthday. Planning for the transition from developmental care to adult healthcare must begin early, ideally with the onset of puberty and adolescence. Promoting this planning is an important role of the child's clinical team and for which the developmental neuropsychologist has a significant role.

The patient–provider relationship. Central to transition is the move from one system of care to another, from developmental healthcare to adult medicine. Each system has its own philosophy, focus, tools, attitudes, and ways of relating among participants. In adult settings, the core framework has traditionally been condition-centered (symptoms, diagnosis, treatment strategies). The primary relationship is typically between the physician (clinician) and the patient. The assumption is that individuals who seek treatment have both a "good-enough" capacity and a willingness to take responsibility for their own healthcare. Psychologically, the adult is presumed to speak for him- or herself. Where children are concerned, parents or caregivers have been the primary decision maker for healthcare. This has two potential consequences: (1) the young adult may not have learned to speak for him- or herself and (2) parents or the caregiver may have difficulty providing opportunities for the young person to take on this responsibility. In the case of adolescents and young adults with neuropsychological limitations in the context of chronic conditions, specific training and practice in this regard is beneficial.

Developmental implications. At the time of transition, an individual's set of competencies is the outcome of developmental experiences shaped by the condition itself and the resources that have been provided to optimize development. However, the individual's neurobehavioral development is incomplete. As he or she assumes the responsibilities of adulthood, the emerging adult is actively engaging in critical developmental tasks of social development and integration, whose mastery may be subject to ongoing challenge.

Developmentally, the dependence-to-autonomy progression from childhood to adolescence to adulthood entails taking responsibility for self as an adult in all relevant societal arenas. This means being able to manage a range of adaptive functional skills needed for daily living, of academic skills relevant for vocational choices, and of self-efficacy skills needed to navigate the social world including the healthcare arena. Successful functioning in all of these is dependent on the achievement of "good-enough" social competencies, executive skills, and regulatory capacities. The adult healthcare team cannot assume these for the individual with a chronic condition. The team needs to deliberately adopt an alternative mindset. As a general rule, the following is likely to be the case: the developmental foundations for behavior have been laid under adverse biological conditions; development trajectories have been derailed across the board and can be expected to interact in nonstandard ways; and the usual expectations for behavior in a person of this age cannot be presumed. Observed behavior may have an atypical neural infrastructure and be relatively inefficient, or fragile, or both, in the face of additional demands—such as the need to understand explanations, follow instructions, track schedules, or remember dosing regimens. The team will need to appreciate that atypical developmental trajectories do not make a person "immature" or "limited" and that individuals likely will react negatively to being treated as such. Atypical trajectories of development may make one inefficient, inflexible, or vulnerable to overload in the face of (ordinary) demands. They may make it difficult for an individual to interact in an accepted fashion, follow conversations, provide a coherent history, describe symptoms effectively, understand explanations and instructions, or remember medications, regimens, and schedules. They may constrain the development of age-expected judgment and insight. All of these limitations can be expected to require a change in the professional behavior and strategies of the clinical team. Of particular concern in this regard is the adolescent or young adult's resistance to complying with instructions and adhering to necessary regimens. This reflects a collision between developmental imperatives for autonomy and what is all too quickly perceived as an authoritarian and controlling stance of the medical establishment that triggers resistance (Drotar, 2000).

Psychological Implications. The core assumption of adult healthcare in the (young) adult, namely that of the individual speaking for self, cannot be made. The members of the adult care team must determine on an individual basis whether this is the case or whether the experience of the health condition has limited the young person's ability to "speak effectively" for self secondary to constraints on the development of expected competencies in understanding, judgment, insight, or executive processing. Limitations on the acquisition of such skills over time can be expected to be significant predictors of adaptive functioning and independence.

Basic principles for the adult care team include the following:

- Don't make assumptions: ask more questions about what the patient understands; find out whether he or she can follow through on treatment regimens (e.g., limitations on memory, sequencing).

- Expect to spend additional time/plan accordingly: more explanation and education will be needed to address neuropsychological limitations on understanding and judgment.
- Develop collaborations: integrate behavioral health specialists into the medical team to aid in the management of behavioral and emotional factors that have the potential to undermine optimal medical care; encourage the patient and family to be members of the team.
- Explore and implement specific adaptations in care (tools): patients may require adapted information resources tailored to their needs (materials at appropriate reading levels, pamphlets and videos matched to the realities of their condition); explicit step-by-step directions and applied teaching of procedures and regimens; and integration of technology to support memory and organizational deficits.
- Recognize and respect the family's history and experiences to date: resist first impressions; allow for initial encounters in which individuals seem demanding, intrusive, and opinionated.

THE NEUROPSYCHOLOGIST'S ROLE IN DEVELOPMENTAL CARE

In both developmental and adult healthcare settings, the neuropsychologist's major contribution is to integrate knowledge of principles of brain–behavior development via his or her central role in neurobehavioral assessment, consultation, and case management. The neuropsychologist makes a specific contribution to ongoing clinical management by educating the child, adolescent, or young adult; family members; and the care team about the neuropsychological underpinnings of behavior in general and the unique behavioral profile of this particular young person.

In the developmental setting, the neuropsychologist is concerned with outcomes. The child's current "package" of skills and compromises is an outcome of the child's developmental course, and the neuropsychologist acts to promote optimal future outcomes, given the expected impact of the condition on subsequent developmental mastery. In an evaluation, the neuropsychologist makes a judgment about the potential integrity of the development course prior to the onset of the insult and considers the impact of premorbid temperament and neuropsychological status/deficits on the child's developmental trajectory. The neuropsychologist will evaluate how these factors may interact with the changed behavioral outcomes secondary to the insult in terms of both ongoing development and more acute recovery. She or he will then determine the child's profile of strengths and compromises in physical capacities (sensory, motor processing), regulatory capacities (arousal, attention, executive processing), and knowledge acquisition (learning, memory, thinking) and relate the patterns of performance to both the developmental course of the new condition and its impact on ongoing development. The outcome of the neuropsychological assessment is thus a comprehensive analysis of developmental, neuropsychological, and psychosocial variables that forms the basis for effective case management and success working with the family and care team around upcoming developmental challenges.

Developmental challenges involve the full range of daily living, vocational, and social demands experienced by all individuals. The neuropsychologist is part of the team that provides education and support around life skills programming, including independent living (self-care and grooming, nutrition, household chores and management, basic financial management skills), development of a social self (social relationships and networks, intimate relationships, sexuality), self in the community (access and use of community based services, academic skills needed to support vocational choices and workplace expectations) (Rey-Casserly & Bernstein, 2008). The degree to which education and/or support is needed in each of these broad domains varies considerably, but all should be considered. It is, for example, not infrequently the case that a family and/or child is focused on performance and services in the educational setting and will fail to understand that the child is not able to look after him- or herself independently with respect to self-care and grooming, interact successfully with other children, or regulate behavior or emotion as expected for age. In all settings, education and support to address issues of self-advocacy and ability to access assistance, awareness of physical limitations that constrain mobility and navigation, and awareness of mental limitations (such as reduced judgment or insight, understanding of safety issues) are needed and will be critical in helping the individual understand the social, regulatory, and legal systems that operate in the adult world.

There are two major areas in which the developmental neuropsychologist is particularly important, and both of these have notable implications for the adult health-care team. First, the developmental task of moving from dependence to autonomy will involve education of both parents and child. The findings of the most current neuropsychological assessment are valuable in shaping the discussion, but the primary emphasis will be on development and developmental outcomes, that is, the child's or adolescent's mastery of critical age-expected capacities across behavioral domains. Central to this will be facilitating an understanding by the parents of the child's developmental needs and what is to be expected as the child gets older. A particular focus is on helping parents to not put their parenting "on hold" for extended periods in which critical development goals must be met. This is education that will be revisited repeatedly throughout childhood and adolescence as the child matures and must tackle each new developmental challenge. As the child moves into adolescence, parents will need information about issues of competency and limitations thereof, as well as the associated needs for guardianship or conservatorship in due course. These are often difficult conversations that need to be revisited regularly throughout adolescence, and parents need support to address the many psychological issues that may be raised. Ideally, this education should be initiated with the entire care team so that everyone is prepared for the transition to responsibility for self at age 18 years. The neuropsychologist's work with the young person and the parents has a primary aim of education about the individual's neuropsychological profile of strengths and limitations and its impact on achievement of life goals. Discussion should include the individual's capacity for autonomy and independence, the degree to which she or he has a realistic understanding of her or his situation (medically, behaviorally, emotionally), the extent of self-knowledge and ability to reflect on goals and aspirations, and the capacity for self-control and personal efficacy, all of which are critical elements in exploring post-adolescence life and living options, identifying needed resources and services, and making relevant choices. These conversations can be difficult. Young people may resist guidance, want to act like others, and lack insight to appreciate their limited options. Sensitivity, respect, and patience by clinical professionals should help young people facing difficult decisions, and discussions must be revisited regularly as part of ongoing care and management.

The second responsibility of the neuropsychologist in the developmental setting is to be the necessary liaison with the education system. School is a child's "job" at which she or he spends multiple hours per day, and adequate neuropsychological functioning is as important in this setting as in places of adult employment. Professional services include diagnosis and management (e.g., recommendations for educational placement, instructional programming, behavior management, social skills support), as well as consultation, psychoeducation, and counseling.

In a pediatric setting, cognitive ability (IQ) tests have a different role than in adult practice. They facilitate access to educational and social services and are necessary to document developmental disabilities and obtain educational services and/or placement, as well as social services and entitlements. However, they are often poorly understood, and education is often needed about the nature and impact of neuropsychological deficits on daily functioning and their relationship to psychological test scores and profiles, an educational role that is uniquely that of the neuropsychologist. There are two primary messages in this regard. The first pertains to the issue of IQ scores and what they measure. Assumptions about IQ scores go in two directions: low IQ scores mean that one is limited in all situations (not necessarily the case); higher IQ scores mean that one is fully intact in all situations (also not the case). Both of these outcomes can be instantiated in individuals with NDD or AcqD. Lowered IQ scores may be an index of significant compromise with respect to everyday functional capacities, justifying a range of services and/or accommodations. However, many individuals maintain IQ scores in an age-expected or higher range in the presence of significant brain injury or compromise. The latter may have a well-developed vocabulary and be quite articulate in conversation but be incapable of independent daily functioning or unable to follow instructions from a physician or other care team member. Even relatively mild insult can result in neuropsychological deficit that has significant ramifications with respect to judgment, insight, inhibitory control, and self-management. For this group of individuals, the major limiting factors are typically those of judgment, insight, and self-control.

Individuals with compromised intellectual capacities due to altered brain development trajectories may be significantly challenged with respect to independent functioning yet able to learn many skills that make them more effective users of the healthcare system. They may demonstrate many basic functional capacities, have access to basic social language, and be good experiential learners able to retain new information where the relevance of the information or instructions to them is explained at a level commensurate with their understanding and when the information load is within their range. However, they may not easily manage more arbitrary and abstract relationships that have no concrete real-world referents and are not supported by structure. The typical problem is an inability to adapt flexibly to novel or changing situations and demands, resulting from disordered attention and insecure or minimally available executive processes as needed for initiating and switching, integrating elements, generalizing concepts, generating problem-solving strategies, and/or controlling information (planning, sequencing, prioritizing, multitasking). The impact on even ordinary events is that of rapid overload; the individual is overwhelmed and stops listening or reacts negatively. Either response can undermine the provider-patient relationship and set up negative expectations. The neuropsychologist plays a major role both in educating the care team and in supporting both patient and team in the face of the mismatch between the patient's presentation and his or her actual competence.

The neuropsychologist may also need to clarify for parents and the healthcare team the source of behaviors that appear "psychological." The individual described as having problems of "motivation," "initiative," "attitude," or "emotional control" may not be demonstrating behaviors that are purely (or even mostly) psychological; these problems may be manifestations of the direct effects of neuropsychological deficit and must be managed accordingly. Therapeutic interventions to address maladaptive behaviors need to be carefully designed to take into account the impact of both neuropsychological deficits and psychological reactions in the observed behavioral failures. For both NDD and AcqD, these clinical decisions must also consider family risk factors for psychiatric conditions and/or the patient's pre-injury temperament/personality status, psychiatric risk, and coping resources. Appreciation of the above can be challenging for the adult care team but can affect the way the team structures and reinforces the provision of healthcare.

THE NEUROPSYCHOLOGIST'S ROLE IN THE ADULT HEALTHCARE SETTING

The primary roles of the neuropsychologist include the management of an individual with a chronic medical condition and education of the individual, involved family members, and medical care team. This is as true of the neuropsychologist's role during the individual's childhood and adolescence as for the transition to the adult healthcare system. In working with the team, the neuropsychologist can help the physician and/or medical team understand how to support the patient (e.g., medical instructions); consult in the development of specific tools or equipment and adaptation of educational materials; and/or educate the team about different components of effective functioning—experiential learning for everyday adaptive skills, acquisition and manipulation of knowledge, regulatory and executive capacities for managing behavior—and their implications for the delivery of healthcare.

In working with the individual, the focus of support is to achieve a better understanding of the roles and responsibilities of personal healthcare in a new system and in the context of a realistic appraisal of the help required by the individual. The range of support for individuals includes the following:

- Education about what the individual must do to meet expectations of the healthcare system.
- Identification of strengths and weaknesses as a basis for developing strategies and/or accommodations to meet specific demands.
- Direct instruction, coaching, and supervision with practice and role-playing in the roles and responsibilities of adulthood with respect to medical care, including such basics as how to talk to clinicians, how to remember and describe symptoms, and timeliness for appointments.
- Preparation for the use of technological aids for making appointments, organizing schedules, tracking medications, and providing reminders.
- Identification of psychological barriers to following through on appointments and treatment strategies.
- Introduction of behavioral strategies for managing anxiety and maximizing coping resources.
- Identification of resources (e.g., community, governmental) to help navigate the requirements of modern healthcare service delivery and social services.

In working with family members, the focus of support is that of validation of what has been an unusual and intense relationship with their child and the clinical team over many years, in the context of a need for everyone to "move on" developmentally to the extent possible. All individuals have a right to autonomy. The primary caretakers of individuals with chronic conditions, usually the parents, may be fully in agreement with this principle. However, they may need major support in "letting go" to allow their child to progress to the next phase of life. Parents are also entitled to progress to the next stage of their own development and may need support to accept and accomplish this.

Letting go typically means that a child moves out of the parental home. This may come about in different forms depending on the young person's skills and needs; the move may be to a college setting, to another independent living situation, or to a supervised group setting. The clinician needs to respect the fact that for some families, letting go is not an option; they have legal guardianship, and the young person lives at home or their family and/or social values require long-term caretaking for disadvantaged family members.

In all contexts and interactions, the important themes to address, and regularly reinforce, include the followng:

- Recognition of the critical role of primary caretakers in the individual's development over a long time; recognition of the loss of a closely bonded developmental care team.
- Recognition and discussion of the caretakers' ongoing developmental needs.
- Support of primary caretakers around the (necessary) changes in their caretaking role and the loss of a social role they have maintained for a long time.
- Realistic appraisal of the individual's need for parental support and of parents' ability to provide different levels of care and support, as well as identification of strategies for letting go.
- Reassurance that resources to support the individual are in place and effective.
- Recognition of the need for legal safeguards with respect to healthcare, demise of primary caretakers, and/or changes in neuropsychological status.

CONCLUSION

The role of the neuropsychologist goes well beyond the needs of the healthcare system alone. All the principles described above will be necessary for education and case management with respect to the integration of individuals with a history of chronic conditions who will enter higher education and vocational settings and access community networks and services. With detailed knowledge of developmental trajectories, brain–behavior relationships, and social contexts and systems, the neuropsychologist is ideally equipped to provide a critical service in promoting the optimal integration of individuals into these wider life opportunities.

REFERENCES

Barker, D. J. P. (2001). Fetal and infant origins of adult disease. *Monatsschrift Kinderheilkunde, 149*, S2–S6. doi: 10.1007/s001120170002

Bauer, A. M., & Boyce, W. T. (2004). Prophecies of childhood: How children's social environments and biological propensities affect the health of populations. *International Journal of Behavioral Medicine, 11*, 164–175. doi: 10.1207/s15327558ijbm1103_5

Blakemore, S. J. (2008). The social brain in adolescence. *Nature Reviews Neuroscience, 9*, 267–277. doi: nrn2353 [pii] 10.1038/nrn2353

Committee on Psychosocial Aspects of Child and Family Health, Committee on Early Childhood Adoption Dependent Care, Section on Developmental Behavioral Pediatrics, Garner, A. S., Shonkoff, J. P., Siegel, B. S.,... Wood, D. L. (2012). Early childhood adversity, toxic stress, and the role of the pediatrician: Translating developmental science into lifelong health. *Pediatrics, 129*, e224–e231. doi: 10.1542/peds.2011-2662

Cooley, W. C., & Sagerman, P. J. (2011). Supporting the health care transition from adolescence to adulthood in the medical home. *Pediatrics, 128*, 182–200. doi: 10.1542/peds.2011-0969

Crouse, N. R., Dahiya, S., & Gutmann, D. H. (2011). Rethinking pediatric gliomas as developmental brain abnormalities. *Current Topics in Developmental Biology, 94*, 283–308. doi: B978-0-12-380916-2.00009-7 [pii] 10.1016/B978-0-12-380916-2.00009-7

Dennis, M. (2011). *Age, plasticity and the immature brain: Historical and current ideas.* Paper presented at the American Psychological Association Annual Convention, Washington, DC.

Dennis, M., & Barnes, M. A. (2010). The cognitive phenotype of spina bifida meningomyelocele. *Developmental Disabilities Research Reviews, 16*, 31–39. doi: 10.1002/ddrr.89

Drotar, D. (Ed.). (2000). *Promoting adherence to medical treatment in chronic childhood Illness. Concepts, methods, and interventions.* Hillsdale, NJ: Lawrence Erlbaum Associates.

Duke, N. N., & Scal, P. B. (2011). Adult care transitioning for adolescents with special health care needs: A pivotal role for family centered care. *Maternal and Child Health Journal, 15*, 98–105. doi: 10.1007/s10995-009-0547-1

Ferriero, D. M. (2004). Neonatal brain injury. *The New England Journal of Medicine, 351*, 1985–1995.

Fox, S. E., Levitt, P., & Nelson, C. A. I. (2010). How the timing and quality of early experiences influence the development of brain architecture. *Child Development, 81*, 28–40. doi: 10.1111/j.1467-8624.2009.01380.x

Hochstein, M., Halfon, N., & Inkelas, M. (1998). Creating systems of developmental health care for children. *Journal of Urban Health: Bulletin of the New York Academy of Medicine, 75*, 751–771. doi: 10.1007/BF02344505

Iuvone, L., Mariotti, P., Colosimo, C., Guzzetta, F., Ruggiero, A., & Riccardi, R. (2002). Long-term cognitive outcome, brain computed tomography scan, and magnetic resonance imaging in children cured for acute lymphoblastic leukemia. *Cancer, 95*, 2562–2570. doi: 10.1002/cncr.10999

Johnston, M. V. (2009). Plasticity in the developing brain: Implications for rehabilitation. *Developmental Disabilities Research Reviews, 15*, 94–101. doi: 10.1002/ddrr.64

Juranek, J., Fletcher, J. M., Hasan, K. M., Breier, J. I., Cirino, P. T., Pazo-Alvarez, P.,... Papanicolaou, A. C. (2008). Neocortical reorganization in spina bifida. *Neuroimage, 40*, 1516–1522. doi: S1053-8119(08)00103-1 [pii] 10.1016/j.neuroimage.2008.01.043

Kuhlthau, K. A., Bloom, S., Van Cleave, J., Knapp, A. A., Romm, D., Klatka, K.,... Perrin, J. M. (2011). Evidence for family-centered care for children with special health care needs: A systematic review. *Academic Pediatrics, 11*, 136–143. doi: 10.1016/j.acap.2010.12.014

Lesnik, P. G., Ciesielski, K. T., Hart, B. L., Benzel, E. C., & Sanders, J. A. (1998). Evidence for cerebellar-frontal subsystem changes in children treated with intrathecal chemotherapy for leukemia: Enhanced data analysis using an effect size model. *Archive of Neurology, 55*, 1561–1568.

McManus, B. M., Carle, A., Acevedo-Garcia, D., Ganz, M., Hauser-Cram, P., & McCormick, M. (2011). Modeling the social determinants of caregiver burden among families of children with developmental disabilities. *American Journal on Intellectual and Developmental Disabilities, 116*, 246–260. doi: 10.1352/1944-7558-116.3.246

Park, D. C., & Reuter-Lorenz, P. (2009). The adaptive brain: Aging and neurocognitive scaffolding. *Annual Review of Psychology, 60*, 173–196. doi: 10.1146/annurev.psych.59.103006.093656

Perrin, J. M., Bloom, S. R., & Gortmaker, S. L. (2007). The increase of childhood chronic conditions in the United States. *Journal of the American Medical Association, 297*, 2755–2759. doi: 297/24/2755 [pii] 10.1001/jama.297.24.2755

Pledger, C. (2003). Discourse on disability and rehabilitation issues. Opportunities for psychology. *American Psychologist, 58*, 279–284.

Rey-Casserly, C., & Bernstein, J. H. (2008). Making the transition to adulthood for individuals with learning disorders. In L. E. Wolf, H. E. Schreiber, & J. Wasserstein (Eds.), *Adult learning disorders: Contemporary issues* (pp. 363–388). New York: Psychology Press.

Rey-Casserly, C., & Meadows, M. E. (2008). Developmental perspectives on optimizing educational and vocational outcomes in child and adult survivors of cancer. *Developmental Disabilities Research Reviews, 14*, 243–250. doi: 10.1002/ddrr.31

Schwartz, L. A., Tuchman, L. K., Hobbie, W. L., & Ginsberg, J. P. (2011). A social-ecological model of readiness for transition to adult-oriented care for adolescents and young adults with chronic health conditions. *Child: Care, Health and Development, 37*, 883–895. doi: 10.1111/j.1365-2214.2011.01282.x

Shonkoff, J. P. (2010). Building a new biodevelopmental framework to guide the future of early childhood policy. *Child Development, 81*, 357–367. doi: 10.1111/j.1467-8624.2009.01399.x

Stein, R. E. (1998). Children with chronic conditions in the 21st century. *Journal of Urban Health, 75*, 732–738. doi: 10.1007/BF02344503

Watson, R., Parr, J. R., Joyce, C., May, C., & Le Couteur, A. S. (2011). Models of transitional care for young people with complex health needs: A scoping review. *Child: Care, Health and Development, 37*, 780–791. doi: 10.1111/j.1365-2214.2011.01293.x

20 Modeling Cognitive Aging Following Early Central Nervous System Injury

Reserve and the Flynn Fffect

M. Douglas Ris and Merrill Hiscock

Developmental factors as they relate to brain disease and injury have long been the essence of pediatric neuropsychological practice. It is also well established that age as a proxy for brain development is an important moderator of the effects of brain insults. Indeed, "plasticity" as a hypothetical construct encompasses the differential effects of brain injury at different stages of development (Johnson, 2009). Yet, how brain development interacts with injury over the lifespan has received considerably less attention by neuropsychologists than is deserved. What may be easily overlooked, especially when working with a population of a confined age, is that there is no point in time when the brain reaches stasis. A fundamental principle is that neurodevelopment is a dynamic process that continues throughout the lifespan, and thus developmental factors always need to be considered. Even in later life, development is likely to be affected by events during the formative years. For this reason, the perspective of the pediatric/child neuropsychologist must extend beyond childhood and adolescence. Likewise, the perspective of the adult neuropsychologist must expand to consider possibly relevant events that occurred at an early age. A truly "lifespan development" perspective is necessary. In 2000, Dennis, Spiegler, and Hetherington wrote, "The new millennium presents the challenge of understanding CNS insult across the lifespan" (p.104). As we progress into the second decade of the millennium, that challenge is even more pressing.

Two questions that naturally arise relative to the content of this volume are: (1) What happens to the various populations of children represented in this volume during the adult years, particularly as they face physical and neurocognitive changes of later adulthood? And, (2) What is different about these children's development and aging compared with those who have been spared significant brain disease or injury in childhood? The ultimate goals of outcomes research are to increase understanding about how to avert or mitigate ill effects, promote optimal growth and function, and, in the process, learn more about the course of development across the lifespan. In this chapter, we attempt to address two major concepts that, we argue, have strong relevance for research of this nature. The first involves hypothetical constructs of increasing popularity—biological reserve (BR) and cognitive reserve (CR) capacity (hereafter referred to collectively as reserve)—as significant explanatory factors in "outcome" following neuropathological changes in the brain. The second, the Flynn effect, explores vexing methodological and inferential challenges to cross-sectional and longitudinal research on cognitive development where cohort effects are likely. Increased appreciation of these constructs will promote this lifespan development agenda.

NORMAL AND ABNORMAL AGING

Microscopic changes are found in the brains of individuals as they age. Whereas early reports were of profound neuronal loss, more recent research indicates that there are more subtle and selective changes in the absence of age-associated diseases, for example, in dendritic branching. The hippocampus and prefrontal cortex appear to be brain regions most at risk (Burke & Barnes, 2006). Raz et al. (2007) reported that association cortex, neostriatum, and cerebellum show age-related effects, while primary visual cortex and entorhinal cortex are relatively spared until very late in life.

How these changes correlate with cognitive changes is only partially understood. For example, Head et al. (2002) found that prefrontal volume loss predicted performance on measures of executive function during early (but not late) skill acquisition. Genetic polymorphisms as predictors of rate of cognitive decline is also an area of active research and likely to yield new insights into the mechanisms of cognitive aging. However, early results suggest complex relationships (Raz, Rodrigue, Kennedy, & Land, 2009).

The term "cognitive aging" has come to refer to the relationship between adult age and cognitive functioning (Salthouse, 2010). There is now a wealth of data demonstrating changes in cognitive functioning over time, but cross-sectional studies and longitudinal studies tell a somewhat different story. These studies indicate stability in some functions and decline in others, but the degree and pattern of decline is not wholly consistent across research methodologies. In cross-sectional analyses, a distinct pattern has been replicated so many times that Salthouse has referred to this as the prototypical aging profile. Across measures of intelligence and neuropsychological tests, there is consistent evidence for stability or even gains well into advanced age in such functions as vocabulary and general information, while measures of processing speed and efficiency start to show declines as early as the fourth decade of life. Rather than a decline in multiple abilities, Salthouse interprets these declines across multiple measures as rooted in a few fundamental capacities (fluid ability, working memory, visual memory) that bear the strongest relationships to a higher-order factor (Salthouse, 2009).

Longitudinal studies, on the other hand, sometimes demonstrate increased scores over time on measures that show declines in cross-sectional studies. Contradictory findings are usually attributed to cohort effects, which are a major confounding potential in cross-sectional studies (to be taken up later in this chapter). Schaie et al. (2004) provide evidence from the Seattle Longitudinal Study (SLS) of significant cohort effects that vary considerably across different functions. Inductive reasoning, verbal meaning, and spatial orientation show positive shifts across birth cohorts spanning the end of the 19th century to the early 1970s. However, number skills have decreased since the 1924 cohort. The effect of this on cross-sectional studies would be to underestimate changes associated with aging in the former domains and overestimate aging effects in number skills. The SLS has identified factors that decrease the risk for age-related decline, including health, environment and stimulation, flexible personality style, high cognitive status of spouse, and maintained high levels of perceptual processing speed. These longitudinal test data have also been found to predict dementia 7–14 years before the diagnosis is made.

Age-associated diseases such as Alzheimer's (AD) are characterized by early and advanced neuropathological changes in the brain with preclinical states up to 20–30 years prior to clinical manifestations of dementia (Small, Kepe, & Barrio, 2006). These neuropathological changes include increased neurofibrillary tangle density, widely distributed and diffuse neuritic plaques, and amyloid body deposits that cause neuronal loss and associated cognitive decline. Even in the absence of clinical dementia, cognitive abilities may show an abnormal course over time that has been termed "accelerated" or "exacerbated" cognitive aging. Risk for such abnormal trajectories has been the subject of conjectures collectively referred to here as "reserve theories."

RESERVE THEORIES

Margin of Safety and Redundancy Models

The "margin of safety" model states that there is an inherent redundancy in the nervous system such that tissue can be lost without apparent consequences (Corkin et al., 1989; Teuber, 1974). However, with decreased redundancy resulting from injury or aging, there can be the appearance of a new deficit or exacerbation of an existing one. Corkin et al. (1989) found support for this in a longitudinal study of World War II veterans suffering penetrating head and peripheral nerve injuries in which the former showed "exacerbated" decline several decades later. Drawing from probability theory and reliability engineering, Glassman (1987) asserted that the human brain may be far larger than it needs to be for short-term survival. Throughout the lifespan, he argued, redundancy and flexibility in simpler behavioral functions decrease in favor of more complex and differentiated functions.

Brain Reserve Capacity

There is mounting evidence that children who suffer brain insults may be susceptible to late-emerging sequelae, much like post-polio syndrome where the loss of lower motor neurons that occurs with normal aging produces new symptoms later in life. Such observations have resulted in increased interest in the aging of populations that have suffered an early insult to the brain, spawning such theoretical formulations as brain reserve capacity (Satz, 1993) and cognitive reserve capacity (Stern, 2002). BR, similar to earlier "margin of safety" and "threshold" concepts,

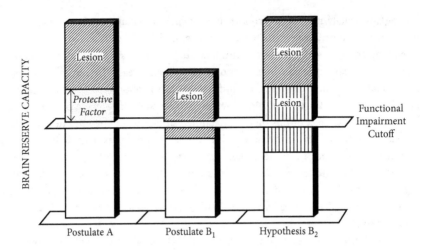

BRAIN RESERVE CAPACITY

Postulate A   Postulate B₁   Hypothesis B₂

FIGURE 20.1

Brain Reserve Capacity. From Satz, (1993). Copyright 1993 by the American Psychological Association Inc.

is based in evidence of redundancy in the central nervous system such that functioning is preserved until a critical threshold of "damage" is reached. Figure 20.1 illustrates how an individual with high BR (postulate A) would be protected as compared to an individual with low BR (postulate B₁) against the effects of comparable lesions. As expressed by Dennis, Spiegler, and Hetherington (2000), prior injury "reduces the options for biological plasticity" (p.103). Biological reserve is typically inferred through anatomic or histologic characteristics of the brain, such as volume, synaptic count, and dendritic elaboration as well as by distal biomarkers, such as head circumference.

Cognitive Reserve Capacity

CR capacity (Stern, 2002) represents an extension of this theory by taking into account cognitive factors that impart protection or vulnerability. CR is typically estimated by measures reflecting accumulated experience, such as socioeconomic status, intelligence quotient (IQ), and years of education. Parent IQ has been used as a proxy for a child's reserve.

Although ultimately CR has a physiological basis, the difference between BR and CR is in the level of analysis. Hence, CR is related to processing efficiency rather than anatomical differences in the brain substrate. This would lead to the prediction that, due to more limited BR (a "hardware" factor) and CR (a "software" factor), individuals sustaining brain injury early in life (therefore having lower reserve) would be vulnerable to increased age-related decline in neuropsychological functioning (corresponding to the "double hit" scenario depicted in Figure 20.1).Evidence supporting theories of BR and CR comes from literature on multi-infarct dementia where more pronounced deficits are seen in patients with a prior history of traumatic brain injury (TBI) (Roth, 1986), as well as studies of age-related decline in memory following traumatic brain injury (Klein, Houx, Jolles, 1996), dementia in Parkinson's disease (Quinn et al., 1986) and acquired immune deficiency syndrome (Nowak et al., 1991).

Reserve has been invoked to explain differential risk of dementia, such as AD, and both age of onset and rate of decline in dementia. In other words, high reserve (HR) in contrast to low reserve (LR) individuals are reported to have lower rates and later age of onset of dementia but faster decline once a clinical diagnosis is reached (Wilson et al., 2004). This is because patients with higher CR sustain greater burden of AD neuropathology for any level of symptomatology. When this neuropathology becomes too advanced, there is no longer sufficient substrate for CR to function. Thus, there is precipitous system collapse in the case of HR compared with an earlier, more gradual decline in LR individuals. Consistent with this, Hall et al. (2007) report that high education was protective in the sense of delaying the onset of memory decline. However, with the approach of incident dementia, the rate of memory decline increased for each year of formal education. These findings were not anticipated by all reserve theorists. For example, according to Dennis, Spiegler, and Hetherington (2000), "Deficits emerge when reserve is depleted, so that markers of cognitive reserve such as larger brain size and high premorbid intelligence are associated with later onset and *slower* (italics added) decline in adult dementia" (p.103).

How do we understand what appears to be different patterns of decline in HR and LR individuals confronting age-related disease like AD in contrast to typical aging? The science of complex systems, which has only recently begun to address functionally interdependent networks, may provide some insights (Buldyrev et al., 2010). Based on mathematical modeling, single networks were found to be more robust when network nodes were more distributed. In the case of interdependent networks, however, broader distribution increased risk of failure. The Sandpile Model, first introduced by Bak et al. in 1987, is often used in the study of cascades and was used by Brummitt, D'Souza, and Leicht (2012) to study "catastrophic cascades" in interdependent systems, such as power grids. They found that there was an optimal degree of interconnectivity that would mitigate the largest avalanches by diverting load to neighboring networks. Too much interconnectivity, though, can increase the risk of large cascades. Extrapolating from this, we could consider CR as based in interconnected networks, with those that are more highly interconnected (i.e., HR) being subject to larger catastrophic failures as "load" increases or as the infrastructure (neural substrate) decays. Therefore, with the increase in robustness of redundant systems, as proposed by Glassman (1987) and others, comes a risk of more precipitous and complete collapse of the system. HR, therefore, imparts both protection and vulnerability.

Differential risk for AD was substantiated in a meta-analysis by Valenzuela and Sachdev (2006) of more than 20 studies involving more than 29,000 individuals where there was a 46% lower risk for dementia in HR individuals. In typical aging, as well, LR individuals (by virtue of deficient education or previous injury) appear to show accelerated or exacerbated cognitive aging. Indeed, there is evidence that low education portends greater functional decline with age (Snowdon et al., 1989), although recent findings from the Victoria Longitudinal Study (Zahodne et al., 2011) challenge this conclusion on methodological grounds (see below).

Raymont et al. (2008) provide some of the strongest evidence for both accelerated cognitive decline and the buffering effects of CR. They studied 199 participants in the Vietnam Head Injury Study who took part in phase 3 of the study. Performance on the American Forces Qualification Test AFQT, a test developed by the US Department of Defense and given at induction to measure a wide range of cognitive abilities, was compared pre-injury, 12–15 years post-injury, and more than 30 years post-injury.

Survivors of penetrating head injuries who tested high initially tended to have higher scores post-injury. Compared to healthy controls, the head injury group also tended to show greater declines in scores with increased age.

Ambiguity in what is meant by "accelerated cognitive aging" contributes to the inconsistency and confusion in this literature. On the one hand, it could be taken to mean a negatively accelerating curve, as may be the case in high reserve AD patients (Wilson et al., 2004). On the other hand, accelerated cognitive aging may refer to earlier onset and higher frequency of dementia, as reported in individuals with Down syndrome (Ward, 2004). Finally, "acceleration" may be seen in the form of divergent curves for HR and LR individuals, with the latter declining faster with age than the former (Richards et al., 2004). These are not alternative ways of describing the same phenomenon and have implications for how cognitive aging is conceptualized in the context of age-related diseases and prior brain injury. As noted earlier, depending upon the sense in which the term is used, HR may be either a protective factor (for onset of dementia) or a risk factor (for rate of decline).

Elaborations on Cognitive Reserve Capacity

Stern (2009) describes BR as "passive" with an inherent fixed "threshold" beyond which functional impairment will occur for everyone. This is in contrast to "active" models of CR that do not assume such a threshold. Still, Stern implies at least a "soft" threshold or "inflection point" that assumes a discontinuous relationship between the underlying pathology and its behavioral manifestations (see pp. 2016–2017) as conveyed in his statement, "Although two patients might have the same amount of brain reserve capacity, the patient with more CR (cognitive reserve) may tolerate a larger lesion than the other patient before clinical impairment is apparent." We will return to the notion of thresholds later in this chapter.

Stern (2003) makes a distinction between CR and "compensation" in the context of brain damage whereby performance is maximized by "using brain structures or networks not engaged when the brain is not damaged" (p. 590). Although theoretically distinguishable, Stern acknowledges that differentiating CR from compensation can be methodologically challenging.

Later (Stern, 2009), CR is defined as being comprised of "neural reserve," which is individual variability in brain and cognitive networks that modulate one's ability to cope with brain pathology, and "neural compensation," which is individual variability in the utilization of brain structures or networks not normally used by individuals with intact brains. As with CR, there are individual differences in compensation, and those with greater CR also tend to have more ability to compensate.

Is CR a unitary or multidimensional construct? In other words, does CR moderate the effects of brain injury in a fairly uniform way across various cognitive functions, or does it have a differential effect? Are some indices of reserve better than others? In a paper published posthumously, Satz et al. (2011) observed that there is a lack of evidence for purported indicators of reserve, and they are critical of the assumption that multiple indicators can serve interchangeably to estimate the hypothetical construct of reserve. The paucity of research addressing construct validity "... weakens the interpretability of specific indicator variables (e.g., education, brain size) hypothesized to represent the construct as well as the predicted/

moderated outcomes" (p. 123). Satz and colleagues propose two models whereby BR and CR form either a single factor (one-factor model) or two separate factors (two-factor model), in addition to a third model in which CR alone consists of four factors (executive function, processing resources, complex mental activity, and "g/intelligence").

Risk and Reserve

Dennis and colleagues (2006) place the concepts of BR and CR into a developmental context by focusing on disorders familiar to pediatric neuropsychologists. They note that "pathological burden" or "load" can be imparted by injury (TBI), treatment (chemotherapy, radiotherapy), or genetic heterogeneity (Down syndrome). Hebb's (1942) principle that fewer resources are required to maintain existing neural systems/capacities than to develop new ones is cited to highlight that, after a brain injury, children will exhibit two kinds of changes—one associated with reconstituting (often incompletely) established systems and the other supporting a trajectory (often abnormal) of new capacities. We would extend this to apply to adult development construed as a constantly changing neural infrastructure in which recovery after a neurological insult places demands upon the system not only to reconstituted acquired abilities but also to support a normal or abnormal trajectory (i.e., cognitive aging). This comports well with the finding of Scarmeas et al., (2003) that networks underlying CR (as measured by positron emission tomography) in old subjects show evidence of reorganization compared to younger subjects, perhaps as a compensatory reaction to age-related atrophy.

Reserve and Neuropathological Conditions of Childhood

The analysis by Dennis et al. (2006) contributes in several important ways to reserve theory, including questioning the appropriateness of "threshold" versus "gradient" models of reserve as applied to conditions of childhood: "Although there may be thresholds of damage that when exceeded, preclude plasticity of function, the concept that reserve varies in degree finds considerable support in the literature" (p. 73). They have also extended the notion of pathological burden to genetic conditions, thereby including many disorders of childhood previously underrepresented in this discussion. It is worth pointing out that when considering both acquired and congenital neuropathological conditions, somewhat different constructs of "reserve" are being estimated by the same proxies. In the case of acquired injuries/diseases, reserve would be the product of recursive brain and cognitive development over the period preceding the injury. So, to some extent, reserve reflects what the child was. In the case of congenital disorders, proxies of reserve are used to estimate what the child's capacity would have been absent the disorder.

What happens in the case of a single insult to the brain during childhood? Presumably, reserve theory would postulate the following: diminished BR capacity and compromised CR capacity, both of which prospectively constrain the development of CR. A child suffering such pathological burden does not benefit from subsequent experience to the same degree, and learning could be considered ecologically impoverished, partly as a result of a compromised ability to make use of experience and partly as a result of being exposed to educational, occupational, social, and other life experiences that are less "rich."

Successive insults to the brain increase pathological burden, thereby further eroding BR, CR, and prospective CR capacity. If the aging of the brain can be conceptualized as a late "insult," as evidenced by pathological changes in the brain with increased age, then serial insults to the brain are inevitable for children suffering from neurogenetic disorders, traumatic brain injury, iatrogenic injury, and the other conditions of childhood that have neuropathological consequences.

Reserve, therefore, is a complex, multidetermined, hypothetical construct. In the context of the remote effects of early disturbances of the central nervous system, HR can be imparted by genetic endowment, healthy development, high-quality experiences that promote cognitive and emotional growth, and long duration of experiences that result in high accumulation of knowledge. LR can be related to the interaction of genetic endowment, disease/injury during development, diminished quality of experiences, and short duration of experiences that result in low accumulation of knowledge. If, as Stern claims, CR is something that accrues over time, the child suffering brain insult not only incurs diminished reserve as a result of the injury or disease but also a diminished capacity to develop reserve post-injury to buffer a second insult or a decline secondary to the aging process. This would be mitigated by a later age at the time of the first insult. Thus, even in cases where the effects of the initial insult were equivalent, susceptibility to the effects of a later insult, or cognitive aging, should be lower when the initial insult occurred at a later age (assuming comparable pre-injury reserve).

REMAINING "COMPLEXITIES"

Threshold Effects

Thresholds are most compatible with nature that can be "cut at the joints," as Plato put it, or that which is a matter of kind rather than magnitude (Meehl, 1995). Also, highly interconnected systems are inclined, as we have seen, to exhibit threshold effects under certain conditions. Reserve theories originated from observations of discontinuity between pathological substrate and clinical symptoms. Thresholds then (whether "hard" or "soft") are fundamental to an explanation of the emergence of manifestations of pathology and their temporal course.

A more linear model would predict that degradation in behavior or cognition of HR and LR individuals would follow parallel trajectories. If one imposes a cutoff of some sort on these curves (such as for incident dementia), then such a cutoff is reached earlier by the LR individual, and HR individuals seem "protected." However, such an effect is inherent to both the nature of the outcome and how it is measured. In a linear model, the degree of degradation in behavior is the same in both cases. Thresholds seem to successfully predict some of the research on categorical entities, such as AD. It is less clear that thresholds are consistent with what is found in outcomes that are more dimensional or systems that are less interconnected. Indeed, notwithstanding the conclusions of some (Corkin et al., 1989; Raymont et al., 2008), LR and HR individuals may approximate linear and parallel trajectories, rather than divergent trajectories, as they age. This leads us to consider some of the methodological complications and confounding factors that could account for contradictory findings.

General Versus Specific Cognitive Effects

What functions are most at risk for accelerated cognitive aging? Dennis et al. (2006) refers to task "challenge" as a risk factor in her model. Corkin et al. (1989) note differences in "task demands" affecting developmental trajectory. Thus, trajectory in later life may be a function of cognitive requirements, characterized as effortful or efficient, as proposed by Stern (2009). In the case of prior brain injury, one could posit differential decline for those abilities most susceptible to aging effects or those abilities most affected by the previous disease or injury. In many cases, there is enough overlap to render this point moot (e.g., processing speed seems to be particularly vulnerable for children treated with cranial radiation for cancer, as well as adults as they age). However, if we consider focal injuries with more specific effects, this question becomes relevant. The findings of Corkin et al. (1989) on veterans with head injuries did not fully support either of these conjectures. Some, but not all, "defective capacities" showed exacerbated decline. Furthermore, the head-injured group showed exacerbated decline on some tasks that were most resistant to aging in the control group. As we have proposed previously, an alternative perspective is that divergent or parallel trajectories for HR and LR individuals could be predicted on the basis of the degree of interconnectivity/interdependence of the systems constituting the neural infrastructure.

Psychometric factors attendant to the issue of measurement of differential cognitive deficits (Chapman & Chapman, 1973; Chapman & Chapman, 2001; Knight & Silverstein, 2001) must also be considered. For example, Himanen et al. (2006) found slight cognitive decline over a 30-year interval in 61 patients who had suffered traumatic brain injury. Interestingly, one function most susceptible to age-related decline, psychomotor speed, was not significantly different from baseline at the 30-year follow-up. However, this may be a spurious finding related to the fact that this ability was significantly impacted by the injury, producing a floor effect and apparent stability over time. So, the differential impact of the injury across multiple functions combined with psychometric scaling differences accounted for the pattern of decline observed in this sample.

Neural Substrate and Reserve Phenotype

According to Dennis et al. (2006), spatial gradients (right-left, up-down, front-back) are also moderators of the effects of brain lesions during childhood and likely play a role in how reserve develops. More specifically, these authors note the particular risk to reserve capacity faced by children with anterior lesions and the functions subserved by these brain systems (inhibitory control and working memory). This is consistent with Stern's (2009) assertion that there are certain cognitive functions (localizable) that are critical substrates for the development of CR capacity. Drawing from an elegant series of imaging studies, Stern (2009) concludes, "Neural reserve recognizes that old and young individuals may use the same networks to mediate task performance, albeit with different levels of efficiency and capacity.... On the other hand, there are clearly situations where older individuals adopt networks that are not used by younger subjects, presumably in response to age-related neural changes" (p. 2027). A network comprised of several areas in the frontal lobe known to be involved in control processes and working memory (bilateral superior frontal, left medial frontal, right medial frontal, and left middle frontal gyri) seemed to be associated with CR in these functional magnetic resonance imaging studies. In the language of complex systems, neural components of CR comprised of these "spanning clusters of nodes" are uniquely situated to support broad function (Buldyrev et al., 2010).

Other research implicates additional regions of the brain. Corkin et al. (1989) found that left hemisphere lesions had a greater impact than right hemisphere lesions on rate of decline with age. Measuring actual change with age, Raymont et al. (2008) found that left parietal and right frontal lobe atrophy predicted greater rate of decline in cognitive functioning on the AFQT, as well as injuries specifically impacting the caudate nucleus, right amygdala, hippocampus, and corpus callosum. So, although frontal/executive control functions are reasonable candidates for the reserve phenotype because of their integrative and cognitive binding roles, this may depend, in part, on the outcome being measured.

Methodological Issues

Practice Effects and Reliable Change

Practice effects, a major concern for longitudinal research, may account for some of the inconsistencies in cross-sectional and longitudinal research, as demonstrated by Ronnlund et al. (2005). For some age spans, the practice adjusted curves for composite memory scores corresponded more closely to cross-sectional curves than longitudinal curves. Ronnlund has also shown practice-related benefits in Tower of London solution time. There remain fundamental differences in how to interpret the longitudinal and cross-sectional data in research on age-related decline. Salthouse argues for the early onset of decline and the strengths of the cross-sectional data. Others have noted that age-related decline is likely to be both heterogeneous across different functions and nonlinear, as evidenced by longitudinal data adjusted for practice (Nilsson, Sternang, Ronnlund, & Nyberg, 2009).

Most of the studies reviewed above involve attempts to capture change through repeated measurements using fallible methods. How one sorts "true" change from error that is inherent in one's instrumentation has been the subject of research over the past two decades. The Reliable Change Index (RCI) was originally developed as a means to measure positive change in the context of psychological treatment (Jacobson & Truax, 1991), although it can also be employed to estimate negative change associated with deterioration resulting from brain disease or injury. Essentially, the RCI uses information about the psychometric properties of the instruments to determine whether change over time is "real" or attributable to measurement artifact. The formula proposed by Jacobson and Truax (1991) is:

$$RC = (x_2 - x_1)/S_{diff}$$

where x_1 is the pretest score, x_2 is the post-test score, and S_{diff} is the standard error of the difference between the two scores ($\sqrt{2}(S_E)^2$). Regression-based approaches were subsequently applied where, for example, repeated administration of memory tests (particularly over short intervals) may result in gains (or mitigated decline) that reflect previous exposure rather than actual changes in memory function (McSweeny et al., 1993).

Regression to the Mean

Another complication in interpreting longitudinal data in this context is the well-known tendency for extreme scores to "regress" upon retesting. So, HR individuals may show declines simply as a result of statistical artifact, as pointed out by Zahodne et al. (2011). Interpretive caution must be exercised, therefore, when dealing with metrics with weak psychometric properties where group membership is defined by extreme scores, be it high (HR) or low (LR). Noting the inconsistent results of studies investigating the relationship between reserve and decline for specific cognitive functions, Zahodne et al. (2011) found no moderating effect of education on four domains of cognitive functioning in a longitudinal study of aging in 1014 participants in the Victoria Longitudinal Study. In other words, declines with age were linear, and slopes were equivalent across education levels. These authors point out that previous studies showing more rapid decline in HR individuals may be an artifact of regression to the mean, which would be even more of a potential confound for instruments with lower reliability.

Regression may represent unrecognized confounding in other studies as well. In the previously cited study by Raymont et al. (2008), close examination of their data would suggest greater decline in those who initially scored higher, and this has also been found in two samples of survivors of childhood medulloblastoma (Ris et al., 2001; Ris et al., in press). Decline over time that is compounded by regression to the mean can be confused with an accelerated course for those with HR and can appear to attenuate decline in those with LR.

COHORT EFFECTS

As noted above in the cross-sectional literature on cognitive aging, complex cohort effects can complicate the interpretation of brain-related changes in cognition over time. In fact, one could argue that the Flynn effect could constitute a risk factor (for at least some functions) in that older cohorts would have less reserve and so be more vulnerable to the deleterious effects of aging than younger cohorts. This is the subject of the next section of this chapter.

THE FLYNN EFFECT AND COGNITIVE RESERVE THEORY

Problems Created by the Flynn Effect

Cohort effects are the bane of cross-sectional developmental research designs. If the investigator wants to determine how spatial ability, for example, changes between the ages of 6 years and 15 years, he or she could sample children at the ages of 6, 9, 12, and 15 years. Development would not be assessed directly, but age group would serve as a proxy for development. This is a classical cross-sectional design, and it is vulnerable to cohort effects. Indeed, each group differs from every other group with respect to the intended independent variable, the passage of time. In addition, each group may differ from every other group with respect to a large number of other variables that may contribute to scores on a test of spatial ability. For instance, probably only the oldest group has been exposed to instruction in geometry. The oldest children might have accumulated more total time playing video games that require visuospatial skill, but younger children may have played more video games at earlier stages of development. These are some of the potential confounding variables, or cohort effects, which complicate interpretation of between-group differences in spatial ability that might be obtained from a cross-sectional study.

The previous hypothetical situation is a modest example of the risks associated with cohort effects. If we modify the example so that the age range under consideration extends from 6 years to 60 years, the cohort effects are likely to increase in number and strength. The differences that could exist between 6-year-olds and 60-year-olds are more numerous and more worrisome than the differences between 6-year-olds and 15-year-olds. Because the damage that can be inflicted on developmental studies by cohort effects is well known in psychology, one might ask why cross-sectional research is still being done. The answer, of course, is that cross-sectional designs demand relatively few resources and yield relatively quick results. Long-term longitudinal (follow-up) studies are more difficult to execute. They require more resources including the infrastructure necessary to track participants over a long interval and the capability of inducing participants to continue their involvement in the study. Above all, long-term longitudinal studies require the luxury of waiting for several years or several decades before meaningful results become available. If cross-sectional studies were to be deemed unacceptable, then the number of developmental studies would be sharply reduced.

Let us disregard, for now, the pragmatic barriers to conducting long-term longitudinal research and imagine that we have the resources, including the time, to undertake a 30-year follow-up study of adolescents who sustained closed head injuries prior to the age of 8 years. We gain access to a sample of 18-year-olds who meet our inclusion criteria, and we plan to track at 10-year intervals these individuals until they are 48 years old. Because we are interested in the trajectory of their general cognitive ability, we decide to administer the fourth edition of the Wechsler Adult Intelligence Scale (WAIS-IV).

We then have to set up a straightforward long-term longitudinal study. Because we have only one cohort, we are confident that there can be no cohort effects. Being aware that the content and format of the Wechsler IQ tests tend to change, sometimes quite markedly, from one edition to the next, we decide to administer the WAIS-IV at each of the four evaluation points. In that way, we can make "apples-to-apples" comparisons. Unfortunately, the decision to stay with the same test over a period of 30 years, even though it obviates the problem of content and format changes, makes the study vulnerable to a cohort effect. How can we have a cohort effect in a pure longitudinal design? The cohort effect is the Flynn effect, and it enters the study through the gradual obsolescence of the norms.

If the initial evaluation takes place in 2012, the WAIS-IV norms already will be 6 years out of date. Our 18-year-old subjects will be compared with individuals who were 18 years old when the test was normed in 2006. In the meantime, those individuals from the standardization sample will have become 24-year-olds whose IQs from 6 years ago are 1.8 points lower than the IQs of the current cohort of 18-year-olds. By 2042, 30 years later, when our subjects are administered the WAIS-IV for the last time, at the age of 48 years, the normative scaled scores for individuals who were 48 years old in 2006 will have become 2.16 points too low and the normative IQs will have become nearly 10.8 points too low. In other words, the IQs that we obtain in 2042 will overestimate actual IQ by nearly 11 points.

This scenario assumes that performance on the Wechsler IQ continues to increase at a steady rate of 3 points per decade. The rate of change may decline in the future or it may accelerate. No one knows what to expect. The important point, for present purposes, is that the Flynn effect can cause a cohort effect to intrude into a longitudinal design. We want to compare our subjects' performance with the norms for their peer group, but we are forced to compare their performance with norms for people who were born 36 years prior to their birth. This is the "virtual" second cohort, and it is not an appropriate comparison group for drawing conclusions about cognitive change in our study group.

Two means for circumventing this problem are available to us, but both solutions come with limitations. First, we could use raw scores to track changes in the performance of our sample of patients with head injuries. Because we no longer would be comparing the patients to any reference group, the virtual cohort effect (Flynn effect) will be eliminated. Although it may be informative to plot the patterns of raw-score change across the decades of our longitudinal study, it will be difficult to determine whether the changes observed in our clinical group are significantly different from changes that would occur in a normal control group, for example, changes associated with aging, declining sensorimotor capability, or deteriorating health. The second solution would be to adjust the normative scores for the passage of time, that is, to apply a correction of 3 IQ points per decade (Flynn, 2007) or a correction that is optimized individually for each subtest (Dickinson & Hiscock, 2010). The shortcoming of this second solution is that it assumes that the magnitude of the Flynn effect will remain constant over the next 30 years. Probably the only fully satisfactory solution is to select a well-matched normal control group at the outset of the study and to follow both the clinical and normal control groups for the duration of the longitudinal study. This would be a good solution from a research design perspective, but it would substantially increase the amount of resources required.

The preceding example, couched in terms of longitudinal research, illustrates problems that are shared by the clinical neuropsychologist who would follow a single patient over a long period of time. If a new edition of the IQ test has been published prior to follow-up testing, the clinician must decide whether to switch to the new edition or to remain with the older version that was used in the earlier evaluation of the patient. Switching means that the patient will be administered a test with somewhat different content and perhaps different format and scoring rules. Direct comparison between performance on at least some subtests from the older and newer tests may not be possible. Remaining with the older version means that comparisons between first and subsequent assessments will be contaminated by the Flynn effect. Whereas both the original version and revised version of the IQ test could be administered in follow-up testing, this would demand considerably more time from both patient and clinician and, in addition, performance on the second test to be administered during the follow-up evaluation is likely to be altered by the immediately prior administration of the first test.

The Flynn Effect and Cognitive Reserve

If average IQ increases from one cohort to the next younger cohort, and if higher IQs provide some protection against the adverse consequences of an acquired brain injury, then one might suspect that the Flynn effect provides at least a modest benefit to the younger child with brain injury. Unfortunately, this is not the case. Average raw scores on some tests will be elevated slightly in young children, relative to scores of older children, but no one is advantaged at all relative to his or her own age group. In fact, the Flynn effect may work to the disadvantage of younger children if the brain injury causes the child to become relatively isolated at an early age from the social and cultural factors that augment cognitive development, that is, the factors that underlie the Flynn effect.

Clinicians who work with brain-injured children recognize the importance of distinguishing between previously acquired skills, which typically are retained or relatively unimpaired by the injury, and new skills, which often are acquired with great difficulty or not at all (Anderson, Northam, Hendy, & Wrennall, 2001). Quite apart from the unresolved question of age-related changes in plasticity (e.g., St. James-Roberts, 1981), the younger child with brain injury is disadvantaged by having to face a future filled with new information to be learned and new skills to be mastered. Though much remains for the older child, adolescent, and adult to learn, there are significant advantages in having already acquired (and retained) the basic cognitive tools of language and calculation prior to the injury. The Flynn effect intensifies the burden of the younger child with brain injury. Because average IQ throughout the culture continues to rise following the injury, the young child must struggle not only to avoid falling farther and farther behind his or her peers but also to function satisfactorily in a society that is gradually increasing its expectations and demands. Translated into the language of CR, the child with an early brain injury may need a greater amount of CR than the older brain-injured individual in order to achieve a comparable outcome.

Education and IQ

The Flynn effect is potentially relevant to the theory of CR in other ways. Education is one nexus between the respective phenomena. Although it would be premature to declare that the rising IQ curve is entirely attributable to increased formal education, that variable appears to be one of the most plausible explanations (Flynn, 2006, 2007). Likewise, although the factors contributing to CR are yet to be established with certainty, education level appears to be one of the strongest and most consistent correlates of risk for dementia onset at a particular age (Bickel & Kurz, 2009; McDowell, Xi, Lindsay, & Tierney, 2007). Numerous other factors have been proposed as putative contributors to both phenomena. Although the analogy between the Flynn effect and cognitive reserve with respect to education ultimately may prove to be imperfect, it would be interesting to know whether the same educational variables contribute to both phenomena.

IQ also has been proposed in the CR literature as a major determinant of long-term cognitive outcomes (Richards & Sacker, 2003; Starr & Lonie, 2008). IQ, of course, is the phenomenon of interest in studies of the Flynn effect (e.g., Flynn, 1999). Cognitive ability is a predictor variable in the CR literature, but it is the primary criterion variable in the Flynn effect literature. Nonetheless, the environmental "multipliers" that are thought to be responsible for the rising IQs (Dickens & Flynn, 2001b; Flynn, 2007) might also contribute to CR. This possibility will be explored in detail in the following sections.

Dissociation

A central issue in neuropsychology is the degree to which cognitive functions are localized in the cerebral cortex. This is a concern that can be traced back to the neuroscience and neurology of the early 19th century (Boring, 1957; Clarke & Jacyna, 1987). The phrenologists suggested that the repertoire of human functions comprises a large number of skills and traits that are precisely localized in different areas of the cortex. Subsequent contributors to 19th-century neuroscience took more conservative stances on localization. Flourens, the influential French neuroscientist, argued that the major parts of the central nervous system (cerebral hemispheres, brain stem, basal ganglia, etc.) are differentially specialized relative to each other, but functions are uniform within each of those structures. He called the specialization of each part *action propre* and the unified action of each part *action commune*. Subsequent contributions by clinicians such as Broca and experimental physiologists such as Fritsch, Hitzig, and Munk established that focal lesions within the cerebral cortex had selective effects on particular functions. Thus, *action commune* could not be entirely correct, but debate continued about the degree to which regions of the forebrain are specialized. Since the latter part of the 19th century, the dominant position on functional specialization has continued to vary from the side of *action propre* (emphasis on localization of functions) to *action commune* (emphasis on unity) and back again, but the positions on both sides of the issue have become progressively less extreme.

Luria (1973) propelled neuropsychology beyond the *action commune* versus *action propre* dichotomy when he pointed out that the degree to which a function can be localized to a specific cortical region depends on the complexity of the function. Simple functions such as limb flexion or perception of a flash of light can be localized quite precisely, but higher mental functions such as language or calculation defy precise localization. Luria advocated a kind of "syndrome analysis" in which lesion effects could be used to decompose higher mental functions into their underlying constituent processes. Sometimes two dissimilar syndromes could be attributed to the same underlying deficit because the syndromes share a component process, and sometimes similar manifestations could be produced by different underlying causes. The perspective of Luria ultimately evolved into the neuropsychological concepts of association and dissociation (e.g., McCarthy & Warrington, 1990).

A parallel dialectic is prominent in the history of intelligence theory. Whereas some theorists such as Spearman (1904) emphasized general intelligence, or *g*, others such as Thurstone (1948) emphasized special abilities American IQ tests such as the various Wechsler and Stanford-Binet tests, with their combinations of component scores and overall IQ, reflect a combination of the two perspectives. Consequently, although there are other points of view (e.g., Gardner, 2006; Goleman, 1995; Sternberg, 1985), the mainstream of intelligence research and application shows a remarkable parallel to the history of functional cerebral localization. In both fields, the longstanding contention between unitary and fractionated models has been resolved by more complex models in which both viewpoints are represented.

Flynn (2006) proposed an explicit parallel between rising IQ scores and the neuropsychological principle of dissociation. His argument rests on evidence that the Flynn effect is not uniform across different cognitive realms but, on the contrary, different IQ subtest scores have been rising at markedly different rates. For example, scores from Wechsler performance subtests have been increasing much more rapidly than scores from most of the verbal subtests (Flynn, 1999) but scores from the Similarities subtest have been increasing much more rapidly than scores from the other verbal subtests (Flynn, 2007). If we assume, as does Flynn, that the differential impact of the Flynn effect is attributable to cultural influences, then both brain damage and cultural variables seem to affect different cognitive abilities to varying degrees. In other words, both brain damage and cultural variables may produce dissociations among mental abilities.

Perhaps the uneven patterns of cognitive aging that we described earlier in this chapter (Salthouse, 2010; Schaie et al., 2004) have counterparts in the uneven patterns of intergenerational increase of various cognitive skills. However, mapping the pattern of cognitive decline in the individual onto the pattern of cognitive improvement in the population—no matter how tempting it may be to try—might be precluded by the aforementioned indeterminacy of the pattern of decline. At present, we can only say that there is an intriguing parallel between the dissociations observed in cognitive aging and those observed in the Flynn effect.

Individual and Social Multipliers

What are the cultural variables that are responsible for the rising IQ scores, and why do those variables influence some cognitive domains more than others? These questions might be especially relevant to the concept of CR and, for that reason, we will address them in some detail. First, it should be pointed out that different authors have offered numerous explanations for the Flynn effect, which range from urbanization and better nutrition to electronic media and mathematics education. Many of those explanations are described in Neisser (1998). Some of the most plausible explanations are based on improvements in education or increased access to education, which will be discussed below. First, however, we want to describe a more general framework in which to consider the action of education and other cultural factors.

Dickens and Flynn (2001b) have constructed a conceptual framework based on "individual multipliers" and "social multipliers." These concepts are summarized in Dickens and Flynn (2001a), Flynn (2006), and Flynn (2007). Individual multipliers are factors that contribute to heterogeneity among people with respect to their skills, knowledge, and accomplishments. Social multipliers are factors that affect a culture or society as a whole. In order to understand how the Flynn effect might relate to CR theory, one has to understand both kinds of multiplier.

Individual multipliers are factors in the child's social environment that tend to amplify individual differences. The starting point is one or more individual characteristics, which may be innate. The next step, which is not unique to the Dickens and Flynn (2001b) model, is the power of those individual characteristics to contribute to the construction of the child's personal environment. Following Bell's (1968) landmark analysis of the child's contribution to the manner in which he or she is parented, the notion of bidirectional socialization effects became influential in developmental psychology and behavioral genetics (e.g., Jensen, 1975; Plomin, 1986; Scarr, 1992). A succinct statement of the idea is that each child makes his or her own environment. Although the outcome is not necessarily advantageous to the child or society, Flynn (2007) has focused on the combination of favorable traits and favorable environments: "... those who have an advantage for a particular trait will become matched with superior environments for that trait" (p. 38).

Dickens and Flynn (2001b) use this argument to demonstrate that individual excellence in a particular domain is not based solely or even largely on the individual's genetic endowment. Whereas "good" genes for IQ and intellectual curiosity may help a child to read well and enable the child to ask intelligent questions, these are but first steps on the path to high achievement. The child's academic aptitude and interest may prompt the teacher to praise the child frequently in the classroom, and the child's enjoyment of reading may cause the school librarian to suggest additional books to be read. Praise and special attention from teachers will motivate the child to devote more time and effort to academic pursuits, which in turn will elicit more praise and special attention. If the parents are told that their child shows unusual aptitude in school, they are likely to stimulate and reward the child, which probably will intensify the child's efforts. These chains of reciprocal actions ultimately may lead to advantageous classroom placements, superior schools, university scholarships, prizes and accolades, and so on. If continued through adolescence and young adulthood, this pattern of interactions will enable the individual to achieve high levels of academic and occupational success. If so, the success is not attributable to genetic endowment per se but to the protracted interaction with the favorable social environment that the child himself or herself has attracted.

Individual multipliers tend to propel certain children toward the upper end of the bell curve but they do not elevate the curve itself and therefore do not account for the Flynn effect. Instead, Flynn (2006, 2007) attributes elevation of the curve to social multipliers, whose effects can be likened to those of the proverbial high tide that floats all boats. As a first approximation, one could conceptualize a social multiplier as an environmental factor that changes an entire culture through a series of feedback loops similar to those hypothesized to underlie individual multipliers. One of Flynn's best examples is the increased skill level at which the game of basketball is played. The advent of television exposed professional basketball to a huge audience, and this mass exposure led to higher salaries for players (and, accordingly, a stronger incentive for boys to aspire to become professional players). The increased popularity of the game led to more activity on playgrounds across America and to improved average skill levels. Higher normative skill levels on the outdoor courts spread to organized teams and leagues. More intense competition stimulated more improvement in skill level and, perhaps, to larger crowds at games, which would facilitate the hiring of better coaches, who in turn would contribute to an additional increase in the average skill level. Although individual multipliers also operated within this milieu, and serve to enhance the skills of elite players such as Michael Jordan, the social multipliers had a positive effect on all players.

An Explanation for the Rising Scores

Flynn (2006, 2007) believes that the social multiplier effect has elevated certain intellectual skills through mechanisms similar to those responsible for elevating skills in certain sports. The key mechanism in both instances is the raising of performance standards. There might not be a specifiable stimulus, such as the televising of basketball, that sets the elevation mechanism into motion, but Flynn has suggested that changes in education have made important contributions to the rising test scores. Flynn has articulated two different scenarios. The first explanation, described in Flynn (2006), involves two phases within the 20th century. In the first phase, prior to 1948 (the time at which the original Wechsler Intelligence Scale for Children [WISC] was published), the increase in IQ scores was attributable to widespread increases in the number of years of formal public education. IQ scores went up because young people spent more time in school and reached higher academic levels. Flynn suggested that something quite different happened during the period following World War II. Beginning about 1948, a societal shift occurred such that on-the-spot problem solving (fluid intelligence) came to be valued more than it had been, while schools began to place less value on traditional "disciplined" learning (crystallized intelligence). As society became more affluent, work environments became more stimulating and more demanding of ad hoc problem solving. At the same time, people were enjoying more opportunities to pursue stimulating hobbies. Accordingly, one's skill at solving novel problems at work or playing chess or video games during one's leisure became more important than memorizing lines from Shakespeare or recalling the battles of the American Revolutionary War. It was as if society was altering people's cognitive profile by reinforcing aspects of nonverbal IQ at the expense of aspects of verbal IQ.

Flynn's second scenario is that IQ scores have been influenced by the pervasiveness of scientific concepts, scientific terminology, and scientific knowledge. Flynn (2006) noticed an especially large increase between 1948 and 2002 in scores on the Similarities subtest of the WISC. Although he initially interpreted this unanticipated increase as an instance of improved ad hoc problem solving, he subsequently regarded it as a prime example of the influence of science (Flynn, 2007). Good (2-point) responses to items from the Similarities subtest of the Wechsler IQ tests typically reflect knowledge of abstractions, such as categories that science imposes on the natural world, rather than the concrete associations that are salient in children's day to-day lives. Flynn suggests that even people who do not know much about science have been influenced profoundly by the abstract concepts and logic of science. Consequently, the children of today are more likely to provide the abstract associations required by the Similarities subtest instead of the more concrete and utilitarian associations that would have been more salient to earlier generations.

Environmental Multipliers and Cognitive Reserve

Both kinds of multiplier—individual and social—are relevant to CR theory in so far as both categories of multiplier effects illustrate the potential strength of environments. Moreover, the important environmental variables are not the traditional sociological variables such as socioeconomic status (SES) and parental education level. Individual multipliers can operate differentially on children within the same family, and social multipliers have a pervasive effect throughout entire cohorts, irrespective of SES, race, and similar factors. (In fact, Dickens and Flynn (2006) have determined that the IQs of black Americans have risen more rapidly than those of white Americans from 1972 to 2002).

The concept of social multipliers also can be applied to CR. Later-born people on average will have more overall CR than earlier-born people (because of their higher average IQ), but the later-born ultimately will lose their advantaged position in the CR distribution as even younger cohorts enter the picture and the normative level continues to move upward. However, if an individual is leading his or her cohort, for example, by having a higher level of education or a better understanding of scientific principles than the average for that cohort, then that individual should have a relatively high level of CR. This, of course, is commensurate with contemporary views about CR (Stern, 2003); if it leads to any novel hypotheses, those hypotheses are not obvious.

According to Flynn (2007), however, the Dickens–Flynn model implies that "current environment has large effects on cognitive skills and that those skills atrophy with disuse" (p. 64). In other words, the effects of cognitive exercise are time limited and equally beneficial at any age. The Dickens–Flynn model thus leads to a seemingly novel perspective on CR. The slope of curves depicting age-related intellectual decline will be identical for the cognitively active person and the cognitively inactive person, but the former will enjoy an advantage at every point. If the cognitive activity begins early in life, it will bestow an advantage that remains constant as long as the cognitive activity is maintained. If the activity begins at an advanced age, it will have the same degree of benefit after it takes effect. If the benefits of being cognitively active include having greater CR, one could infer that the amount of CR would decline if the individual ceases to be active. However, the CR could be reinstated if the individual became active again.

From this interpretation of CR as both a perishable and a renewable resource—similar to physical fitness—certain predictions can be made. For example, a societal trend (such as solving Sudoku puzzles), if capable of increasing the CR of young adults, would have an equivalent effect on older adults. If the cognitive exercise engages older adults to the degree that it engages younger adults—and this may be a difficult condition to satisfy—it follows from Flynn's position that the magnitude of any beneficial effect on CR would be equal in both age groups. Once Sudoku grows out of favor, however, the CR engendered by its practice will abate, and this abatement presumably will occur in both age groups.

As noted in our previous discussion of the principle of dissociation, the Flynn effect is selective for certain cognitive domains. This selectivity is important for at least two reasons. For Flynn (2007), it is especially important because the skills that have increased most dramatically are not those that have the highest correlations with general intelligence (*g*). Instead, "What dominates depends on what seizes control of powerful multipliers" (Flynn, 2007, p. 41). This finding encourages new perspectives on the fundamental questions about the nature of intelligence. The selectively of the Flynn effect also is important because the so-called culture-free or culture-reduced tests have been affected more than tests such as verbal tests that are subject to culture-specific learning. We are forced to conclude that environmental effects are not always direct or predictable. Selectivity, or dissociation, also carries implications for CR theory. In the previous scenario involving Sudoku puzzles, for instance, it is possible that proficiency in Sudoku would protect Sudoku skills from deterioration with age or brain insult but would have little or no protective effect on other skills.

Both individual and social multipliers are inherently selective for cognitive domains. The potential relevance of individual multipliers to CR is illustrated by the following anecdote. Flynn (2007) cites the case of a man named Richard Wetherill, a remarkably skilled chess player who played the game at a high level until his rather sudden death, after which a postmortem examination revealed signs of advanced Alzheimer's disease (see Melton, 2005). Although Mr. Wetherill had complained about a diminution of his chess abilities about 2 years prior to his death, a thorough battery of tests administered at that time revealed no indication of dementia. Yet, 2 years later his brain contained numerous neurofibrilliary tangles and senile plaques. In the words of Melton, "The anatomical evidence indicated advanced disease, with a level of physical damage that would have reduced most people to a state of total confusion. Yet for Wetherill the only impact was that he could no longer play chess to high standards" (p. 32).

Flynn points out that intense cognitive activity did not prevent Mr. Wetherill's cognitive decline. It is impossible to be sure that the cognitive activity even slowed the progression of the mental decline once it began. Perhaps Mr. Wetherill's CR was so great that, despite a normal rate of decline, his abilities remained above the threshold for obvious impairment. Paradoxically, it was only in his realm of extraordinary expertise—chess—that he noticed deterioration. Perhaps in this realm, and only in this realm, his expectations of high performance made him particularly sensitive to a loss of skill.

One interpretation of Mr. Wetherill's story is that it exemplifies the potential of extraordinary individual multipliers (in the domain of chess, in this instance) to augment CR. That augmented CR seems to have allowed Mr. Wetherill, despite a severely compromised brain, to function at a high level in his domain of special skill and quite normally in domains assessed in a dementia evaluation. Nonetheless, his subjective complaints arose from his perception that his special skill was diminished. It could be argued, of course, that the cognitive demands of competitive chess are greater than those of everyday living and that is why Mr. Wetherill noticed only the erosion of his chess skills. However, it is also likely that he valued his performance in chess more than his ability to remember to pick up items at the grocery store or to recall a news story that he had read in the morning newspaper. Perhaps people are sensitive to adverse changes in a highly developed skill only because they monitor their performance very closely in a realm of special importance to them.

The remarkable case of Mr. Wetherill leaves many questions unanswered, and some of them can be parlayed into testable research questions. First, how confident can we be that this man's resistance to cognitive deterioration is attributable to his intense cognitive activity in the domain of chess? Perhaps his CR would have been unusually great irrespective of his chess playing. His extraordinary skill in chess may have been merely one manifestation of a man who possessed extraordinary intellectual ability in certain domains. Second, can we extrapolate the case of Mr. Wetherill, with his long history of individual multipliers in the realm of chess, to other people who have no extraordinary skill but maintain a high level of cognitive activity through activities such as reading, crossword puzzles, or Sudoku? Finally, would we expect to see evidence of a high degree of CR in the typical person who engages in no deliberate cognitive exercise but is subject to the social multipliers that affect nearly everyone in a particular time and place?

Let's imagine a culture in which chess—instead of basketball—has captivated nearly everyone for several decades. An ordinary person might have acquired an impressive amount of expertise in chess because the level of competition has been pushed to a high level by social multipliers. Would that ordinary person possess more CR than another ordinary person who has chosen not to play chess and who engages in no other challenging cognitive activity? How much CR would be expected in an ordinary person who acquires chess expertise early in life and then abandons the game or in another ordinary person who develops expertise by playing the game later in life?

Some of these questions can be addressed by studying bilingualism (Bialystok, Craik, Green, & Golan, 2009). It has been reported that bilinguals and multilinguals manifest symptoms of dementia onset 4 or 5 years later than comparable monolinguals (Bialystok, Craik, & Freedman, 2007; Chertkow et al., 2010; Craik, Bialystok, & Freedman, 2010). An interpretation in terms of cognitive reserve is strongly supported by computed tomography (CT-scan) findings that the brains of bilingual patients showed more temporal lobe atrophy than the brains of monolinguals despite comparable cognitive functioning (Schweizer, Ware, Fischer, Craik, & Bialystok, 2012). The cognitive skills of bilinguals were better preserved despite their more advanced brain deterioration.

The study of bilingualism allows not only comparisons between bilinguals and monolinguals but also comparisons of bilinguals on numerous variables such as age of second-language acquisition, proficiency in the second language, and degree to which the second language currently is used. By isolating different dimensions of bilingualism, it should be possible to address many of the questions raised by the Wetherill case. For instance, does enhancement of CR depend on a high degree of proficiency in the second language or on current use of the second language? Does a second language acquired later in life bestow the same beneficial effect on CR as a second language acquired early in life? Is CR in bilinguals correlated with their performance on experimental tasks that yield a bilingual advantage? Experiments with bilinguals could be used to test Flynn's (2007) prediction that mental activity has an ephemeral effect, that is, dementia onset is delayed by bilingualism only if the individual has continued to communicate in both languages until the time when deteriorative changes are occurring in the brain. Early bilingualism followed by disuse of the secondary language should convey no protection against dementia or other neurological insult.

Final Comments on the Flynn Effect

Although we have portrayed the Flynn effect as an increase in IQ, evidence is accumulating to suggest that the Flynn effect applies not only to IQ but also to memory (Baxendale, 2010; Rönnlund & Nilsson, 2009) and at least some of the other abilities that are measured in the neuropsychological evaluation (Connor, Spiro, Obler, & Albert, 2004; Dickinson & Hiscock, 2011). If the Flynn effect applies to skills that lie outside the traditional and somewhat arbitrary set of skills represented in IQ tests, then the potential relevance of the Flynn effect to CR theory is increased. This would make it more plausible that the environmental multipliers known to affect the skills required by certain Wechsler IQ subtests might also affect chess, Sudoku, and other skilled activities that, in turn, could be related to CR.

But one must keep in mind that the impact of the Flynn effect varies across specific abilities. Average scores on the Digit Symbol and Similarities subtests increase in adults by as much as 0.3 standard deviation per decade, while scores on Digit Span and Arithmetic subtests show little or no increase (Dickinson & Hiscock, 2010). For Flynn (2007) this variability across component tests (which we have previously referred to as "dissociation") is important because it undermines the construct of general intelligence (g). If some combination of environmental variables is raising some cognitive skills quite dramatically while failing to raise others, then how is it possible to maintain that these various cognitive skills are all related to each other as different facets of g? Flynn's solution to this conundrum is to differentiate intelligence into three "levels": the level of individual differences, the level of society, and the level of the brain.

Flynn (2007) argues that intelligence simultaneously can act as a highly correlated set of abilities at the level of individual differences (as reflected in g) while acting as a collection of functionally independent abilities at the level of society (as revealed by the domain specificity of the Flynn effect). The factor structure of intellect may account for individual differences in fluid and crystallized intelligence but it cannot account for the pattern of cognitive skills that are targeted for enhancement by changes in societal values. Consequently, hypotheses based on psychometrics at the individual-differences level should not be imposed on the society level.

While acknowledging that common factors (e.g., blood supply, neurotransmitters) may affect brain functioning globally so as to produce individual differences in general intelligence, Flynn reminds us that "skills swimming feely of *g* also have a physiological substratum" (p. 60). Here he is referring to the cognitive skills favored by social selection, which must also be represented in the brain. Flynn ultimately settles on a hybrid model of intelligence at the brain level that is organized according to a combination of common factors and specialized factors. In effect, he has rediscovered the *action commune* and *action propre* of Flourens. Unlike Flourens, however, Flynn chooses to emphasize the specialized factors, which he considers to be the skills that respond to "specialized cognitive exercise" (p. 56).

The Flynn effect and the Dickens–Flynn interpretation of the Flynn effect reinforce and broaden several prevalent themes in neuropsychology. Brain injury, even when the cause is endogenous, often can be construed as an environmental effect that is imposed on a previously normal brain. Likewise, the Flynn effect demonstrates that the social environment impacts the normal brain. Although both categories of environmental effects are capable of producing changes in general mental ability, the more dramatic changes tend to be domain specific. The magnitude of these environmental effects varies across individuals, and the heterogeneity in the degree of impact on different individuals is not predictable on the basis of general intelligence, nor has it been shown to be predictable on the basis of brain characteristics. Activity in a particular cognitive realm may provide protection against the adverse effects of brain injury, and this phenomenon might depend on mechanisms that are similar or identical to the mechanisms that underlie the individual multipliers of the Dickens–Flynn model.

Of greatest potential importance to CR theory is the organization of cognitive abilities into three autonomous levels. Flynn (2007) cautions us to avoid "conceptual imperialism," in which hypotheses derived from the organizing scheme of one level are applied to another level. Just as the general intelligence concept of the individual differences level fails to predict which skills will be selected for elevation by the Flynn effect, general intelligence may not predict the abilities that will be most resistant to impairment following brain injury. Although Flynn believes that "functional autonomy" in the brain matches the pattern shown by IQ gains over time, it is quite possible that specialization of functions in different brain regions will not closely resemble functional specialization at either the individual-differences or society levels. Indeed, the organizing principles of CR theory could differ from those of any of the three Dicken–Flynn levels. Nonetheless, if one digs beneath the surface of CR theory and the Flynn effect, one will find parallels that justify continuing cross-fertilization between the two fields of enquiry.

OVERALL CONCLUSIONS

This chapter has addressed the matter of early injury to the brain superimposed on lifespan development. Does a prior injury or compromised early development of the brain always portend a more malignant course of cognitive aging later in life? If so, what are the factors that determine the severity of the accelerated decline? To what degree do premorbid individual differences account for the cognitive outcomes? To what extent can the individual's subsequent environment alter the cognitive outcomes? Can principles derived from the Flynn effect be helpful in constructing a theoretical basis for understanding the effects of societal and individual environmental variables on normal and deviant cognitive development?

Researchers face formidable methodological and conceptual hurdles when attempting to answer these questions. Neither our capability for tracking normal and perturbed cognitive development across the lifespan nor our ability to integrate and interpret the evidence is sufficient to lead us to robust and definitive conclusions. As is often the case in science, simple answers are elusive, and the closer one looks, the more complicated the matter becomes. The complexities discussed here suggest the need for improved precision and conceptual clarity with respect to constructs such as accelerated cognitive aging. Also needed is more precise specification of the diverse outcomes we are modeling (e.g., age-related diseases, cognitive functions), along with additional research to establish the validity of manifest variables that are purported to measure latent constructs such as BR capacity and CR capacity. The evidence reviewed here also suggests the need for two different models, one discontinuous and one continuous, to account for the relationship between reserve and function in disease as compared to typical aging.

Among the more relevant methodological challenges facing the researcher is a powerful cohort effect, that is, the Flynn effect, that reflects surprisingly rapid changes in societal milieu in which cognitive development occurs. In the absence of proper controls, the Flynn effect is capable of confounding the interpretation of both longitudinal and cross-sectional investigations of neuropsychological development over the lifespan. At the same time, attempts to understand the Flynn effect have yielded some novel insights into the nature of cognitive skills and the environmental "multipliers" that shape those skills. Similar to neuropsychological formulations in some respects, and quite different in others, ideas derived from the Flynn effect have the potential to add an essential environmental context to the concepts of BR and CR.

REFERENCES

Anderson, V., Northam, E., Hendy, J., & Wrennall, J. (2001). *Developmental neuropsychology: A clinical approach*. Hove, UK: Psychology Press.

Bak, P., Tang, C., & Wiesenfeld, K. (1987). Self-organizing criticality: An explanation of 1/f noise. *Physical Review Letters, 59*, 381–384.

Baxendale, S. (2010). The Flynn effect and memory function. *Journal of Clinical and Experimental Neuropsychology, 32*, 699–703.

Bell, R. Q. (1968). A reinterpretation of the direction of effects in studies of socialization. *Psychological Review, 75*, 81–95.

Bialystok, E., Craik, F. I. M., Green, D. W., & Gollan, T. H. (2009). Bilingual minds. *Psychological Science in the Public Interest, 10*, 89–129.

Bialystok, E., Craik, F. I. M., & Freedman, M. (2007). Bilingualism as a protection against the onset of symptoms of dementia. *Neuropsychologia, 45*, 459–464.

Bickel, H., & Kurz, A. (2009). Education, occupation, and dementia: The Bavarian School Sisters Study. *Dementia and Geriatric Cognitive Disorders, 27*, 548–556.

Boring, E. G. (1957). *A history of experimental psychology* (2nd ed.). New York: Appleton-Century-Crofts.

Brummitt, C. D., D'Souza, R. M., & Leicht, E. A. (2012). Suppressing cascades of load in interdependent networks. *Proceedings of the National Academy of Sciences, 109*, E680–E689. Published on line February 21, 2012.

Buldyrev, S. V., Parshani, R., Paul, G., Stanley, E., & Havlin, S. (2010). Catastrophic cascade of failures in interdependent networks. *Nature, 464,* 1025–1028.

Burke, S. N., & Barnes, C. A. (2006). Neural plasticity in the ageing brain. *Nature Reviews Neuroscience, 7,* 30–40.

Chapman, L. J., & Chapman, J. P. (1973). Problems in the measurement of cognitive deficit. *Psychological Bulletin, 79,* 380–385.

Chapman, L. J., & Chapman, J. P. (2001). Commentary on two articles concerning generalized and specific cognitive deficits. *Journal of Abnormal Psychology, 110,* 31–39.

Chertkow, H. Whitehead, V., Phillips, N., Wolfson, C., Atherton, J., & Bergman, H. (2010). Multilingualism (but not always bilingualism) delays the onset of Alzheimer disease: Evidence from a bilingual community. *Alzheimer Disease and Associated Disorders, 24,* 118–125.

Clarke, E., & Jacyna, L. S. (1987). *Nineteenth-century origins of neuroscientific concepts.* Berkeley, CA: University of California Press.

Connor, L. T., Spiro, A. III, Obler, L. K., & Albert, M. L. (2004). Change in object naming ability during adulthood. *Journals of Gerontology: Psychological Sciences, 59B,* 203–209.

Corkin, S., Rosen, T. J., Sullivan, E. V., & Clegg, R. A. (1989). Penetrating head injury in young adulthood exacerbates cognitive decline in later years. *The Journal of Neuroscience, 9,* 3876–3883.

Craik, F. I. M., Bialystok, E., & Freedman, M. (2010). Delaying the onset of Alzheimer's disease: Bilingualism as a form of cognitive reserve. *Neurology, 75,* 1726–1729.

Dennis, M., Spiegler, B. J., & Hetherington, R. (2000). New survivors for the new millennium: Cognitive risk and reserve in adults with childhood brain insults. *Brain and Cognition, 42,* 102–105.

Dennis, M., Yeates, K. O., Taylor, H. G., & Fletcher, J. M. (2006). Brain reserve capacity, cognitive reserve capacity, and age-based functional plasticity after congenital and acquired brain injury in children. In Y. Stern (Ed.), *Cognitive reserve: Theory and application* (pp. 53–83). Hove, UK: Taylor and Francis.

Dickens, W. T., & Flynn, J. R. (2001a). Great leap forward: A new theory of intelligence. *New Scientist,* April 21, 44–47.

Dickens, W. T., & Flynn, J. R. (2001b). Heritability estimates versus large environmental effects: The IQ paradox resolved. *Psychological Review, 108,* 346–369.

Dickens, W. T., & Flynn, J. R. (2006). Black Americans reduce the racial IQ gap: Evidence from standardization samples. *Psychological Science, 17,* 913–920.

Dickinson, M. D., & Hiscock, M. (2010). Age-related IQ decline is reduced markedly after adjustment for the Flynn effect. *Journal of Clinical and Experimental Neuropsychology, 32,* 865–870.

Dickinson, M. D., & Hiscock, M. (2011). The Flynn effect in neuropsychological assessment. *Applied Neuropsychology, 18,* 136–142.

Flynn, J. R. (1999). Searching for justice: The discovery of IQ gains over time. *American Psychologist, 54,* 5–20.

Flynn, J. R. (2006). Efeito Flynn: Repensando a inteligência e seus efeitos [The Flynn effect: Rethinking intelligence and what affects it]. In C. Flores-Mendoza & R. Colom (Eds.), *Introdução à psicologia das diferenças individuais* [Introduction to the psychology of individual differences] (pp. 387–411). Porto Alegre, Brasil: ArtMed. (English trans. available from jim.flynn@stonebow.otago.ac.nz).

Flynn, J. R. (2007). *What is intelligence?* Cambridge, UK: Cambridge University Press.

Gardner, H. (2006). *Multiple intelligences: New horizons* (2nd ed.). New York: Basic Books.

Glassman, R. B. (1987). An hypothesis about redundancy and reliability in the brains of higher species: Analogies with genes, internal organs, and engineering systems. *Neuroscience & Biobehavioral Reviews, 11,* 275–285.

Goleman, D. P. (1995). *Emotional intelligence*. New York: Bantam.

Hall, C. B., Derby, C., LeValley, A., Katz, M. J., Verghese, J., & Lipton, R. B. (2007). Education delays accelerated decline on a memory test in persons who develop dementia. *Neurology, 69*, 1657–1664.

Head, D., Raz, N., Gunning-Dixon, F., Williamson, A., & Acker, J. D. (2002). Age-related differences in the course of cognitive skill acquisition: The role of regional cortical shrinkage and cognitive resources. *Psychology and Aging, 17*, 72–84.

Hebb, D. O. (1942). The effect of early and late brain injury upon test scores, and the nature of normal adult intelligence. *Proceedings of the American Philosophical Society, 85*, 275–292.

Himanen, L., Portin, R., Isoniemi, H., Helenius, H., Kurki, T., & Tenovuo, O. (2006). Longitudinal cognitive changes in traumatic brain injury: A 30-year follow-up study. *Neurology, 66*, 187–192.

Jacobson, N. S., & Truax, P. (1991). Clinical significance: A statistical approach to defining meaningful change in psychotherapy research. *Journal of Consulting and Clinical Psychology, 59*, 12–19.

Jensen, A. R. (1975). The meaning of heritability in the behavioral sciences. *Educational Psychologist, 11*, 171–183.

Johnson, M. V. (2009). Plasticity in the developing brain: Implications for rehabilitation. *Developmental Disabilities Research Reviews, 15*, 94–101.

Klein, M., Houx, P. J., & Jolles, J. (1996). Long-term persistent cognitive sequelae of traumatic brain injury and the effect of age. *Journal of Nervous and Mental Diseases, 184*, 459–467.

Knight, R. A., & Silverstein, S. M. (2001). A process-oriented approach for averting confounds resulting from general performance deficiencies in schizophrenia. *Journal of Abnormal Psychology, 110*, 15–30.

Luria, A.R. (1973). *The working brain: An introduction to neuropsychology* (B. Haigh, Trans.). New York: Basic Books.

McDowell, I., Xi, G., Lindsay, J., & Tierney, M. (2007). Mapping the connections between education and dementia. *Journal of Clinical and Experimental Neuropsychology, 29*, 127–141.

McCarthy, R. A., & Warrington, E. K. (1990). *Cognitive neuropsychology: A clinical introduction*. San Diego: Academic Press.

McSweeny, A. J., Naugle, R. I., Chelune, G. J., & Luders, H. (1993). T scores for change: An illustration of a regression approach to depicting change in clinical neuropsychology. *The Clinical Neuropsychologist, 7*, 300–312.

Meehl, P. E. (1995). Bootstraps taxometrics: Solving the classification problem in psychopathology. *American Psychologist, 50*, 266–274.

Melton, L. (2005). Use it, don't lose it. *New Scientist, 188*, 32–35.

Neisser, U. (Ed.) (1998). *The rising curve: Long-term gains in IQ and related measures*. Washington, DC: American Psychological Association.

Nilsson, L. G., Sternang, O., Ronnlund, M., & Nyberg, L. (2009). Challenging the notion of an early—onset of cognitive decline. *Neurobiology of Aging, 30*, 521–524.

Nowak, M. A., Anderson, R. M., McLean, A. R., Wolfs, T. F., Goudsmit, J., & May, R. M. (1991). Antigenic diversity thresholds and the development of AIDS. *Science, 254*, 963–969.

Plomin, R. (1986). *Development, genetics, and psychology*. Hillsdale, NJ: Lawrence Erlbaum Associates.

Quinn, N. P., Rosser, M. N., & Marsden, C. D. (1986). Dementia and Parkinson's disease-pathological and neurochemical considerations. *British Medical Bulletin, 42*, 86–90.

Raz, N., Rodrigue, K. M., Kennedy, K. M., & Acker, J. D. (2007). Vascular health and longitudinal changes in brain and cognition in middle-aged and older adults. *Neuropsychology, 21*, 149–157.

Raz, N., Rodrigue, K. M., Kennedy, K. M., & Land, S. (2009). Genetic and vascular modifiers of age-sensitive cognitive skills: Effects of COMT, BDNF, Ape, and hypertension. *Neuropsychology, 23*, 105–116.

Raymont, V., Greathouse, A., Redding, K., Lipsky, R., Salazar, A., & Grafman, J. (2008). Demographic, structural and genetic predictors of late cognitive decline after penetrating head injury. *Brain, 131*, 543–558.

Richards, M., & Sacker, A. (2003). Lifetime: Antecedents of cognitive reserve. *Journal of Clinical and Experimental Neuropsychology, 25*, 614–624.

Richards, M., Shipley, B., Fuhrer, R., & Wadsworth, M. E. J. (2004). Cognitive ability in childhood and cognitive decline in mid-life: Longitudinal birth cohort study. *BMJ, 328*, 552. doi:10.1136/bmj.37972.513819.EE (published 3 February 2004).

Ris, M. D., Packer, R., Goldwin, J., Jones- Wallace, D., & Boyett, J. M. (2001). Intellectual outcome after reduced-dose radiation therapy plus adjuvant chemotherapy for medulloblastoma: A Children's Cancer Group study. *Journal of Clinical Oncology, 19*, 3470–3476.

Ris, M. D., Walsh, K., Wallace, D., Armstrong, F. D., Holmes, E., Gajjar, A.,... Packer, R. J. (in press). Intellectual and academic outcome following two chemotherapy regimens and radiotherapy for Average Risk medulloblastoma: COG A9961. *Pediatric Blood and Cancer.*

Rönnlund, M., & Nilsson, L.-G. (2009). Flynn effects on sub factors of episodic and semantic memory: Parallel gains over time and the same set of determining factors. *Neuropsychologia, 47*, 2174–2180.

Ronnlund, M., Nyberg, L., Beckman, L, & Nilsson, L.-G. (2005). Stability, growth, and decline in adult life-span development of declarative memory: Cross-sectional and longitudinal data from a population-based sample. *Psychology and Aging, 20*, 3–18.

Roth, M. (1986). The association of clinical and neurological findings and its bearings on the classification and etiology of Alzheimer's disease. *British Medical Bulletin, 42*, 42–50.

Salthouse, T. A. (2009). Decomposing age correlations on neuropsychological and cognitive variables. *Journal of the International Neuropsychological Society, 15*, 650–661.

Salthouse, T. A. (2010). Selective review of cognitive aging. *Journal of the International Neuropsychological Society, 16*, 754–760.

Satz, P. (1993). Brain reserve capacity on symptom onset after brain injury: A formulation and review of evidence for threshold theory. *Neuropsychology, 7*, 273–295.

Satz, P., Cole, M. A., Hardy, D. J., & Rassovsky, Y. (2011). Brain and cognitive reserve: Mediator(s) and construct validity, a critique. *Journal of Clinical and Experimental Neuropsychology, 33*, 121–130.

Scarmeas, N., Zarahn, E., Anderson, K., Hilton, J., Flynn, J., Van Heertum, R., Sackheim, H., & Stern, Y. (2003). Cognitive reserve modulates functional brain responses during memory tasks: A PET study in healthy young and elderly subjects. *Neuroimage, 19*, 1215–1227.

Schaie, W. K., Willis, S. L., & Caskie, G. I. L. (2004). The Seattle longitudinal study: Relationship between personality and cognition. *Aging, Neuropsychology and Cognition, 11*, 304–324.

Scarr, S. (1992). Developmental theories for the 1990s: Development and individual differences. *Child Development, 63*, 1–19.

Schweizer, T. A., Ware, J., Fischer, C. E., Craik, F. I. M., & Bialystok, E. (2012). Bilingualism as a contributor to cognitive reserve: Evidence from brain atrophy in Alzheimer's disease. *Cortex, 48*, 991–996.

Small, G. W., Kepe, V., & Barrio, J. R. (2006). Seeing is believing: Neuroimaging adds to our understanding of cerebral pathology. *Current Opinion in Psychiatry, 19*, 564–569.

Snowdon, D. A., Ostwald, S. K., & Kane, R. L. (1989). Education and survival and interdependence in elderly Catholic sisters, 1936–1988. *American Journal of Epidemiology, 130*, 999–1012.

Spearman, C. (1904). "General intelligence," objectively determined and measured. *American Journal of Psychology, 15*, 201–293.

Starr, J. M., & Lonie, J. (2008). Estimated pre-morbid IQ effects on cognitive and functional outcomes in Alzheimer disease: A longitudinal study in a treated cohort. *BMD Psychiatry, 8 (Electronic)*. doi: 10.1186/1471-244X-8-27

St. James-Roberts, I. (1981). A reinterpretation of hemispherectomy data without functional plasticity of the brain. I. Intellectual function. *Brain and Language, 13*, 31–53.

Stern, Y. (2003). The concept of cognitive reserve: A catalyst for research. *Journal of Clinical and Experimental Neuropsychology, 25*, 589–593.

Stern, Y. (2002). What is cognitive reserve? Theory and research application of the reserve concept. *Journal of the International Neuropsychological Society, 8*, 448–460.

Stern, Y. (2009). Cognitive reserve. *Neuropsychologia, 47*, 2015–2028.

Sternberg, R. J. (1985). *Beyond IQ: A triarchic theory of human intelligence.* Cambridge, UK: Cambridge University Press.

Teuber, H. L. (1974). Recovery of function after lesions of the central nervous system: History and prospects. *Neuroscience Research Program Bulletin, 12*, 197–211.

Thurstone, L. L. (1948). Psychological implications of factor analysis. *American Psychologist, 3*, 402–408.

Valenzuela, M. J., & Sachdev, P. (2006). Brain reserve and dementia: A systematic review. *Psychological Medicine, 36*, 441–454.

Ward, L. (2004). Risk factors for Alzheimer's disease in Down syndrome. In L. M. Giddon (Ed.), *International review of research in mental retardation* (Vol. 29, pp. 62–117). San Diego, CA: Academic Press.

Wilson, R. S., Li, Y., Aggarwal, N. T., Barnes, L. L., McCann, J. J., Gilley, D. W., & Evans, D. A. (2004). Education and the course of cognitive decline in Alzheimer's disease. *Neurology, 63*, 1198–1202.

Zahodne, L. B., Glymour, M. M., Sparks, C., Bontempo, D., Dixon, R. A., MacDonald, S. W. S., & Manly, J. J. (2011). Education does not slow cognitive decline with aging: 12-year evidence from the Victoria Longitudinal Study. *Journal of the International Neuropsychological Society, 17*, 1039–1046.

Index

Printed in the USA/Agawam, MA
July 24, 2018

679480.072